THE WASHINGTON MANUAL™ OF CRITICAL CARE

3rd Edition

Marin H. Kollef, MD
Virginia E. and Sam J. Golman
Chair in Respiratory Intensive Care Medicine
Professor of Medicine
Division of Pulmonary & Critical Care Medicine
Director, Critical Care Research
Director, Respiratory Care Services
Washington University School of Medicine
Barnes-Jewish Hospital
St. Louis, Missouri

Warren Isakow, MD
Associate Professor of Medicine
Division of Pulmonary and Critical Care Medicine
Director, Medical Intensive Care Unit
Washington University School of Medicine
Barnes-Jewish Hospital
St. Louis, Missouri

A. Cole Burks, MD
Instructor of Medicine
Division of Pulmonary and Critical Care Medicine
Washington University School of Medicine
Barnes-Jewish Hospital
St. Louis, Missouri

Vladimir N. Despotovic, MD
Assistant Professor of Medicine
Division of Pulmonary and Critical Care Medicine
Washington University School of Medicine
Barnes-Jewish Hospital
St. Louis, Missouri

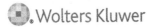
. Wolters Kluwer

Philadelphia · Baltimore · New York · London
Buenos Aires · Hong Kong · Sydney · Tokyo

Acquisitions Editor: Keith Donnellan
Editorial Coordinator: Dave Murphy
Marketing Manager: Dan Dressler
Production Project Manager: Bridgett Dougherty
Design Coordinator: Joan Wendt
Manufacturing Coordinator: Beth Welsh
Prepress Vendor: Aptara, Inc.

9 8 7 6

Printed in the United States of America

Library of Congress Cataloging-in-Publication Data

Names: Kollef, Marin H., editor. | Isakow, Warren, editor. | Washington
   University (Saint Louis, Mo.). School of Medicine.
Title: The Washington manual of critical care / [edited by] Marin H. Kollef,
   Warren Isakow.
Other titles: Manual of critical care
Description: Third edition. | Philadelphia : Wolters Kluwer, [2018] |
   Includes bibliographical references and index.
Identifiers: LCCN 2017042759 | ISBN 9781496328519
Subjects: | MESH: Critical Care–methods | Critical Illness–therapy |
   Handbooks
Classification: LCC RC86.8 | NLM WX 39 | DDC 616.02/8–dc23
LC record available at https://lccn.loc.gov/2017042759

To purchase additional copies of this book, call our customer service department at (800) 638-3030 or fax orders to (301) 223-2320. International customers should call (301) 223-2300.

Visit Lippincott Williams & Wilkins on the Internet: at LWW.com. Lippincott Williams & Wilkins customer service representatives are available from 8:30 am to 6 pm, EST.

We dedicate this manual to all health care providers
involved in the care of critically ill patients and their families.
We acknowledge their efforts and sacrifices and hope
this manual can assist them in some meaningful way.
We also acknowledge our families for their support and to
the critical care community of Washington University and
Barnes-Jewish Hospital for their commitment to the education
and well-being of trainees.

Contributors

Luigi Adamo, MD
Fellow
Cardiovascular Division
Washington University School of Medicine
Barnes-Jewish Hospital
St. Louis, Missouri

Patrick R. Aguilar, MD
Assistant Professor of Medicine
Division of Pulmonary and Critical Care
  Medicine
Washington University School of Medicine
Barnes-Jewish Hospital
St. Louis, Missouri

Jennifer Alexander-Brett, MD, PhD
Assistant Professor of Medicine
Division of Pulmonary and Critical Care
  Medicine
Washington University School of Medicine
Barnes-Jewish Hospital
St. Louis, Missouri

Adam Anderson, MD
Assistant Professor of Medicine
Division of Pulmonary and Critical Care
  Medicine
Washington University School of Medicine
Barnes-Jewish Hospital
St. Louis, Missouri

Baback Arshi, MD
Assistant Professor of Neurology and
  Neurosurgery
Division of Neurocritical Care
University of Illinois at Chicago
Chicago, Illinois

Jason G. Bill, MD
Fellow
Division of Gastroenterology
Washington University School of
  Medicine
Barnes-Jewish Hospital
St. Louis, Missouri

Pierre Blais, MD
Fellow
Division of Gastroenterology
Washington University School of
  Medicine
Barnes-Jewish Hospital
St. Louis, Missouri

Morey A. Blinder, MD
Professor of Medicine, Pathology and
  Immunology
Division of Hematology
Washington University School of
  Medicine
Barnes-Jewish Hospital
St. Louis, Missouri

Alan C. Braverman, MD
Alumni Endowed Professor in
  Cardiovascular Diseases
Director, Marfan Syndrome Clinic
Director, Inpatient Cardiology Firm
Washington University School of
  Medicine
Barnes-Jewish Hospital
St. Louis, Missouri

Steven L. Brody, MD
Dorothy R. and Hubert C. Moog Professor
Division of Pulmonary and Critical Care
   Medicine
Washington University School of Medicine
Barnes-Jewish Hospital
St. Louis, Missouri

A. Cole Burks, MD
Assistant Professor of Medicine
Division of Pulmonary Diseases &
   Critical Care Medicine
University of North Carolina at Chapel
   Hill
Chapel Hill, North Carolina

Jason P. Burnham, MD
Instructor of Medicine
Division of Infectious Diseases
Washington University School of Medicine
Barnes-Jewish Hospital
St. Louis, Missouri

Derek E. Byers, MD, PhD, FCCP
Associate Professor of Medicine
Chair, Washington University IRB
Director, Pulmonary Morphology Core
Division of Pulmonary and Critical Care
   Medicine
Washington University School of Medicine
Barnes-Jewish Hospital
St. Louis, Missouri

Mirnela Byku, MD, PhD
Assistant Professor of Medicine
Advanced Heart Failure and Transplant
   Cardiology
University of North Carolina in Chapel
   Hill
Chapel Hill, North Carolina

Amy Cacace, MD
Fellow
Division of Pulmonary and Critical Care
   Medicine
Washington University School of Medicine
Barnes-Jewish Hospital
St. Louis, Missouri

Mario Castro, MD, MPH
Alan A. and Edith L. Wolff Professor of
   Pulmonary and Critical Care Medicine
Professor of Medicine, Pediatrics, and
   Radiology
Washington University School of
   Medicine
Barnes-Jewish Hospital
St. Louis, Missouri

Murali M. Chakinala, MD, FCCP
Professor of Medicine
Division of Pulmonary and Critical Care
   Medicine
Washington University School of Medicine
Barnes-Jewish Hospital
St. Louis, Missouri

Stephanie H. Chang, MD
Medical Resident
Department of Surgery
Washington University School of Medicine
Barnes-Jewish Hospital
St. Louis, Missouri

Alexander C. Chen, MD
Associate Professor of Medicine
Director of Interventional Pulmonology
Division of Pulmonary and Critical Care
   Medicine
Washington University School of
   Medicine
Barnes-Jewish Hospital
St. Louis, Missouri

Steven Cheng, MD
Associate Professor of Medicine
Division of Nephrology
Washington University School of Medicine
Barnes-Jewish Hospital
St. Louis, Missouri

Matthew J. Chung, MD
Interventional Cardiology Fellow
Cardiovascular Division
Washington University School of Medicine
Barnes-Jewish Hospital
St. Louis, Missouri

William E. Clutter, MD
Associate Professor of Medicine
Division of Endocrinology, Metabolism,
and Lipid Research
Washington University School of
Medicine
Barnes-Jewish Hospital
St. Louis, Missouri

Shayna N. Conner, MD, MSCI
Assistant Professor
Department of Obstetrics and Gynecology
Division of Maternal Fetal Medicine
Washington University School of Medicine
Barnes-Jewish Hospital
St. Louis, Missouri

Daniel H. Cooper, MD
Associate Professor of Medicine
Cardiovascular Division
Washington University School of Medicine
Barnes-Jewish Hospital
St. Louis, Missouri

Jeffrey S. Crippin, MD
Bornefeld Chair in Gastrointestinal
Research and Treatment
Professor of Medicine
Division of Gastroenterology
Washington University School of Medicine
Barnes-Jewish Hospital
St. Louis, Missouri

Paulina Cruz Bravo, MD
Instructor of Medicine
Division of Endocrinology, Metabolism
and Lipid Research
Washington University School of
Medicine
Barnes-Jewish Hospital
St. Louis, Missouri

Julianne S. Dean, DO
Critical Care Fellow
BC-Emergency Medicine
Washington University School of
Medicine
Barnes-Jewish Hospital
St. Louis, Missouri

Jessica M. Despotovic, MD
Instructor in Clinical Obstetrics and
Gynecology
Department of Obstetrics and Gynecology
Washington University School of Medicine
Barnes-Jewish Hospital
St. Louis, Missouri

Vladimir N. Despotovic, MD
Assistant Professor of Medicine
Division of Pulmonary and Critical Care
Medicine
Washington University School of Medicine
Barnes-Jewish Hospital
St. Louis, Missouri

Rajat Dhar, MD
Associate Professor
Division of Neurocritical Care
Department of Neurology
Washington University School of
Medicine
Barnes-Jewish Hospital
St. Louis, Missouri

Erik R. Dubberke, MD, MSPH
Associate Professor of Medicine
Director, Section of Transplant Infectious
Diseases
Washington University School of
Medicine
Barnes-Jewish Hospital
St. Louis, Missouri

Fahad Edrees, MD
Fellow
Division of Nephrology
Washington University School of Medicine
Barnes-Jewish Hospital
St. Louis, Missouri

Gregory A. Ewald, MD
Associate Professor of Medicine
Medical Director, Cardiac Transplant
Program
Cardiovascular Division
Washington University School of Medicine
Barnes-Jewish Hospital
St. Louis, Missouri

Kristen Fisher, MD
Fellow
Division of Pulmonary and Critical Care
  Medicine
Washington University School of Medicine
Barnes-Jewish Hospital
St. Louis, Missouri

Yuka Furuya, MD
Fellow
Division of Pulmonary and Critical Care
  Medicine
Washington University School of Medicine
Barnes-Jewish Hospital
St. Louis, Missouri

Seth Goldberg, MD
Assistant Professor of Medicine
Division of Nephrology
Washington University School of Medicine
Barnes-Jewish Hospital
St. Louis, Missouri

Mollie Gowan, PharmD
Clinical Pharmacist
Medical Intensive Care Unit
Washington University School of Medicine
Barnes-Jewish Hospital
St. Louis, Missouri

Jonathan M. Green, MD, MBA
Professor of Medicine, Pathology and
  Immunology
Associate Dean for Human Studies and
  Executive Chair of the IRB
Washington University School of Medicine
Barnes-Jewish Hospital
St. Louis, Missouri

C. Prakash Gyawali, MD
Professor of Medicine
Division of Gastroenterology
Washington University School of Medicine
Barnes-Jewish Hospital
St. Louis, Missouri

Kevin Haas, MD
Associate Program Director for
  Interventional Pulmonology
University of Illinois at Chicago
Chicago, Illinois

Chase Hall, MD
Fellow
Division of Pulmonary and Critical Care
  Medicine
Washington University School of Medicine
Barnes-Jewish Hospital
St. Louis, Missouri

Theresa Human, PharmD
Clinical Pharmacist
Neurology Intensive Care Unit
Washington University School of Medicine
Barnes-Jewish Hospital
St. Louis, Missouri

Amy M. Hunter, RN, BSN, MHS, CIC
Director, Patient Safety and Quality
Washington University School of
  Medicine
Barnes-Jewish Hospital
St. Louis, Missouri

Warren Isakow, MD
Associate Professor of Medicine
Director, Medical Intensive Care Unit
Division of Pulmonary and Critical Care
  Medicine
Washington University School of Medicine
Barnes-Jewish Hospital
St. Louis, Missouri

Tracy L. Ivy, MD
Assistant Professor of Pediatrics
Division of Allergy, Immunology, and
  Pulmonary Medicine
Washington University School of Medicine
Barnes-Jewish Hospital
St. Louis, Missouri

Ronald Jackups, Jr., MD, PhD
Assistant Professor
Assistant Medical Director, BJH Blood
  Bank and Hematology Laboratory
Division of Pathology and Immunology
Washington University School of Medicine
Barnes-Jewish Hospital
St. Louis, Missouri

Paul Juang, PharmD, BCPS, BCCCP, FASHP, FCCM
Clinical Specialist, MICU
Washington University School of
    Medicine
Barnes-Jewish Hospital
Professor of Pharmacy Practice
St. Louis College of Pharmacy
St. Louis, Missouri

Andrew M. Kates, MD
Professor of Medicine
Cardiovascular Division
Washington University School of Medicine
Barnes-Jewish Hospital
St. Louis, Missouri

Salah G. Keyrouz, MD, FAHA
Associate Professor of Neurology
Medical Director, Neurology/
    Neurosurgery ICU
Washington University School of
    Medicine
Barnes-Jewish Hospital
St. Louis, Missouri

Eric Knoche, MD
Assistant Professor of Medicine
Division of Medical Oncology
Washington University School of
    Medicine
Barnes-Jewish Hospital
St. Louis, Missouri

Marin H. Kollef, MD
Virginia E. and Sam J. Golman
    Chair in Respiratory Intensive
    Care Medicine
Professor of Medicine
Division of Pulmonary & Critical Care
    Medicine
Director, Critical Care Research
Director, Respiratory Care Services
Washington University School of
    Medicine
Barnes-Jewish Hospital
St. Louis, Missouri

Kevin M. Korenblat, MD
Professor of Medicine
Division of Gastroenterology
Washington University School of
    Medicine
Barnes-Jewish Hospital
St. Louis, Missouri

Tobias B. Kulik, MD
Assistant Professor of Neurology and
    Neurological Surgery
Department of Neurology
University of New Mexico Health
    Sciences Center
Albuquerque, New Mexico

Terrance T. Kummer, MD, PhD
Assistant Professor of Neurology
Division of Neurocritical Care
Washington University School of
    Medicine
Barnes-Jewish Hospital
St. Louis, Missouri

Gabriel D. Lang, MD
Assistant Professor of Medicine
Division of Gastroenterology
Washington University School of Medicine
Barnes-Jewish Hospital
St. Louis, Missouri

Shane J. LaRue, MD
Assistant Professor of Medicine
Cardiovascular Division
Washington University School of Medicine
Barnes-Jewish Hospital
St. Louis, Missouri

Stephen Y. Liang, MD, MPHS
Assistant Professor of Medicine
Divisions of Infectious Diseases and
    Emergency Medicine
Washington University School of Medicine
Barnes-Jewish Hospital
St. Louis, Missouri

Caline S. Mattar, MD
Instructor in Medicine
Director, Global Health Track for
  Infectious Diseases
Director, Global Health Scholars
  Pathway in Internal Medicine
Washington University School of
  Medicine
Barnes-Jewish Hospital
St. Louis, Missouri

Rachel McDonald, MD
Critical Care Fellow
Division of Pulmonary and Critical Care
  Medicine
Washington University School of
  Medicine
Barnes-Jewish Hospital
St. Louis, Missouri

Jesse L. Mecham, MD
Attending Physician
Department of Emergency Medicine
Missouri Baptist Medical Center
St. Louis, Missouri

Claire Meyer, MD
Assistant Professor of Medicine
Division of Gastroenterology
Washington University School of Medicine
Barnes-Jewish Hospital
St. Louis, Missouri

Scott T. Micek, PharmD
Associate Professor
Division of Pharmacy Practice
St. Louis College of Pharmacy
St. Louis, Missouri

Daniel K. Mullady, MD, FASGE
Associate Professor of Medicine
Director of Interventional Endoscopy
Washington University School of
  Medicine
Barnes-Jewish Hospital
St. Louis, Missouri

Lemuel R. Non, MD
Instructor of Medicine
Division of Infectious Diseases
Washington University School of Medicine
Barnes-Jewish Hospital
St. Louis, Missouri

Nadia M. Obeid, MD
Instructor
Department of Surgery
Washington University School of
  Medicine
Barnes-Jewish Hospital
St. Louis, Missouri

Zaher K. Otrock, MD
Clinical Pathologist
Department of Pathology
Henry Ford Hospital
Detroit, Michigan

Rupa R. Patel, MD, MPH, DTM&H
Assistant Professor of Medicine
Division of Infectious Diseases
Washington University School of
  Medicine
Barnes-Jewish Hospital
St. Louis, Missouri

Varun Puri, MD, MSCI
Associate Professor of Surgery
Division of Cardiothoracic Surgery
Washington University School of
  Medicine
Barnes-Jewish Hospital
St. Louis, Missouri

Nandini Raghuraman, MD
Clinical Fellow
Department of Obstetrics and
  Gynecology
Division of Maternal Fetal Medicine
Washington University School of
  Medicine
Barnes-Jewish Hospital
St. Louis, Missouri

Britney M. Ramgopal, MD
Fellow
Division of Pulmonary and Critical Care
  Medicine
Washington University School of
  Medicine
Barnes-Jewish Hospital
St. Louis, Missouri

Krunal Raval, MD
Fellow
Division of Infectious Diseases
Washington University School of
  Medicine
Barnes-Jewish Hospital
St. Louis, Missouri

Ian R. Ross, MD
Instructor of Medicine
Department of Medicine
Washington University School of
  Medicine
Barnes-Jewish Hospital
St. Louis, Missouri

Tonya D. Russell, MD
Associate Professor of Medicine
Division of Pulmonary and Critical Care
  Medicine
Washington University School of
  Medicine
Barnes-Jewish Hospital
St. Louis, Missouri

Joel C. Schilling, MD, PhD
Assistant Professor of Medicine
Cardiovascular Division
Washington University School of
  Medicine
Barnes-Jewish Hospital
St. Louis, Missouri

**Douglas J.E. Schuerer, MD,
FACS, FCCM**
Professor of Surgery
Department of Surgery
Washington University School of
  Medicine
Barnes-Jewish Hospital
St. Louis, Missouri

Sandeep S. Sodhi, MD, MBA
Electrophysiology Fellow
Division of Cardiovascular Medicine
Washington University School of Medicine
Barnes-Jewish Hospital
St. Louis, Missouri

Shweta Sood, MD, MS
Fellow
Division of Pulmonary and Critical Care
Washington University School of Medicine
Barnes-Jewish Hospital
St. Louis, Missouri

Andrej Spec, MD
Assistant Professor of Medicine
Division of Infectious Diseases
Washington University School of Medicine
Barnes-Jewish Hospital
St. Louis, Missouri

Molly J. Stout, MD, MSCI
Assistant Professor, Obstetrics and
  Gynecology
Division of Maternal-Fetal Medicine
Washington University School of Medicine
Barnes-Jewish Hospital
St. Louis, Missouri

**Carol J. Sykora, MBA, MEd,
MT(ASCP), CIC, FAPIC**
Infection Prevention Specialist
Department of Patient Safety and
  Quality
Washington University School of Medicine
Barnes-Jewish Hospital
St. Louis, Missouri

Beth E. Taylor, DCN, RDN-AP, CNSC, FCCM
Research/Education Clinical Nutrition
  Specialist
Surgical/Trauma Unit
Clinical Faculty, ACGME ACCM
  Fellowship Program
Washington University School of
  Medicine
Barnes-Jewish Hospital
St. Louis, Missouri

Lorene A. Temming, MD, MSCI, FACOG
Assistant Professor, Maternal and Fetal
  Medicine
Department of Obstetrics and
  Gynecology
Carolinas HealthCare System
Charlotte, North Carolina

Dany Thekkemuriyil, MD
Physician
SSM Health Medical Group
St. Louis, Missouri

Garry S. Tobin, MD
Professor of Medicine
Director, Washington University Diabetes
  Center
Division Endocrinology, Metabolism,
  and Lipid Research
Washington University School of
  Medicine
Barnes-Jewish Hospital
St. Louis, Missouri

Abhaya P. Trivedi, MD
Assistant Professor of Medicine
Rush University Medical Center
Chicago, Illinois

Tracy Trupka, MD
Fellow
Division of Pulmonary and Critical Care
  Medicine
Washington University School of
  Medicine
Barnes-Jewish Hospital
St. Louis, Missouri

Tyson Turner, MD, MPH
Clinical Fellow
Cardiovascular Division
Washington University School of
  Medicine
Barnes-Jewish Hospital
St. Louis, Missouri

Anitha Vijayan, MD
Professor of Medicine
Division of Nephrology
Washington University School of
  Medicine
Barnes-Jewish Hospital
St. Louis, Missouri

David K. Warren, MD, MPH
Professor of Medicine
Division of Infectious Diseases
Washington University School of
  Medicine
Barnes-Jewish Hospital
St. Louis, Missouri

Brian T. Wessman, MD, FACEP, FCCM
Associate Professor of Anesthesiology and
  Emergency Medicine
Section Chief, EM/CCM Section
Washington University School of
  Medicine
Barnes-Jewish Hospital
St. Louis, Missouri

Chad A. Witt, MD
Assistant Professor of Medicine
Division of Pulmonary and Critical Care
  Medicine
Washington University School of
  Medicine
Barnes-Jewish Hospital
St. Louis, Missouri

Keith F. Woeltje, MD, PhD
Professor of Medicine
Division of Infectious Diseases
Washington University School of
  Medicine
Barnes-Jewish Hospital
St. Louis, Missouri

Usman Younus, MD
Clinical Fellow
Division of Nephrology
Washington University School of
  Medicine
Barnes-Jewish Hospital
St. Louis, Missouri

Roger D. Yusen, MD, MPH
Associate Professor of Medicine
Division of Pulmonary and Critical Care
  Medicine
Washington University School of
  Medicine
Barnes-Jewish Hospital
St. Louis, Missouri

Preface

This is the third edition of *The Washington Manual™ of Critical Care*, building on the long tradition of *The Washington Manual™ of Medical Therapeutics*, and the two prior Critical Care manuals. This project was originally inspired by the expanding knowledge base in critical care medicine and the demands this places on health care professionals treating critically ill patients. Our primary goal in preparing this manual is to provide clinicians and students with comprehensive and current treatment algorithms for the bedside diagnosis and management of the most frequently encountered illnesses and problems encountered in the intensive care unit (ICU) setting. Since the last edition we have included new chapters on extracorporeal membrane oxygenation and the management of the transplant patient in the ICU. We have also revamped most of the existing chapters to keep them up to date with the expanding medical literature. The chapters were written by Washington University faculty physicians and experts in their fields from the Departments of Internal Medicine, Neurology, Surgery, Obstetrics and Gynecology, and Anesthesiology, often with the assistance of subspecialty fellows and residents. The tables and algorithms that accompany each chapter are meant as guides and may not be appropriate for all patients. Further reading of the literature is always encouraged and this manual is expected to be used in conjunction with trained critical care clinicians. We would especially like to give our sincerest thanks to Becky Light for her tireless efforts in preparing chapters and for acting as the liaison between the Pulmonary and Critical Care Department, the chapter's authors, and Lippincott Williams & Wilkins.

Contents

1

Introduction to Shock

Marin H. Kollef

Shock is a common problem in the intensive care unit, requiring immediate diagnosis and treatment. It is usually defined by a combination of hemodynamic parameters (mean blood pressure <60 mm Hg, systolic blood pressure <90 mm Hg), clinical findings (altered mentation, decreased urine output), and abnormal laboratory values (elevated serum lactate, metabolic acidosis). The first step is to identify the cause of shock, as each condition will require different interventions. The overall goal of therapy is to reverse tissue hypoperfusion as quickly as possible in order to preserve organ function. Table 1.1 and Algorithms 1.1 and 1.2 offer an approach for determining the main cause of shock. Specific management of the various shock states is presented in the following chapters. Early evaluation with echocardiography, intraesophageal aortic waveform assessment, or right heart catheterization will allow determination of the cause of shock and will assist in management.

TABLE 1.1	Hemodynamic Patterns Associated with Specific Shock States[a]							
Type of Shock	CI	SVR	PVR	SvO_2	RAP	RVP	PAP	PAOP
Cardiogenic (e.g., myocardial infarction or cardiac tamponade)	↓	↑	N	↓	↑	↑	↑	↑
Hypovolemic (e.g., hemorrhage, intravascular volume depletion)	↓	↑	N	↓	↓	↓	↓	↓
Distributive shock (e.g., septic, anaphylaxis)	N-↑	↓	N	N-↑	N-↓	N-↓	N-↓	N-↓
Obstructive (e.g., pulmonary embolism)	↓	N-↑	↑	N-↓	↑	↑	↑	N-↓

[a]Equalization of RAP, PAOP, diastolic PAP, and diastolic RVP indicates cardiac tamponade.
CI, cardiac index; SVR, systemic vascular resistance; PVR, pulmonary vascular resistance; SvO_2, mixed venous oxygen saturation; RAP, right arterial pressure; RVP, right ventricular pressure; PAP, pulmonary artery pressure; PAOP, pulmonary artery occlusion pressure; ↑, increased; ↓, decreased; N, normal.

ALGORITHM 1.1 Main Causes of Shock

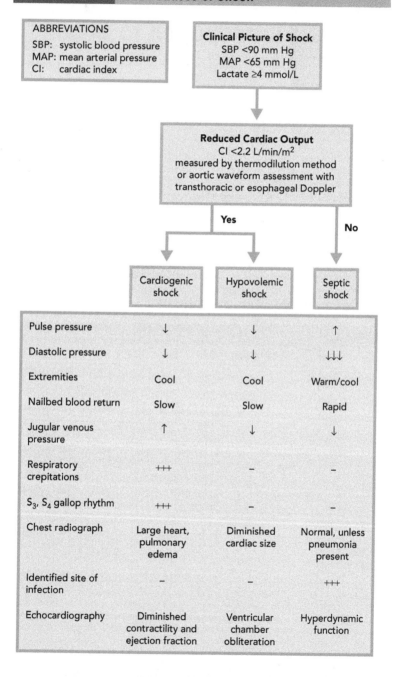

ABBREVIATIONS
SBP: systolic blood pressure
MAP: mean arterial pressure
CI: cardiac index

Clinical Picture of Shock
SBP <90 mm Hg
MAP <65 mm Hg
Lactate ≥4 mmol/L

Reduced Cardiac Output
CI <2.2 L/min/m²
measured by thermodilution method
or aortic waveform assessment with
transthoracic or esophageal Doppler

Yes → **No**

Cardiogenic shock | Hypovolemic shock | Septic shock

	Cardiogenic shock	Hypovolemic shock	Septic shock
Pulse pressure	↓	↓	↑
Diastolic pressure	↓	↓	↓↓↓
Extremities	Cool	Cool	Warm/cool
Nailbed blood return	Slow	Slow	Rapid
Jugular venous pressure	↑	↓	↓
Respiratory crepitations	+++	−	−
S₃, S₄ gallop rhythm	+++	−	−
Chest radiograph	Large heart, pulmonary edema	Diminished cardiac size	Normal, unless pneumonia present
Identified site of infection	−	−	+++
Echocardiography	Diminished contractility and ejection fraction	Ventricular chamber obliteration	Hyperdynamic function

ALGORITHM 1.2 Miscellaneous Causes of Shock

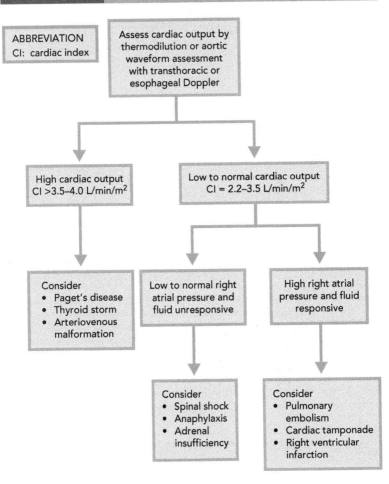

ABBREVIATION
CI: cardiac index

Assess cardiac output by thermodilution or aortic waveform assessment with transthoracic or esophageal Doppler

High cardiac output
CI >3.5–4.0 L/min/m²

Low to normal cardiac output
CI = 2.2–3.5 L/min/m²

Consider
- Paget's disease
- Thyroid storm
- Arteriovenous malformation

Low to normal right atrial pressure and fluid unresponsive

High right atrial pressure and fluid responsive

Consider
- Spinal shock
- Anaphylaxis
- Adrenal insufficiency

Consider
- Pulmonary embolism
- Cardiac tamponade
- Right ventricular infarction

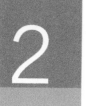

Hypovolemic Shock

Marin H. Kollef

Hypovolemic shock occurs as a result of decreased circulating blood volume, most commonly from acute hemorrhage. It may also result from heat-related intravascular volume depletion or fluid sequestration within the abdomen. Table 2.1 provides a classification of hypovolemic shock based on the amount of whole blood volume lost. In general, the greater the loss of whole blood, the greater the resultant risk of mortality. However, it is important to note that other factors can influence the outcome of hypovolemic shock including age, underlying comorbidities (e.g., cardiovascular disease), and the rapidity and adequacy of the fluid resuscitation.

Lactic acidosis occurs during hypovolemic shock because of inadequate tissue perfusion. The magnitude of the serum lactate elevation is correlated with mortality in hypovolemic shock and may be an early indicator of tissue hypoperfusion, despite near-normal–appearing vital signs. The treatment of lactic acidosis depends on reversing organ hypoperfusion. This is reflected in the equation for tissue oxygen delivery shown here. Optimizing oxygen delivery to tissues requires a sufficient hemoglobin concentration to carry oxygen to tissues. Additionally, ventricular preload is an important determinant of cardiac output. Providing adequate intravascular volume will ensure that stroke volume and cardiac output are optimized to meet tissue demands for oxygen and other nutrients. If, despite adequate preload, cardiac output is not sufficient for the demands of tissues, then dobutamine can be employed to further increase cardiac output and oxygen delivery.

TABLE 2.1	Classification of Hypovolemic Shock	
Category	Whole Blood Volume Loss (%)	Pathophysiology
Mild (compensated)	<20	Peripheral vasoconstriction to preserve blood flow to critical organs (brain and heart)
Moderate	20–40	Decreased perfusion of organs such as the kidneys, intestine, and pancreas
Severe (uncompensated)	>40	Decreased perfusion to brain and heart

ALGORITHM 2.1 Management of Hypovolemic Shock

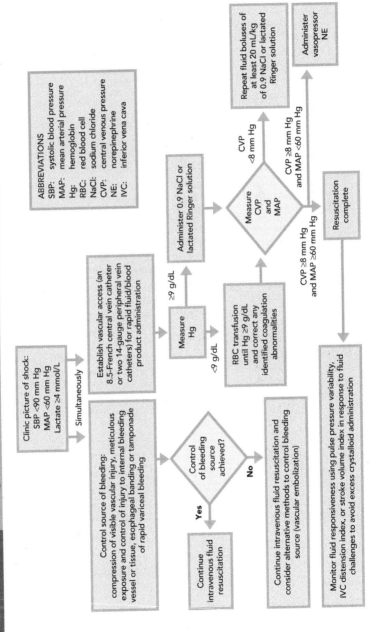

Clinic picture of shock:
SBP <90 mm Hg
MAP <60 mm Hg
Lactate ≥4 mmol/L

Simultaneously

Establish vascular access (an 8.5-French central vein catheter or two 14-gauge peripheral vein catheters) for rapid fluid/blood product administration

Measure Hg

≥9 g/dL → Administer 0.9 NaCl or lactated Ringer solution

<9 g/dL → RBC transfusion until Hg ≥9 g/dL and correct any identified coagulation abnormalities

Measure CVP and MAP

CVP <8 mm Hg → Repeat fluid boluses of at least 20 mL/kg of 0.9 NaCl or lactated Ringer solution

CVP ≥8 mm Hg and MAP <60 mm Hg → Administer vasopressor NE

CVP ≥8 mm Hg and MAP ≥60 mm Hg → **Resuscitation complete** → Monitor fluid responsiveness using pulse pressure variability, IVC distension index, or stroke volume index in response to fluid challenges to avoid excess crystalloid administration

Control source of bleeding: compression of visible vascular injury, meticulous exposure and control of injury to internal bleeding vessel or tissue, esophageal banding or tamponade of rapid variceal bleeding

Control of bleeding source achieved?

Yes → Continue intravenous fluid resuscitation

No → Continue intravenous fluid resuscitation and consider alternative methods to control bleeding source (vascular embolization)

ABBREVIATIONS
SBP: systolic blood pressure
MAP: mean arterial pressure
Hg: hemoglobin
RBC: red blood cell
NaCl: sodium chloride
CVP: central venous pressure
NE: norepinephrine
IVC: inferior vena cava

TABLE 2.2 | Adjunctive Therapies for Hypovolemic Shock

Therapy	Rationale
Airway control	To provide appropriate gas exchange in the lungs and to prevent aspiration
Cardiac/hemodynamic monitoring	To identify dysrhythmias and inadequate fluid resuscitation (Algorithm 2.1)
Platelet/fresh-frozen plasma administration	Required because of dilutional effects of crystalloid and blood administration as well as consumption from ongoing bleeding The prothrombin time and partial thromboplastin time should be corrected and the platelet count should be kept >50,000/mm^3 with ongoing bleeding
Activated factor VII and/or antifibrinolyic agents (tranexamic acid)	Should be considered in the presence of diffuse or nonoperative ongoing hemorrhage when clotting abnormalities have been corrected
Calcium chloride, magnesium chloride	To reverse ionized hypocalcemia and hypomagnesemia resulting from the administration of citrate with transfused blood, which binds ionized calcium and magnesium
Rewarming techniques (e.g., warm fluids, blankets, radiant lamps, head covers, warmed humidified air, heated body cavity lavage)	Hypothermia is a common consequence of massive blood transfusion that can contribute to cardiac dysfunction and coagulation abnormalities
Monitor for and treat for transfusion-related complications including transfusion-related acute lung injury (TRALI) and transfusion reactions	These are immunologically mediated, requiring appropriate use of mechanical ventilation with positive end-expiratory pressure for TRALI and bronchodilators and corticosteroids for severe bronchoconstriction, subglottic edema, and anaphylaxis
Antibiotics	When open dirty or contaminated wounds are present to prevent and treat bacterial infections
Corticosteroids	For patients presumed to have adrenal injury and patients unable to mount an appropriate stress response

$$\dot{D}O_2 = CaO_2 \times CO$$
$$CaO_2 = (Hb \times 1.34 \times SaO_2) + 0.0031\ PaO_2$$
$$CO = SV \times HR$$

where $\dot{D}O_2$ = oxygen delivery, CaO_2 = arterial oxygen content, CO = cardiac output, Hb = hemoglobin concentration, SaO_2 = arterial hemoglobin oxygen saturation, PaO_2 = arterial oxygen tension, SV = stroke volume, and HR = heart rate.

The treatment goals in hypovolemic shock are to control the source of hemorrhage and to administer adequate intravascular volume replacement. Control of the source of hemorrhage may be as simple as placing a pressure dressing on an open bleeding wound, or it may require urgent operative exploration to identify and control the bleeding source from an intra-abdominal or intrathoracic injury. Angiographic embolization of a bleeding vessel may also be helpful for bleeding injuries that are not amenable to surgical intervention (e.g., multiple pelvic fractures with ongoing hemorrhage). Therefore, most episodes of hypovolemic shock are managed by trauma specialists, usually in the emergency department setting. However, all clinicians caring for critically ill patients should be able to recognize the early clinical manifestations of hypovolemic shock and to initiate appropriate fluid management.

An algorithm for the fluid management of hypovolemic shock is provided in Algorithm 2.1. At least two large bore (14 to 16 gauge or larger) peripheral vein catheters and/or an 8.5-French central vein catheter should be placed to allow rapid blood product and crystalloid administration. A mechanical rapid transfusion device should also be used to decrease the time required for each unit of blood or liter of crystalloid to be infused. In a patient with ongoing hemorrhage, initial administration of 2 to 4 L of crystalloid (0.9 NaCl or lactated Ringer's solution) and group O blood should be given. Most hospitals will employ four units of Rh-positive O blood for men and women who are not in childbearing age and Rh-negative O blood for women who are in childbearing age. Type-specific blood is usually administered after the first four units of nontyped blood are given. The goal of blood transfusion therapy during ongoing hemorrhage is to maintain the hemoglobin value above 8 g/dL.

In addition to the initial administration of crystalloid and red blood cells, other therapies will be required in patients with hypovolemic shock. These are summarized in Table 2.2 and are especially important for patients requiring massive transfusions or those with ongoing blood loss.

SUGGESTED READINGS

Ausset S, Glassberg E, Nadler R, et al. Tranexamic acid as part of remote damage-control resuscitation in the prehospital setting: a critical appraisal of the medical literature and available alternatives. *J Trauma Acute Care Surg.* 2015;78(6 suppl 1):S70–S75.
  Reviews the evidence supporting the use of various hemorrhage control therapies to include tranexamic acid.
Chatrath V, Khetarpal R, Ahuja J. Fluid management in patients with trauma: restrictive versus liberal approach. *J Anaesthesiol Clin Pharmacol.* 2015;31(3):308–316.
  Provides up-to-date recommendations for fluid resuscitation in patients with hemorrhagic shock.
Duchesne JC, McSwain NE Jr, Cotton BA, et al. Damage control resuscitation: the new face of damage control. *J Trauma.* 2010;69(4):976–990.
  A concise review on strategies for optimizing damage control resuscitation in trauma.
Holcomb JB, Tilley BC, Baraniuk S, et al. Transfusion of plasma, platelets, and red blood cells in a 1:1:1 vs a 1:1:2 ratio and mortality in patients with severe trauma: the PROPPR randomized clinical trial. *JAMA.* 2015;313(5):471–482.
  Results from a trial showing no mortality benefit, but more patients in the 1:1:1 group achieved hemostasis and fewer experienced death due to exsanguination by 24 hours. Even though there was an increased use of plasma and platelets transfused in the 1:1:1 group, no other safety differences were identified between the two groups.

3 Sepsis and Septic Shock

Marin H. Kollef and Scott T. Micek

Sepsis is a life-threatening organ dysfunction caused by a dysregulated host response to infection. In the United States, approximately 750,000 cases of sepsis occur each year. The mortality associated with sepsis ranges from 30% to 50%, with mortality increasing with advancing age. Although complex, the pathophysiology of sepsis involves a series of interacting pathways involving immune stimulation, immune suppression, hypercoagulation, and hypofibrinolysis. Cardiovascular management plays an important role in the treatment of sepsis and septic shock. Hypotension occurs because of failure of vasoconstriction by vascular smooth muscle resulting in peripheral vasodilation. Cardiovascular resuscitation has been demonstrated to be an important determinant of survival in patients with septic shock. In addition to cardiovascular management, appropriate initial antimicrobial treatment of patients with sepsis also appears to be an important determinant of patient outcome. Table 3.1 provides the new consensus definitions for sepsis and septic shock.

The unscrambling of the complex pathophysiology associated with sepsis and septic shock has made much progress. Unfortunately, no proven agent targeting the pathways involved in septic shock is currently available. Table 3.2 highlights the supportive medications most commonly used in septic shock. The challenge for clinicians is the integration of these pharmacotherapies to confer the recognized survival benefit into critical care practice. The Surviving Sepsis Campaign has teamed with the Institute for Healthcare Improvement to create the Sepsis Bundles, which are designed in an effort to optimize the timing, sequence, and goals of the individual elements of care as delineated in the Surviving Sepsis Guidelines. The benefits associated with the use of comprehensive treatment protocols integrating goal-directed hemodynamic stabilization, early appropriate antimicrobial therapy, and associated adjunctive sepsis therapies initiated in the emergency department and continued in the intensive care unit have been reported in several earlier prospective trials (Algorithms 3.1 and 3.2). However, more recent trials evaluating goal-directed therapy in septic shock have shown no benefit compared to current standard practice which includes administering intravenous antibiotics and adequate fluid resuscitation. An important issue with these new trials is that the current standard of practice has evolved over the years incorporating many of the elements of early goal-directed resuscitation of septic shock.

The significance of early, aggressive, volume resuscitation and hemodynamic stabilization was demonstrated in a randomized, controlled, single-center trial in patients who presented to the emergency department with signs of septic shock, as published by Rivers et al. Administration of crystalloids, red blood cell transfusions, vasopressors, and inotropes

TABLE 3.1	Consensus Definition of Sepsis
Sepsis	Life-threatening organ dysfunction caused by a dysregulated host response to infection
Organ dysfunction	Increase in the Sequential Organ Failure Assessment (SOFA) score ≥2
Septic shock	Vasopressors to maintain a mean arterial pressure ≥65 mm Hg and lactate >2 mmol/L in absence of hypovolemia
Poor outcomes for sepsis (at least two of the following)	Quick SOFA • Respiratory rate ≥22/min • Altered mentation • Systolic blood pressure ≤100

based on aggressive monitoring of intravascular volume and a tissue oxygen marker within 6 hours of presentation to the emergency department resulted in a 16% decrease in absolute 28-day mortality. The major differences in treatment between the intervention and control groups were in the volume of intravenous fluids received, the number of patients transfused packed red blood cells, the use of dobutamine, and the presence of a dedicated study team for the first 6 hours of care.

The implementation of treatment pathways mimicking the interventions of the well-scripted, carefully performed procedures employed by Rivers et al. has been put into practice in the clinical setting. Micek et al. employed standardized order sets

TABLE 3.2	Medications Commonly Used in Septic Shock		CO	MAP	SVR
I. Vasopressors					
Norepinephrine		0.05–0.5 mcg/kg/min	–/+	++	+++
Dopamine		5–20 mcg/kg/min	++	+	++
Epinephrine		0.05–2 mcg/kg/min	++	++	+++
Phenylephrine		2–10 mcg/kg/min	0	++	+++
Vasopressin		0.04 units/min	0	+++	+++
II. Inotrope					
Dobutamine		2.5–10 mcg/kg/min	+++	–/+	–/0
III. Corticosteroids[a]					
Hydrocortisone (+/– fludrocortisone 50 mcg daily)		50 mg every 6 hrs			
IV. Antibiotic management (see Algorithm 3.2)					

[a]The benefits of corticosteroids in septic shock are limited to patients with vasopressor-dependent septic shock despite adequate fluid resuscitation.
CO, cardiac output; MAP, mean arterial blood pressure; SVR, systemic vascular resistance.

ALGORITHM 3.1 Fluid Management of Septic Shock

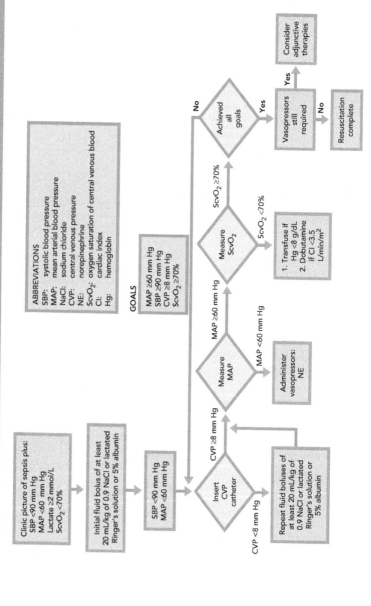

Clinic picture of sepsis plus:
SBP <90 mm Hg
MAP <60 mm Hg
Lactate ≥2 mmol/L
ScvO₂ <70%

Initial fluid bolus of at least 20 mL/kg of 0.9 NaCl or lactated Ringer's solution or 5% albumin

SBP ≥90 mm Hg
MAP <60 mm Hg

Insert CVP catheter

CVP <8 mm Hg

Repeat fluid boluses of at least 20 mL/kg of 0.9 NaCl or lactated Ringer's solution or 5% albumin

CVP ≥8 mm Hg

Measure MAP

MAP <60 mm Hg → Administer vasopressors: NE

MAP ≥60 mm Hg

Measure ScvO₂

ScvO₂ <70% →
1. Transfuse if Hg <8 g/dL
2. Dobutamine if CI <3.5 L/min/m²

ScvO₂ ≥70%

Achieved all goals

No

Yes → Vasopressors still required

Yes → Consider adjunctive therapies

No → Resuscitation complete

GOALS
MAP ≥60 mm Hg
SBP ≥90 mm Hg
CVP ≥8 mm Hg
ScvO₂ ≥70%

ABBREVIATIONS
SBP: systolic blood pressure
MAP: mean arterial blood pressure
NaCl: sodium chloride
CVP: central venous pressure
NE: norepinephrine
ScvO₂: oxygen saturation of central venous blood
CI: cardiac index
Hg: hemoglobin

ALGORITHM 3.2 **Antibiotic Management of Sepsis and Septic Shock**

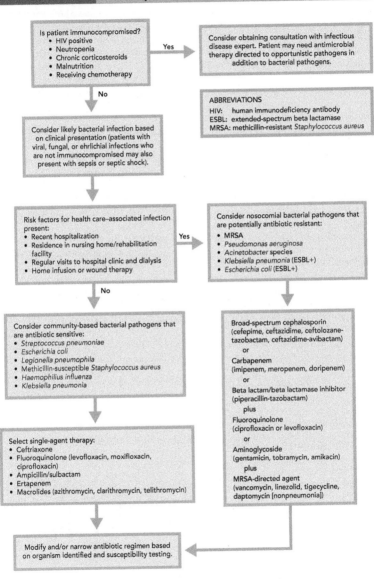

Is patient immunocompromised?
- HIV positive
- Neutropenia
- Chronic corticosteroids
- Malnutrition
- Receiving chemotherapy

→ Yes → Consider obtaining consultation with infectious disease expert. Patient may need antimicrobial therapy directed to opportunistic pathogens in addition to bacterial pathogens.

No ↓

ABBREVIATIONS
HIV: human immunodeficiency antibody
ESBL: extended-spectrum beta lactamase
MRSA: methicillin-resistant *Staphylococcus aureus*

Consider likely bacterial infection based on clinical presentation (patients with viral, fungal, or ehrlichial infections who are not immunocompromised may also present with sepsis or septic shock).

↓

Risk factors for health care–associated infection present:
- Recent hospitalization
- Residence in nursing home/rehabilitation facility
- Regular visits to hospital clinic and dialysis
- Home infusion or wound therapy

→ Yes → Consider nosocomial bacterial pathogens that are potentially antibiotic resistant:
- MRSA
- *Pseudomonas aeruginosa*
- *Acinetobacter* species
- *Klebsiella pneumonia* (ESBL+)
- *Escherichia coli* (ESBL+)

No ↓

Consider community-based bacterial pathogens that are antibiotic sensitive:
- *Streptococcus pneumoniae*
- *Escherichia coli*
- *Legionella pneumophila*
- Methicillin-susceptible *Staphylococcus aureus*
- *Haemophilius influenza*
- *Klebsiella pneumonia*

↓

Broad-spectrum cephalosporin (cefepime, ceftazidime, ceftolozane-tazobactam, ceftazidime-avibactam)
or
Carbapenem (imipenem, meropenem, doripenem)
or
Beta lactam/beta lactamase inhibitor (piperacillin-tazobactam)
plus
Fluoroquinolone (ciprofloxacin or levofloxacin)
or
Aminoglycoside (gentamicin, tobramycin, amikacin)
plus
MRSA-directed agent (vancomycin, linezolid, tigecycline, daptomycin [nonpneumonia])

Select single-agent therapy:
- Ceftriaxone
- Fluoroquinolone (levofloxacin, moxifloxacin, ciprofloxacin)
- Ampicillin/sulbactam
- Ertapenem
- Macrolides (azithromycin, clarithromycin, telithromycin)

↓

Modify and/or narrow antibiotic regimen based on organism identified and susceptibility testing.

that focused on intravenous fluid administration and the appropriateness of initial antimicrobial therapy for sepsis and septic shock. Patients managed in this manner were more likely to receive intravenous fluids >20 mL/kg of body weight prior to vasopressor administration, and consequently were less likely to require vasopressor administration at the time of transfer to the intensive care unit. Patients managed with this approach were also more likely to be treated with an appropriate initial antimicrobial regimen. As a result of the aggressive management initiated in the emergency department and continued in the intensive care unit, patients managed via the sepsis order sets had statistically shorter hospital lengths of stay and a lower risk for 28-day mortality. Similar results have been reported from a multicenter study coordinated by the Surviving Sepsis Campaign Group and supported by a recently performed meta-analysis.

The ProMISe, ARISE, and ProCESS trials all failed to show that goal-directed protocolized resuscitation of septic shock improved outcome. It is important to recognize that the patients in these three trials were not as ill as those in the original Rivers trial as manifested by lower mortality in the control arms (29%, 19%, 19%, respectively vs. 46% in the Rivers trial) and higher central venous oxygen saturation (ProMISe 74%, ARISE 76% vs. Rivers 49%). As a result, these trials do not exclude a survival benefit of early goal-directed resuscitation in patients with septic shock.

In summary, the initial management of patients with septic shock appears to be critical in terms of determining outcome. Institution of standardized physician order sets, or some other systematic timely approach, for the management of patients with severe infections appears to consistently improve the delivery of recommended therapies and, as a result, may improve patient outcomes. Given that evidence-based treatment pathways typically have no additional risks and are associated with little to no acquisition costs, their implementation should become the standard of care for the management of septic shock. Moreover, emerging clinical experience suggests that achievement of negative fluid balance after the initial resuscitation phase, and stabilization of the patient with septic shock, confers additional survival benefit.

SUGGESTED READINGS

ARISE Investigators; ANZICS Clinical Trials Group, Peake SL, et al. Goal-directed resuscitation for patients with early septic shock. *N Engl J Med.* 2014;371(16):1496–1506.
   The Australia/New Zealand trial examining goal-directed therapy of septic shock.
Chen C, Kollef MH. Conservative fluid therapy in septic shock: an example of targeted therapeutic minimization. *Crit Care.* 2014;18(4):481.
   A meta-analysis reviewing the evidence in support of goal-directed therapy for septic shock.
Dellinger RP, Levy MM, Rhodes A, et al; Surviving Sepsis Campaign Guidelines Committee including the Pediatric Subgroup. Surviving sepsis campaign: international guidelines for management of severe sepsis and septic shock: 2012. *Crit Care Med.* 2013;41(2): 580–637.
   Evidence-based recommendations for the initial resuscitation and treatment of patients with septic shock and sepsis.
Levy MM, Dellinger RP, Townsend SR, et al. The Surviving Sepsis Campaign: results of an international guideline-based performance improvement program targeting severe sepsis. *Intensive Care Med.* 2010;36(2):222–231.
   A multicenter experience instituting an algorithm to improve the outcomes of patients with sepsis.

Martin-Loeches I, Levy MM, Artigas A. Management of severe sepsis: advances, challenges, and current status. *Drug Des Devel Ther.* 2015;9:2079–2088.

Discusses the current approaches to the management of septic shock including controversial issues such as corticosteroids and innovative therapies.

Micek ST, Roubinian N, Heuring T, et al. Before-after study of a standardized hospital order set for the management of septic shock. *Crit Care Med.* 2006;34(11):2707–2713.

A before-after study demonstrating improvements in 28-day mortality and length of stay for patients with septic shock managed with a standardized order set in the emergency department.

Micek ST, Welch EC, Khan J, et al. Empiric combination antibiotic therapy is associated with improved outcome against sepsis due to gram-negative bacteria: a retrospective analysis. *Antimicrob Agents Chemother.* 2010;54(5):1742–1748.

Discusses importance of combination antibiotic therapy to appropriately treat resistant pathogens.

Mouncey PR, Osborn TM, Power GS, et al; ProMISe Trial Investigators. Trial of early, goal-directed resuscitation for septic shock. *N Engl J Med.* 2015;372(14):1301–1311.

The UK trial examining goal-directed therapy of septic shock.

ProCESS Investigators, Yealy DM, Kellum JA, et al. A randomized trial of protocol-based care for early septic shock. *N Engl J Med.* 2014;370(18):1683–1693.

The US trial examining goal-directed therapy of septic shock.

Rivers E, Nguyen B, Havstad S, et al; Early Goal-Directed Therapy Collaborative Group. Early goal-directed therapy in the treatment of sepsis and septic shock. *N Engl J Med.* 2001;345:1368–1377.

Randomized trial demonstrating the survival benefit of a goal-directed approach to the initial resuscitation of patients with sepsis and septic shock.

Singer M, Deutschman CS, Seymour CW, et al. The Third International Consensus Definitions for Sepsis and Septic Shock (Sepsis-3). *JAMA.* 2016;315(8):801–810.

Highlights the new consensus definition of sepsis and septic shock.

Cardiogenic Shock

Mirnela Byku and Joel C. Schilling

Cardiogenic shock occurs when there is inadequate circulation and compromised organ perfusion primarily due to cardiac dysfunction. Low cardiac output, despite adequate or even elevated filling pressures is the defining feature of cardiogenic shock. If untreated, this results in a failure of global oxygen delivery to meet oxygen consumption, resulting in tissue hypoperfusion, which leads to multisystem failure and death. Cardiogenic shock is characterized by prolonged hypotension (systolic blood pressure [SBP] <90 mm Hg for at least 30 minutes) in the setting of decreased cardiac output (typically <1.8 L/min/m² without support and <2.2 L/min/m² with support) despite adequate left ventricular (LV) preload (LV end-diastolic pressure >18 mm Hg and/or pulmonary artery occlusion pressure >15 mm Hg). Cool, mottled extremities; altered mentation; and oliguria are clinical manifestations of systemic hypoperfusion. These signs may not always be present, however, it is important to note that low cardiac output and mild hypotension are not cardiogenic shock without evidence of end-organ hypoperfusion. The mortality rate from cardiogenic shock remains high despite advances in revascularization and hemodynamic support strategies. Among patients hospitalized with an acute myocardial infarction (AMI) complicated by cardiogenic shock, the 30-day mortality rate remains between 40% and 50%, despite the increasing rates of early reperfusion by primary percutaneous coronary intervention (PCI) and advances in temporary mechanical support.

ETIOLOGY

Cardiogenic shock can occur in decompensated patients with long-standing cardiomyopathy or can be the result of an acute process. There are many known causes of cardiac injury that can result in shock physiology, with acute myocardial dysfunction in setting of AMI being the most common (see Table 4.1). The incidence of cardiogenic shock in setting of AMI has more recently been reported to occur in 5% to 8% of patients, with this number having been as high as 20% in the past. Patients who develop cardiogenic shock in the setting of AMI typically have extensive myocardial damage to the anterior LV wall due to an ischemic insult (>40% of myocardium) or have multivessel coronary artery disease (CAD). The severity of shock from LV infarction is generally related to the quantitative loss of functional myocardium. Complications of AMI, such as arrhythmias, ventricular septal defects, papillary muscle dysfunction, or myocardial rupture causing pericardial tamponade, may also trigger the onset of shock. Shock is more likely to occur in those with advanced age (>70 years), a history of diabetes mellitus, prior myocardial infarction (MI), or known congestive heart failure.

TABLE 4.1	Causes of Cardiogenic Shock

Acute myocardial infarction
    Left ventricular pump failure
        Large infarction
        Smaller infarction with pre-existing LV dysfunction
    Mechanical complications
        Free wall rupture/tamponade
        Papillary muscle dysfunction/rupture
        Right ventricular infarction
        Ventricular septal defect
        Aortic dissection

Severe cardiomyopathy/congestive heart failure
    Dilated cardiomyopathy
    Stress-induced or Takotsubo cardiomyopathy

Acute myocarditis (infectious, toxin/drug, transplant rejection)

Myocardial contusion

Calcium channel or beta-blocker overdose

Acute/severe valvular insufficiency
    Acute mitral regurgitation (e.g., chordal rupture)
    Acute aortic insufficiency

Obstruction to left ventricular outflow
    Hypertrophic obstructive cardiomyopathy
    Aortic stenosis

Obstruction to ventricular filling
    Pericardial effusion/tamponade
    Mitral stenosis
    Left atrial myxoma

Additionally, cardiogenic shock is seen in the setting of severe cardiomyopathy due to hypertrophy, stress-induced cardiomyopathy, acute myocarditis, severe valvular disease, and ischemic, dilated, or peripartum cardiomyopathy. Cardiogenic shock due to acute-on-chronic decompensated heart failure is also rising, with a reported incidence of 4% in this population.

PATHOPHYSIOLOGY

Cardiogenic shock generally occurs when myocardial dysfunction exceeds a critical threshold of cardiac injury either from a single large MI (typically considered to involve >40% of the myocardium), a cumulative amount of damage from multiple infarctions, or from diffuse myocardial injury from other inciting factors. With shock, there is increasing myocardial oxygen demand due to elevated end-diastolic ventricular pressure along with decreasing oxygen supply from hypotension and falling cardiac output. This results in a self-perpetuating spiral of progressive ischemia and cardiac dysfunction, which can ultimately culminate in death. Therapeutic

ALGORITHM 4.1 Pathophysiology of Cardiogenic Shock

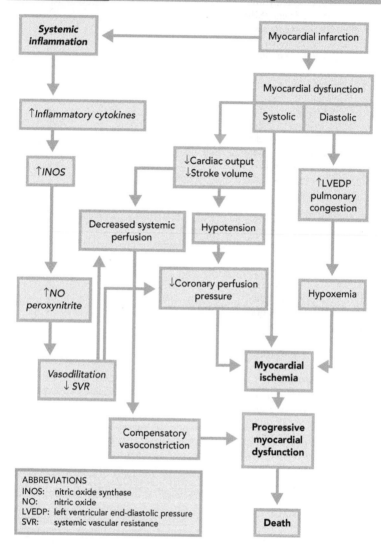

approaches for cardiogenic shock strive to interrupt this spiral at various steps in the pathophysiology of this disorder (Algorithm 4.1).

It is important to note that shock can develop even when the LV EF is not severely depressed (>30%), suggesting that there are other factors contributing to the development of end-organ hypoperfusion. Further support of this notion comes from data demonstrating that in many cases of AMI with shock, systemic vascular resistance (SVR) can be unexpectedly low, as a consequence of an associated systemic inflammatory response syndrome (SIRS). This response is initiated by myocardial necrosis and hypoperfusion and is associated with high levels of cytokines and systemic/vascular nitric oxide, which have both negative inotropic and vasodilatory effects, contributing to end-organ hypoperfusion.

PATIENT CHARACTERISTICS

Shock is more likely to develop in the setting of AMI among patients who are older, female, and those who have more comorbid conditions (diabetes, prior known CAD, history of cerebrovascular disease, history of renal insufficiency, and pre-existing heart failure). Cardiogenic shock can complicate ST elevation MI or non-ST elevation MI and it is more common in patients with anterior location of MI. By angiography, the left anterior descending artery is most commonly the culprit vessel, but patients with cardiogenic shock frequently have multivessel CAD. Signs and symptoms of cardiogenic shock usually develop after hospital admission (median, 6.2 hours after initial MI symptoms) and the majority of patients develop shock within the first 24 hours of AMI. A significant minority (~25%) of patients may develop cardiogenic shock after 24 hours, possibly due to recurrent ischemia. It should be noted that a subset of cardiogenic shock patients who present with poor cardiac output and evidence of systemic hypoperfusion but without frank hypotension has been described. These so-called normotensive cardiogenic shock patients have a lower mortality than their hypotensive counterparts (43% vs. 66%, respectively) but their risk of death is still much higher than AMI patients without hypoperfusion.

EVALUATION AND DIAGNOSIS

Prompt recognition of cardiogenic shock is essential for management, as timely and appropriate treatment can significantly reduce mortality. Patients with low blood pressure (BP) (<90 mm Hg) should be quickly assessed for the presence of pulsus paradoxus (suggestive of cardiac tamponade), signs of congestive heart failure (elevated jugular venous pressure, pulmonary edema, and S3 gallop), and evidence of end-organ hypoperfusion (cool, mottled extremities; weak pulses; altered mental status; and reduced urine output). A careful cardiac examination should be performed to assess for the presence of valvular disease or mechanical complications. It is important to keep in mind that in the setting of low cardiac output, the murmurs of mitral regurgitation, critical aortic stenosis or insufficiency may be diminished or virtually inaudible, therefore prompt imaging with an echocardiogram is often necessary. An electrocardiogram should be obtained without delay to look for evidence of acute ischemia or infarction, and to assist in triage for emergency reperfusion when indicated. Serum cardiac biomarkers should be measured at presentation and serially to diagnose acute myocardial injury even when the electrocardiogram is nondiagnostic. Obtaining rapid echocardiography is imperative and should be performed as soon as possible to assess for LV or right ventricular (RV) dysfunction, valvular pathology, and to exclude AMI-related mechanical complications (papillary muscle rupture, ventricular wall rupture, and ventricular septal defect) or cardiac tamponade, given that primary therapy for such conditions requires immediate invasive treatment, such as emergency surgical intervention.

When the etiology remains unclear, bedside pulmonary artery catheterization can be helpful in differentiating cardiogenic from other forms of shock. However, in cases of shock due to suspected acute myocardial ischemia or infarction, such studies should not delay definitive evaluation by left heart catheterization and coronary angiography. In addition to assisting with diagnosis, pulmonary artery catheter monitoring can help guide the use of vasopressor and inotropic medications and gauge hemodynamic stability, which allows for early implementation of additional support when necessary. This is particularly useful to guide treatment in patients with pre-existing cardiomyopathy and chronic heart failure who present with "mixed" shock (cardiogenic, septic, and hypovolemic shock).

TREATMENT

Initial Medical Management

The primary driver of cardiogenic shock, except when the aforementioned mechanical complications are present, is impaired LV function. Patients with cardiogenic shock require immediate intervention to stabilize their hemodynamics and interrupt the viscous cycle of tissue hypoperfusion. This can limit the development of multisystem organ failure and irreversible organ damage (Algorithm 4.2). These patients typically need intensive care level of monitoring with central venous access, continuous monitoring of arterial pressure and urine output, and often mechanical ventilation. In general it is important that patients are treated in a hospital environment where advanced management options, such as PCI, mechanical circulatory assist devices, and cardiac surgery are readily available. Optimal management of cardiogenic shock is directed by the etiology of myocardial injury, a crucial concept that is discussed in the following sections.

Shock Associated with AMI

Similar to any patient with an acute coronary syndrome, patients with cardiogenic shock who have evidence of acute ischemia or infarction should receive full-dose aspirin and early consideration of an adenosine diphosphate (ADP) receptor blocker, unless contraindicated. Thienopyridines may be withheld until coronary anatomy is defined and the possible need for emergent surgical intervention has been determined, given the potential for increased perioperative bleeding. Once plans are made to proceed with PCI, thienopyridines should be administered as early as possible. Beta blockers and angiotensin-converting enzyme (ACE) inhibitors should be avoided until hemodynamic stability is achieved. In the absence of overt pulmonary congestion, as seen in shock due to RV infarct and failure, fluid resuscitation may help reverse hypotension and maintain adequate perfusion. Systemic hypotension may initially require treatment with vasopressors, although the lowest dose needed to support organ perfusion should be used as these agents can increase afterload and oxygen demand for the failing myocardium. The evidence guiding first-line pressor selection in cardiogenic shock is limited, however, both norepinephrine (starting dose, 1 to 40 mcg/min) and dopamine (starting dose, 5 to 20 mcg/kg/min) can be used and titrated to hemodynamic effect. Depending on the dose, dopamine has combined inotropic and vasopressor effects and can theoretically improve renal perfusion

ALGORITHM 4.2 **Management of Suspected Cardiogenic Shock**

Suspected CS
- SBP <90 mm Hg
- Signs of low cardiac output (oliguria, poor MS, pulmonary edema)

ABBREVIATIONS
CS: cardiogenic shock
SBP: systolic blood pressure
MS: mental status
ECG: electrocardiogram
AMI: acute myocardial infarction
BP: blood pressure
MAP: mean arterial pressure
LV/RV: left ventricular/right ventricular
IABP: intra-aortic balloon counterpulsation
MR: mitral regurgitation
VSD: ventricular septal defect
PA: pulmonary artery
PCI: percutaneous coronary intervention
CABG: coronary artery bypass surgery
LVAD: left ventricular assist device

Initial evaluation and rapid stabilization immediate ECG
Look for evidence of AMI
(ST elevation, LBBB (new), suspected posterior MI)
Supplemental O₂ / Mech ventilation *(for hypoxia)*
BP support
SBP <90 mm Hg
Dopamine (5–15 µg/kg/min)
SBP <80 mm Hg (w Dopa)
Norepinephrine (1–20 µg/min)
Goal MAP >65 mm Hg
All patients on vasopressors should have intra-arterial pressure monitoring

If ECG(+)

Immediate reperfusion therapy

Thrombolysis/IABP
Only if Cath Lab not immediately available

Then transfer for

Cardiac catheterization
- <36 hrs from onset of AMI
- <12–18 hrs from onset of shock
No other contraindication to anticoagulation
IABP support

If ECG(–)

Emergent echocardiogram
Evaluate LV/RV function
r/o mechanical complications resulting in CS
- Acute MR/papillary muscle rupture, VSD, Free wall rupture, RV infarction
PA catheter monitoring
Confirm cardiac etiology
CI <2.2 L/min/m²
PCWP >15 mm Hg

No revascularization possible continued medical support
if BP stable consider
Inotropic support
Dobutamine (2.5–10 µg/min)
Milrinone (0.375–0.75 µg/kg/min)
Avoid in hypotension, renal failure (Milrinone)

Suitable for revascularization
PCI *(infarct artery only)*
Rec. use of stents and abciximab
or Emergent CABG
(3V dz, L Main dz, or PCI not possible)

Refractory shock
Consider LVAD, transplant evaluation

by mesenteric vasodilation at low doses. A downside of dopamine utilization is the high rate of tachyarrhythmias that can occur. Of note, dopamine was associated with a significantly higher rate of adverse events and of 28-day mortality compared with norepinephrine in a recent subgroup analysis of 280 patients with cardiogenic shock randomized to either therapy. Other options include the combination of an inotrope, such as dobutamine, with norepinephrine to improve cardiac output. In general, milrinone should be avoided during the acute phase of cardiogenic shock due to its potential to worsen hypotension and to accumulate with renal dysfunction. As mentioned previously, AMI with cardiogenic shock may be associated with SIRS and relatively low SVR. In this setting, traditional measures of cardiogenic shock treatment, such as inotropes, that involve decreasing SVR and increasing cardiac output may not always be beneficial. If a patient develops refractory hypotension despite the use of pressors and inotropes, temporary mechanical circulatory assist devices may be necessary (detailed below).

A fundamental concept of current treatment of cardiogenic shock in patients with obstructive CAD and AMI is the recognition that early revascularization is key to reduce mortality. Patients with evidence of an acute coronary syndrome and cardiogenic shock should be referred for urgent left heart catheterization and revascularization if coronary anatomy is suitable. Results from the randomized SHOCK trial comparing early revascularization with conservative management showed that patients <75 years of age with AMI and cardiogenic shock had ~20% relative risk reduction in mortality with early PCI or coronary artery bypass surgery, defined as revascularization within 2 days of presentation. Therefore, current guidelines recommend early revascularization, when feasible, for patients who are within 36 hours of the onset of AMI. Of note, 36% of the patients in the SHOCK trial who underwent revascularization received coronary artery bypass surgery, an observation that reflects the complex and extensive CAD in these high-risk patients. Nonrandomized data show there may also be a benefit from early revascularization in patients >75 years old. Current guidelines recommend that such patients should be considered for early revascularization on an individual basis. Randomized trials of reperfusion for ST-elevation MI have suggested that pharmacologic reperfusion by thrombolytic therapy alone is less effective than primary PCI in the presence of cardiogenic shock. Therefore, timely PCI is the preferred method of reperfusion, when available, for patients with AMI and cardiogenic shock. Delayed reperfusion is associated with a significant increase in mortality even in a time frame as short as minutes to hours. Therefore, for patients who cannot undergo timely coronary intervention, there is limited data that thrombolysis combined with intra-aortic balloon counterpulsation may benefit patients as a temporizing measure to definitive revascularization.

Shock in Setting of Cardiomyopathy

The combination of improved medical treatment for heart failure, rapid revascularization post-MI, and the use of internal cardiac defibrillators, has led to a steady increase in the number of patients with chronic, advanced heart failure. These patients are at risk of deterioration and can present with cardiogenic shock. Worsening ischemic heart disease, infection, arrhythmia, pulmonary embolism, or progression of their underlying cardiomyopathy can precipitate cardiac compromise in these patients. Clinically, such patients typically present with evidence of multiorgan dysfunction, including elevated liver function tests (LFTs), rising creatinine, decreasing urine output and lactic acidosis. They also have evidence of increased SVR and hypoperfusion with cold extremities, nausea and vomiting, as well as altered mental status. Patients with cardiogenic shock due to advanced heart failure frequently have low BP, low cardiac output, and high SVR, in contrast to some cases of shock due to AMI where the SVR may not be as elevated due to a SIRS response.

Early management should focus on the use of inotropes such as dobutamine (2.5 to 10 mcg/min) or milrinone (0.375 to 0.75 mcg/kg/min, with or without a loading dose of 50 mcg/kg) to restore perfusion. Both of these agents increase contractility and have a vasodilatory effect (milrinone > dobutamine). Because of its potential for peripheral vasodilation, dobutamine and milrinone should be used with caution in patients with significant hypotension (SBP <80 mm Hg). In this case, the combination with norepinephrine or epinephrine may be useful to maintain BP and perfusion. As noted above, milrinone should also be used with great caution in patients with worsening renal function due to the potential accumulation of vasoactive metabolites that produce arrhythmias and hypotension.

In cardiogenic shock related to hypertrophic cardiomyopathy with severe diastolic dysfunction and outflow tract obstruction requires preservation of afterload to prevent worsening of the outflow tract obstruction and hypotension. This results in a seemingly paradoxical need to avoid inotropes and intra-aortic balloon counterpulsation (as described below) because inotropic agents and balloon pumps decrease afterload and increase contractility, resulting in worse outflow obstruction and thus, hypotension. Therefore, these approaches should be avoided in hypertrophic cardiomyopathy with severe diastolic dysfunction and the selective peripheral vasoconstrictor phenylephrine should be the pressor of choice when these patients present with shock.

Cardiac Tamponade

Cardiac tamponade represents a unique cause of shock in which external compression of the heart significantly restricts filling and limits cardiac output. Because it is rapidly reversible with pericardiocentesis, prompt recognition is essential. Cardiac tamponade remains a clinical diagnosis. Important clinical signs on examination include the presence of exaggerated pulsus paradoxus (where the inspiratory fall in SBP exceeds ~10 mm Hg), distended jugular veins, and muffled heart sounds. The most common cause is a significant pericardial effusion, although more unusual causes of impaired filling—such as a localized thrombus compressing the left atrium following cardiac surgery—are possible. Echocardiography may demonstrate the classic findings of a pericardial effusion with evidence of diastolic compression of the right side of the heart and exaggerated respiratory variation in Doppler-measured mitral inflow velocities. When hypotension is present, rapid infusion of intravenous fluids may help maintain BP, but removal of the offending pericardial fluid by percutaneous pericardiocentesis or surgical drainage is the definitive treatment. If the diagnosis is in question, pulmonary artery catheterization may be useful to confirm hemodynamic evidence of tamponade, suggested by equalization of elevated right atrial (RA), RV diastolic, pulmonary artery diastolic, and pulmonary artery wedge pressures.

Mechanical Support for Cardiogenic Shock

In addition to pharmacologic measures, treatment with mechanical circulatory support (MCS) devices should be considered in more severe forms of circulatory failure. The aim of MCS is to support the failing heart and maintain perfusion when pharmacologic approaches are failing. MCS should be employed in refractory cardiogenic shock to prevent the development of multiorgan failure. Ideally, temporary mechanical support is used as a bridge to recovery or to other more durable therapies such as a surgically implanted left ventricular assist device (LVAD) or heart transplantation. In cardiac arrest patients, MCS enables treatment of the underlying cause while maintaining adequate perfusion. There are many options for temporary MCS, including intra-aortic balloon pump (IABP), Impella™, and extracorporeal membrane oxygenation (ECMO), which can be utilized in patients with cardiogenic shock, and will be discussed in detail in the following section.

Circulatory Assist Devices in Cardiogenic Shock

Intra-Aortic Balloon Counterpulsation. The IABP is the most extensively studied and utilized form of MCS for cardiogenic shock. The device is placed via an accessible artery, usually the femoral artery, into the descending aorta. During diastole, the balloon inflates with helium gas, which augments diastolic pressure and increases coronary perfusion. During systole, the balloon deflates rapidly, creating a temporary vacuum that reduces afterload and improves LV ejection. Balloon pump counterpulsation is the only means to augment central aortic pressure and vital organ perfusion (including coronary blood flow) while simultaneously reducing afterload and myocardial oxygen demand. Early IABP support can be beneficial as a bridge to revascularization, to recovery following transient myocardial stunning, or en route to more advanced support devices or cardiac transplantation. It should be considered as an early intervention for patients with cardiogenic shock in whom there are none of the following contraindications: severe aortic insufficiency, severe peripheral vascular disease, aortic dissection, bleeding diathesis, or sepsis. Complications include bleeding, vascular injury (limb ischemia), thrombocytopenia, and infection.

Currently, IABP usage in cardiogenic shock has declined from a class I recommendation to a class IIb recommendation in the American guidelines and a class III recommendation in the European guidelines. The primary driver of this change was the results of the SHOCK II trial, published in 2012. SHOCK II was a randomized controlled trial of 600 patients with cardiogenic shock complicating AMI, expected to undergo early revascularization and managed with optimized medical therapy (OMT), randomized to IABP (301 patients) versus no IABP (299 patients). There was no difference between groups in 30-day mortality, the primary end point. Secondary end points, such as time to hemodynamic stabilization, ICU length of stay, lactic acidosis, renal function, vasopressor dose, and treatment duration, were also similar between groups. On the other hand, the IABP group had similar rates of major bleeding, peripheral ischemic complication, stroke and sepsis to the control group, therefore meeting safety parameters. As a result, there is currently no sufficient data to either strongly support or deny the use of IABPs in cases of severe refractory shock complicating AMI. It is important to note that the patients studied were very ill, with multiple comorbidities and all had ischemic heart disease, making overall mortality very high and therefore harder to see any beneficial effect of the intervention. Further studies may be necessary to evaluate IABP use in patients who are not yet in refractory shock and with fewer comorbidities.

Percutaneous and Surgical Ventricular Assist Devices

When OMT and IABP support are inadequate to stabilize vital organ perfusion, more advanced forms of support may be necessary and should be considered before irreversible end-organ damage occurs. Temporary LVADs can be inserted surgically or percutaneously and provide improved cardiac output and LV unloading. In a suitable patient with cardiogenic shock, a temporary LVAD is used to "bridge" the patient to recovery or a definitive treatment such as a durable LVAD or orthotopic heart transplantation. The percutaneous transvalvular LVADs (Impella™ 2.5 and 5.0; Abiomed, Inc.) and percutaneous left atrial-to-femoral artery ventricular assist device (Tandem-Heart™; CardiacAssist, Inc.) may be better tolerated in patients not stable enough for surgically implanted devices. The Impella™ works on the principle of an Archimedes screw. A large bore pig tail catheter with a miniature impeller pump is percutaneously inserted in the femoral artery and advanced across the aortic valve. The inlet at the distal catheter is positioned in the left ventricle and the device can continuously pump up to 2.5 to 5.0 L/min of blood (depending on model catheter size) into the ascending aorta. The TandemHeart™ System involves a large bore venous catheter inserted into the left atrium via transseptal puncture for withdrawal of oxygenated blood and an arterial catheter placed in the femoral artery for blood return, with an intervening extracorporeal centrifugal pump that can provide up to 5.0 L/min of flow.

While experience with temporary LVADs is growing, their impact on clinical outcomes in patients with cardiogenic shock remains limited. In a small randomized comparison involving only 26 patients, a percutaneously inserted Impella™ 2.5 compared favorably with an IABP with respect to improved hemodynamic indices, while there was no difference in the 30-day mortality rate (although the study was not powered to assess a difference in this end point). More recently, the Impella™ versus IABP reduces mortality in STEMI patients treated with PCI in severe cardiogenic shock (IMPRESS) trial results were published. The IMPRESS trial was a randomized controlled trial of 48 patients with severe cardiogenic shock complicating AMI randomized to Impella™ CP ($n = 24$) or IABP ($n = 24$). There was no difference in the primary end point of 30-day mortality between the groups. Six-month mortality was also similarly very high between the groups at 50%. Therefore, although theoretically appealing, further outcome data using these devices in cardiogenic shock are needed. Contraindications to Impella™ insertion include aortic regurgitation, aortic dissection/aneurysm, severe peripheral vascular disease, bleeding diathesis, LV thrombus, and sepsis. Device-related complications, including bleeding, vascular compromise, thromboembolic events, and infections, pose continued challenges to management in this critically ill patient population.

Extracorporeal Life Support with Extracorporeal Membrane Oxygenation. ECMO is a modified form of cardiopulmonary bypass designed to support both cardiac and pulmonary function. Technologic improvements have made this technique more readily accessible and its use has increased dramatically over the past few years, especially in patients with refractory cardiogenic shock or circulatory arrest.

ECMO involves the use of a centrifugal pump to drive blood from the patient's venous system through an externalized membrane oxygenator system, then returning it to the patient's arterial system. Venoarterial (VA) ECMO is the configuration utilized for cardiogenic shock. For peripheral ECMO the cannulation sites are typically the femoral artery and vein or internal jugular vein. Central ECMO requires a partial sternotomy with placement of the venous catheter in the RA or vena cava with arterial cannulation in the aorta. In addition to assisting in gas exchange, VA ECMO can augment cardiac output and typically provide up to 5 L/min of support. Advantages of ECMO over other temporary assist devices include the ability to oxygenate blood in hypoxemic states and provide support for both left and right ventricles. Peripheral ECMO can be placed at the bedside, making it useful in cases of circulatory arrest. Complications include risk of limb ischemia, bleeding, and hemolysis. The American Heart Association Guidelines for Cardiopulmonary Resuscitation state that ECMO is reasonable to perform and its benefit outweighs risk in the setting of cardiac arrest or shock because of a potentially reversible condition, such as myocarditis. It is important to note that the VA ECMO circuit "bypasses" the heart and therefore the introduction of oxygenated blood into the ascending aorta leads to increased LV afterload. The increased afterload prevents efficient LV ejection leading to stagnation of blood in the ventricle and high LV filling pressures, which can lead to thrombus formation and pulmonary edema, respectively. As a result, unloading the LV with an LV vent may be necessary. The LV vent can either be placed percutaneously, such as an Impella™, or surgically via central LA or LV cannula. The use of an LV vent is critical when native LV contractility and pulsatility are significantly reduced (e.g., the aortic valve is mostly closed).

CONCLUSION

- Cardiogenic shock is a condition that occurs as a consequence of profound cardiac dysfunction leading to multisystem organ hypoperfusion.
- The most common cause of cardiogenic shock is significant cardiac injury in the setting of AMI.
- Mortality remains high in the acute phase of shock and prompt diagnosis and appropriate treatment are paramount to improve the chances of survival.
- A bedside echocardiogram is required as soon as possible to evaluate for mechanical complications resulting in shock, such as acute valvular abnormality, free wall rupture, acute ventricular septal defect (VSD), cardiac tamponade, etc., which necessitate emergent surgical evaluation.
- The use of early PCI for AMI improves outcomes, therefore rapid diagnosis and referral for left heart catheterization is necessary.
- Optimal management requires early recognition and aggressive medical treatment with pressors and inotropes.
- Special cases of cardiogenic shock exist and have distinct treatment strategies, such as:
  - RV infarct—fluid resuscitation, transvenous pacing
  - Hypertrophic cardiomyopathy—fluid resuscitation and phenylephrine
  - Cardiac tamponade—fluid resuscitation and urgent pericardiocentesis
- In cases of severe and refractory shock, temporary mechanical support with IABP, Impella™, and/or ECMO should be considered as a bridge to further durable therapy such as LVADs or cardiac transplantation.

SUGGESTED READINGS

Cave DM, Gazmuri RJ, Otto CW, et al. Part 7: CPR techniques and devices: 2010 American heart association guidelines for cardiopulmonary resuscitation and emergency cardiovascular care. *Circulation.* 2010;122(18 suppl 3):S720–S728.

Cheng JM, den Uil CA, Hoeks SE, et al. Percutaneous left ventricular assist devices vs. intra-aortic balloon counterpulsation for treatment of cardiogenic shock: a meta-analysis of controlled trials. *Eur Heart J.* 2009;30(17):2102–2108.

De Backer D, Biston P, Devriendt J, et al. Comparison of dopamine and norepinephrine in the treatment of shock. *N Engl J Med.* 2010;362(9):779–789.

Results of the randomized SOAP II trial showing higher adverse event rates and 28-day mortality associated with dopamine use among the subgroup of patients with cardiogenic shock.

Gilotra NA, Stevens GR. Temporary mechanical circulatory support: a review of the options, indications, and outcomes. *Clin Med Insights Cardiol.* 2015;8(suppl 1):75–85.

Review of currently used temporary mechanical assist devices in the treatment of cardiogenic shock.

Hochman JS. Cardiogenic shock complicating acute myocardial infarction: expanding the paradigm. *Circulation.* 2003;107(24):2998–3002.

A review of cardiogenic shock including newer information regarding pathophysiology and management.

Hochman JS, Sleeper LA, Webb JG, et al. Early revascularization in acute myocardial infarction complicated by cardiogenic shock. SHOCK Investigators. Should we emergently revascularize occluded coronaries for cardiogenic shock. *N Engl J Med.* 1999;341(9):625–634.

Published results of the landmark SHOCK trial showing reduced mortality for patients (less than age 75) randomized to a strategy of early revascularization versus conservative management.

Hollenberg SM, Kavinsky CJ, Parrillo JE. Cardiogenic shock. *Ann Intern Med.* 1999;131(1):47–59.

A general review of cardiogenic shock and evidence-based management.

Ouweneel DM, Eriksen E, Sjauw KD, et al. Impella CP versus intra-aortic balloon pump in acute myocardial infarction complicated by cardiogenic shock: The IMPRESS trial. *J Am Coll Cardiol.* 2016; doi: 10. 1016/j.jacc. 10.022.

Study comparing Impella versus IABP in the management of cardiogenic shock complicating AMI.

Reynolds HR, Hochman JS. Cardiogenic shock: Current concepts and improving outcomes. *Circulation.* 2008;117(5):686–697.

Seyfarth M, Sibbing D, Bauer I, et al. A randomized clinical trial to evaluate the safety and efficacy of a percutaneous left ventricular assist device versus intra-aortic balloon pumping for treatment of cardiogenic shock caused by myocardial infarction. *J Am Coll Cardiol.* 2008; 52(19):1584–1588.

Two articles regarding use of percutaneous left ventricular assist devices compared with IABP counterpulsation in the management of cardiogenic shock.

Thiele H, Zeymer U, Werdan K, et al; IABP-SHOCK II Trial Investigators. *N Engl J Med.* 2012;367(14):1287–1296.

The published results of SHOCK II trial.

Various Authors. *J Am Coll Cardiol.* 2000;36(3, suppl 1).

JACC supplement with several publications on clinically relevant substudies from the SHOCK trial and Registry.

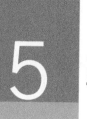

Anaphylactic Shock

Marin H. Kollef

Anaphylaxis refers to the characteristic and often life-threatening clinical manifestations of the immunoglobulin E (IgE)–mediated immediate hypersensitivity reaction, involving mast cell and basophil degranulation with release of histamine, tryptase, prostaglandins, and leukotrienes, that occurs following exposure to various substances. Anaphylactoid reactions are clinically indistinguishable from anaphylaxis but are not IgE mediated. They are thought to result from direct mast cell degranulation independent of IgE or from alterations in arachidonic acid metabolism. The substances that trigger anaphylaxis and anaphylactoid reactions differ and are outlined in Table 5.1.

Reactions can develop within minutes, but usually <1 hour, after exposure to a triggering substance. More rapid reactions occur with parenteral exposure. Initial symptoms include flushing, pruritus, and a sense of doom. Characteristic clinical manifestations of varying severity develop involving the skin, eyes, respiratory and gastrointestinal tracts, and cardiovascular and central nervous systems, as listed in Table 5.2. Cardiovascular collapse (shock) occurs in approximately 30% of cases and results from (a) hypovolemia induced by increased vascular permeability and loss of intravascular volume, (b) hypotension from peripheral vasodilation, (c) myocardial depression, and (d) bradycardia. Up to 50% of patients describe respiratory symptoms, which can progress to respiratory failure from severe upper airway edema, bronchospasm, and cardiogenic and noncardiogenic pulmonary edema. Biphasic reactions occur in up to 20% of patients, characterized by a second round of symptoms 1 to 8 hours after the initial reaction (although up to 72 hours have been reported).

Diagnosis is clinical and involves a broad differential diagnosis including urticaria, status asthmaticus, "red man" syndrome (vancomycin), scromboidosis (histamine-like compound in spoiled fish such as tuna, mackerel, mahi-mahi, and blue fish), carcinoid, pheochromocytoma, mastocytosis, monosodium glutamate ingestion, and panic attacks. Serum levels of tryptase (especially the beta subtype) and histamine, when elevated, support the diagnosis. Tryptase levels are elevated for 1 to 6 hours after the event, but serum histamine levels fall within 30 to 60 minutes. A 24-hour urine n-methyl histamine level compared to a later baseline can be a helpful alternative. Patients should be questioned about exposure to potential triggers, but no substance is identified in up to 60% of cases.

Treatment is outlined in Algorithm 5.1 and is based on the joint recommendations of the American Academy of Allergy, Asthma, and Immunology and the American College of Allergy, Asthma, and Immunology. Pharmacologic therapy involves epinephrine to reverse the respiratory and cardiovascular effects and blocking the effects of histamine with histamine 1 and 2 receptor blockers. There are no

TABLE 5.1	Causes of Anaphylaxis (Substances Are Paired with the Most Common Associated Mechanism)

Anaphylaxis (IgE mediated)
  Foods (especially nuts, eggs, fish, shellfish, and cow's milk)
  Antibiotics (especially penicillin; 4% positive by allergy testing also test positive to cephalosporins)
  Vaccines
  Anesthetics
  Insulin and other hormones
  Antitoxins
  Blood and blood products
  Insect stings and bites (bee, wasp, and ant)
  Snake bites
  Latex
  Allergy immunotherapy

Anaphylactoid reactions (direct mast cell degranulation, altered AA metabolism)
  Nonsteroidal anti-inflammatory drugs (especially aspirin)
  Opiates
  Sulfites
  Radiocontrast media
  Neuromuscular blocking agents (curoniums and succinylcholine)
  Gamma globulin
  Antisera
  Exercise

IgE, immunoglobulin E; AA, arachidonic acid.

TABLE 5.2	Clinical Manifestations of Anaphylaxis and Laboratory Tests

Clinical Manifestations:

Eyes
  Pruritus
  Lacrimation
  Conjunctival erythema
  Periorbital edema
	Skin
	  Pruritus
	  Flushing
	  Urticaria
	  Angioedema

Cardiovascular
  Hypotension
  Tachycardia (bradycardia when severe)
  Arrhythmias
  Cardiac arrest
  Paradoxical hypertension (in presence of beta-adrenergic blockers)
	Respiratory
	  Dyspnea
	  Stridor/wheezing/hoarseness
	  Difficulty swallowing
	  Pulmonary edema

Gastrointestinal
  Nausea/vomiting
  Diarrhea
  Abdominal pain
	Neurologic
	  Anxiety and "sense of doom"
	  Presyncope and syncope
	  Seizures

Laboratory Tests:
  Total serum or plasma tryptase
  Mature beta tryptase
	Plasma histamine
	Platelet-activating factor

ALGORITHM 5.1 **Acute Treatment of Patients with Anaphylaxis**

Immediate treatment is indicated for all patients with significant respiratory, cardiac, or gastrointestinal symptoms as symptoms can progress rapidly to shock, respiratory failure, and death, and there are **NO absolute contraindications to epinephrine.**

Suspected impending respiratory collapse (stridor, wheezing, tachypnea, dyspnea, difficulty swallowing)

No — **Yes**

Place patient in recumbent position. Obtain large bore IV access (but do not delay next step). Continuous monitoring of blood pressure, heart rate, oxygen saturation, and respiratory symptoms.

Immediate intubation as delay may increase difficulty of endotracheal intubation. Cricothyroidotomy may be necessary if severe airway edema.

IM epinephrine 0.3–0.5 mg 1:1000 to anterior or lateral thigh, preferably. Repeat after 5 minutes as needed (up to 70% can require second dose). **FOR SEVERE SYMPTOMS OR POOR RESPONSE TO IM GIVE** IV epinephrine 0.1–0.2 mg (1 mL 1:1000 in 10 cc 0.9% NaCl [0.1 mg/cc]) every 1–2 minutes until response or epinephrine infusion (1 mg in 250 mL 5% dextrose water [4 mcg/mL]) at 2–10 mcg/min **IF HYPOTENSIVE GIVE;** 1–2 L IV 0.9% NaCl rapid infusion.

Treat all patients with histamine 1 and 2 (H1, H2) blockers.
1) Diphenhydramine (H1) 25–50 mg IV **and**
1) Ranitidine (H2) 50 mg IV or
2) Famotidine (H2) 20 mg IV

Clinical response?

Yes

No

If patient taking home beta blocker;
1) Glucagon 1–2 mg IV/IM q5min to effect
For continued hypotension;
1) Start continuous IV epinephrine (Levophed) infusion at 5–10 mcg/min titrated to effect.
2) Continued aggressive fluid resuscitation (via rapid transfuser if available).
For continued respiratory symptoms, if not intubated;
1) Inhaled beta agonists (albuterol) 0.5 mL 0.5% in 2.5 cc 0.9% NaCl nebulized q15min.

If patient is pregnant;
1) Fetal monitoring
2) Position on left side
3) Maintain SBP ≥90 mm Hg
4) Supplemental oxygen
5) Consider emergent cesarean delivery for persistent fetal distress

ABBREVIATIONS
IV: intravenous
IM: intramuscular
SBP: systolic blood pressure

contraindications to the use of epinephrine, and numerous studies have shown that it is underused in emergency treatment, with delay resulting in shock and respiratory failure. In a study by Korenblat et al., 70% of patients with severe symptoms required at least two epinephrine injections. Intramuscular injection of epinephrine has been associated with fewer complications in several studies compared to intravenous administration. Intravenous steroids have no role in the acute treatment of anaphylaxis but may prevent phase 2 reactions that can occur up to 72 hours after initial presentation. Steroids are given as an initial dose of 1 to 2 mg/kg of intravenous methylprednisolone, or equivalent, and continued for up to 4 days (intravenously or orally). On discharge, patients should be referred to an allergist for testing and monitoring and provided with home epinephrine self-injectors (EpiPen).

SUGGESTED READINGS

Campbell RL, Bellolio MF, Knutson BD, et al. Epinephrine in anaphylaxis: higher risk of cardiovascular complications and overdose after administration of intravenous bolus epinephrine compared with intramuscular epinephrine. *J Allergy Clin Immunol Pract.* 2015;3:76–80.
An observational cohort study showing that patients who received intravenous bolus epinephrine administration were more likely to experience an overdose and adverse cardiovascular complications.

Fleming JT, Clark S, Camargo CA Jr, et al. Early treatment of food-induced anaphylaxis with epinephrine is associated with a lower risk of hospitalization. *J Allergy Clin Immunol Pract.* 2015;3:57–62.
Retrospective review of 384 emergency department visits for food-induced anaphylaxis demonstrating that those individuals receiving epinephrine therapy prior to emergency department arrival were less likely to require hospitalization.

Korenblat P, Lundie MJ, Dankner RE, et al. A retrospective study of epinephrine administration for anaphylaxis: how many doses are needed? *Allergy Asthma Proc.* 1999;20:383–386.
Retrospective review of 105 anaphylactic episodes to determine the level of severity and corresponding number of epinephrine injections required for symptom reversal.

Lieberman P, Nicklas RA, Oppenheimer J, et al. The diagnosis and management of anaphylaxis practice parameter: 2010 update. *J Allergy Clin Immunol.* 2010;126:477–480.
Joint recommendations on the definition, causes, manifestations, diagnosis, and treatment for patients with anaphylaxis and anaphylactoid reactions.

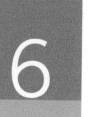

6

Mechanical Causes of Shock

Patrick R. Aguilar

Mechanical shock can be precipitated by an array of syndromes that produce an acute loss of pulmonary vascular cross-sectional area, either by direct obstruction of pulmonary vasculature or through vasoconstriction driven by vasoactive mediators. The end result is an acute rise in pulmonary vascular resistance (PVR), which leads to right ventricular (RV) strain, RV failure, and shock. *Mechanical shock* is also called *obstructive shock*; these terms are used interchangeably in the literature. Cardiac tamponade, discussed in Chapter 4, can also be considered a mechanical cause of shock. However, its pathophysiology is distinct from the other forms of shock discussed here. Although the various etiologies of shock are discussed in isolation in this manual, it is important to recognize that several forms of shock may be present at the same time.

This discussion will focus on four major etiologies of mechanical shock: (1) massive pulmonary embolism (PE), (2) air embolism, (3) fat embolism, and (4) amniotic fluid embolism. The degree of hemodynamic compromise caused by any of these causes of mechanical shock is determined by (1) the magnitude of pulmonary arterial vascular obstruction and/or vasoconstriction, (2) RV performance and reserve, and (3) pre-existing cardiopulmonary disease (CPD). For example, a segmental pulmonary embolus normally survivable in an otherwise healthy postpartum patient may produce mechanical shock in a patient with pre-existing pulmonary arterial hypertension and marginal RV function.

The pulmonary circulation is normally a high-capacitance, low-resistance circuit. In general, a right ventricle cannot acutely compensate for a mean pulmonary arterial pressure (mPAP) greater than 40 mm Hg. Therefore, the finding of mPAP values greater than 40 mm Hg without clinical signs of RV failure suggests a subacute or chronic cause of pulmonary arterial hypertension. In the absence of pre-existing CPD, the increase in RV afterload and mPAP is directly proportional to the magnitude of pulmonary vascular obstruction and/or vasoconstriction. Echocardiographic findings of acute RV dysfunction may be evident following a 25% to 30% reduction in pulmonary vascular cross-sectional area. However, the degree of obstruction necessary to cause hemodynamic compromise and shock may be much lower in a patient with pre-existing CPD.

Without aggressive intervention, an acute elevation in PVR beyond the capacity of RV compensation precipitates a deleterious chain of events that ends in refractory shock, circulatory collapse, and death. Algorithm 6.1 illustrates the interdependent nature of the multiple factors that contribute to obstructive shock. Successful management of mechanical shock syndromes requires early recognition and rapid initiation

ALGORITHM 6.1 Pathophysiology of Mechanical Shock

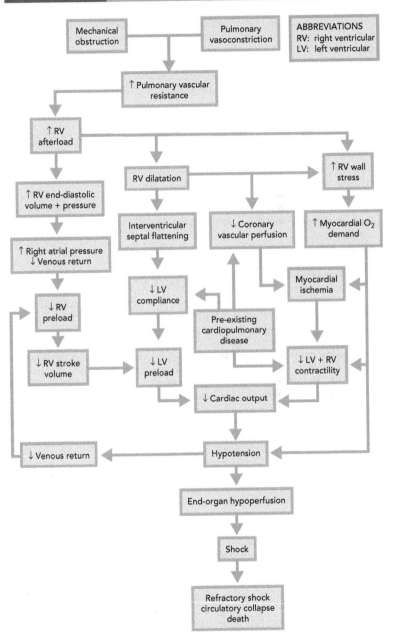

of supportive measures to restore hemodynamic stability and prevent end-organ dysfunction.

Common clinical findings in mechanical shock states include tachycardia, hypotension, and signs of end-organ hypoperfusion (i.e., decreased urine output, cool and mottled extremities, and altered mental status). Physical examination should reveal signs of decompensated RV failure, including jugular venous distention, tricuspid regurgitation murmur, accentuated P2, hepatojugular reflux, and Kussmaul's sign. Dysregulation of ventilation–perfusion matching results in hypoxemia and tachypnea. In catastrophic cases, ventricular fibrillation, pulseless electrical activity, or asystole may be the initial presentation.

Diagnostically, sinus tachycardia is frequently seen on EKG, with or without changes suggestive of RV strain and myocardial ischemia. Echocardiographic signs of RV dysfunction, including RV dilatation, hypokinesis, tricuspid regurgitation, and flattening of the interventricular septum, may also be present. Common laboratory findings include hyponatremia, elevated serum brain natriuretic peptide (BNP), and markers of myocardial injury (troponin T or I).

The following sections discuss the unique features, pathophysiology, and management of four common mechanical shock syndromes. Table 6.1 contains a list of risk factors and presenting signs and symptoms for each syndrome.

PULMONARY EMBOLISM

Venous thromboembolism (VTE) is a common complication in critically ill medical and surgical patients. Most intensive care unit (ICU) patients have multiple major risk factors for VTE, including trauma, prolonged immobilization, malignancy, and indwelling vascular access devices. Clinical studies in medical ICUs have shown up to one-third of patients not receiving deep venous thrombosis prophylaxis will eventually develop VTE at some point during their hospital course. Approximately 5% to 10% of patients with VTE develop PE, with approximately 10% of these cases causing hemodynamically significant or massive PE. The presence of shock in the setting of PE is associated with a five- to sevenfold increase in mortality. Patients presenting with cardiopulmonary arrest have mortality rates exceeding 65%.

Bedside 2D echocardiography is a useful diagnostic tool for evaluating hemodynamic status in patients with suspected massive PE. Alternative diagnoses, such as cardiomyopathy, valvular disease, cardiac tamponade, and aortic dissection, can be quickly excluded from the differential diagnosis. McConnell's sign, a classic echocardiographic sign of massive PE, is characterized by global RV hypokinesis with relative sparing of the apical segments.

Initiation of therapy should not be delayed for confirmatory diagnostic testing. Treatment should be focused on (1) restoring hemodynamic stability, (2) maintaining adequate oxygenation, and (3) reducing clot burden and preventing recurrent embolus. A management algorithm for massive PE is shown in Algorithm 6.2.

Multiple randomized controlled trials have addressed the role of thrombolytic (fibrinolytic) therapy versus anticoagulation with unfractionated or low–molecular-weight heparin as initial treatment for PE. In patients with hemodynamic instability, thrombolytic therapy has been associated with faster recovery of RV function and improvement in hemodynamic status. Among patients with "moderately severe" pulmonary emboli, the use of half-dose tPA has been associated with decreased incidence of pulmonary hypertension after 28 months of follow-up. Additionally, a

TABLE 6.1	Risk Factors and Common Manifestations of Mechanical Shock States	
	Risk Factors	**Common Signs and Symptoms**
Massive pulmonary embolism	• Immobilization • Surgery within last 3 months • Prior history of VTE • Malignancy • Chronic cardiopulmonary disease • Trauma • Obesity • Central venous catheters • Hypercoagulable state	• Pleuritic chest pain • Respiratory distress • Cough • Wheezing • Hemoptysis • Hypoxemia • Cyanosis • Fever
Air embolism syndrome	• Open surgical site above RA (craniotomy, cesarean section) • Use of medical gases in laparoscopic or endoscopic procedures • Volume depletion • Barotrauma • Pulmonary vasodilators • Biopsy of airway or lung parenchyma • Venous access devices • Contrast injection • Trauma	• Anxiety • Sense of impending doom • Chest pain • Respiratory distress • Wheezing • Cyanosis • Hypoxemia • Gasp reflex • Mill-wheel murmur on auscultation • Agitation, delirium, seizure activity (arterial gas embolization)
Fat embolism syndrome	• Blunt force trauma resulting in long bone and pelvic fractures • Orthopedic procedures • Extensive rib fractures • Burn injury • Acute pancreatitis • Diabetes mellitus • Sickle cell anemia • Liposuction • Parenteral lipid infusion	• Agitation • Delirium • Seizure activity • Fevers and chills • Chest pain • Respiratory distress • Wheezing • Cyanosis • Hypoxemia • Petechial rash involving axilla and upper trunk
Amniotic fluid embolism syndrome	• Pregnancy • Peripartum • Postpartum (up to 48 hrs) • Difficult labor • Use of labor induction agents • Amniocentesis • First or second trimester abortion • Trauma	• Agitation and delirium • Seizure activity • Fevers and chills • Nausea and vomiting • Respiratory distress • Wheezing • Chest pain • Cyanosis • Hypoxemia • Profuse hemorrhage with no obvious structural cause • Fetal bradycardia or late decelerations

ALGORITHM 6.2 Management Algorithm for Massive Pulmonary Embolism

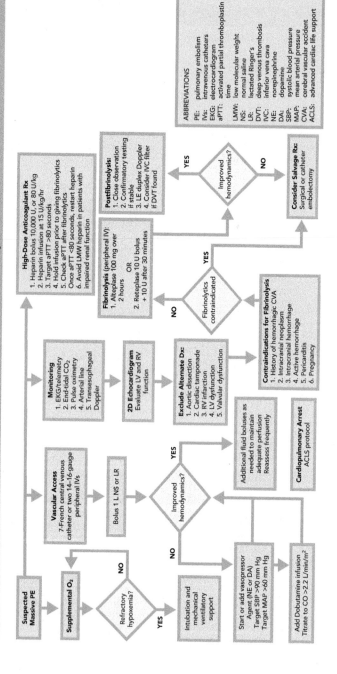

recent meta-analysis demonstrated a decrease in all-cause mortality associated with the combined use of therapeutic anticoagulation and thrombolysis when compared to the use of therapeutic anticoagulation alone. The risk of major bleeding was increased with thrombolysis, though this association was only significant in patients older than 65 years of age. Accordingly, in patients with moderately severe pulmonary emboli without absolute contraindications to thrombolysis, the early use of thrombolytics should be considered. In those with hemodynamic instability, and no contraindications, this should be considered even more strongly. For patients with major contraindications to thrombolytic therapy or unresponsive to pharmacologic thrombolysis, catheter thrombectomy or open surgical embolectomy may be attempted. Although no randomized, controlled trials have evaluated its effect, the use of extracorporeal membrane oxygenation (ECMO) in patients with hemodynamic instability after acute PE has been shown in a recent systematic review to be associated with a 70% overall survival, regardless of what specific treatment option was used to address the embolism. While more data are needed to guide decision-making, this therapy should be considered in patients with severe shock from pulmonary emboli.

Once hemodynamic stability is restored, definitive diagnosis can be established by computed tomographic angiography or pulmonary angiography. An evaluation for deep venous thrombosis by duplex Doppler ultrasound should be performed with consideration of inferior vena cava filter placement in patients with marginal cardiac function and high clot burden.

AIR EMBOLISM

Air embolism syndrome (AES) occurs when gas enters the arterial or venous circulation driven by a pressure gradient favoring entrainment of gas, or through direct injection. Arterial gas embolization may occur through anatomic shunts (e.g., patent foramen ovale, vascular malformations), pulmonary vasodilator administration, or if the filtration capacity of the pulmonary circulation is overwhelmed by a large volume of gas entering the venous circulation. Indeed, each case of venous air embolism is a potential case of arterial air embolism. Arterial AES typically does not cause mechanical shock. However, gas entering the coronary circulation may cause myocardial ischemia and cardiogenic shock.

Gas enters the venous circulation when there is a negative intrathoracic pressure in the presence of an open central or peripheral vein, or if the open vein is elevated above the right atrium. Even a seemingly small pressure gradient of -5 cm H_2O is sufficient to allow gas to enter the venous circulation at up to 100 mL/s through a 14-gauge peripheral IV. In the setting of volume depletion and decreased central venous pressure, or if the extravascular environment is under positive pressure (e.g., CO_2 insufflation during laparoscopic surgery), the risk of venous gas embolism increases significantly. Animal studies have shown that sudden, large-volume gas embolism is lethal. On the other hand, slow, continuous small-volume gas embolism is survivable, even if the cumulative volume of gas is large. In humans, the estimated lethal dose in venous AES is approximately 200 to 300 mL, and up to 500 mL if gas is entrained slowly. However, acute embolism of as little as 50 mL of gas may be sufficient to cause hemodynamic compromise.

Venous AES produces mechanical shock mainly through obstruction of the RV outflow tract. The severity of hemodynamic and gas exchange abnormalities depends on (1) total volume of gas entrained, (2) the rate at which gas enters the pulmonary arterial circulation, (3) pre-existing CPD, and (4) severity of the inflammatory response triggered by the gas deposited in the pulmonary circulation. Unlike embolism of solid materials such as thrombus or fat, gas entering the pulmonary arterial circulation is eliminated continuously by diffusion across alveolar capillaries. Thus, if the portal of gas entry is eliminated, and if RV performance is capable of compensating for the elevated PVR, AES-induced mechanical shock should resolve as the embolized gas is cleared.

AES should be considered in the differential diagnosis for patients presenting with acute hemodynamic instability and gas exchange abnormalities in the proper clinical setting. Table 6.1 lists common risk factors for AES. Mechanical shock induced by AES may be difficult to distinguish from other etiologies of shock. If arterial air embolism occurs and air enters the coronary arterial circulation, cardiogenic shock is added to the picture. Early assessment of hemodynamic function using 2D echocardiography, transesophageal Doppler, or PA catheter can determine the predominant cause of shock. Therapy for AES is supportive and should focus on (1) eliminating the portal of gas entry, (2) restoring hemodynamic stability, and (3) promoting clearance of the entrained gas. A management algorithm for AES is shown in Algorithm 6.3.

Although there is no randomized clinical trial data, air aspiration from the RV through a central venous catheter has been reported to remove up to 50% of the embolized gas, producing rapid hemodynamic improvement. The patient is placed in the left lateral decubitus position, elevating the RV above its outflow tract and promoting migration of entrained air back into the RV. A central venous catheter is then placed with the tip approximately 2 cm below the superior vena cava/right atrial junction, and air is aspirated through the distal port. In the setting of refractory cardiopulmonary arrest, emergency thoracotomy, cardiac massage, and direct aspiration of air through the right ventricle may be attempted as a last resort.

Emphasis should be placed on prevention of gas embolization during surgical and medical procedures through adequate hydration, proper patient positioning, avoidance of barotrauma, and observing proper procedures for vascular access insertion and removal. Patients at high risk for AES should be closely monitored via capnography or precordial Doppler ultrasound to detect gas embolization during surgical procedures. Early detection and prompt supportive treatment of AES can dramatically improve outcomes.

FAT EMBOLISM

Fat embolism syndrome (FES) occurs when fat from necrotic bone marrow or adipocytes is released into the venous circulation following trauma or tissue injury, causing mechanical obstruction of the pulmonary vascular bed and triggering a systemic inflammatory response. Approximately 90% of cases of FES occur following blunt trauma resulting in pelvic and long bone fractures. The risk of developing FES rises with the severity of the injury and the number of large marrow-containing bones involved.

The pathobiology of FES remains incompletely understood. Studies have shown circulating fat in blood specimens collected from patients undergoing orthopedic surgery. This observation suggests the presence of fat in the circulation is necessary but not sufficient to precipitate FES. The severity of FES-induced mechanical shock probably depends on multiple factors, including (1) the total volume and rate of fat

ALGORITHM 6.3 Management Algorithm for Air Embolism Syndrome

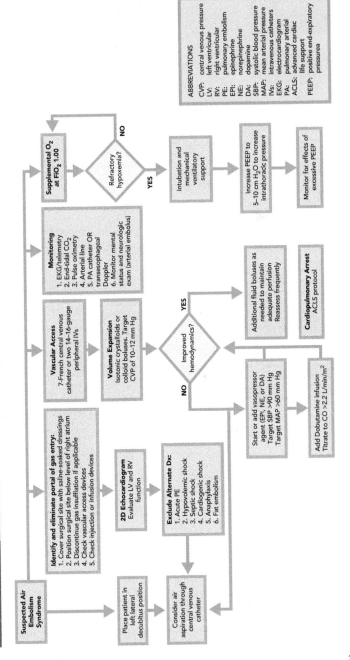

Suspected Air Embolism Syndrome

Place patient in left lateral decubitus position

Consider air aspiration through central venous catheter

Identify and eliminate portal of gas entry:
1. Cover surgical site with saline-soaked dressings
2. Position surgical site below level of right atrium
3. Discontinue gas insufflation if applicable
4. Check vascular access devices
5. Check injection or infusion devices

2D Echocardiogram
Evaluate LV and RV function

Exclude Alternate Dx:
1. Acute PE
2. Hypovolemic shock
3. Septic shock
4. Cardiogenic shock
5. Anaphylaxis
6. Fat embolism

Vascular Access
7-French central venous catheter or two 14–16-gauge peripheral IVs

Volume Expansion
Isotonic crystalloids or colloid boluses. Target CVP of 10–12 mm Hg

Monitoring
1. EKG/telemetry
2. End-tidal CO₂
3. Pulse oximetry
4. Arterial line
5. PA catheter OR transesophageal Doppler
6. Monitor mental status and neurologic exam (arterial embolus)

Supplemental O₂ at FiO₂ 1.00

Refractory hypoxemia?

NO → Supplemental O₂ at FiO₂ 1.00

YES → Intubation and mechanical ventilatory support

Increase PEEP to 5–10 cm H₂O to increase intrathoracic pressure

Monitor for effects of excessive PEEP

Improved hemodynamics?

YES → Additional fluid boluses as needed to maintain adequate perfusion. Reassess frequently

Cardiopulmonary Arrest
ACLS protocol

NO → Start or add vasopressor agent (EPI, NE, or DA). Target SBP >90 mm Hg. Target MAP >60 mm Hg

Add Dobutamine infusion. Titrate to CO >2.2 L/min/m²

ABBREVIATIONS

CVP:	central venous pressure
LV:	left ventricular
RV:	right ventricular
PE:	pulmonary embolism
EPI:	epinephrine
NE:	norepinephrine
DA:	dopamine
SBP:	systolic blood pressure
MAP:	mean arterial pressure
IVs:	intravenous catheters
EKG:	electrocardiogram
PA:	pulmonary arterial
ACLS:	advanced cardiac life support
PEEP:	positive end-expiratory pressure

37

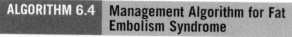

ALGORITHM 6.4 — Management Algorithm for Fat Embolism Syndrome

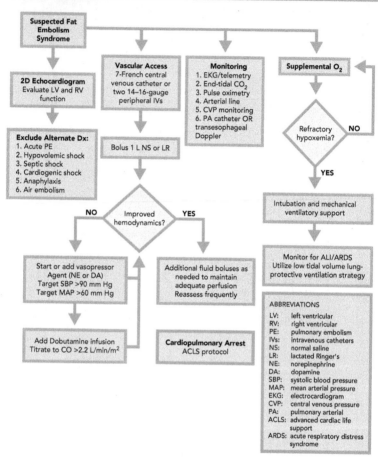

Suspected Fat Embolism Syndrome

2D Echocardiogram
Evaluate LV and RV function

Exclude Alternate Dx:
1. Acute PE
2. Hypovolemic shock
3. Septic shock
4. Cardiogenic shock
5. Anaphylaxis
6. Air embolism

Vascular Access
7-French central venous catheter or two 14–16-gauge peripheral IVs

Bolus 1 L NS or LR

Improved hemodynamics? **NO** / **YES**

Monitoring
1. EKG/telemetry
2. End-tidal CO₂
3. Pulse oximetry
4. Arterial line
5. CVP monitoring
6. PA catheter OR transesophageal Doppler

Supplemental O₂

Refractory hypoxemia? **NO** / **YES**

Intubation and mechanical ventilatory support

Monitor for ALI/ARDS Utilize low tidal volume lung-protective ventilation strategy

Start or add vasopressor Agent (NE or DA) Target SBP >90 mm Hg Target MAP >60 mm Hg

Additional fluid boluses as needed to maintain adequate perfusion Reassess frequently

Add Dobutamine infusion Titrate to CO >2.2 L/min/m²

Cardiopulmonary Arrest ACLS protocol

ABBREVIATIONS

LV:	left ventricular
RV:	right ventricular
PE:	pulmonary embolism
IVs:	intravenous catheters
NS:	normal saline
LR:	lactated Ringer's
NE:	norepinephrine
DA:	dopamine
SBP:	systolic blood pressure
MAP:	mean arterial pressure
EKG:	electrocardiogram
CVP:	central venous pressure
PA:	pulmonary arterial
ACLS:	advanced cardiac life support
ARDS:	acute respiratory distress syndrome

embolization, (2) immunogenicity of the embolized material, (3) intensity of the host inflammatory response, and (4) pre-existing CPD.

Shock in the early phase of FES is mainly caused by mechanical obstruction of the pulmonary vasculature causing RV failure. Within 24 to 72 hours of the initial insult, toxic-free fatty acid metabolites cause systemic inflammation, acute lung injury, and end-organ dysfunction with hemodynamic derangements similar to those found in septic shock. A classic triad of clinical findings consisting of hypoxemia, neurologic dysfunction, and petechial rash involving the upper trunk and axilla may be found in some patients.

No specific diagnostic test is available for FES. Treatment is supportive and should be focused on (1) restoring hemodynamic stability and (2) maintaining adequate oxygenation to avoid end-organ dysfunction. There is some evidence for prophylactic administration of corticosteroids in patients at high risk for FES. However, there is no evidence to support corticosteroid use after the FES has occurred. A management algorithm for FES is shown in Algorithm 6.4. A high clinical index of suspicion and early institution of supportive care is necessary to improve outcomes for patients with FES.

AMNIOTIC FLUID EMBOLISM

Amniotic fluid embolism syndrome (AFES) occurs when amniotic fluid (AF) enters the maternal circulation during labor and delivery or in the postpartum period due to cervical, uterine wall, or placental membrane disruption. Classic findings include the acute onset of shock, hypoxemia, encephalopathy, coagulopathy, and disseminated intravascular coagulation. A fulminant presentation of AES can lead to circulatory collapse and death within a matter of hours. Survivors of this devastating syndrome are frequently left with severe neurologic impairment.

The pathogenesis of AFES remains incompletely understood. AF contains a heterogeneous mixture of water, electrolytes, hormones, and fetal components. AF components are routinely found in blood specimens from asymptomatic pregnant women, suggesting that entry of AF components into the maternal circulation is necessary but not sufficient to cause AFES. The development of AFES is likely determined by multiple factors, including (1) absolute volume of AF and its rate of entry into the maternal circulation, (2) AF composition, which affects its immunogenicity and vasoactive properties, (3) maternal immune response, and (4) pre-existing maternal CPD.

The etiology of AFES-induced shock is often multifactorial and temporally heterogeneous. The early phase of AFES is dominated by severe acute left ventricular (LV) systolic dysfunction and cardiogenic shock. This may be accompanied by arrhythmias including bradycardia, ventricular fibrillation, pulseless electrical activity, or even asystole. Deposition of AF in the pulmonary circulation triggers intense pulmonary vasoconstriction, RV failure and precipitates mechanical shock. The late phase of AFES, typically occurring 1 to 2 hours later, is frequently complicated by distributive shock caused by the severe systemic inflammatory response triggered by immunogenic AF components. Cardiogenic and obstructive shock may persist into the late phase of AFES, but usually improve over time. Disseminated intravascular coagulation and coagulopathy may add hemorrhagic shock to the picture.

The acute onset of agitation, altered mental status, dyspnea, and hemodynamic instability in a pregnant or peripartum woman should raise clinical suspicion for AFES. No specific diagnostic test is available for diagnosing AFES. Management of AFES is supportive and consists of the following goals: (1) restoring and maintaining maternal hemodynamic stability, (2) maintaining adequate oxygenation to prevent maternal and fetal hypoxia, (3) correcting anemia and coagulopathy, (4) treating neurologic manifestations, and (5) expediting delivery of the fetus. A management algorithm for AFES is shown in Algorithm 6.5.

Bedside 2D echocardiography is a useful modality for rapidly assessing LV and RV function. As multiple etiologies of shock are commonly encountered during the course of AFES, a transesophageal Doppler or pulmonary arterial (PA) catheter is useful for monitoring changing hemodynamic status and for guiding fluid resuscitation and titration of vasopressors and inotropes. Successful management of AFES requires early recognition, prompt initiation of supportive measures, and close coordination between the intensivist, obstetrician, and anesthesiologist.

ALGORITHM 6.5 Management Algorithm for Amniotic Fluid Embolism Syndrome

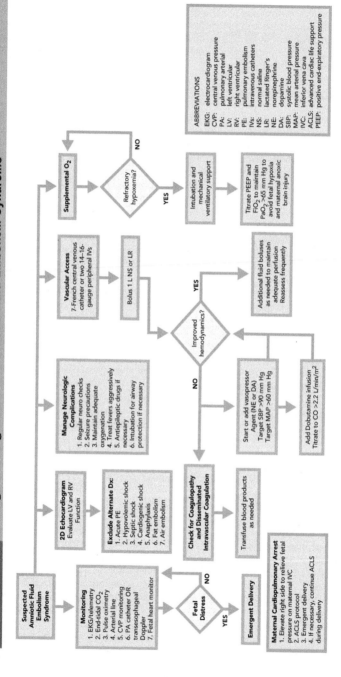

Suspected Amniotic Fluid Embolism Syndrome

Monitoring
1. EKG/telemetry
2. End-tidal CO$_2$
3. Pulse oximetry
4. Arterial line
5. CVP monitoring
6. PA catheter OR transesophageal Doppler
7. Fetal heart monitor

Fetal Distress?
- NO
- YES

Emergent Delivery

Maternal Cardiopulmonary Arrest
1. Elevate right side to relieve fetal pressure on maternal IVC
2. ACLS protocol
3. Emergent delivery
4. If necessary, continue ACLS during delivery

2D Echocardiogram
Evaluate LV and RV Function

Exclude Alternate Dx:
1. Acute PE
2. Hypovolemic shock
3. Septic shock
4. Cardiogenic shock
5. Anaphylaxis
6. Fat embolism
7. Air embolism

Check for Coagulopathy and Disseminated Intravascular Coagulation

Transfuse blood products as needed

Manage Neurologic Complications
1. Regular neuro checks
2. Seizure precautions
3. Maintain adequate oxygenation
4. Treat fevers aggressively
5. Antiepileptic drugs if necessary
6. Intubation for airway protection if necessary

Vascular Access
7-French central venous catheter or two 14-16-gauge peripheral IVs

Bolus 1 L NS or LR

Improved hemodynamics?
- NO
- YES

Additional fluid boluses as needed to maintain adequate perfusion. Reassess frequently

Start or add vasopressor Agent (NE or DA)
Target SBP >90 mm Hg
Target MAP >60 mm Hg

Add Dobutamine infusion
Titrate to CO >2.2 L/min/m^2

Supplemental O$_2$

Refractory hypoxemia?
- NO
- YES

Intubation and mechanical ventilatory support

Titrate PEEP and FiO$_2$ to maintain PaO$_2$ >65 mm Hg to avoid fetal hypoxia and maternal anoxic brain injury

ABBREVIATIONS
EKG: electrocardiogram
CVP: central venous pressure
PA: pulmonary arterial
LV: left ventricular
RV: right ventricular
PE: pulmonary embolism
IVs: intravenous catheters
NS: normal saline
LR: lactated Ringer's
NE: norepinephrine
DA: dopamine
SBP: systolic blood pressure
MAP: mean arterial pressure
IVC: inferior vena cava
ACLS: advanced cardiac life support
PEEP: positive end-expiratory pressure

SUGGESTED READINGS

Agnelli G, Becattini C. Current concepts: acute pulmonary embolism. *N Engl J Med.* 2010; 363:266–274.

Review of diagnostic strategy and management of acute PE, including risk stratification for hemodynamically stable patients with PE.

Chatterjee S, Chakraborty A, Weinberg I, et al. Thrombolysis for pulmonary embolism and risk of all-cause mortality, major bleeding and intracranial hemorrhage: a meta-analysis. *JAMA.* 2014;311(23):2414–2421.

Goldhaber SZ. Echocardiography in the management of pulmonary embolism. *Ann Intern Med.* 2002;136(9):691–700.

Review of common echocardiographic findings in pulmonary embolism.

Jorens PG, Van Marck E, Snoeckx A, et al. Nonthrombotic pulmonary embolism. *Eur Respir J.* 2009;34(2):452–474.

Review of various nonthrombotic etiologies that can produce mechanical shock.

Mellor A, Soni N. Fat embolism. *Anaesthesia.* 2001;56(2):145–154.

A review of etiology, diagnosis, and treatment of fat embolism syndrome.

Mirski MA, Lele AV, Fitzsimmons L, et al. Diagnosis and treatment of vascular air embolism. *Anesthesiology.* 2007;106(1):164–177.

Moore J, Baldisseri MR. Amniotic fluid embolism. *Crit Care Med.* 2005;33(10 suppl):S279–S285.

Thorough discussion of pathogenesis, diagnosis, and treatment of the amniotic fluid embolism syndrome.

Piazza G, Golhaber SZ. The acutely decompensated right ventricle: pathways for diagnosis and management. *Chest.* 2005;128(3):1836–1852.

Overview of the signs and symptoms and general management strategy for acute right ventricular decompensation.

Sharifi M, Bay C, Skrocki L, et al. Moderate pulmonary embolism treated with thrombolysis (from the "MOPETT" trial). *Am J Cardiol.* 2013;111(2):273–277.

Wood KE. Major pulmonary embolism: review of a pathophysiologic approach to the golden hour of hemodynamically significant pulmonary embolism. *Chest.* 2002;121(3):877–905.

Comprehensive review of the pathogenesis, diagnosis, and management of hemodynamically significant pulmonary embolism.

Yusuff HO, Zochios V, Vuylsteke A. Extracorporeal membrane oxygenation in acute massive pulmonary embolism: a systematic review. *Perfusion.* 2015;30(8):611–616.

MANAGEMENT OF RESPIRATORY DISORDERS

7

An Approach to Respiratory Failure

Warren Isakow

Respiratory failure is a common reason for intensive care unit admission and is the final pathway for a number of diseases of differing pathophysiology. A mechanism-based approach enables the clinician to identify the most likely cause for the respiratory failure and to treat appropriately. In general, patients with respiratory failure may be classified into four groups, depending on the component of the respiratory system that is involved.

- Hypercapnic respiratory failure is a consequence of ventilatory failure and is recognized by an elevated $PaCO_2$ above normal (>45 mm Hg at sea level). This pattern of respiratory failure can result from many differing etiologies and generally denotes failure of the respiratory pump mechanism with normal lungs or as a consequence of airways disease or very severe parenchymal lung disease.
- Hypoxemic respiratory failure is a consequence of gas exchange failure and is recognized by hypoxemia (PaO_2 <60 mm Hg), with or without widening of the alveolar-arterial oxygen gradient. Most patients with this form of respiratory failure have ventilation–perfusion (V/Q) mismatch or shunt physiology as the predominant mechanisms for the hypoxemia. Most of these patients will have an abnormal chest x-ray and a process affecting the pulmonary parenchyma; however, intracardiac and intrapulmonary shunts can also present in this manner.
- Mixed respiratory failure with components of multiple pathophysiologic processes that can contribute to both hypoxemia and hypercarbia.
- Type 4 respiratory failure occurs in postoperative patients with a normal respiratory pump and normal lungs, who are sedated or paralyzed or when the metabolic demands of the body are too high for the patient to compensate for. This is common in patients with sepsis and profound metabolic derangements like metabolic acidosis.

HYPERCAPNIC RESPIRATORY FAILURE

The hallmark of hypercapnic respiratory failure is an elevated $PaCO_2$ above 45 mm Hg.

$$PaCO_2 = K \times \frac{VCO_2}{(1 - Vd/Vt) \times VA}$$

where $PaCO_2$ = the partial pressure of carbon dioxide in the blood, K = constant, VCO_2 = carbon dioxide production, Vd/Vt = dead space ratio of each tidal volume breath, and VA = minute ventilation.

ALGORITHM 7.1 Causes of Hypercapnic Respiratory Failure Based on Components of the Respiratory Pump

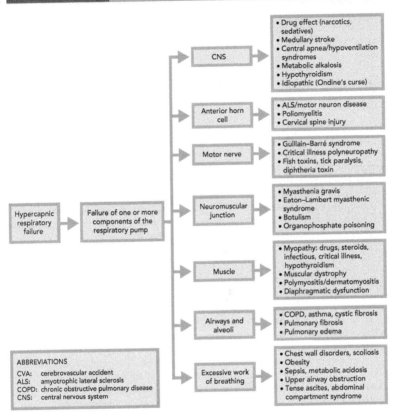

CNS
- Drug effect (narcotics, sedatives)
- Medullary stroke
- Central apnea/hypoventilation syndromes
- Metabolic alkalosis
- Hypothyroidism
- Idiopathic (Ondine's curse)

Anterior horn cell
- ALS/motor neuron disease
- Poliomyelitis
- Cervical spine injury

Motor nerve
- Guillain–Barré syndrome
- Critical illness polyneuropathy
- Fish toxins, tick paralysis, diphtheria toxin

Neuromuscular junction
- Myasthenia gravis
- Eaton–Lambert myasthenic syndrome
- Botulism
- Organophosphate poisoning

Muscle
- Myopathy: drugs, steroids, infectious, critical illness, hypothyroidism
- Muscular dystrophy
- Polymyositis/dermatomyositis
- Diaphragmatic dysfunction

Airways and alveoli
- COPD, asthma, cystic fibrosis
- Pulmonary fibrosis
- Pulmonary edema

Excessive work of breathing
- Chest wall disorders, scoliosis
- Obesity
- Sepsis, metabolic acidosis
- Upper airway obstruction
- Tense ascites, abdominal compartment syndrome

Hypercapnic respiratory failure → Failure of one or more components of the respiratory pump

ABBREVIATIONS
CVA: cerebrovascular accident
ALS: amyotrophic lateral sclerosis
COPD: chronic obstructive pulmonary disease
CNS: central nervous system

Analysis of the previous equation shows that hypercapnia can occur from three processes: (a) an increase in CO_2 production, which is extremely uncommon clinically as a sole cause for hypercarbia, (b) a decrease in minute ventilation by either a reduced tidal volume or respiratory rate, and (c) an increase in dead-space ventilation. Understanding of the "respiratory pump" enables the clinician to systematically consider the cause of hypercapnic respiratory failure in different patients, as depicted in Algorithm 7.1.

The acuity of onset of the hypercapnia is also an important determinant of management. An acute change in $PaCO_2$ of 10 mm Hg will change the blood pH by 0.08 in the opposite direction. In patients with chronic hypercapnia, renal compensation occurs by bicarbonate retention and tends to correct the pH toward normal. In these cases, a change in $PaCO_2$ of 10 mm Hg is reflected by a change of 0.03 in the blood pH in the opposite direction. Recognition of acute hypercapnia or acute-on-chronic hypercapnia is vitally important, as it is a harbinger of an imminent respiratory arrest and potential development of severe hypoxemia.

Important principles in managing patients with hypercapnia are:

- Rapidly institute adequate ventilation: In carefully selected patients, noninvasive ventilation can be tried prior to intubation and mechanical ventilation.
- Cautious use of supplemental oxygen is necessary as oxygen can worsen hypercapnia by a number of mechanisms: worsening of V/Q matching, the Haldane effect, and suppression of central hypoxemic drive. Enough supplemental oxygen should be given to keep the hemoglobin saturation in the 90% to 92% range in most hypercarbic patients with underlying severe obstructive lung disease.
- Sedatives and narcotics can be hazardous and can worsen ventilation and oxygenation in patients with hypercapnia, particularly those with neuromuscular weakness and severe obstructive lung disease.

HYPOXEMIC RESPIRATORY FAILURE

Hypoxemic respiratory failure occurs because of impaired gas exchange or hypoventilation and is defined by a PaO_2 of <60 mm Hg. The first step in ascertaining a cause is looking for concomitant hypercapnia, as would occur with hypoventilation or severe intrinsic lung disease with increased dead-space ventilation, and calculating the alveolar–arterial oxygen gradient by using the alveolar gas equation. The approach to hypoxemic respiratory failure is summarized in Algorithm 7.2.

The alveolar gas equation follows:

$$PAO_2 = FiO_2 (PB - PH_2O) - \frac{PaCO_2}{R}$$

where PAO_2 = alveolar partial pressure of oxygen, FiO_2 = fraction of inspired oxygen, PB = barometric pressure (760 mm Hg at sea level), PH_2O = water vapor pressure (47 mm Hg), $PaCO_2$ = partial pressure of carbon dioxide in the blood, and R = respiratory quotient, assumed to be 0.8.

The alveolar–arterial oxygen gradient = $PAO_2 - PaO_2$. The normal value is between 10 and 15 mm Hg and is influenced by age, increasing by approximately 3 mm Hg every decade after the age of 30 years. For an FiO_2 = 21%, it should be 5 to 25 mm Hg and for an FiO_2 = 100%, it should be <150 mm Hg. Hypoxemic respiratory failure with a widened alveolar–arterial oxygen gradient is caused by V/Q mismatching or shunt pathophysiology. These two processes can be differentiated by improvement of the hypoxemia with supplemental oxygen, in the case of V/Q mismatch, and no improvement in cases with shunt. Diseases that cause airspace flooding, atelectasis, airway disease, or pulmonary vascular problems are common causes of hypoxemic respiratory failure.

Management principles for patients with hypoxemic respiratory failure include:

- Rapid restoration of an adequate arterial saturation, which often requires intubation and mechanical ventilation. Patients with hypoxemia and pulmonary infiltrates as a group, generally respond less well to noninvasive ventilation.
- Use of adequate amounts of positive end-expiratory pressure to reduce FiO_2 to nontoxic levels (FiO_2 <60%).
- A low tidal volume strategy with permissive hypercapnia in patients with acute lung injury/acute respiratory distress syndrome.
- General supportive care in the intensive care unit while the patient's pulmonary process resolves.

ALGORITHM 7.2 General Approach to Hypoxemic Respiratory Failure

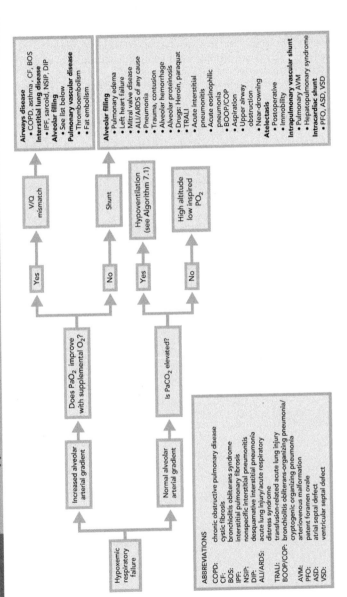

Hypoxemic respiratory failure

→ **Increased alveolar arterial gradient**

→ **Does PaO₂ improve with supplemental O₂?**

Yes → **V/Q mismatch**

Airways disease
- COPD, asthma , CF, BOS

Interstitial lung disease
- IPF, sarcoid, NSIP, DIP

Alveolar filling

Pulmonary vascular disease
- Thromboembolism
- Fat embolism

No → **Shunt**

Alveolar filling
- Pulmonary edema
- Left heart failure
- Mitral valve disease
- ALI/ARDS of any cause
- Pneumonia
- Trauma, contusion
- Alveolar hemorrhage
- Alveolar proteinosis
- Drugs: Heroin, paraquat
- TRALI
- Acute interstitial pneumonitis
- Acute eosinophilic pneumonia
- BOOP/COP
- Aspiration
- Upper airway obstruction
- Near-drowning

Atelectasis
- Postoperative
- Immobility

Intrapulmonary vascular shunt
- Pulmonary AVM
- Hepatopulmonary syndrome

Intracardiac shunt
- PFO, ASD, VSD

Normal alveolar arterial gradient

→ **Is PaCO₂ elevated?**

Yes → **Hypoventilation (see Algorithm 7.1)**

No → **High altitude low inspired PO₂**

ABBREVIATIONS

COPD:	chronic obstructive pulmonary disease
CF:	cystic fibrosis
BOS:	bronchiolitis obliterans syndrome
IPF:	interstitial pulmonary fibrosis
NSIP:	nonspecific interstitial pneumonitis
DIP:	desquamative interstitial pneumonia
ALI/ARDS:	acute lung injury/acute respiratory distress syndrome
TRALI:	transfusion-related acute lung injury
BOOP/COP:	bronchiolitis obliterans-organizing pneumonia/cryptogenic organizing pneumonia
AVM:	arteriovenous malformation
PFO:	patent foramen ovale
ASD:	atrial septal defect
VSD:	ventricular septal defect

45

It is worthwhile to note that hypoxia refers to an oxygen deficit at a tissue level and depends on oxygen delivery. Therefore, cellular hypoxia can be a result of any process that affects oxygen delivery to the tissues, and includes:

- Hypoxic hypoxia (low arterial oxygen saturation and a low PaO_2)
- Anemic hypoxia (low circulating hemoglobin with impaired oxygen delivery)
- Circulatory hypoxia (low cardiac output states)
- Histotoxic hypoxia (poisoning with cyanide where oxygen is delivered to the tissues but cannot be used)

$$Oxygen\ Delivery = Cardiac\ Output \times Arterial\ Oxygen\ Content$$
$$DO_2 = CO \times CaO_2$$
$$DO_2 = CO \times (1.39 \times [Hb\ (g/dL)] \times SaO_2) + (0.003 \times PaO_2)$$

SUGGESTED READINGS

Lanken PN. Approach to acute respiratory failure. In: Lanken PN, ed. *The Intensive Care Unit Manual.* 2nd ed. Philadelphia, PA: Saunders; 2014:3–13.

    A superb concise chapter focusing on developing a pathophysiologic approach to all patients with respiratory failure.

Wood LDH. The pathophysiology and differential diagnosis of acute respiratory failure. In: Hall JB, Schmidt GA, Wood LDH, et al., eds. *Principles of Critical Care.* New York: McGraw Hill; 2005:417–426.

    Another superb textbook chapter focusing on pathophysiology.

Initial Ventilator Setup

Warren Isakow

The initiation of mechanical ventilation is a critical period during the course of a patient's stay in the intensive care unit. The clinician is encouraged to monitor the patient closely during initiation of mechanical ventilation, as this period often provides important answers regarding a patient's underlying pathophysiologic abnormality. This simple bedside process allows for verification of the underlying cause of the decompensation requiring ventilatory support, assessment of severity of the disease process, and the likely response to standard therapies. Simple observations during this time can often lead to appreciation of the major reason for clinical deterioration.

- What is the shape of the capnogram? Is it sloped and consistent with airways disease? If the patient is hypercarbic and the capnogram shape looks normal, the potential cause for hypercarbia is more likely to be extrathoracic, neurologic, or obesity related.
- What is the absolute value of the end-tidal CO_2 ($ETCO_2$)? Is it extremely high initially (due to hypercarbia) or is it very low (likely a metabolic problem with compensatory respiratory alkalosis or a marker of sepsis and tachypnea)?
- In a patient post cardiac arrest and resuscitation, is there adequate perfusion (a sustained and elevated $ETCO_2$ >15 mm Hg)?
- Is there a large gradient between the $PaCO_2$ obtained from an arterial blood gas and the $ETCO_2$, reflecting dead space ventilation? Even more useful is absence of a significant gradient which makes clinically significant acute pulmonary embolism extremely unlikely and can save a trip to the CT scanner.
- What was the patient's minute ventilation prior to intubation and is the ventilator set appropriately to match this? If not, a patient can become acidotic extremely rapidly if the patient's own respiratory compensation for a profound metabolic process is not taken into account by the clinician. This is very important in patients with septic shock, diabetic ketoacidosis, renal failure, salicylate toxicity, and lactic acidosis. The reverse can also occur. In patients with chronic CO_2 retention, if the minute ventilation is set too high, either by an excessive tidal volume or respiratory rate, they can become alkalotic from an excessive acute reduction in $PaCO_2$ (post-hypercapnic alkalosis).
- Is the endotracheal tube (ETT) appropriately positioned and document the distance from the tube tip to the patient's front teeth? A rough guide is 22 cm at the teeth for a female and 23 cm for a male. This approach, together with careful chest auscultation, can avoid the complications of right mainstem intubation prior to the confirmatory chest x-ray being performed.

- What do the secretions look like? Are there purulent secretions, bloody secretions, or vomitus in the airway?
- Was the patient paralyzed for the intubation with a nondepolarizing neuromuscular blocker? If so, ensure adequate analgesia and sedation during the next hour.
- What are the airway pressures?
  - Obtain a sense of the patient's baseline initial airway pressures which will help should any respiratory deterioration develop, such as a pneumothorax or changing lung compliance.
  - Is the peak airway pressure too high, signifying possible ETT malposition in the right mainstem, kinking of the tube or a patient who is biting and undersedated, or an airway resistance problem such as bronchospasm or secretions.
  - Is the plateau pressure high, signifying a compliance problem with the respiratory system which could be due to an intrinsic pulmonary process (auto-PEEP, pulmonary edema, pneumonia) or an extrathoracic cause (tense ascites, abdominal compartment syndrome)?
  - Is the patient trapping air and at risk for auto-PEEP and dynamic hyperinflation? The best way to diagnose this is with auscultation (patient still exhaling when the next breath starts) combined with monitoring the ventilator waveform flows (returning back to baseline?) as well as performing an expiratory pause.
- What sedation strategy is likely to work best with this patient, knowing their underlying physiology, hemodynamics, and anticipated duration of ventilation?
- Does the patient appear comfortable on the ventilator or are they flow/air hungry? Do the ventilator waveforms look smooth and am I meeting the patient's ventilatory demand?

Table 8.1 provides a general guideline to the initial ventilator settings in different clinical circumstances. The table is simply a guide, and the reader should understand that every patient is unique and should have the ventilator adjusted according to the individual's clinical status.

Algorithm 8.1 is a management algorithm for troubleshooting the situation of a patient with persistent high peak airway pressures, a common ventilator-related problem in the intensive care unit. Table 8.2 provides potential causes for an alarm resulting from a low exhaled tidal volume/low minute ventilation.

TABLE 8.1 Guidelines for Initial Ventilator Settings in Different Clinical Scenarios

Indication for Mechanical Ventilation	Mode of Choice	Respiratory Rate (Breaths/min)	Tidal Volume (mL/kg)	FiO$_2$	PEEP	Additional Ventilator Issues	Adjunctive Therapies	Additional Comments
Airway protection, spontaneously breathing patient (e.g., hepatic encephalopathy, upper airway obstruction)	AC (volume) SIMV PSV	10–14	8–10	100%, obtain ABG and wean for sats >92% to goal FiO$_2$ of 40%	5	Peak flow 60 L/min Trigger sensitivity— 2 cm H$_2$O	DVT GI	Maintain on MV until upper airway issues resolved Patients with hepatic encephalopathy are prone to develop a respiratory alkalosis, so TV may need to be reduced
Asthma exacerbation	AC (volume)	Set rate low, 8–12	6–8	100%, obtain ABG and wean for sats >92% to goal FiO$_2$ of 40%	0–5	Set peak flows high, allow adequate expiratory time Consider square wave ventilation Use flow-by for easier triggering	BD ST AB SDN DVT GI	Tolerate hypercarbia, higher peak airway pressures Monitor for auto-PEEP and barotrauma Do not ventilate for a "normal" ABG Apply external PEEP to overcome intrinsic PEEP when triggering Often need heavy sedation initially Once bronchospasm and acute issues adequately resolved, do not do prolonged weaning trials, consider trial of extubation

(continued)

TABLE 8.1 Guidelines for Initial Ventilator Settings in Different Clinical Scenarios *(Continued)*

Indication for Mechanical Ventilation	Mode of Choice	Respiratory Rate (Breaths/min)	Tidal Volume (mL/kg)	FiO_2	PEEP	Additional Ventilator Issues	Adjunctive Therapies	Additional Comments
COPD exacerbation	AC (volume)	Set rate low, 8–12	6–8	100%, obtain ABG and wean for sats >92% to goal FiO_2 of 40%	0–5	Set peak flows high, allow adequate E time. Use flow-by for easier triggering	BD ST AB DVT NUTR	Monitor for auto-PEEP Avoid posthypercapnic alkalosis Tolerate hypercarbia; do not ventilate for a "normal" ABG Monitor for barotrauma Apply external PEEP to overcome intrinsic PEEP when triggering Consider extubation to NIPPV
Hypoxemic respiratory failure with pneumonia or pulmonary edema	AC (volume)	Often need high rates, 16–24 because of high V_E requirements	6–8	100%, obtain ABG and wean for sats >92% to goal FiO_2 of 40%	5–10	Often have high V_E requirements	BD AB DVT GI NUTR	Secretion management is important In septic patients, allow full MVS to divert CO from the respiratory muscles to other vital organs Follow improvement clinically as improved pulmonary compliance

Condition	Mode	Rate	TV	FiO₂	PEEP	Settings	Prophylaxis	Comments
ALI/ARDS	AC (volume) PCV, high-frequency oscillator, APRV	Often need high rates, up to 30, because of high V_E requirements	6	100%, obtain ABG and wean for sats >92% for "safe" FiO_2 of <60%	5–15	May need I:E of 1:1 or 1.5:1 (IRV) Need higher mean airway pressures Allow permissive hypercarbia to pH of 7.20	BD DVT GI NUTR SDN	Consider nebulized prostacyclin, nitric oxide Early trial of prone ventilation Monitor for barotrauma Often require heavy sedation Consider early neuromuscular blockade for 72 hours Consider adjunctive steroids based on etiology Monitor for septic complications
Postoperative respiratory failure	AC (volume)	Set rate at 10–16	8–10	100%, wean rapidly for sats >92% to goal FiO_2 of 30%	5	Verify placement of all lines, tubes placed in OR Peak flow 60 L/min	DVT GI	Await sedatives, paralytics to be cleared, and perform weaning rapidly Prone to hypoventilation after extubation Prone to atelectasis and splinting due to pain which can cause hypoxemia
Hypoventilation from CNS depression, neuromuscular weakness	AC (volume)	Set rate at 10–16	8–10	100%, obtain ABG and wean rapidly for sats of >92% to goal FiO_2 of 30%	5	Peak flow 60 L/min	GI DVT NUTR	Avoid sedatives Prone to atelectasis Follow NIF in patients with weakness

PEEP, positive end-expiratory pressure; AC, assist control; SIMV, synchronized intermittent mandatory ventilation; PSV, pressure support ventilation; ABG, arterial blood gas; sats, hemoglobin oxygen saturation; DVT, deep venous thrombosis prophylaxis; GI, gastrointestinal prophylaxis; MV, mechanical ventilation; TV, tidal volume; BD, bronchodilator regimen; ST, steroids; AB, antibiotics; SDN, sedation; COPD, chronic obstructive pulmonary disease; NIPPV, noninvasive positive pressure ventilation; V_E, minute ventilation; MVS, mechanical ventilator support; CO, cardiac output; PCV, pressure control ventilation; I:E, expiratory time ratio; IRV, inverse ratio ventilation; NUTR, nutritional support; OR, operating room; NIF, negative inspiratory force; APRV, airway pressure release ventilation.

ALGORITHM 8.1 Management Algorithm for High Peak Airway Pressures

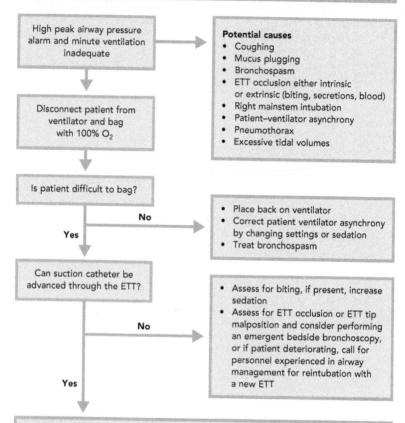

High peak airway pressure alarm and minute ventilation inadequate

Potential causes
- Coughing
- Mucus plugging
- Bronchospasm
- ETT occlusion either intrinsic or extrinsic (biting, secretions, blood)
- Right mainstem intubation
- Patient–ventilator asynchrony
- Pneumothorax
- Excessive tidal volumes

Disconnect patient from ventilator and bag with 100% O_2

Is patient difficult to bag?

No
- Place back on ventilator
- Correct patient ventilator asynchrony by changing settings or sedation
- Treat bronchospasm

Yes

Can suction catheter be advanced through the ETT?

No
- Assess for biting, if present, increase sedation
- Assess for ETT occlusion or ETT tip malposition and consider performing an emergent bedside bronchoscopy, or if patient deteriorating, call for personnel experienced in airway management for reintubation with a new ETT

Yes

Potential causes	Physical examination	Treatment
• Bronchospasm	• Wheezing	• Bronchodilators, steroids
• Tracheal obstruction	• No air entry bilaterally	• Emergent bronchoscopy
• Right mainstem intubation	• No air entry on left side	• Pull back ETT
• Pneumothorax	• Hyperresonance and diminished air entry on affected side	• Decompress with large bore needle in second ICS, midclavicular line, followed by chest tube placement

ABBREVIATIONS
ETT: endotracheal tube
ICS: intercostal space

TABLE 8.2	Potential Causes for a Low Exhaled Tidal Volume/Low Minute Ventilation Alarm

Leak in the circuit
- Tracheal cuff leak
- Patient inadvertently extubated or endotracheal tube tip high, causing a leak
- Ventilator circuit disconnected at any point from the patient to the ventilator
- Large bronchopleural fistula with leak through a chest tube

In patients on pressure support ventilation
- Worsening respiratory system compliance
- Decreased patient effort
- Decreased patient respiratory rate
- Inadequate pressure support being provided

In patients on pressure control ventilation
- Worsening respiratory system compliance

SUGGESTED READINGS

Goligher EC, Ferguson ND, Brochard LJ. Clinical challenges in mechanical ventilation. *Lancet.* 2016;387:1856–1866.

  Review of common clinical problems pertaining to mechanical ventilation.

Reily DJ, Lanken PN. Ventilator alarm situations. In: Lanken PN, ed. *The Intensive Care Unit Manual.* Philadelphia, PA: Saunders; 2001:553–561.

  A practical chapter with clinical information on how to deal with common ventilator alarms.

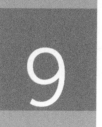

9 Upper Airway Obstruction

Warren Isakow

Acute upper airway obstruction is a medical emergency that requires rapid evaluation of the patient with simultaneous therapy to ensure adequate oxygenation and ventilation of the patient. Prompt recognition of premonitory symptoms and signs may enable the physician to buy precious time for evaluation and planning patient care. Common symptoms include cough, hoarseness, shortness of breath, stridor, nasal flaring, use of accessory muscles, intercostal retractions with progression to cyanosis, and unresponsiveness. Stridor in particular is a serious sign, signifying at least 25% narrowing of the airway. When the patient is in distress, the airway is likely at least 50% narrowed. The common causes of upper airway obstruction are presented in Table 9.1 and an algorithm for the rapid assessment and management of the patient is presented in Algorithm 9.1. It is important to note that with most patients, upper airway obstruction is a clinical diagnosis that does not allow significant time for laboratory testing, arterial blood gas analysis, or even imaging in the acute setting, and all resources should be directed to preventing cardiorespiratory arrest and securing the airway. Figures 9.1 to 9.3 review the anatomic landmarks of the upper airway, a basic cricothyroidotomy set and illustrate practical aspects of performing emergent surgical airway access.

Some common etiologies and their management will be briefly reviewed.

INFECTIOUS EPIGLOTTITIS AND LARYNGITIS

Routine pediatric vaccination against *Haemophilus influenzae* has now made epiglottitis more common in adults than in children. The potential pathogens include *H. influenzae* and *Haemophilus parainfluenzae, Streptococcus pneumoniae, Streptococcus pyogenes, Staphylococcus aureus,* and occasionally anaerobes, while laryngitis is often caused by viruses and rarely *Corynebacterium diphtheriae*, which is more common in unvaccinated individuals.

The classic presentation is of an adult who is drooling, appears toxic, and is sitting upright in the tripod position. These patients have a high potential for complete occlusion of the airway and should be treated with empiric intravenous (IV) antibiotics (options include ceftriaxone, 2 g IV every 24 hours, or TMP-SMX, 10 mg/kg/day divided every 6 hours if allergic to penicillin). Personnel with experience in handling difficult airways should be called in to evaluate the patient, and an emergency tracheostomy set should be brought into the examining room. If an examination is to be performed fiberoptically, preferentially this should be done with a backup plan and equipment in place should the patient require conversion to a surgical airway.

TABLE 9.1	Etiology and Specific Therapy of Upper Airway Obstruction by Site	
Site of Obstruction	**Etiology**	**Specific Therapy**
Nasopharynx	Nasal polyps	Nasal steroids, surgery
	Nasal tumors, lymphoma	Radiation, surgery, chemotherapy
	Adenoidal hypertrophy	Adenoidectomy
	Trauma	Fracture reduction, incise hematomas
	Nasal packing	Prophylactic antibiotics for sinusitis, humidified oxygen
Oropharynx	Ludwig's angina	Antibiotics, drainage, may need tracheotomy
	Odontogenic abscess	
	Retropharyngeal abscess	Antibiotics and drainage
	Peritonsillar abscess	Antibiotics and drainage
	Tonsillar enlargement	Tonsillectomy
	Macroglossia	Supportive, tracheotomy
	Angioedema	Antihistamines, steroids, epinephrine (see text)
	Stevens–Johnson syndrome	Supportive care, tracheotomy
	Burkitt lymphoma	Chemoradiation
	Salivary tumors	Resection
	Le Fort fractures 2 and 3	Tracheotomy, fixation
	Obstructive sleep apnea	CPAP, UPPP, tracheotomy
Laryngopharynx	Epiglottitis	Antibiotics
	Acute bacterial laryngotracheitis (diphtheria)	Antibiotics
	Neoplasms: SCC, papillomatosis	Resection, laser removal
	Angioedema	Antihistamines, steroids, epinephrine (see text)
	Rheumatoid arthritis	Corticosteroids, tracheotomy
	Relapsing polychondritis	Corticosteroids, tracheotomy
	Wegener's granulomatosis	Corticosteroids, cyclophosphamide, tracheotomy
	Midline granuloma	Radiation
	ETT injury: subglottic stenosis	Resection, dilation, cryotherapy
	Trauma, burns, inhalation injury	Tracheotomy
	Hemangiomas	Laser, intralesional steroids, tracheotomy
	Foreign body aspiration, dislodged tooth	Endoscopy
	Iatrogenic: laryngospasm, epistaxis	Supportive

CPAP, continuous positive airway pressure; UPPP, uvulopalatopharyngoplasty; SCC, squamous cell carcinoma; ETT, endotracheal tube.

ALGORITHM 9.1 — Algorithm for the Management of a Patient with Airway Obstruction

Airway obstruction suspected by history and physical examination:

- Inspiratory stridor: lesion at or above glottis
- Biphasic stridor and wheeze: subglottic lesion or below the glottis
- Impaired phonation
- Poor air entry
- Suprasternal retractions
- Universal choking sign
- Respiratory distress
- Tachycardia
- Agitation
- Angioedema
- Wheezing
- Neck swelling

ABBREVIATION
ENT: ear, nose, and throat specialist

Patient awake and breathing

- Attempt to localize cause by history and examination
- Assemble help with personnel experienced in difficult airways (anesthesia, ENT)
- Assemble intubation equipment and a tracheostomy tray
- Consider transfer to the operating room to optimize available equipment and personnel
- Careful performance of indirect laryngoscopy or fiberoptic nasopharyngolaryngoscopy

- Management based on diagnosis
- Can use heliox or BiPAP if etiology not progressive
- Close monitoring

Patient unconscious or signs of impending respiratory arrest

- Call for help to assemble personnel experienced in difficult airways (anesthesia and/or ENT)
- Head tilt-chin lift
- Jaw thrust (if C-spine unstable)
- Insert an oral or nasal airway
- Ventilate with a bag-valve mask
- Attempt direct laryngoscopy and endotracheal intubation
- Surgical airway (bedside tracheostomy)
- Cricothyroidotomy or needle cricothyrotomy if personnel not available to perform a bedside surgical airway

- Additional management based on etiology

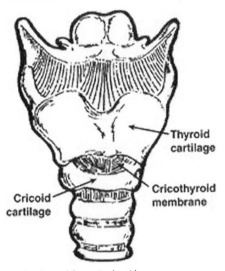

Figure 9.1. Anatomic landmarks used for a cricothyroidotomy.

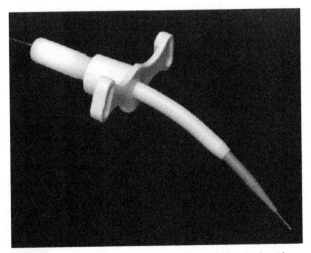

Figure 9.2. A typical Seldinger technique commercially available cricothyroidotomy set with guidewire, dilator, and cricothyroidotomy device. (Used with permission from Nina Singh-Radcliff. 5-Minute Anesthesia Consult. Philadelphia, PA: Wolters Kluwer/Lippincott Williams & Wilkins, 2013.)

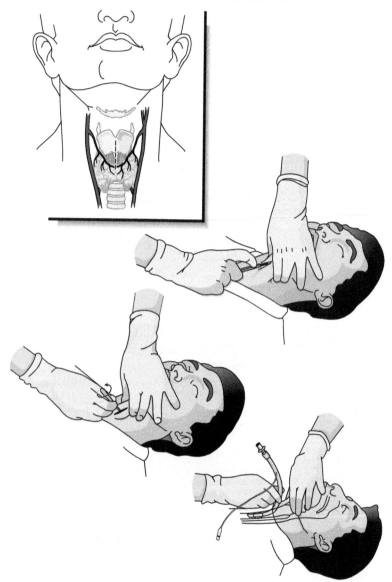

Figure 9.3. Basic steps in performing a cricothyroidotomy. (Credit: LifeART image copyright © 2016. Lippincott Williams & Wilkins. All rights reserved.)

The examination needs to be performed cautiously so as not to precipitate further narrowing of the airway.

In cases of epiglottitis, the epiglottis appears swollen and beefy. Diphtheria is characterized by a gray pseudomembrane covering the posterior pharynx. Blood cultures may occasionally be positive for bacteria, and a lateral radiograph of the neck may show the swollen epiglottis. The patient should not be sent out of the intensive care unit for any studies and should not be left alone. Most patients improve rapidly with antibiotics and failure to improve should raise concern for development of a soft tissue abscess in the parapharyngeal space. Patients with diphtheria should also receive equine antitoxin and a macrolide antibiotic.

ANGIOEDEMA

Angioedema can occur through a variety of mechanisms and results in painless swelling of the soft tissues of the face. The common precipitants are angiotensin-converting enzyme inhibitors, immunoglobulin E–mediated allergic reactions to foods or medications, and complement activation through an inherited or acquired C1 esterase inhibitor deficiency/impairment.

Patients are treated with antihistamines, steroids, and epinephrine, with airway management as noted in the algorithm. Of note, these pharmacologic interventions do not impact the bradykinin pathway, and are therefore of questionable efficacy, but are routinely administered due to occasional diagnostic uncertainty, and clinical concern for anaphylaxis. Patients with hereditary deficiency of C1 esterase inhibitor respond to early therapy with icatibant (a selective bradykinin B2 receptor antagonist). Additional options for these patients include fresh frozen plasma (which contains small amounts of C1 esterase inhibitor), purified C1 inhibitor concentrate, or Ecallantide (a kallikrein inhibitor).

POSTEXTUBATION STRIDOR

Stridor occurs in up to 15% of patients after extubation, and most cases are caused by laryngeal edema. Laryngospasm and secretions in the airway are less common causes of stridor in this situation.

Risk factors for the development of postextubation laryngeal edema include female gender, prolonged intubation, use of larger bore endotracheal tubes, history of difficult intubation, and high endotracheal tube cuff pressures.

Prevention of postextubation laryngeal edema includes measures to choose the appropriate size endotracheal tube for the patient's airway and monitoring of endotracheal tube cuff pressures to keep the cuff pressure below 25 mm Hg. In addition, attention should be paid to the patients CXR to ensure that the cuff is not positioned in the subglottic space, but rather in the more distal trachea.

Pre-extubation assessment of airway patency can be performed by utilizing a cuff leak test, a simple, noninvasive bedside test, utilizing the difference in inhaled tidal volumes and exhaled tidal volumes, with the cuff deflated. The patient's upper airway should be thoroughly suctioned prior to the test and the trachea suctioned after cuff deflation to avoid aspiration of secretions from the oropharynx and accumulated secretions above the endotracheal tube cuff. The sensitivity and specificity of this test varies greatly in clinical trials and depends on the leak cutoff value chosen. Overall, the cuff leak test is useful in identifying patients at low risk for postextubation laryngeal edema (high negative predictive value). Additional methods of airway evaluation include use of ultrasound to assess air column width, and video laryngoscopy or flexible endoscopy; however, these techniques have not been validated in large patient populations.

In patients who do not have a leak and have additional risk factors for postextubation laryngeal edema as noted above, at least 2 doses of prophylactic steroids, with the first dose given from 4 hours to preferably at least 12 hours pre-extubation is recommended. This strategy has reduced the risk of postextubation laryngeal edema.

In a patient where there is significant concern for airway patency after extubation, an airway exchange catheter can be left in place after extubation. These catheters provide for the ability to replace the endotracheal tube over the catheter in case intubation is difficult and some devices allow for provision of supplemental oxygen and limited ventilation. Experience in the use of these devices is important with particular attention paid to depth of insertion to avoid pneumothoraces.

Immediate management of the patient who develops acute postextubation laryngeal edema should consist of nebulized racemic epinephrine, which will cause local vasoconstriction and reduce edema. Most physicians also use short courses (48 hours) of IV corticosteroids; however, there are no randomized data to support this treatment. In patients who exhibit signs of respiratory distress, the safest option is reintubation to secure the airway. Additional options to consider in patients who are not in distress include heliox, which lowers airway resistance and may reduce work of breathing, allowing time for steroids to work. The use of noninvasive ventilation in carefully selected patients has been described, however, in patients who exhibit signs of distress and who have progressive airway narrowing, delaying intubation can be hazardous and these strategies should be used with caution.

SUGGESTED READINGS

Aboussouan LS, Stoller JK. Diagnosis and management of upper airway obstruction. *Clin Chest Med.* 1994;15(1):35–53.
  An excellent review article on the topic.
Bas M, Greve J, Stelter K, et al. A randomized trial of icatibant in ACE-inhibitor-induced angioedema. *N Engl J Med.* 2015;372:418–425.
  Subcutaneous icatibant resulted in faster resolution of angioedema compared to patients who only received steroids and antihistamines.
Gehlbach B, Kress JP. Upper airway obstruction. In: Hall JB, Schmidt GA, Wood LDH, eds. *Principles of Critical Care.* 3rd ed. New York: McGraw Hill; 2005:455–464.
  An excellent review article on the topic.
Goodenberger D. Medical emergencies. In: Carey CF, Lee HH, Woeltje KF, eds. *The Washington Manual of Medical Therapeutics.* 29th ed. Philadelphia, PA: Lippincott, Williams & Wilkins; 1998:494–526.
  An excellent concise chapter on the management of common emergencies in the ICU.
Jaber S, Chanques G, Matecki S, et al. Post extubation stridor in intensive care unit patients: risk factors, evaluation and importance of the cuff leak test. *Intensive Care Med.* 2003;29: 69–74.
  Risks for stridor include increased severity of illness, medical cause for intubation, traumatic and difficult intubations, a history of self-extubation, overdistended endotracheal tube cuffs, and a prolonged period of intubation.
Khosh MM, Lebovics RS. Upper airway obstruction. In: Parillo JE, Dellinger RP, eds. *Critical Care Medicine.* 2nd ed. St Louis, MO: Mosby; 2001:808–825.
  A thorough textbook chapter which divides etiologies into anatomic location.

Nzeako UC, Frigas E, Tremaine WJ. Hereditary angioedema. A broad review for clinicians. *Arch Intern Med*. 2001;161:2417–2429.

Reviews the genetic forms of the disease, the clinical presentation, diagnosis and therapeutic options as well as options for prophylaxis.

Pluijms WA, van Mook WN, Wittekamp BH, et al. Postextubation laryngeal edema and stridor resulting in respiratory failure in critically ill adults: updated review. *Critical Care*. 2015;19:295.

An excellent review article with a nice section on the cuff leak test as well as an algorithm for patients with postextubation stridor.

Zuraw BL. Hereditary angioedema. *N Engl J Med*. 2008;359:1027–1036.

Case vignette followed by review of treatment strategies and formal guidelines.

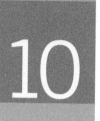

The Acute Respiratory Distress Syndrome

Marin H. Kollef

Acute lung injury (ALI) and the acute respiratory distress syndrome (ARDS) are life-threatening examples of acute pulmonary edema. Although a distinction between ALI and ARDS was originally conceived as representing a spectrum of severity (ALI less severe than ARDS), overlap between the two entities is sufficiently great that most experts no longer believe the distinction is clinically important.

The incidence of ARDS in the United States is estimated to be 200,000 cases per year, with a mortality rate of 35% to 40%, which has significantly decreased from a rate of 65% to 70% in the early 1980s. While the major physiologic consequence of ARDS is hypoxia, most patients ultimately die from the underlying cause (e.g., sepsis) or associated complications (e.g., multiorgan failure) rather than from refractory hypoxemia per se. Current therapy for ARDS centers around treatment of the underlying cause, a pressure-targeted strategy of low tidal volume ventilation aimed at preventing further lung injury, and appropriate fluid management.

In 1994, the American-European Consensus Conference (AECC) on ARDS convened to develop a set of diagnostic criteria for ARDS. With these criteria, in conjunction with the more recent view that there is little importance in the distinction between ALI and ARDS, along with evolving changes in the use of hemodynamic monitoring (see later discussion), the diagnosis of ARDS should be considered whenever the following criteria are met (Algorithm 10.1): (a) an appropriate clinical setting (i.e., a likely underlying cause), (b) the development of bilateral alveolar and/or interstitial infiltrates of acute onset (<72 hours) on frontal chest radiograph, (c) a ratio of the pulmonary arterial oxygen pressure in millimeters of mercury (PaO_2) divided by the fraction of inspired oxygen (FiO_2) of <300, and (d) no clinical evidence that left ventricular failure or intravascular volume overload is the principle cause for the acute radiographic pulmonary infiltrates. In 2012, a modified definition of ARDS called the Berlin Definition was developed and validated as shown in Table 10.1, addressing a number of limitations of the prior AECC definition and eliminating the term ALI.

ARDS can arise from direct injury to the lung parenchyma or from indirect systemic insults transmitted to the lung by the pulmonary circulation (Table 10.2). Direct causes of ARDS include pneumonia, gastric aspiration, blunt chest trauma, near drowning, and toxic inhalations. Common indirect causes include sepsis, large-volume blood transfusions (typically >15 Units), massive tissue trauma, lung transplantation, reperfusion after cardiopulmonary bypass, drug overdoses, and pancreatitis. Although more than 60 conditions have been associated with ARDS, the most frequent cause is sepsis, followed by pneumonia and aspiration.

ALGORITHM 10.1 **Ventilator Management in Acute Lung Injury/Acute Respiratory Distress Syndrome**

Acute hypoxic respiratory failure with the following
- Appropriate clinical setting
- Bilateral patchy, diffuse, or homogenous pulmonary infiltrates on frontal radiograph
- PaO_2/FiO_2 ≤300

Is there suspicion of left heart failure?

ABBREVIATIONS
PaO_2: Partial pressure arterial oxygen in mm Hg
FiO_2: Fraction inspired oxygen for example, room air = 0.21
PBW: Predicted body weight
VT: Tidal volume
PEEP: Positive end-expiratory pressure in cm H_2O
RR: Respiratory rate
PP: Plateau pressure in cm H_2O
A/C: Assist/control mode of mechanical ventilation

No **Yes**

Calculate PBW in kilogram
- Men = 50 + 2.3 (height in inches – 60)
- Women = 45.5 + 2.3 (height in inches – 60)

Cardiogenic pulmonary edema supported by
- Clinical signs
- Pulmonary capillary wedge pressure >18 mm Hg
- Esophageal Doppler ultrasonography with decreased cardiac index and increased corrected flow time
- Echocardiographic evidence of left heart failure

Start mechanical ventilation in A/C mode with the following initial parameters
- VT 6 mL/kg PBW
- PEEP 5–10 cm H_2O
- RR ≤35

Mechanical ventilation goals
- PaO_2 55–80 mm Hg or SaO_2 ≥88%
- PP ≤30 cm H_2O
- FiO_2 <0.6
- pH goal 7.30–7.35

*Obtain PP at least every 4 hours with 0.5 second end-inspiratory pause

GOALS MET?

No **Yes**

Go to Algorithm 10.2

- If PP >30 cm H_2O; decrease VT 1 mL/kg PBW to as low as 4 mL/kg to achieve PP ≤30 cm H_2O
- If PP <25 cm H_2O and TV <6 mL/kg PBW; increase TV by 1 mL/kg until PP >25 cm H_2O or TV = 6 mL/kg
- Increase PEEP using minimal amount necessary to maintain FiO_2 <0.6 (see **Table 10.4**)*
- If pH 7.15–7.30 increase RR until pH >7.30 or $PaCO_2$ <25 (consider $NaHCO_3$ if RR = 35 and $PaCO_2$ <25)
- If pH <7.15 increase RR to 35; if pH remains <7.15 and $NaHCO_3$ used or considered, increase TV by 1 mL/kg until pH >7.15 (may exceeded PP)

* Some experts prefer PEEP of 10–15 cm H_2O during the first 48–96 hours of ARDS if other parameters, like PP, remain within acceptable limits

No **Yes**

Go to Table 10.5 **GOALS MET?**

TABLE 10.1	The Berlin Definition of Acute Respiratory Distress Syndrome (ARDS)
Timing/onset:	Within 1 wk of a known clinical insult (see Table 10.2) or new or worsening respiratory symptoms
Chest radiograph/ computed tomography:	Bilateral opacities not fully explained by effusions, lobar collapse, or nodules
Origin of edema/ opacities:	Cannot fully be explained by cardiac pump failure or fluid overload. Needs objective measure (e.g., echocardiography, transthoracic/esophageal Doppler, pulmonary artery catheter) to exclude hydrostatic edema if no risk factors for ARDS present
Impaired oxygenation:	Mild: 200 mm Hg < PaO_2/FiO_2 ≤300 mm Hg with PEEP or CPAP ≥5 cm H_2O Moderate: 100 mm Hg < PaO_2/FiO_2 ≤200 mm Hg with PEEP ≥5 cm H_2O Severe: PaO_2/FiO_2 ≤100 mm Hg with PEEP ≥5 cm H_2O

CPAP, continuous positive airway pressure; PEEP, positive end-expiratory pressure; PaO_2, partial pressure of arterial oxygen; FiO_2, fraction of inspired oxygen.

The pathogenesis of ARDS starts with a pulmonary or systemic insult that triggers an inflammatory response within the lungs. The resulting "noncardiogenic, increased permeability" form of pulmonary edema follows a predictable clinical and pathologic course that has been separated into three clinically meaningful phases. The exudative phase occurs immediately and lasts approximately 3 to 7 days. Pathologically, it is characterized by "diffuse alveolar damage," the cardinal features of which are: (a) the accumulation of extravascular lung water, protein, and inflammatory cells (primarily neutrophils) in the interstitial and alveolar spaces, precipitates of which result in the characteristic intra-alveolar "hyaline membranes," (b) type 1 alveolar cell necrosis, and (c) intra-alveolar hemorrhage. The physiologic consequences of filling alveoli with edema and cellular debris are reduced alveolar ventilation, intrapulmonary

TABLE 10.2	Common Causes of ARDS	
Direct Causes		**Indirect Causes**
Pneumonia		Sepsis
Aspiration		Severe traumatic shock
Inhalation injuries		Large-volume blood transfusions (>15 Units) (TRALI)
Blunt pulmonary trauma		Pancreatitis
Near drowning		Reperfusion after cardiopulmonary bypass
Drug toxicities/overdoses; narcotics, tricyclic antidepressants, chemotherapeutic agents, fat emulsion, amiodarone		

TRALI, transfusion-related acute lung injury.

TABLE 10.3	Conditions Mimicking Acute Respiratory Distress Syndrome
Cardiogenic pulmonary edema	Acute eosinophilic pneumonia
Diffuse alveolar hemorrhage	Miliary tuberculosis
Acute interstitial pneumonia	Cryptogenic organizing pneumonia
Acute pulmonary alveolar proteinosis	Disseminated cancer

shunting, and reduced lung compliance with increased work of breathing. The clinical consequences are a need for mechanical ventilatory support to reduce the work of breathing, a high FiO_2 to achieve an acceptable PaO_2, and positive airway pressure throughout the respiratory cycle to improve alveolar ventilation.

Overlapping with the late exudative phase is a proliferative phase, which usually lasts another 2 to 3 weeks, and is characterized by increased numbers of type 2 pneumocytes, clearing of alveolar edema and debris, improving gas exchange, and, eventually, liberation from the ventilator.

Finally, some patients may progress after 2 to 3 weeks to a clinically obvious fibrotic phase. These patients develop progressive interstitial and alveolar fibrosis, occasionally with large emphysematous bullae prone to rupture, and prolonged ventilator dependency with increased morbidity and mortality. Progression to fibrosis has decreased with the use of lung protective modes of ventilation.

ARDS must be distinguished from cardiogenic pulmonary edema and other less common causes of diffuse pulmonary infiltrates due to differences in treatment. If the underlying cause of the acute pulmonary infiltrates is not certain, then computed tomography, bronchoalveolar lavage, or other diagnostic tests should be performed to exclude such entities as diffuse alveolar hemorrhage, acute interstitial pneumonia, disseminated cancer, acute eosinophilic pneumonia, miliary tuberculosis, and cryptogenic organizing pneumonia (Table 10.3). Although radiographically and physiologically similar, diffuse alveolar damage is not a prominent pathologic feature of these disease entities.

The evidence base for a particular strategy of mechanical ventilatory support for ARDS was greatly strengthened in 2000 by the landmark ARMA clinical trial, conducted by the National Institutes of Health ARDS Network. This trial demonstrated a 22% relative reduction in mortality when tidal volumes of 6 mL/kg of predicted body weight (PBW) were used rather than more traditional volumes of 12 mL/kg. The lower tidal volumes are thought to prevent microscopic barotrauma to relatively normal alveoli, which can worsen the extent and/or severity of inflammatory pulmonary edema, an outcome sometimes described as *ventilator-induced lung injury.*

The other major aspect of mechanical ventilatory support concerns the use of positive end-expiratory pressure (PEEP). PEEP increases the amount of aerated lung, thereby improving oxygenation by decreasing the shunt fraction, allowing a lower FiO_2 to be used. However, it can also be associated with barotrauma and depressed cardiovascular function. Because of these potentially conflicting effects, another major clinical trial (ALVEOLI) was conducted by the ARDS Network to determine the relative benefit of high versus low PEEP. The results of this study showed no difference in outcomes between higher PEEP (mean, 13.2 cm H_2O) and lower PEEP

TABLE 10.4	Suggested Combinations of FiO_2 and PEEPS in ARDS		
FiO_2	0.3	0.4	0.5	0.6
PEEP	5	5–8	8–10	10
FiO_2	0.7	0.8	0.9	1.0
PEEP	10–14	14	14–18	18–23

(mean, 8.3 cm H_2O) levels. Thus, some recommend that the lowest level of PEEP be used to support oxygenation and to maintain an FiO_2 at or below 0.6. However, a meta-analysis of three trials examining lower versus higher levels of PEEP found a survival advantage in the subset of ARDS patients ($PaO_2/FiO_2 \leq 200$ mm Hg) who received higher levels of PEEP. Therefore, some experts favor higher (10 to 15 cm H_2O) rather than lower (5 to 10 cm H_2O) PEEP during the early phase of ARDS (Table 10.4). More recently, an analysis of 3562 patients with ARDS demonstrated that driving pressure (plateau pressure – PEEP), a measure where tidal volume is normalized to functioning lung size, best stratified risk in ARDS. Driving pressure reductions accomplished with ventilatory setting adjustments were also strongly associated with survival.

Other ventilation strategies can be used as "rescue" therapies when oxygenation is inadequate despite the previously mentioned approach to ventilatory support, or when patients require unacceptable levels of FiO_2 or airway pressure. These include prone ventilation, inverse ratio ventilation, airway pressure release ventilation, neuromuscular blockade, high-frequency ventilation, extracorporeal membrane oxygenation (ECMO), or inhalational prostacyclin or nitric oxide (Table 10.5). Among these, only prone ventilation, neuromuscular blockade, and ECMO have been associated with mortality improvement in specific patient populations.

The benefit or harm of using glucocorticoids in ARDS appears to depend on dose, duration, and timing. A prospective, randomized, double-blind, placebo-controlled clinical trial in 2007 by Meduri et al. of moderate-dose methylprednisolone (1 mg/kg for 2 weeks followed by a taper during 2 weeks) reported significantly reduced duration of mechanical ventilation (5 vs. 9.5 days; $p = 0.002$), length of intensive care unit (ICU) stay (7 vs. 14.5 days; $p = 0.007$), and pulmonary and extrapulmonary organ dysfunction in the methylprednisolone-treated group. There was also significantly reduced ICU mortality with a strong trend ($p = 0.07$) toward reduced hospital mortality. Finally, the corticosteroid treatment group also had a significantly lower rate of infections ($p = 0.0002$).

Two prospective, randomized, double-blind, placebo-controlled clinical trials of corticosteroid administration have also been conducted in patients with unresolving (>7 days) ARDS (one by the Meduri et al. group with 24 patients and conducted at four medical centers, and the other by the multicenter National Institutes of Health-sponsored ARDS Network with 180 patients). Both studies showed significant improvements in ventilator-free days, shock-free days, and ICU-free days. The study by Meduri et al. reported improved ICU ($p = 0.002$) and in-hospital ($p = 0.03$) mortality, but the ARDS Network study did not. Indeed, in the latter study, there was a trend toward increased mortality in patients administered glucocorticoids >2 weeks after the onset of ARDS. Possible confounding factors in the latter study, however,

TABLE 10.5	Rescue Therapies and Steroids in Acute Respiratory Stress Syndrome

Rescue therapies indicated when PaO$_2$ <55 mm Hg or SaO$_2$ <88% with
- FiO$_2$ >0.7 or
- PP >30 cm H$_2$O

Inhaled pharmacologic agents^a
- Inhaled epoprostenol
- Inhaled nitric oxide
- Inhaled iloprost (prostaglandin I$_2$)

Prone ventilation^b
- Contraindications:
  - Open wounds/burns on the ventral body surface
  - Unstable fractures
  - Spinal instability
  - Increased intracranial pressure
  - Hemodynamic instability
- Caution if tracheostomy, chest tubes, obesity, ascites
- Maintain in prone position for 18–20 hrs of every 24

Other adjunctive/salvage ventilator strategies:
- Inverse ratio ventilation (inspiratory time > expiratory time)
- High-frequency ventilation
- Airway pressure release ventilation
- Extracorporeal membrane oxygenation^c
- Neuromuscular blockade^b

Steroids (Controversial)
- 1–7 days but ideally ≤72 hrs;
  - No role yet identified unless documented adrenal insufficiency.
  - Give methylprednisolone (or equivalent) 1 mg/kg IV bolus, then 1 mg/kg/day continuous IV infusion for 14 days.
  - If receiving paralytics, delay use until concomitant use of paralytic agents is not required.
  - If no clear physiologic or radiologic benefit in 3–5 days, discontinue.
  - After 14 days or successful patient extubation, decrease to 0.5 mg/kg/day IV and continue for 7 days, then decrease to 0.25 mg/kg/day IV and continue for 7 days, then stop.
- 7–14 days, if steroids were not started earlier;
  - Benefit less certain, but in select cases may try the same protocol as above. If no clear physiologic or radiologic benefit in 3–5 days, discontinue.
- 14 days
  - Probably no role for steroid use in these cases (may cause increased mortality if used routinely in this time course). However, a trial may still be considered in select cases.

---

^{a}These agents should not be given IV as they may worsen shunting by vasodilating capillaries in nonaerated alveoli.
^{b}Recent trials suggest survival advantage.
^{c}Should be considered in case of severe single organ dysfunction such as ARDS following influenza infection.
PaO$_2$, arterial oxygen pressure in millimeters of mercury; SaO$_2$, oxygen saturation in percent; FiO$_2$, fraction inspired oxygen; PP, plateau pressure in centimeters of H$_2$O; IV, intravenously.

include a greater use of paralytic agents in the treated group and a shortened course of therapy compared with the Meduri et al. protocol.

Overall, the data from these various studies support the use of moderate-dose steroids for ARDS patients of duration <2 weeks (Table 10.5). Steroids should be withheld until it is certain that paralytic agents are not required concomitantly. Because physiologic and radiologic parameters appear to improve substantially within 3 to 5 days after beginning steroid use, it may be reasonable to discontinue steroids after this time in those patients who fail to show any significant response. In those who do respond, however, steroids should be continued for up to 4 weeks (Table 10.5).

Corticosteroids should not be *routinely* started in patients with unresolving ARDS more than 2 weeks after onset. However, they may be considered in selected cases; here again, a 3- to 5-day course should at least establish whether there will be physiologic or radiologic improvement before longer trials are considered. Recently, Papazian et al. demonstrated that neuromuscular blockers in ARDS were associated with a survival advantage. Clinicians should carefully weigh the advantages and disadvantages of combining corticosteroids and neuromuscular blockers, especially since both agents are associated with the development of critical illness myopathy and polyneuropathy.

The injured lung during ARDS is also highly vulnerable to worsening pulmonary edema by high pulmonary capillary pressures. However, until recently, fluid management during ARDS often emphasized the need to maintain intravascular volume to optimize hemodynamic performance, even at the risk of worsening pulmonary edema. Even though hemodynamic stability and organ perfusion need to be maintained, another trial by the ARDS Network from 2006 (FACTT) showed that minimizing pulmonary capillary pressures without compromising systemic organ perfusion could be accomplished, with a decreased duration of mechanical ventilation and ICU stay as the result (Algorithm 10.2). However, no mortality benefit was shown.

The FACTT study also showed no improvement in survival or organ function if hemodynamic management was guided with pulmonary artery catheters (PACs) instead of with simple central venous pressure monitoring in patients with established ARDS, and PACs were associated with increased complications. Thus, the routine use of PACs for hemodynamic management of ARDS can no longer be recommended. Moreover, growing evidence is mounting that more optimal use of ventilator parameters (tidal volume ≤6 mL/PBW) and achievement of neutral to negative net fluid balance can prevent the occurrence of ARDS in high-risk patients.

Numerous studies have examined the long-term outcome of patients who survive ARDS. In one study, the average stay in the ICU from ARDS was 25 days. At discharge, patients had lost 18% of their body weight, and had significant functional limitations. At 1 year, patients had persistent functional limitations due to muscle wasting and weakness. Lung volume and spirometric measurements in survivors were normal or near normal by 6 months to 1 year (defined as >80% of predicted amounts), and most patients did not require supplemental oxygen.

In summary, ARDS is a severe life-threatening form of pulmonary edema with characteristic clinical, radiologic, and physiologic consequences. Beyond treating the inciting event, current ARDS management centers on volume- and pressure-limited lung protective ventilation, conservative fluid management, and possibly the early use of moderate-dose corticosteroids. Rescue therapies are reserved for those patients who remain hypoxic despite ventilator and fluid management. However, the use

ALGORITHM 10.2 Fluid Management in Acute Lung Injury/ Acute Respiratory Distress Syndrome

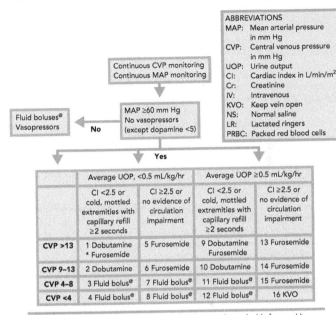

ABBREVIATIONS
MAP: Mean arterial pressure in mm Hg
CVP: Central venous pressure in mm Hg
UOP: Urine output
CI: Cardiac index in L/min/m²
Cr: Creatinine
IV: Intravenous
KVO: Keep vein open
NS: Normal saline
LR: Lactated ringers
PRBC: Packed red blood cells

Continuous CVP monitoring
Continuous MAP monitoring

MAP ≥60 mm Hg
No vasopressors
(except dopamine <5)

Fluid boluses@
Vasopressors

No

Yes

	Average UOP, <0.5 mL/kg/hr		Average UOP ≥0.5 mL/kg/hr	
	CI <2.5 or cold, mottled extremities with capillary refill ≥2 seconds	CI ≥2.5 or no evidence of circulation impairment	CI <2.5 or cold, mottled extremities with capillary refill ≥2 seconds	CI ≥2.5 or no evidence of circulation impairment
CVP >13	1 Dobutamine * Furosemide	5 Furosemide	9 Dobutamine Furosemide	13 Furosemide
CVP 9–13	2 Dobutamine	6 Furosemide	10 Dobutamine	14 Furosemide
CVP 4–8	3 Fluid bolus@	7 Fluid bolus@	11 Fluid bolus@	15 Furosemide
CVP <4	4 Fluid bolus@	8 Fluid bolus@	12 Fluid bolus@	16 KVO

For Cell # 1, 5, 6 furosemide 20 mg IV bolus, or IV infusion at 3 mg/hr. **HOLD** if Cr >3, or Cr 0–3 with labs consistent with renal failure, or vasopressor/fluid bolus in last 12 hours.

Reassess in 1 hour; double furosemide dose hourly until UOP >0.5 mg/hr or maximum of 24 mg/hr or 160 mg bolus.

For Cell # 9, 13, 14, 15 furosemide 20 mg IV bolus, or IV infusion at 3 mg/hr. **HOLD** if Cr >3, or Cr 0–3 with labs consistent with renal failure, or vasopressor/fluid bolus in last 12 hours.

Reassess in 4 hours; if still in cell where furosemide is indicated give same dose if UOP >3 mL/kg/hr, double if ≤3 mL/kg/hr, to a maximum of 24 mg/hr or 160 mg bolus.

For Cell # 3, 4, 7, 8 give a NS, plasmalyte, or LR bolus of 15 mL/kg, 1 Unit PRBCs, or 25 g 25% albumin.

Reassess in 1 hour.

Administer up to 3 boluses in 24 hours if indicated by Cell #.

For Cell # 11, 12 give a NS, plasmalyte, or LR bolus of 15 mL/kg, 1 Unit PRBCs, or 25 g 25% albumin.

Reassess in 4 hours.

Additional boluses at physician discretion

For Cell # 1, 2, 9, 10 Dobutamine, start at 5 mcg/kg/min

Increase by 5 mcg/kg/min until CI >2.5

* If furosemide not available can use bumetanide with a dose equivalency of 40:1 (Lasix 40 mg = bumetanide 1 mg).
@Fluid boluses should ideally only be administered to patients demonstrating fluid responsiveness using an objective dynamic measure to minimize the unnecessary use of crystalloid or oncotic solutions. Patients are considered fluid responsive if pulse pressure variability decreased to <13%, inferior vena cava distention index with respiration decreased to <18%, and the stroke volume index difference increased to >10%. (Adapted from the 2006 FACTT trial, this complex algorithm may not be appropriate for all patients and in all clinical settings and should be used with physician discretion and judgment.)

of specific interventions such as ECMO is increasingly utilized in certain high-risk populations (see Chapter 86). At 1 year, survivors of ARDS often must endure some degree of functional disability from muscle weakness and wasting, but lung function measurements can be expected to approach normal values.

SUGGESTED READINGS

Amato MB, Meade MO, Slutsky AS, et al. Driving pressure and survival in the acute respiratory distress syndrome. *N Engl J Med.* 2015;372(8):747–755.

An analysis of 3562 patients with ARDS demonstrating that reductions in driving pressure (Plateau pressure – PEEP) were associated with survival.

ARDS Definition Task Force, Ranieri VM, Rubenfeld GD, et al. Acute respiratory distress syndrome: the Berlin Definition. *JAMA.* 2012;307(23):2526–2533.

The Berlin Definition attempts to make the definition of ARDS more objective and offers severity categorization based on the degree of impaired oxygenation.

Bernard GR, Artigas A, Brigham KL, et al. The American-European Consensus Conference on ARDS: definitions, mechanisms, relevant outcomes and clinical trial coordination. *Am J Respir Crit Care Med.* 1994;149(3 Pt 1):818–824.

The American-European Consensus Conference on ARDS was established in 1992 between the American Thoracic Society and the European Society of Intensive Care Medicine. The goals of the Committee were to form a uniform definition of ALI and ARDS, better define the mechanism of acute lung injury, identify risk factors, prevalence, and outcomes, and to promote clinical study coordination.

Briel M, Meade M, Mercat A, et al. Higher vs lower positive end-expiratory pressure in patients with acute lung injury and acute respiratory distress syndrome: systematic review and meta-analysis. *JAMA.* 2010;303(9):865–873.

Analysis of three trials comparing outcome in patients receiving higher PEEP versus lower PEEP levels. Overall, no difference in hospital survival was found. However, higher PEEP levels were associated with improved survival among the subgroup of patients with ARDS.

Brower RG, Lanken PN, MacIntyre N, et al; The National Heart, Lung, and Blood Institute ARDS Clinical Trials Network. Higher versus lower positive end-expiratory pressures in patients with the acute respiratory distress syndrome. *N Engl J Med.* 2004;351(4): 327–336.

The "ALVEOLI" trial was conducted by the ARDS Network at 23 affiliated centers. The trial compared mechanical ventilation with higher PEEP (mean 13.2 ± 3.5 cm H2O) versus lower PEEP (mean 8.3 ± 3.2) when tidal volumes of 6 mL/kg PBW were used. The trial was stopped after 549 patients were enrolled when no significant difference was found between the two groups for death.

Guerin L, Monnet X, Teboul JL. Monitoring volume and fluid responsiveness: from static to dynamic indicators. *Best Pract Res Clin Anaesthesiol.* 2013;27(2):177–185.

An up to date review on determining the presence or absence of fluid responsiveness using objective parameters.

Guérin C, Reignier J, Richard JC, et al; PROSEVA Study Group. Prone positioning in severe acute respiratory distress syndrome. *N Engl J Med.* 2013;368(23):2159–2168.

A randomized trial demonstrating a survival advantage with prone positioning.

Herridge MS, Cheung AM, Tansey CM, et al; Canadian Critical Care Trials Group. One-year outcomes in survivors of the acute respiratory distress syndrome. *N Engl J Med.* 2003;348(8):683–693.

This longitudinal study was conducted at four medical-surgical intensive care units in Toronto, Canada. At the time of discharge, patients had lost 18% of their body weight, with 71% returning to their baseline body weight by 1 year. Lung volume and spirometric measurements were normal by 6 months, defined as being within 80% predicted.

Meduri GU, Golden E, Freire AX, et al. Methylprednisolone infusion in early severe ARDS: results of a randomized controlled trial. *Chest.* 2007;131(4):954–963.

> *Randomized, double-blinded, placebo-controlled trial of moderate-dose methylprednisolone in early ARDS conducted in the surgical and medical intensive care units at five medical centers in Memphis, TN, randomizing patients 2:1 to methylprednisolone versus placebo (n = 63 vs. 28) and treating patients for up to 28 days, showing a significant reduction in duration of mechanical ventilation, length of ICU stay, and organ dysfunction in the treatment group.*

Meduri GU, Headley AS, Golden E, et al. Effect of prolonged methylprednisolone therapy in unresolving acute respiratory distress syndrome: a randomized controlled trial. *JAMA.* 1998;280(2):159–165.

> *Randomized, double-blinded, placebo-controlled clinical trial conducted at four medical centers in Memphis, TN of 24 patients with ARDS that did not show improved lung injury scores by day 7 assigned 2:1 to receive methylprednisolone (initially 2 mg/kg/day and continued for 32 days) versus placebo. The study showed significant improvement in the primary outcomes of lung injury, MODS scores, and ICU and in-hospital mortality in the methylprednisolone-treated patients.*

Papazian L, Forel JM, Gacouin A, et al; ACURASYS Study Investigators. Neuromuscular blockers in early acute respiratory distress syndrome. *N Engl J Med.* 2010;363(12):1107–1116.

> *Survival improvement was associated with the use of neuromuscular blockers early on in ARDS.*

Serpa Neto A, Simonis FD, Barbas CS, et al. Association between tidal volume size, duration of ventilation, and sedation needs in patients without acute respiratory distress syndrome: an individual patient data meta-analysis. *Intensive Care Med.* 2014;40(7):950–957.

> *A meta-analysis showing that lung protective ventilator setting including tidal volume ≤6 mL/kg predicted body weight was associated with a survival advantage.*

Steinberg KP, Hudson LD, Goodman RB, et al; The National Heart, Lung, and Blood Institute Acute Respiratory Distress Syndrome Clinical Trials Network. Efficacy and safety of corticosteroids for persistent acute respiratory distress syndrome. *N Engl J Med.* 2006; 354(16):1671–1684.

> *The "LaSRS" trial was a double-blind randomized controlled clinical trial conducted by the ARDS Network at 25 affiliated centers. The study enrolled 180 patients with ARDS of at least 7 to 28 days duration and randomly assigned them to receive either methylprednisolone (2 mg/kg bolus then 0.5 mg/kg every 6 hours for 14 days, 0.5 mg/kg every 12 hours for 7 days, and then tapered over 4 days), or placebo. The study found no difference in 60-day mortality between those treated with corticosteroids versus placebo (29.2% vs. 28.6%) but did identify significant physiologic and radiologic improvements favoring corticosteroids. Some have criticized the trial for too rapid withdrawal of steroids and for significant differences in the use of paralytics between groups.*

The Acute Respiratory Distress Syndrome Network, Brower RG, Matthay MA, et al. Ventilation with lower tidal volumes as compared with traditional tidal volumes for acute lung injury and the acute respiratory distress syndrome. *N Engl J Med.* 2000;342(18):1301–1308.

> *The "ARMA" trial was conducted at 10 university centers in the ARDS Network. The trial enrolled patients with ARDS and compared ventilation with traditional tidal volumes (mean 11.8 ± 0.8 mL/kg PBW) versus low tidal volumes (mean 6.2 ± 0.8 mL/kg PBW). The trial was stopped after enrolling 861 patients after the lower tidal volume group had significantly lower mortality (31% vs. 39%).*

The National Heart, Lung, and Blood Institute Acute Respiratory Distress Syndrome (ARDS) Clinical Trials Network, Wiedemann HP, Wheeler AP, et al. Comparison of two fluid-management strategies in acute lung injury. *N Engl J Med.* 2006;354(24):2564–2575.

> *The "FACTT" trial was a randomized controlled clinical trial conducted by the ARDS Network at 20 affiliated centers. The study enrolled 1000 patients with ARDS of less than 48 hours duration and randomly assigned them to a conservative versus liberal fluid management strategy for 7 days. Patients were also randomly assigned to treatment guided by PAC versus CVP monitoring (see the following citation). The study found no*

difference in 60-day mortality (25.5% vs. 28.4%) but did identify significant differences in ventilator time and ICU stay favoring the conservative fluid management strategy.

The National Heart, Lung, and Blood Institute Acute Respiratory Distress Syndrome (ARDS) Clinical Trials Network. Pulmonary artery versus central venous catheter to guide treatment of acute lung injury. *N Engl J Med.* 2006;354:2213–2224.

The "FACTT" study also yielded this paper based on outcome among the 1000 patients with ARDS who were randomly assigned to conservative versus liberal fluid management for 7 days. Patients were randomly assigned to treatment guided by pulmonary versus central venous catheter monitoring. The study found no difference between the PAC and CVP groups in 60-day mortality (27.4% vs. 26.3%).

Zielinski MD, Jenkins D, Cotton BA, et al; AAST Open Abdomen Study Group. Adult respiratory distress syndrome risk factors for injured patients undergoing damage-control laparotomy: AAST multicenter post hoc analysis. *J Trauma Acute Care Surg.* 2014;77(6):886–891.

One of several recent reports linking fluid balance with the development of ARDS in high-risk surgical patients.

11 Status Asthmaticus

Chase Hall and Mario Castro

Asthma is a common disorder affecting approximately 300 million worldwide and 24 million Americans. It is a chronic inflammatory disease of the airways characterized by airway hyperreactivity and inflammation, bronchoconstriction, and mucus hypersecretion. Asthma exacerbations result in nearly 13.6 million unscheduled emergency department (ED)/physician office visits, 500,000 hospitalizations, and 3600 deaths in the United States. In school-aged children, asthma accounts for nearly 13 million missed school days per year. In adults, nearly 10.1 million days of work are missed because of asthma. The economic impact of asthma is estimated to be $56 billion annually.

Approximately 10% of patients hospitalized with asthma are admitted to the intensive care unit (ICU), and 2% are intubated. Mortality rates range from 0.5% to 3% in hospitalized patients. Morbidity and mortality from asthma disproportionately affect the economically disadvantaged, women, and minorities, especially African Americans and Hispanics from Puerto Rico. The Nationwide Inpatient Sample, a study looking at >80,000 US hospital admissions for asthma, reported a hospital mortality rate of 0.5%. The majority of asthma-related deaths occurred in patients older than 35 years. The study found no significant differences in hospitalized mortality rates in regard to race, suggesting that the disproportionate effect on minorities may be the result of prehospital factors such as access to health care, inadequate preventive therapy, or delay in seeking medical treatment. Risk factors for death from asthma are listed in Table 11.1.

Patients at risk of future exacerbations can be identified in the clinic using objective measures of asthma control such as the Asthma Control Test™ (ACT) or the Asthma Control Questionnaire (ACQ). Patients with a low ACT (<19) or high ACQ (>1.25) have inadequately controlled asthma and are at risk of future exacerbations. Acutely, patients present with dyspnea, cough, chest tightness, and wheezing which fails to respond to standard asthma therapy such as bronchodilators. In severe asthma episodes, airway obstruction, respiratory muscle fatigue due to work of breathing, and altered V/Q relationships can lead to hypercapnia and hypoxemic respiratory failure. This chapter will focus on the initial hospital and ICU management, as well as ventilator strategies for patients with status asthmaticus.

Status asthmaticus is defined as a prolonged severe episode of asthma that is unresponsive to initial standard therapy that may lead to respiratory failure. The episodes may be rapid onset (in a matter of hours) or, more typically, progress during several hours to days. The former is often referred to as *asphyxic* asthma and occurs in a minority of cases. Rapid-onset status asthmaticus is more common in men, and is oftentimes triggered by exposure to allergens, irritants, exercise, psychosocial stress,

TABLE 11.1	Risk Factors for Death from Asthma

Lower socioeconomic status
Female gender
African-American or Puerto Rican race
Smoking
"Labile asthma," high degree of variability in peak expiratory flow
Blood eosinophilia
Poor perception of dyspnea: alexithymia, a psychological trait characterized by difficulty in perceiving and expressing emotions and body sensations
History of sudden severe exacerbations (asphyxic asthma)
History of intubation for asthma
History of ICU admission for asthma
Two or more hospitalizations for asthma within the past year
Three or more ED visits for asthma in the past year
Hospitalization or ED visit for asthma within past month
Use of more than two canisters per month of inhaled short-acting β_2-agonists
Current use or recent withdrawal of oral corticosteroids
Poor perception of airflow obstruction
Comorbid cardiovascular disease
Sensitivity to Alternaria

ICU, intensive care unit; ED, emergency department.

and inhaled illicit drugs. It may also develop after exposure to aspirin, nonsteroidal anti-inflammatory drugs, or β-blockers in susceptible individuals. This form of status asthmaticus represents a more "bronchospastic" pathophysiology, and is associated with rapid resolution with treatment. More commonly, asthma episodes develop during several hours to days, and may be triggered by viral or atypical infection. Airway obstruction in these cases is due to airway inflammation, bronchoconstriction, and mucus plugging.

In both forms, the pathologic processes result in airway obstruction and expiratory airflow limitation. Insufficient expiratory time results in air trapping, dynamic hyperinflation (DHI), and persistent positive end-expiratory alveolar pressure, also referred to as *intrinsic positive end-expiratory pressure* (iPEEP). This alters lung mechanics by increasing the work of breathing while simultaneously placing the diaphragm at a mechanical disadvantage. The increased work load placed on the respiratory muscles results in increased O_2 consumption and CO_2 production, setting up a vicious cycle.

DHI adversely affects cardiovascular function because of the dramatic fluctuations in intrathoracic pressure during inspiration and expiration (evident on physical examination as pulsus paradoxus). During inspiration, there can be exaggerated right ventricular filling and paradoxic interventricular septal motion, resulting in impaired left ventricular filling. During expiration, the increased intrathoracic pressure impairs ventricular diastolic filling, resulting in decreased cardiac output and compromised diaphragmatic blood flow, exacerbating metabolic acidosis and respiratory muscle fatigue. This downward spiral from the multiple pathophysiologic processes results in hypoxemic and hypercapnic respiratory failure (Algorithm 11.1).

ALGORITHM 11.1 Status Asthmaticus Pathophysiology

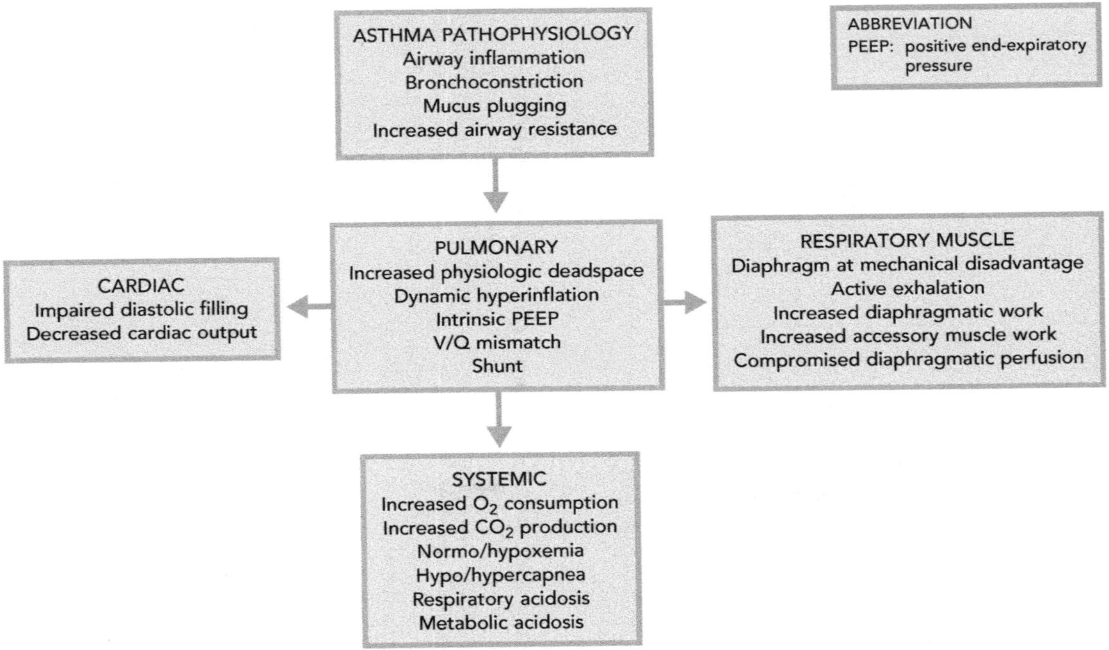

ASTHMA PATHOPHYSIOLOGY
Airway inflammation
Bronchoconstriction
Mucus plugging
Increased airway resistance

PULMONARY
Increased physiologic deadspace
Dynamic hyperinflation
Intrinsic PEEP
V/Q mismatch
Shunt

RESPIRATORY MUSCLE
Diaphragm at mechanical disadvantage
Active exhalation
Increased diaphragmatic work
Increased accessory muscle work
Compromised diaphragmatic perfusion

CARDIAC
Impaired diastolic filling
Decreased cardiac output

SYSTEMIC
Increased O_2 consumption
Increased CO_2 production
Normo/hypoxemia
Hypo/hypercapnea
Respiratory acidosis
Metabolic acidosis

ABBREVIATION
PEEP: positive end-expiratory pressure

TABLE 11.2	Differential Diagnoses to Consider

Upper airway obstruction
Tumor
Epiglottitis
Vocal cord dysfunction
Foreign body aspiration
Endobronchial lesion (e.g., amyloid, carcinoid, stricture)
Congestive heart failure
Chronic obstructive pulmonary disease
Bronchiolitis obliterans
Pulmonary embolism
Churg–Strauss syndrome
Gastroesophageal reflux
Obstructive sleep apnea
Tracheobronchomalacia
Herpetic tracheobronchitis
Mitral stenosis
Aspirin sensitivity
Adverse drug reaction
   Angiotensin-converting enzyme inhibitor
   β_2-Adrenergic antagonist
   Inhaled pentamidine

Rapid evaluation of the patient presenting with status asthmaticus is essential, focusing on key points of the history such as duration of symptoms, potential inciting exposures, medication use, and previous history of severe attacks. Patients should be questioned regarding the presence of symptoms suggestive of comorbid, complicating, or similarly presenting conditions (Table 11.2). Key historical and physical examination findings are listed in Table 11.3.

TREATMENTS

Standard Treatment for All Patients

Oxygen

- Supplemental oxygen to maintain SaO_2 >92%.

Inhaled Bronchodilators

- β_2-Agonists administered via metered-dose inhalers (MDIs) or nebulized bronchodilators. They increase cyclic adenosine monophosphate (c-AMP)-mediated bronchodilation. Albuterol (2.5 to 5 mg) nebulization every 20 minutes (or four to eight puffs of MDI with spacer) within the first hour.
- Alternatively, albuterol may be given as a continuous nebulization at a dose of 10 to 15 mg during 1 hour with telemetry monitoring. A Cochrane review of 165 randomized controlled trials supports the use of continuous nebulization versus intermittent MDI in patients with severe acute asthma who present to the ED to increase their pulmonary functions and reduce hospitalization.

TABLE 11.3 Typical Physical Examination and Laboratory Findings in Asthma by Severity

Finding	Mild	Moderate	Severe	Respiratory Arrest Imminent
Breathless	Walking Can lie down	Talking Prefers sitting	At rest Hunched forward	
Speaks in	Sentences	Phrases	Words	
Alertness	May be agitated	Usually agitated	Usually agitated	Drowsy or confused
Respiratory rate	Increased	Increased	>30 breaths/min	
Accessory muscle use and retractions	Usually not	Usually	Usually	
Wheeze	Moderate, often end expiratory	Loud	Usually loud	Absent
Pulse (beats/min)	<100	100–120	>120	Bradycardia (<60)
Pulsus paradoxus	Absent (<10 mm Hg)	May be present (10–25 mm Hg)	Often present (>25 mm Hg)	Absence suggests respiratory muscle fatigue
PEF	>80%	60–80%	<60%	
PaO_2	Normal	>60 mm Hg	<60 mm Hg	
$PaCO_2$	<45 mm Hg	<45 mm Hg	>45 mm Hg	
SaO_2	>95%	91–95%	<90%	

PEF, peak expiratory flow.

- Levalbuterol (1.25 mg) nebulized every 20 minutes within the first hour, then every 1 to 4 hours as needed can be used in place of albuterol, although there are no data to support its superiority over albuterol.
- Initial treatment should include ipratropium 0.5 mg nebulized every 20 minutes, given concomitantly with albuterol (shown to improve airflow limitation in acute asthma exacerbations in first 36 hours). This antagonizes cyclic guanosine monophosphate (cGMP)-mediated bronchoconstriction.
- In the case of intubated patients, bronchodilators should be given via MDI (e.g., albuterol along the inspiratory circuit or between a Y-piece and the endotracheal tube).
- Long-acting β_2-agonists (salmeterol, formoterol, vilanterol) are not indicated for the treatment of acute asthma. Long-acting β_2-agonists may be continued as add-on therapy in the hospitalized patient and in the outpatient setting.

- The administration of intravenous β_2-agonists is no more effective and potentially more toxic than delivery via aerosol and is therefore not recommended.

Corticosteroids

- Initial dose of methylprednisolone, 125 mg intravenously once, or equivalent oral dose if the patient is able to tolerate oral administration. Corticosteroids decrease inflammatory response and upregulate β-receptors.
- Subsequently, methylprednisolone, 40 to 60 mg intravenously every 6 to 12 hours (usually 2 mg/kg/day or less) or equivalent dose given orally if there is no suspected impairment in gastrointestinal absorption.
- Consider tapering dose after 36 to 48 hours, depending on clinical response.

Additional Therapeutic Considerations

Antibiotics

- Not recommended routinely for uncomplicated asthma exacerbation.
- Justified if patients have fever, purulent sputum, or if there is evidence of pneumonia or bacterial sinusitis complicating the asthma exacerbation.

Magnesium

- IV magnesium (2 g infused during 20 minutes) is relatively safe but does not appear to be more effective than standard therapy. Thought to antagonize calcium-mediated bronchoconstriction. No supporting data beyond administration of initial dose in ED.
- Less data available regarding use of inhaled magnesium but may improve lung function in severe asthma exacerbations (forced expiratory volume in 1 second [FEV1] less than 50% predicted) when added to inhaled bronchodilators.

Methylxanthines

- Not recommended for initial treatment in acute asthma.
- Equivalent bronchodilator properties as β_2-agonists but with increased potential of toxicity (tachyarrhythmia).

Epinephrine

- No proven advantage over inhaled bronchodilator therapy, but with added potential for toxicity, especially in hypoxemic patients.
- Consider in patients who do not respond or are unable to cooperate with intensive inhaled bronchodilator treatment.
- Dosing: 0.5 mg of a 1:1000 dilution given subcutaneously every 20 minutes three times if needed.

Heliox

- The use of helium–oxygen (HeO_2) mixtures in severe obstructive airway disease is based on the decreased density of heliox compared with air, resulting in more laminar rather than turbulent airflow.
- Use either 60%:40% or 70%:30% heliox (helium:oxygen) mixtures.
- Limited data suggest improved delivery of aerosolized bronchodilators (albuterol) when given with heliox rather than oxygen.
- The use of heliox in the mechanically ventilated patient should only be considered in those institutions that have significant experience and familiarity with its use

because of potential technical complications regarding volume and pressure monitoring with standard ventilators.

Ventilator Strategies

The goal of management in status asthmaticus is to unload the respiratory muscles, correct hypoxemia, provide adequate ventilation, and minimize lung injury, particularly from DHI, while treating the underlying airway inflammation and bronchoconstriction.

Noninvasive Ventilation

- Although the concept of treating acute asthma (an air trapping disease) with additional airway pressure at the end of expiration seems counterintuitive, a number of studies have indicated that it may actually reduce the work of breathing during exacerbations of bronchospasm. Bilevel positive airway pressure (BiPAP) also enhances the bronchodilator effect of albuterol.
- Noninvasive positive pressure ventilation (NIPPV) in an acute exacerbation may prevent the need for intubation.
- NIPPV with either continuous positive airway pressure or BiPAP may be considered as initial treatment of patients presenting to the ED with status asthmaticus who are alert, cooperative, and able to protect their airways while tolerating a full face mask.
- Initial BiPAP settings, IPAP (inspiratory positive airway pressure) of 8 and EPAP (expiratory positive airway pressure) of 5, are adjusted promptly to achieve patient comfort and compliance and decrease work of breathing (decreased respiratory rate, increased tidal volume) without exceeding IPAP of 15 and EPAP of 5.
- Aerophagia with subsequent vomiting and aspiration are potential complications of NIPPV, and patients should be closely monitored and kept in nothing by mouth status.
- Clinical improvement after initiation of NIPPV (decreased respiratory rate, improved air movement, decreased $PaCO_2$) should be documented shortly after initiation of NIPPV and pharmacologic treatment (within 30 minutes).
- Lack of improvement should prompt the clinician to the need for intubation and mechanical ventilation. Once deemed necessary, intubation should not be delayed.
- NIPPV is contraindicated in patients with decreased mental status and hemodynamic instability.

Invasive Ventilation

Ventilator strategies should concentrate on allowing adequate expiratory time to avoid DHI and barotrauma. Mechanical ventilation with volume-controlled ventilation is preferable. Suggested initial settings are listed in Table 11.4. A lung protective and permissive hypercapnia strategy should be employed, targeting a plateau pressure <30 cm H_2O. iPEEP should be monitored by performing an end-expiratory hold maneuver. The iPEEP is equal to total PEEP minus set PEEP (set on ventilator) (Fig. 11.1). The goal should be to maintain iPEEP <20 cm H_2O. This often can be achieved by reducing the respiratory rate (typically not below 10 to 14 breaths/min) or decreasing the tidal volume (typically 6 to 8 mL/kg). Increasing the flow rate (≥100 L/min) or square waveform has minimal impact on DHI once the minute ventilation has been limited.

TABLE 11.4	Initial Ventilator Settings in Status Asthmaticus
Parameter	Setting
Mode	Volume controlled
Minute ventilation	10 L
Tidal volume	6–8 mL/kg
Respiratory rate	10–14 breaths/min
Inspiratory flow rate	60–80 LPM
I:E	1:3 up to 1:5
PEEP	5 cm H_2O
FIO_2	Titrate to keep SpO_2 >90%

LPM, liters per minute; PEEP, positive end-expiratory pressure.

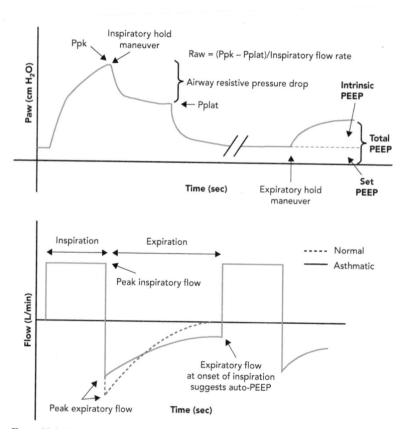

Figure 11.1. Intrinsic positive end-expiratory pressure (PEEP). Ppk, peak pressure; Pplat, plateau pressure.

INTUBATION CONSIDERATIONS

Preparation for intubation is crucial and the procedure should be performed by a skilled intensivist or anesthesiologist. Patients should be intubated with a size 8.0-mm tube to decrease resistance and to allow adequate room for suctioning and bronchoscopy, if needed. Complications include arrhythmias, laryngospasm, aspiration, and pneumothorax due to excessive bagging. Propofol, etomidate, and ketamine are appropriate induction agents using rapid sequence induction. Hypotension during or postintubation is common in status asthmaticus because of multiple factors, including the application of positive pressure throughout the respiratory cycle in patients with pre-existing DHI and iPEEP, hypovolemia, and sedation. It should be managed with sedatives and liberal IVF (intravenous fluids) as well as the aforementioned ventilator strategies to minimize DHI. If needed, with close monitoring of SpO_2, the patient can be disconnected from the ventilator circuit to allow adequate exhalation of trapped gas and decrease intrathoracic pressure.

OTHER CONSIDERATIONS

Combination of propofol (or benzodiazepine) with fentanyl should be considered for sedation to minimize patient–ventilator dyssynchrony and to enforce controlled hypoventilation. Ketamine can be considered for sedation due to its anesthetic as well as bronchodilatory properties. Neuromuscular blockade should be considered in patients with status asthmaticus on mechanical ventilation who demonstrate considerable patient–ventilator dyssynchrony with unacceptably high plateau pressures and iPEEP despite adequate sedation and analgesia. Neuromuscular blocking agents should be given as intermittent boluses with neuromuscular (train of four) monitoring. Administration of neuromuscular blocking agents as continuous infusions should be avoided because of the increased risk of myopathy associated with concurrent corticosteroid use.

For refractory cases, inhaled anesthetics (sevoflurane, isoflurane, and halothane) have been used. In some cases, bronchoscopy has been used to remove impacted mucus to improve ventilation. Extracorporeal carbon dioxide removal ($ECCO_2R$) as well as extracorporeal membrane oxygenation (ECMO) has been used successfully in case reports for severe respiratory acidosis that is refractory to maximal medical and ventilator management, however, larger clinical trials are needed.

SUGGESTED READINGS

Abrams D, Brodie D. Emerging indications for extracorporeal membrane oxygenation in adults with respiratory failure. *Ann Am Thorac Soc.* 2013;10(4):371–377.
  Review of ECMO for respiratory failure, including asthma.
American Lung Association, Epidemiology & Statistics Unit, Research and Program Services. Trends in Asthma Morbidity and Mortality, September 2012.
  A resource for asthma statistics.
Barr RG, Woodruff PG, Clark S, et al. Sudden-onset asthma exacerbations: clinical features, response to therapy, and a 2-week follow-up. Multicenter Airway Research Collaboration (MARC) investigators. *Eur Respir J.* 2000;15(2):266–273.
  A nice article that reviews the clinical features of sudden-onset asthma.

Brenner K, Abrams DC, Agerstrand CL, et al. Extracorporeal carbon dioxide removal for refractory status asthmaticus: experience in distinct exacerbation phenotypes. *Perfusion.* 2014;29(1):26–28.
A review of ECCO₂R and a few case presentations.

Brenner B, Corbridge T, Kazzi A. Intubation and mechanical ventilation of the asthmatic patient in respiratory failure. *Proc Am Thorac Soc.* 2009;6(4):371–379.
A review of mechanical ventilation in asthma.

British Guideline on the Management of Asthma. British Thoracic Society & Scottish Intercollegiate Guidelines Network. 2016. www.brit-thoracic.org.uk
A broad overview of asthma and the evidence behind management techniques.

Camargo CA, Jr, Spooner CH, Rowe BH. Continuous versus intermittent beta-agonists in the treatment of acute asthma. *Cochrane Database Syst Rev.* 2003;(4):CD001115.
A meta-analysis comparing continuous versus intermittent albuterol in acute asthma.

Cates CJ, Welsh EJ, Rowe BH. Holding chambers (spacers) versus nebulisers for beta-agonist treatment of acute asthma. In: Cates CJ, editor. *Cochrane Database Syst Rev.* Chichester, UK: John Wiley & Sons, Ltd; 2013. http://doi.wiley.com/10.1002/14651858.CD000052. pub3. Accessed July 25, 2017.
Meta-analysis comparing spacers versus nebulizers for delivery of albuterol in acute asthma.

Centers for Disease Control and prevention (CDC). *Asthma–Most Recent Asthma Data.* https:// www.cdc.gov/asthma/most_recent_data.htm. Accessed July 25, 2017.
Updated CDC asthma statistics.

Chung KF, Wenzel SE, Brozek JL, et al. International ERS/ATS guidelines on definition, evaluation and treatment of severe asthma. *Eur Respir J.* 2014;43(2):343–373.
A nice resource specifically focused on evaluation and management of the severe asthma patient.

Global Strategy for Asthma Management and Prevention. Global Initiative for Asthma (GINA). 2016. www.ginasthma.com. Accessed July 25, 2017.
Review of scientific literature by an international panel of experts on the GINA Science Committee.

Guidelines for the Diagnosis and Management of Asthma—expert panel report 3. National Asthma Education and Prevention Program, National Institutes of Health, National Heart, Lung and Blood Institute. www.nhlbi.nih.gov/guidelines/asthma/index.htm. Accessed July 25, 2017.
EPR-3 guidelines for the diagnosis and management of asthma.

Gupta D, Keogh B, Chung KF, et al. Characteristics and outcome for admissions to adult, general critical care units with acute severe asthma: a secondary analysis of the ICNARC case mix program database. *Crit Care.* 2004;8(2):R112–R121.
A secondary analysis of asthma admissions to the ICU from a high-quality clinical database across England, Wales, and Northern Ireland.

Kao CC, Jain S, Guntupalli KK, et al. Mechanical ventilation for asthma: a 10-year experience. *J Asthma.* 2008;45(7):552–556.

Kenyon N, Zeki AA, Albertson TE, et al. Definition of critical asthma syndromes. *Clin Rev Allergy Immunol.* 2015;48(1):1–6.
A review of outcomes for patients requiring intubation for severe asthma over a 10-year period.

Krishnan V, Diette GB, Rand CS, et al. Mortality in patients hospitalized for asthma exacerbations in the United States. *Am J Respir Crit Care Med.* 2006;174(6):633–638.
A review of mortality in patients hospitalized for asthma exacerbations in the United States.

Leatherman JW. Mechanical ventilation for severe asthma. *Chest.* 2015;147(6):1671–1680.
An excellent resource on ventilator management for intubated asthma patients.

Lim W, Mohammad AR, Carson K, et al. Non-invasive positive pressure ventilation for treatment of respiratory failure due to severe acute exacerbations of asthma. *Cochrane database Syst Rev.* 2012;12:CD004360.
Cochrane review of NIPPV in asthma.

Louie S, Morrissey BM, Kenyon NJ, et al. The critically ill asthmatic–from ICU to discharge. *Clin Rev Allergy Immunol.* 2012;43(1–2):30–44.
An excellent article that reviews the hospital management of acutely ill asthmatic patients.

Marini JJ. Dynamic hyperinflation and auto-positive end-expiratory pressure: lessons learned over 30 years. *Am J Respir Crit Care Med.* 2011;184(7):756–762.
A review of DHI and auto-PEEP.

McFadden ER. Acute severe asthma. *Am J Respir Crit Care Med.* 2003;168(7):740–759.
A review of acute severe asthma that spans epidemiology to management.

Rodrigo GJ, Castro-Rodriguez JA. Anticholinergics in the treatment of children and adults with acute asthma: a systematic review with meta-analysis. *Thorax.* 2005;60(9):740–746.
A meta-analysis on the use of anticholinergics in acute asthma.

Rodrigo GJ, Castro-Rodriguez JA. Heliox-driven β2-agonists nebulization for children and adults with acute asthma: a systematic review with meta-analysis. *Ann Allergy, Asthma Immunol.* 2014;112(1):29–34.
Meta-analysis of Heliox-driven nebulization of β2-agonists in acute asthma.

Rodrigo GJ, Rodrigo C, Pollack CV, et al. Use of helium-oxygen mixtures in the treatment of acute asthma: a systematic review. *Chest.* 2003;123(3):891–896.
A review of Heliox in the management of acute asthma.

Turner MO, Noertjojo K, Vedal S, et al. Risk factors for near-fatal asthma. A case-control study in hospitalized patients with asthma. *Am J Respir Crit Care Med.* 1998;157:1804–1809.
A review of risk factors for near-fatal asthma.

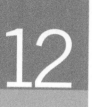

12

Acute Exacerbations of Chronic Obstructive Pulmonary Disease

Shweta Sood and Chad A. Witt

Chronic obstructive pulmonary disease (COPD) is projected to be the fifth leading cause of morbidity and third leading cause of mortality worldwide by 2020. COPD accounted for more than 8 million office visits, 1.5 million ER visits, 700,000 hospitalizations, and over 130,000 deaths in 2009. Approximately $50 billion was spent on COPD management in 2010. The vast majority of costs and mortality were related to acute exacerbations of COPD (AECOPD). An estimated 12.7 million adults in the United States were diagnosed with COPD in 2011. The number of patients with COPD is expected to rise with the aging of the population.

COPD is defined by chronic inflammation of small airways (bronchitis) and alveolar destruction (emphysema) that both contribute to airflow obstruction associated with obstructive lung disease. Symptoms include dyspnea and chronic cough with or without sputum production in patients with known risk factors for developing COPD (such as smoking or environmental exposures). Spirometry is mandatory for initial diagnosis with a forced expiratory volume in 1 second/forced vital capacity (FEV_1/FVC) value of less than 70% and an FEV_1 value less than 70%. The severity of COPD is based on spirometry, symptoms as assessed by Modified Medical Research Council (MMRC) or COPD Assessment Test (CAT) questionnaires, and the frequency of exacerbations. These are best summarized by COPD classification model illustrated in Figure 12.1.

AECOPD is a purely clinical diagnosis. It is defined by worsening respiratory symptoms including (1) increased shortness of breath at rest or with activity from baseline, (2) increased cough from baseline, and/or (3) increased sputum production from baseline. Triggers for acute COPD exacerbation include infections (viral and bacterial) and environmental exposures. However, nearly one-third of COPD exacerbations do not have identifiable cause. The diagnosis can be challenging as underlying comorbidities such as heart failure, arrhythmias, and extrapulmonary infections can mimic or exacerbate COPD symptoms. Physical exam findings, laboratory data, and imaging can help diagnose AECOPD but do not define an exacerbation. Signs such as tachypnea, tachycardia, wheezing, and accessory muscle use support diagnosis of AECOPD. Patients may have leukocytosis with positive sputum cultures, respiratory viral panels, or blood cultures. Arterial blood gases (ABG) can be useful in detecting worsening hypercarbia ($PaCO_2$ >50 mm Hg) or hypoxemia (PaO_2 <60 mm Hg). Chest radiographs can be useful in detecting an infiltrate or other etiologies for dyspnea such as volume overload (Algorithm 12.1).

The medical management of AECOPD has been evaluated in numerous clinical trials. Management involves bronchodilator therapy, systemic corticosteroids, antibiotics, and oxygen through noninvasive ventilation and mechanical ventilation.

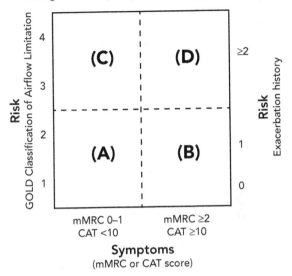

Figure 12.1. COPD severity assessment. The severity of COPD can be assessed using GOLD staging (based on FEV$_1$), symptoms (using validated screening questionnaires such as mMRC and CAT), and exacerbation history (0, 1, or greater than or equal to 2 per year).
Group A: Low risk, less symptoms. GOLD 1-2, 0-1 exacerbation/year AND mMRC 0–1 or CAT <10
Group B: Low risk, more symptoms. GOLD 1-2, 0-1 exacerbation/year AND mMRC >0–1 or CAT >10
Group C: High risk, less symptoms. GOLD 3-4 >2, exacerbation/year AND mMRC <0–1 or CAT <10
Group D: High risk, more symptoms. GOLD 3-4, >2, exacerbation/year AND mMRC >0–1 or CAT >10

Short-acting bronchodilators are important in the initial management of AECOPD, reducing symptom intensity by dilating constricted bronchioles. Short-acting anticholinergic agents (ipratropium) can be used in combination with short-acting β$_2$-adrenergic receptor agonists (albuterol, levalbuterol). Both metered-dose inhalers and nebulizer treatments are equally efficacious. However, if patients are unable to inspire deeply in the midst of AECOPD, then nebulizer treatments may be preferred. Inhaled bronchodilators are superior to systemic bronchodilators. The side effect profile of inhaled bronchodilators is generally well tolerated. Inhaled short-acting β$_2$-adrenergic receptor agonists can cause lactic acidosis in high concentrations. Overall, the side effect profile of anticholinergic agents is favorable compared with β$_2$-adrenergic receptor agonists, making anticholinergic agents a reasonable first option. If the patient is not improving with maximum doses of anticholinergic treatment, the addition of a short-acting β$_2$-agonist has been shown to be beneficial.

Systemic corticosteroid treatment for AECOPD has been demonstrated to be beneficial. Corticosteroids decrease recovery time and reduce relapses within the first 30 days after an exacerbation. Furthermore, corticosteroids have been associated with shorter hospital length of stay in nonmechanically ventilated patients. Oral corticosteroids are recommended; parenteral corticosteroids have no demonstrated additional benefit but should be considered in patients with poor oral intake or limited gut absorption. Prednisone 30 to 60 mg daily, or equivalent formulations can be used. The optimal duration of corticosteroid course is unclear, however, recent studies suggest 5 days of treatment are noninferior to 14 days.

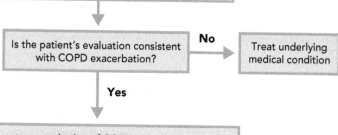

ALGORITHM 12.1 Initial Evaluation and Medical Management of Acute Exacerbations of Chronic Obstructive Pulmonary Disease (COPD)

Initial Evaluation:
- Initial clinical evaluation, including history and physical exam
  - Triggers for COPD exacerbation
  - Increased cough, sputum production, or dyspnea
  - Prior hospitalizations or ICU admissions
  - Tachypnea, tachycardia, accessory muscle use, and wheezing
- Basic laboratory studies, including complete blood cell count and basic metabolic panel
- Chest radiography
- Arterial blood gas analysis

Is the patient's evaluation consistent with COPD exacerbation? — **No** → Treat underlying medical condition

Yes

Treat acute exacerbation of COPD:
- Oxygen therapy by nasal cannula or face mask
  - Titrate PaO_2 to >60 mm Hg or SaO_2 >90%, with care not to over correct hypoxemia and precipitate hypercapnia
- Bronchodilator therapy (Table 12.1)
- Corticosteroid therapy (Table 12.1)
- Antibiotic therapy (Table 12.1 and as per local antibiotiogram)
- Proceed with mechanical ventilatory support if needed (Algorithm 12.2)

Antibiotics are beneficial in AECOPD. Antibiotics reduce sputum production, reduce treatment failure, and improve mortality. Common organisms associated with COPD exacerbations include *Streptococcus pneumoniae, Moraxella catarrhalis,* and *Haemophilus influenzae*. Additionally, *Pseudomonas aeruginosa* is increasingly seen in patients with advanced COPD (GOLD stage 3 or 4). Community-acquired respiratory viruses including influenza virus, parainfluenza virus, rhinovirus, respiratory syncytial virus, and human metapneumovirus can trigger infections as well. Sputum cultures, nasopharyngeal respiratory viral panel assessment (most commonly by polymerase chain reaction (PCR) or direct antigen testing), and blood cultures are helpful in narrowing antibiotic selection. Many antibiotics have been studied, including, but not limited to amoxicillin, trimethoprim-sulfamethoxazole, tetracycline, clarithromycin, azithromycin, ciprofloxacin, levofloxacin, and moxifloxacin. There have been limited studies evaluating the use of newer, broader-spectrum antibiotics compared to the older, narrower-spectrum antibiotics, and to date there is no evidence that broader-spectrum antibiotics decrease mortality. However, because of concern of antibiotic resistance, broader-spectrum agents are frequently used now. Initial broad-spectrum antibiotic coverage based on local antimicrobial resistance patterns is appropriate for most ICU patients with AECOPD. Cultures, including sputum, respiratory viral panel, and blood cultures, can often help narrow coverage after 48 hours. The duration of antibiotic therapy is not well established but suggested to be between 5 and 10 days.

There are other medical therapies that have been used to treat AECOPD, including mucolytic agents, chest physiotherapy (CPT), and methylxanthine bronchodilators. There is no evidence to support the use of these therapies, in fact the latter two may be detrimental. No study has ever shown benefit of CPT for AECOPD, and some studies have shown a transient decrease in FEV_1 after treatment, thus raising the possibility that CPT may be harmful. Given the frequent and significant side effect profile of methylxanthines, and the lack of evidence demonstrating improved outcomes with these agents, the routine use of methylxanthines for AECOPD is not recommended (Table 12.1).

Oxygen therapy has not been as rigorously studied because the benefit has been inferred. Oxygen should be administered by nasal cannula or face mask to improve PaO_2 >60 mm Hg or SaO_2 to 88% to 92%. Improving oxygenation above 92% is not helpful and in patients with chronic hypercarbic respiratory failure hypoxemia can worsen V/Q matching and precipitate worsening hypercarbia.

Often despite early diagnosis or treatment with bronchodilators, systemic corticosteroids, antibiotics, and oxygen, patients with AECOPD can continue to decompensate. This decompensation manifests clinically as increased work of breathing, worsening hypercarbia and respiratory acidosis, and worsening hypoxemia. Frequent clinical assessment of patients with AECOPD is necessary to identify patients that are failing therapy and who require higher levels of support as early as possible.

Noninvasive positive pressure ventilation (NIPPV) has been shown to improve dyspnea, hypercarbia, and acidosis in AECOPD. Furthermore, studies show NIPPV decreases intubation rates, improves mortality, and shortens length of hospital stay. Serial ABG should be measured after initiation of NIPPV. A lack of improvement in symptoms or ABG showing worsening hypercarbia, respiratory acidosis, or hypoxemia despite NIPPV suggests the need for intubation and invasive mechanical ventilation (Algorithm 12.2).

Mechanical ventilation should be considered in any patient with cardiopulmonary arrest, hemodynamic instability despite adequate resuscitation, altered mental status, aspiration or emesis, copious secretions, inability to tolerate NIPPV, or patients who have failed a trial of NIPPV. Initial ventilator setting in patients with AECOPD should focus on a sufficient expiratory time with an ideal inspiratory to expiratory ratio of 1:4. Maneuvers that prolong expiratory time include low respiratory rate, adequate but not excessive tidal volumes, minimal positive end-expiratory pressure (PEEP), and high flow rates. Volume assist control ventilation is commonly used with rate 10 to 12 breaths/min; tidal volume, 6 to 8 mL/kg; PEEP of 0 to 5 cm H_2O; and an adequate FiO_2 to keep the hemoglobin saturation near 92%.

TABLE 12.1	Medications Commonly Used for Acute Exacerbations of Chronic Obstructive Pulmonary Disease	
Medication	**Dose and Route**	**Frequency**
Bronchodilators		
Anticholinergic agent		
Ipratropium bromide	0.5 mg nebulized or 18–36 mcg metered-dose inhaler	Every 4–6 hrs
β_2-Adrenergic receptor agonist		
Albuterol	2.5–5 mg nebulized 180 mcg metered-dose inhaler	Every 4–6 hrs
Corticosteroids		
Methylprednisolone	125 mg intravenously	Every 6 hrs for 3 days then
	60 mg by mouth	Every day for 4 days then
	40 mg by mouth	Every day for 4 days then
	20 mg by mouth	Every day for 4 days
Prednisone	30–60 mg by mouth	Every day for 5–7 days or longer course with taper
Oral antibiotics		
Trimethoprim-sulfamethoxazole	160/800 mg by mouth	Every 12 hrs for 5–10 days
Amoxicillin	250 mg by mouth	Every 6 hrs for 5–10 days
Doxycycline	200 mg by mouth	First day followed by
	100 mg by mouth	Every 12 hrs for 5–10 days
Azithromycin	500 mg by mouth	First day followed by
	250 mg by mouth	Every day for 4 days OR
	500 mg by mouth	Every day for 3 days

These patients require high flows (peak flow 75 to 90 L/min) to allow for an inspiratory to expiratory ratio of 1:4. The initial settings should be adjusted by assessing the patient's comfort level and synchrony with the ventilator and serial ABG. Sedation is often needed to ensure synchrony. The patient should not be ventilated to a normal $PaCO_2$, but instead to a normal pH at the patient's baseline $PaCO_2$.

It is also important to monitor the patient for the development of auto-PEEP, also called intrinsic PEEP, while undergoing mechanical ventilation. This can be detected by monitoring capnograph tracing, ventilator waveforms, or measuring intrinsic PEEP. Capnography, or end-tidal carbon dioxide ($EtCO_2$), will often show prolongation of phase 2 of the $EtCO_2$ waveform. This is often called "shark finning" of the $EtCO_2$ waveform and indicates obstruction with expiration. Ventilator waveforms will indicate failure of flow to return baseline before initiation of subsequent inspiration. Intrinsic PEEP can also be measured by initiating an expiratory pause maneuver on the ventilator. Auto-PEEP can occur with inadequate flows, excessive tidal volume, and high respiratory rates. Auto-PEEP results in increased intrathoracic pressure, decreased venous return, and systemic hypotension. Furthermore, auto-PEEP

ALGORITHM 12.2 Mechanical Ventilation in Acute Exacerbations of Chronic Obstructive Pulmonary Disease

Are there reasons why patient cannot tolerate noninvasive ventilation?

- Acute respiratory failure
- Agitation or decreased mental status
- Hemodynamic instability
- Excessive secretions
- Structural abnormality precluding mask fitting
- Extreme obesity
- Aspiration or emesis

ABBREVIATION

BiPAP: bilevel positive airway pressure

No　　**Yes**

- Initiate BiPAP therapy in a setting prepared to perform endotracheal intubation if necessary

- Titrate PaO$_2$ to >60 mm Hg or SaO$_2$ >90% with care not to hyperventilate and reduce pCO$_2$ significantly below patient's baseline.

Proceed with endotracheal intubation

Is patient improving?

No

Yes

Continue periodic BiPAP treatments until patient's respiratory status has stabilized.

increases the work of breathing by causing dynamic hyperinflation, thus making it more difficult for the patient to trigger the ventilator. Extrinsic PEEP can be added to offset this effect. While on mechanical ventilation, patients with AECOPD should also receive adequate deep venous thrombosis and stress ulcer prophylaxis. Nutritional support is vitally important in these patients, but should not contain excessive carbohydrates as this can increase CO_2 production.

Survival from AECOPD is variable and dependent on numerous factors. In one study, older age, low Glasgow Coma score, and lower pH were associated with increased risk of mortality in ICU patients with AECOPD. Mortality can be reduced with early diagnosis of AECOPD based on symptoms and supported with physical exam, laboratory data, and/or imaging studies. Early treatment with bronchodilators, systemic corticosteroids, antibiotics, and oxygen can yield better outcomes. NIPPV is beneficial but should not delay intubation and mechanical ventilation in patients with worsening respiratory failure.

One of the biggest predictors of future AECOPD admissions is prior AECOPD admissions. For this reason, prior to discharge from the hospital, all patients with AECOPD should be medically optimized with appropriate inhaler therapy. This includes long-acting anticholinergic agents (tiotropium) and short-acting β_2-agonists (albuterol). In certain COPD patients, combinations of inhaled long-acting β-agonist, long-acting anticholinergic agents, and inhaled corticosteroids are beneficial. After discharge, a short course of antibiotics and corticosteroids may be helpful for most patients as described above. Patients with severe COPD and recurrent hospitalizations despite medical optimizations and compliance can be considered for roflumilast. Influenza and pneumococcal vaccinations should be up to date prior to discharge. Resting and walking oxygen evaluation should be done prior to discharge to evaluate home oxygen needs. Smoking cessation counseling should be provided to all patients who continue to smoke. Pulmonary rehabilitation should be considered for patients with moderate or severe COPD who have had an AECOPD within the past 4 weeks. Nutrition counseling should be done for patients with extremes in BMI. Patient education on inhaler technique, medication compliance, and monitoring for worsening symptoms can help ensure better outcomes as well.

SUGGESTED READINGS

Bach PB, Brown C, Gelfand SE, et al. Management of acute exacerbations of chronic obstructive pulmonary disease: a summary and appraisal of published evidence. *Ann Intern Med.* 2001;134(7):600–620.

Review of studies guiding management of acute exacerbations of COPD including evidence for or against oxygen therapy, bronchodilators, corticosteroids, antibiotics, and noninvasive ventilation.

Brochard L, Mancebo J, Wysocki M, et al. Noninvasive ventilation for acute exacerbations of chronic obstructive pulmonary disease. *N Eng J Med.* 1995;333(13):817–822.

Randomized study showing that noninvasive ventilation for acute exacerbations of COPD reduced the need for endotracheal intubation, reduced hospital stay, and reduced in-hospital mortality.

Chandra D, Stamm JA, Taylor B, et al. Outcomes of noninvasive ventilation for acute exacerbations of chronic obstructive pulmonary disease in the United States, 1998–2008. *Am J Respir Crit Care Med.* 2012;185(2):152–159.

A retrospective analysis to determine the prevalence and trends of noninvasive ventilation for AECOPD.

Criner GJ, Bourbeau J, Diekemper RL, et al. Executive summary: prevention of acute exacerbation of COPD: American College of Chest Physicians and Canadian Thoracic Society guideline. *Chest.* 2015;147(4):883–893.

Executive summary outlining current state of knowledge regarding the prevention of AECOPD from chest.

Leuppi JD, Schuetz P, Bingisser R, et al. Short-term vs. conventional glucocorticoid therapy in acute exacerbations of chronic obstructive pulmonary disease: the REDUCE randomized clinical trial. *JAMA.* 2013;309(21):2223–2231.

Randomized trial showing 5-day treatment with systemic glucocorticoids was noninferior to 14-day treatment with regard to reexacerbation within 6 months of follow-up.

Lightowler JV, Wedzicha JA, Elliot MW, et al. Non-invasive positive pressure ventilation to treat respiratory failure resulting from exacerbations of chronic obstructive pulmonary disease: Cochrane systematic review and meta-analysis. *BMJ.* 2003;326:185–189.

Systematic review of randomized controlled trials showing that the use of noninvasive positive pressure ventilation should be first-line therapy to decrease the need for endotracheal intubation and decrease mortality in patients with acute exacerbations of COPD.

Llor C, Moragas A, Hernández S, et al. Efficacy of antibiotic therapy for acute exacerbations of mild to moderate chronic obstructive pulmonary disease. *Am J Respir Crit Care Med.* 2012;186(8):716–723.

Randomized trial showing treatment of ambulatory exacerbation of mild to moderate COPD with antibiotics prolongs time to next exacerbation.

McCrory DC, Brown C, Gelfand SE, et al. Management of acute exacerbations of COPD: a summary and appraisal of published evidence. *Chest.* 2001;119(4):1190–1209.

Review of available data on the evaluation, risk stratification, and management of patients with acute exacerbation of COPD.

Niewoehner D, Erbland M, Deupree RH, et al. Effect of systemic glucocorticoids on exacerbations of chronic obstructive pulmonary disease. *N Eng J Med.* 1999;340:1941–1947.

Randomized controlled trial showing clinical benefit of systemic glucocorticoids for acute exacerbations of COPD, as well as showing that there was no benefit to an 8-week course of corticosteroids over a 2-week course.

Nouira S, Marghli S, Boukef R, et al. Standard versus newer antibacterial agents in the treatment of severe acute exacerbation of chronic obstructive pulmonary disease: a randomized trial of trimethoprim-sulfamethoxazole versus ciprofloxacin. *Clin Infect Dis.* 2010;51(2):143–149.

Randomized controlled trial demonstrating that trimethoprim-sulfamethoxazole was not inferior to ciprofloxacin in the treatment of acute exacerbations of COPD.

Saginer A, Aytemur ZA, Cirit M, et al. Systemic glucocorticoids in severe exacerbations of COPD. *Chest.* 2001;119(3):726–730.

Randomized trial showing that patients receiving 10 days of glucocorticoid treatment instead of 3 days had significant improvements in arterial oxygen tension, FEV_1, and dyspnea on exertion.

Singanayagam A, Schembri S, Chalmers JD. Predictors of mortality in hospitalized adults with acute exacerbation of chronic obstructive pulmonary disease. A systematic review and meta-analysis. *Ann Am Thorac Soc.* 2013;10(2):81–89.

A literature review to identify clinically important factors that predict mortality after hospitalization for AECOPD.

Snow V, Lascher S, Mottur-Pilson C, et al. Evidence base for management of acute exacerbations of chronic obstructive pulmonary disease. *Ann Intern Med.* 2001;134(7):595–599.

Review of evidence concerning risk stratification, diagnostic testing, and therapeutic interventions for management of acute exacerbation of COPD.

Stefan MS, Rothberg MB, Shieh M, et al. Association between antibiotic treatment and outcomes in patients hospitalized with acute exacerbation of COPD treated with systemic steroids. *Chest.* 2013;143(1):82–90.

A retrospective cohort study showing that the addition of antibiotics to a regimen that includes steroids may have a beneficial effect on short-term outcomes for patients hospitalized with AECOPD.

Stoller JK. Clinical practice. Acute exacerbations of chronic obstructive pulmonary disease. *N Engl J Med.* 2002;346:988–994.

> *Review of treatment of acute exacerbations of COPD, including medical management and ventilatory support.*

Vestbo J, Hurd SS, Agustí AG, et al. Global strategy for the diagnosis, management, and prevention of chronic obstructive pulmonary disease. *Am J Respirat Crit Care Med.* 2013;187(4): 347–365.

> *Executive summary summarizing strategies to manage diagnosis and manage COPD, including AECOPD, from ATS.*

Walters JA, Tan DJ, White CJ, et al. Systemic corticosteroids for acute exacerbations of chronic obstructive pulmonary disease. *Cochrane Database of Syst Rev.* 2014;(9):CD001288.

> *A literature review of randomized control trials showing oral and parenteral corticosteroids both equally reduced treatment failure, relapse, and hospital length of stay in nonventilated patients.*

13 Sleep-Disordered Breathing in the Intensive Care Unit

Tracy L. Ivy and Tonya D. Russell

Sleep has a range of effects on respiratory physiology in healthy patients, as outlined in Table 13.1. In patients with underlying comorbidities such as severe chronic obstructive pulmonary disease or neuromuscular disease, these changes in respiratory physiology can lead to compromise of the patient's cardiopulmonary status. In addition, there are sleep-related breathing disorders that can lead to respiratory failure, in which the main pathophysiology occurs during sleep, such as obstructive sleep apnea (OSA), central sleep apnea (CSA), and sleep-related obesity hypoventilation.

Apneic events during sleep can either be obstructive or central in nature. Obstructive events are associated with ongoing respiratory effort, while there is minimal to no respiratory effort present with central apneas. OSA occurs when there is narrowing of the upper airway during sleep due to excessive soft tissue or structural abnormalities, resulting in limitation or cessation of airflow, which can be associated with arousals or oxygen desaturations. OSA has been associated with increased risk of excessive daytime somnolence, hypertension, stroke, and heart failure. The severity of OSA can be quantified by the number of events per hour (apnea–hypopnea index) or by the severity of sleepiness, as shown in Table 13.2.

The prevalence of obstructive sleep apnea–hypopnea syndrome (OSAHS), in which OSA is associated with daytime sleepiness, has been estimated to be 4% of men and 2% of women. However, recent studies suggest that this may underestimate the prevalence given the increasing age and BMI of the population, as well as the fact that approximately 70% to 80% of patients remain undiagnosed. Although it has not been extensively studied, the prevalence of sleep apnea in the intensive care unit (ICU) is likely even higher, given that patients with sleep apnea frequently have comorbid conditions that are common in patients admitted to the ICU such as obesity, diabetes mellitus, hypertension, ischemic heart disease, heart failure, and cerebrovascular disease. Recognizing and treating OSA is important because in certain hospitalized patients, such as those in the postoperative period, it has been associated with a significant increase in risk of respiratory failure, cardiac events, and transfer to the ICU.

CSA can occur in the setting of severe heart failure (Cheyne–Stokes respirations [CSRs]), stroke, or narcotic use. CSRs are characterized by central apneas followed by crescendo–decrescendo periods of hyperventilation. It occurs in approximately 40% of patients with congestive heart failure (CHF) and is even more prevalent in decompensated CHF inpatients. The cause of this breathing pattern in CHF is increased chemosensitivity to carbon dioxide, as well as circulatory delay to the chemoreceptors. Treatment of the underlying heart failure is important, but positive airway pressure, whether applied through a ventilator or noninvasively, has the potential to improve CSR.

TABLE 13.1	Effects of Sleep on Respiratory Physiology

Decreased hypoxic ventilatory response
Decreased hypercapnic ventilatory response
Increased muscle hypotonia
Increased airway resistance
Increased arousal threshold from events related to increased airway resistance
(NREM > REM)

NREM, nonrapid eye movement; REM, rapid eye movement.

Obesity hypoventilation syndrome (OHS) is frequently used to describe hypoventilation during sleep occurring in obese patients, which results in daytime hypercapnia. The prevalence of OHS is not clear, and the definition of OHS in the literature is variable. However, the American Academy of Sleep Medicine (AASM) Task Force has made recommendations for diagnostic criteria for sleep hypoventilation syndrome, of which OHS is a part, as shown in Table 13.3. It is apparent that hypercapnia can occur in the setting of severe OSA alone, sleep-related hypoventilation without apneic or hypopneic events (OHS), or in combination.

OSA and OHS should be considered in patients with hypercapnic respiratory failure who have any of the signs and symptoms listed in Table 13.4. CSA should also be considered if there is a history of CHF, stroke, or narcotic use. In patients with hypercapnia related to OSA alone, continuous positive airway pressure (CPAP), at a pressure that resolves the obstructive events, should correct the hypercapnia. However, in patients in whom there is a component of sleep-related hypoventilation, bilevel positive airway pressure (BiPAP) is usually required. The expiratory positive airway pressure (EPAP) setting is used to maintain the airway patency, while the inspiratory positive airway pressure (IPAP) setting is used to ventilate the patient. The larger the difference between the IPAP and EPAP, the larger the tidal volume the patient should receive.

Treatment of CSA typically requires BiPAP with a set backup respiratory rate. Although CPAP or BiPAP may be effective to treat some patients with combined obstructive and central sleep apnea, there is an additional ventilator mode (adaptive servo ventilation or ASV) that is effective at treating patients with both types of

TABLE 13.2	Severity of Obstructive Sleep Apnea	
Severity	AHI[a]	Level of Impairment[b]
Mild	5–15	Sedentary activities requiring minimal attention (i.e., watching television, reading, passenger in a car)
Moderate	15–30	Activities requiring some attention (i.e., meetings, concerts)
Severe	>30	Activities requiring active attention (i.e., conversation, eating, driving)

[a]AHI (apnea–hypopnea index), number of apneas and hypopneas per hour; apnea is defined as cessation of airflow; hypopnea is defined as ≥30% reduction in airflow associated with a 3% oxygen desaturation; all events must be at least 10 seconds.
[b]Extent of daytime somnolence.

TABLE 13.3	Diagnostic Criteria for Sleep Hypoventilation Syndrome[a]
Signs and Symptoms	**Monitoring**
Cor pulmonale Pulmonary hypertension Unexplained excessive daytime somnolence Erythrocytosis Waking hypercapnia ($PaCO_2$ >45 mm Hg)	Increase in $PaCO_2$ during sleep >10 mm Hg from awake supine values Oxygen desaturations during sleep not associated with apneas or hypopneas

[a]Must meet at least one criterion from each column.

apnea. ASV provides an adjustable EPAP, adjustable inspiratory pressure support, and an auto backup rate. However, a recent study demonstrated increased cardiovascular mortality in heart failure patients with a reduced ejection fraction who were treated with ASV compared to controls. The AASM therefore recommends that ASV not be prescribed to these patients if their ejection fraction ≤45%.

Unfortunately, there is not much guidance in the literature for empirically picking pressures for CPAP or BiPAP in the setting of sleep-disordered breathing and sleep-related hypoventilation. In the outpatient setting, a split sleep study is performed, in which the first part of the study allows for the diagnosis of the sleep-disordered breathing and the second part of the study allows for the titration of CPAP or BiPAP. In patients with only OSA and no serious comorbid conditions, auto-titrating positive airway pressure (APAP), in which the machine automatically adjusts the pressure to overcome obstructive events, may be appropriate. If an inpatient sleep study is available, this would be the best way to establish a diagnosis of OSA, CSA, or OHS and the best way to determine the necessary pressures required to treat the disorder. However, if a patient requires initiation of therapy without the benefit of a sleep study, it should be initiated in a closely monitored setting such as an ICU or step-down unit.

TABLE 13.4	Signs and Symptoms of Obstructive Sleep Apnea–Hypopnea Syndrome and Obesity Hypoventilation Syndrome
Obesity Snoring Awakening snorting or gasping Witnessed apneas Excessive daytime somnolence Morning headaches Large neck circumference Unrefreshing sleep Poorly controlled hypertension Craniofacial abnormalities (micrognathia, retrognathia, macroglossia) Nocturnal oxygen desaturations Hypercapnia not explained by other etiology Hypothyroidism	

ALGORITHM 13.1 Proposed Evaluation and Treatment Guideline for Intensive Care Unit Patients Suspected of Having Severe Obstructive Sleep Apnea–Hypopnea Syndrome (OSAHS), Central Sleep Apnea (CSA), or Obesity Hypoventilation Syndrome (OHS)

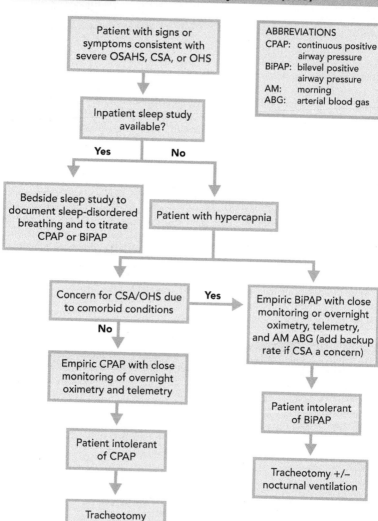

TABLE 13.5	Common Complications and Side Effects of Continuous Positive Airway Pressure or Bilevel Positive Airway Pressure
Nasal/oral dryness	
Eye dryness	
Mask leak	
Aerophagia/gastric distension	
Skin irritation	
Rhinitis/rhinorrhea	

Patients who are morbidly obese or have very severe OSA will frequently require high pressures to resolve the sleep-disordered breathing. If the empiric pressure is too low, then the apnea events or hypoventilation may not be fully resolved, leading to prolonged hypoxemia. Severe hypoxemia has been reported to occur during the empiric use of CPAP. If the empiric pressure is too high, then the patient may experience other complications related to positive pressure, as outlined in Table 13.5, which may decrease the patient's ability to comply with CPAP or BiPAP.

In patients who cannot tolerate CPAP or BiPAP, tracheotomy is the gold standard for treatment of OSA because it allows for the area of upper airway obstruction to be bypassed. However, some morbidly obese patients may require custom tracheotomy tubes in order to fully resolve the obstruction. In addition, if there is a component of CSA or sleep-related hypoventilation not solely due to OSA, then nocturnal ventilation through the tracheotomy tube is required. Algorithm 13.1 demonstrates a proposed algorithm for the evaluation and treatment of patients in the ICU who are suspected of having severe OSA or sleep-related hypoventilation.

SUGGESTED READINGS

American Academy of Sleep Medicine Task Force. Sleep related breathing disorders in adults: recommendations for syndrome definitions and measurement techniques in clinical research. *Sleep.* 1999;22:667–689.
  Reviews recommended definitions for sleep-disordered breathing.
Aurora RN, Bista SR, Casey KR, et al. Updated adaptive servo-ventilation recommendations for the 2012 AASM guideline: "The treatment of central sleep apnea syndromes in adults: practice parameters with an evidence-based literature review and meta-analyses." *J Clin Sleep Med.* 2016;12:757–761.
  Practice recommendations for the use of ASV in patients with central sleep apnea.
Berger KI, Ayappa I, Chatr-Amontri B, et al. Obesity hypoventilation syndrome as a spectrum of respiratory disturbances during sleep. *Chest.* 2001;120:1231–1238.
  Retrospective review of 23 patients with daytime hypercapnia and excessive daytime somnolence.
Bolona E, Hahn PY, Afessa B. Intensive care unit and hospital mortality in patients with obstructive sleep apnea. *J Crit Care.* 2015;30:178–180.
  Evaluates the prevalence of OSA in the ICU and its association with mortality.
Douglas NJ. Respiratory physiology: control of ventilation. In: Kryger MH, Roth T, Dement WC, eds. *Principles and Practices of Sleep Medicine.* Philadelphia, PA: WB Saunders; 2000:221–228.
  Review of respiratory physiology in sleep.

Hai F, Porhomayon J, Vermont L, et al. Postoperative complications in patients with obstructive sleep apnea: a meta-analysis. *J Clin Anesth.* 2014;26:591–600.

Reviews complications of OSA in the postoperative period.

Krieger J. Respiratory physiology: breathing in normal subjects. In: Kryger MH, Roth T, Dement WC, eds. *Principles and Practices of Sleep Medicine.* Philadelphia, PA: WB Saunders; 2000:229–241.

Review of respiratory physiology in sleep.

Kreiger J, Weitzenblum E, Monassier JP, et al. Dangerous hypoxaemia during continuous positive airway pressure treatment of obstructive sleep apnoea. *Lancet.* 1983;322:1429–1430.

Report of a patient with severe hypoxemia occurring with empiric CPAP use for obstructive sleep apnea.

Meoli AL, Casey KR, Clark RW, et al. Hypopnea in sleep-disordered breathing in adults. *Sleep.* 2001;24:469–470.

Reviews recommended definitions of apnea and hypopnea.

Peppard PE, Young T, Barnet JH, et al. Increased prevalence of sleep-disordered breathing in adults. *Am J Epidemiol.* 2013;177:1006–1014.

Reviews increasing prevalence of sleep-disordered breathing in the population.

Sands SA, Owens RL. Congestive heart failure and central sleep apnea. *Crit Care Clin.* 2015; 31:473–495.

Reviews the relationship between congestive heart failure and central sleep apnea.

Shamsuzzaman AS, Gersh BJ, Somers VK. Obstructive sleep apnea—implications for cardiac and vascular disease. *JAMA.* 2003;290:1906–1914.

Report of MEDLINE review of 154 peer-reviewed studies assessing cardiovascular complications associated with obstructive sleep apnea.

Thorpy M, Chesson A, Sarkis D, et al. Practice parameters for the treatment of obstructive sleep apnea in adults: the efficacy of surgical modification of the upper airway. *Sleep.* 1996;19:152–155.

Reviews indications and efficacy of surgical treatment of obstructive sleep apnea.

Young T, Palta M, Dempsey J, et al. The occurrence of sleep disordered breathing among middle-aged adults. *N Engl J Med.* 1993;328:1230–1235.

A random sample of state employees of Wisconsin who underwent polysomnograms to evaluate the prevalence of sleep-disordered breathing.

14 Pulmonary Hypertension and Right Ventricular Failure in the Intensive Care Unit

Abhaya P. Trivedi and Murali M. Chakinala

Decompensated right ventricular failure (DRVF) is a less common cause of shock, which is frequently underdiagnosed, and recognizing its presence requires vigilance for a constellation of symptoms and signs. The treatment of this condition also differs somewhat from the routine shock management guidelines as elucidated elsewhere in this book. Most often, DRVF occurs in the setting of chronic pulmonary hypertension (PH) (i.e., mean pulmonary artery [PA] pressure ≥25 mm Hg) with an inciting acute illness that converts a compensated right ventricle (RV) into DRVF and a hemodynamically unstable emergency.

PATHOPHYSIOLOGY OF RV FAILURE

The RV is a thin-walled chamber that empties by sequential contraction into a low-resistance, high-capacitance pulmonary vascular circuit over the entire period of RV systole. Despite a three- to fourfold increase in cardiac output, there is no increase in pulmonary pressure and RV workload, thanks to pulmonary vasodilation and recruitment of pulmonary vasculature. But when faced with an acute rise in afterload (e.g., massive pulmonary embolism), the RV can decompensate rapidly, leading to shock (Algorithm 14.1). But in the setting of chronic PH, the RV has an innate but limited ability to undergo myocardial hypertrophy, thus reducing wall tension and maintaining contractility for a finite period of time. Even then, a hypertrophied and compensated RV can deteriorate rapidly in the setting of acute pressure and/or pressure overload (Algorithm 14.1).

CAUSES OF DRVF

Table 14.1 lists causes of acute RV failure. Table 14.2 lists the etiology of acute-on-chronic decompensation in patients with known PH.

DIAGNOSIS OF DRVF

Clinical Presentation

DRVF typically manifests as shock due to a low flow state. A history of PH raises the possibility for an acute-on-chronic decompensation due to any of the causes listed in Table 14.2. Signs and symptoms of DRVF are shown in Table 14.3.

ALGORITHM 14.1 Pathophysiology of Decompensated Right Ventricular Failure

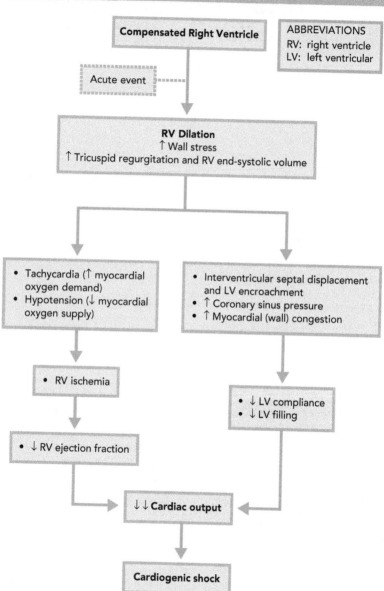

TABLE 14.1	Etiology of Right Ventricular (RV) Failure

Left ventricular dysfunction
RV infarct or perioperative injury
Cardiac tamponade (mimicker of RV failure)
Tricuspid valve disease (regurgitation, stenosis)
Acute massive pulmonary embolus (thrombus, fat, air, or amniotic fluid)
Acute lung injury/adult respiratory distress syndrome
Sickle cell chest syndrome
Congenital heart disease (e.g., atrial septal defect, anomalous pulmonary venous return, Ebstein anomaly)
Acute decompensation of chronic pulmonary arterial hypertension (Table 14.2)

TABLE 14.2	Causes of Acute Hemodynamic Instability in Chronic Pulmonary Arterial Hypertension

Acute medication failure (e.g., noncompliance, interruption of parenteral vasodilator therapy)
Dietary or fluid indiscretion
Increased metabolic demands (e.g., infection, fever, environmental heat, pregnancy)
Venous thromboembolism (submassive or massive)
Induction of general anesthesia
Surgery (left-sided valvular repair, pulmonary thromboendarterectomy, lung transplantation, lobectomy, or pneumonectomy)
Dysrhythmias
Endocrinopathies (e.g., thyroid disorders, adrenal insufficiency)

TABLE 14.3	Signs and Symptoms	
Symptoms	Signs

Symptoms	Signs
Syncope, dizziness	Decreased pulses
RUQ pain	Cool extremities
Abdominal distention	Lower extremity edema
Weight gain	Elevated jugular venous pulsation (without auscultatory crackles)
Early satiety	Right-sided S3
	Pulsatile liver
	Hepatojugular reflux
	Ascites

RUQ, right upper quadrant.

TABLE 14.4	Electrocardiographic Changes in Right Ventricular Failure

Sinus tachycardia
Atrial dysrhythmias (e.g., fibrillation, flutter, reentry tachycardia)
Right axis deviation
Right atrial enlargement
Right ventricular hypertrophy
Right bundle branch block
QR pattern in lead V1
S1 Q3 T3 pattern (RV strain)

Diagnostic Testing

Radiology

Plain radiographs may show enlarged central pulmonary arteries with peripheral pruning if chronic PH is present. Chronic RV enlargement manifests with filling of the retrosternal air space on a lateral chest x-ray. Right-sided pleural effusions rarely may be present but pleural effusions typically indicate left ventricular (LV) dysfunction. If an acute pulmonary embolism is suspected, lower extremity Doppler examinations and either VQ scan or pulmonary embolism protocol computed tomography should be obtained.

Electrocardiogram

Table 14.4 shows the RV changes that can be seen by electrocardiography.

Laboratory Data

In keeping with a low-output state, typical laboratory values of tissue/organ hypoperfusion may be encountered, including anion gap metabolic acidosis, low central venous or mixed venous oxygen saturation, elevated lactate, (prerenal) blood urea nitrogen to creatinine ratio, and low urine sodium. Hepatic congestion results in elevated liver enzymes and hyperbilirubinemia. RV strain can result in significantly elevated B-type natriuretic peptide, while an elevated troponin I level would indicate RV infarction.

Echocardiography

Cardiac echocardiography is arguably the most useful examination in this scenario by establishing RV failure and preserved left-sided cardiac function. Table 14.5 lists echocardiographic findings in DRVF. It provides rapid and important data for diagnosing RV failure, elucidating precipitating causes, and triaging patients into three groups: RV failure with elevated PA pressures, RV failure without elevated pressures, and pericardial disease (Algorithm 14.2).

Pulmonary Artery Catheter

A complementary diagnostic tool in the management of DRVF is the pulmonary artery catheter (PAC). Indications for use of a PAC include differentiating "pump failure" from other causes of shock or assisting with management of DRVF (i.e., optimizing volume status, use of inotropes, and assessing response to pulmonary vasodilators). Challenges to using PAC in DRVF include difficulty introducing the

TABLE 14.5	Echocardiographic Findings in Right Ventricular (RV) Failure

RV hypertrophy (in chronic pulmonary hypertension)
RV dilation and hypokinesis
  McConnell's sign—akinesis of mid-RV free wall with preserved apical wall
    function is a specific (~95%) sign of acute pulmonary embolism
  60/60 sign—discordancy between mean PAP (estimated by RV outflow tract
    acceleration time) and PASP (estimated by tricuspid regurgitation jet)
Paradoxic septal motion due to RV pressure overload
Right atrial enlargement
Hyperdynamic left ventricle due to underfilling (ventricular interdependence)
D-shaped left ventricle and late diastolic left ventricular filling
Pericardial effusion
Tricuspid regurgitation
Elevated pulmonary arterial systolic pressure
Pulmonary artery dilatation
Dilated inferior vena cava or lack of inspiratory collapse
Markers of RV function:
  Reduced tricuspid annular plane systolic excursion (TAPSE: normal ≥2.0 cm)
  Elevated Tei index (normal ≤0.3)

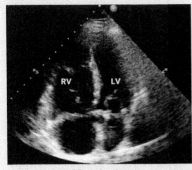

Apical four-chamber view

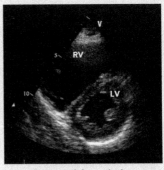

Parasternal short axis view

catheter, increased risk of PA rupture from "overwedging" the distal balloon tip, and poor tolerance of arrhythmias. The characteristic pattern of DRVF includes elevated central venous, RV, and PA pressures with reduced cardiac output, stroke volume, and mixed venous oxygen saturation. With end-stage RV failure or in the setting of RV infarction, the PA pressure may decline, as the RV is unable to generate enough force to eject blood into the pulmonary vasculature. The PA occlusion pressure is typically low but may be elevated as LV compliance worsens. Cardiac output should be measured by the Fick method as tricuspid regurgitation or intracardiac shunts make the thermodilution method unreliable. One should place more emphasis on trends gleaned from PAC readings rather than one-time absolute values. Lack of skill in evaluation of waveforms can lead to poor interpretation of collected data and inappropriate management decisions. The use of the PA catheter in managing critically ill patients has not shown an improvement in mortality. Its use in patients

ALGORITHM 14.2 Diagnostic Pathway in Suspected Right Ventricular (RV) Failure

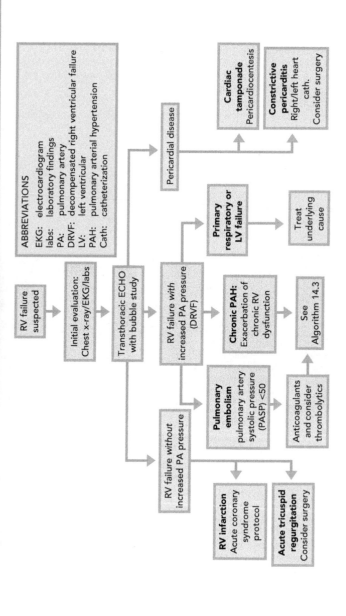

ABBREVIATIONS

EKG: electrocardiogram
labs: laboratory findings
PA: pulmonary artery
DRVF: decompensated right ventricular failure
LV: left ventricular
PAH: pulmonary arterial hypertension
Cath: catheterization

RV failure suspected

Initial evaluation: Chest x-ray/EKG/labs

Transthoracic ECHO with bubble study

Pericardial disease

Cardiac tamponade
Pericardiocentesis

Constrictive pericarditis
Right/left heart cath, Consider surgery

RV failure with increased PA pressure (DRVF)

Primary respiratory or LV failure

Treat underlying cause

Chronic PAH: Exacerbation of chronic RV dysfunction

See Algorithm 14.3

Pulmonary embolism pulmonary artery systolic pressure (PASP) <50

Anticoagulants and consider thrombolytics

RV failure without increased PA pressure

RV infarction Acute coronary syndrome protocol

Acute tricuspid regurgitation Consider surgery

with acute DRVF failure with established PH has not been proven to be beneficial. Risks and benefits need to be weighed carefully, and the procedure should be performed and interpreted by skilled individuals.

TREATMENT OF ACUTE DECOMPENSATED RV FAILURE

The treatment of acute DRVF (Algorithm 14.3) includes:

- Identify and correct precipitating factors
- Correct hypoxemia (maybe uncorrectable if right-to-left intracardiac shunt exists)
- Reverse hypotension and restore circulation
- Treat volume overload and RV encroachment

Identify and Correct Precipitating Factors

In patients with known PH and chronic RV dysfunction, identification of precipitating factors (Table 14.2) must be sought and corrected. Maintain a high index of suspicion for occult infection in patients with chronic indwelling venous catheters; empiric therapy to treat bacteremia is appropriate. Sepsis will be poorly tolerated but fluid resuscitation has to be tempered by not aggravating RV dilation and LV compression. Atrial tachyarrhythmias should be slowed with digoxin, amiodarone, or cardioversion. Nodal blockers that also have negative inotropic effects or systemic vasodilatory effects (e.g., Verapamil, Diltiazem) should not be used. Bradycardias may require temporary pacing as the situation demands.

Correct Hypoxemia

Oxygen is a potent pulmonary vasodilator, and liberal oxygen administration to correct alveolar hypoxia will minimize hypoxic vasoconstriction. If positive pressure ventilation is needed, employ the lowest plateau pressures, through low tidal volume and positive end-expiratory pressure, in order to limit RV afterload (from intra-alveolar vessel compression) and decreases in venous return, while still maintaining adequate oxygenation and avoiding respiratory acidosis. Hypotension and poor ventilation during intubation can also have profound hemodynamic consequences. Ketamine or etomidate should be considered as induction agents and propofol should be avoided to decrease the risk of hypotension. Vasopressors should be immediately available and in some instances initiated prior to induction or uptitrated prior to administration of induction medications if the patient is already hypotensive. Once intubated, permissive hypercapnia should be avoided as hypoxic pulmonary vasoconstriction is augmented in hypercarbic conditions. Bronchospasm and agitation are frequently overlooked causes of elevated pulmonary vascular resistance (PVR) in ventilated patients and should be managed aggressively.

Reverse Hypotension and Restore Circulation

Factors governing RV stroke volume are the same as those for the LV: preload, afterload, and myocardial contractility. Treatment of DRVF encompasses all three parameters.

Preload

Insufficient preload is generally not an issue in DRVF. If shock is due to decreased preload (i.e., central venous pressure <5 mm Hg) cautious volume challenges of crystalloid should be employed until central venous pressure is 10 to 12 mm Hg or serial cardiac output assessments should be monitored. Overexuberant volume

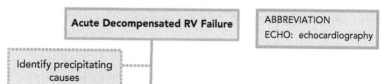

ALGORITHM 14.3 Management of Decompensated Right Ventricular (RV) Failure

Acute Decompensated RV Failure

ABBREVIATION
ECHO: echocardiography

Identify precipitating causes

Correct hypoxemia, *if able*
- Caution with positive pressure ventilation and positive end-expiratory pressure (PEEP)
- Avoid hypercarbia and acidemia

Reverse hypotension and restore circulation
- Rapid assessment of volume status: measure central venous pressure (CVP), ECHO, or pulmonary artery catheter >> *modest fluid challenges if CVP <5*
- Assess organ perfusion: measure lactate, venous saturation >> *early vasopressor use*

↑ **RV contractility**
- Dobutamine
- Milrinone

Pulmonary vasodilator
- Inhaled nitric oxide or inhaled epoprostenol
- *If not hypotensive,* intravenous prostacyclin analog or sildenafil

If refractory, consider atrial septostomy, Potts shunt, ECLS

After stabilization
- Remove excess volume
- Transition to chronic pulmonary vasodilator

administration can worsen RV distention and encroach on the LV, further reducing cardiac output and worsening hypotension.

Systemic Hypotension

A low systemic diastolic pressure coupled with elevated RV end-diastolic pressure (common in DRVF) narrows the myocardial perfusion gradient, leading to RV ischemia. Thus vasopressors have an important role in restoring systemic blood pressure to maintain organ perfusion and minimize RV ischemia. While no agent is superior, norepinephrine has both inotropic and peripheral vasopressor properties without major pulmonary vascular constriction. Dopamine, which may result in marked tachycardia, is also a reasonable choice given its positive inotropic and peripheral vasoconstrictive effects. The lowest doses of pressors should be used to minimize tachycardia, dysrhythmias, myocardial oxygen consumption, and pulmonary vasoconstriction.

Contractility

In *normotensive* patients with persistently unmet peripheral metabolic needs, the next step is addition of an inotrope. There is no ideal inotrope that increases RV contractility without worsening systemic blood pressure. Options include dobutamine at 2 to 5 mcg/kg/min or the longer-acting milrinone, which requires dosage reduction in renal insufficiency.

Afterload Reduction

Selective pulmonary arterial dilation is a critical therapeutic step in breaking the spiral of RV decompensation. Inhaled agents preferentially lower PVR with minimal decreases in systemic vascular resistance and also minimize ventilation–perfusion mismatching and hypoxemia. Two available agents are inhaled nitric oxide and inhaled epoprostenol. Inhaled nitric oxide up to 40 ppm is administered via face mask or endotracheal tube, but methemoglobin levels must be followed. Inhaled epoprostenol (5000 to 20,000 ng/mL) can be delivered as a continuous nebulization. Once cardiac output and blood pressure have improved, the patient can be transitioned to more conventional and longer-term options (e.g., parenteral or longer-acting inhaled prostacyclin analogs). Nonselective vasodilators such as nitroprusside, nitrates, hydralazine, and calcium channel antagonists must be avoided, as they preferentially cause peripheral vasodilation and aggravate hypotension.

Treat Volume Overload and RV Encroachment

Once circulation is restored and the patient has stabilized, excess volume can then be removed. Severe right heart failure can be associated with diuretic resistance, due to poor intestinal absorption, decreased glomerular filtration rate with poor renal arterial perfusion, renal venous congestion from elevated central venous pressures, and intense neurohormonal activation. A suggested stepwise approach is:

1. Loop diuretic (e.g., furosemide, bumetanide) by intravenous bolus or continuous infusion. The latter maintains a continuous renal threshold of drug with constant diuresis and less ototoxicity.
2. If loop diuretic is insufficient, a thiazide diuretic (e.g., chlorothiazide [IV or PO] or metolazone [PO]) can be added.
3. Spironolactone is effective to counter the intense neurohormonal pathway and can be added unless hyperkalemia is present.

4. Finally, mechanical fluid removal with slow continuous venovenous ultrafiltration may be appropriate.

MECHANICAL SUPPORT

Patients that are refractory to optimal pharmacologic therapies should be considered for extracorporeal life support (ECLS). Mechanical support is increasingly considered as an option to bridge to definitive treatment, such as advanced chronic pulmonary vasodilator therapy (e.g., Epoprostenol), lung transplantation and pulmonary thromboendarterectomy in the setting of chronic thromboembolic disease. Prior to initiation of such measures, it is most important to address the patient's bridging potential. Some of the contraindications to initiation of ECLS include major contraindication for anticoagulation, irreversible end-organ damage, and irreversible cardiopulmonary failure in a patient that is not a transplant candidate. There are several modes of mechanical support for RV failure, but venoarterial (VA) extracorporeal membrane oxygenation (ECMO) is typically required. The decision to initiate mechanical support should be made by a multidisciplinary team comprised of an intensivist, pulmonologist/cardiologist, and cardiothoracic surgeon.

SURGICAL INTERVENTIONS

Atrial septostomy, which is the percutaneous creation of a right-to-left shunt in the interatrial septum, allows for right-sided decompression and improved left-sided filling. Although right-to-left shunting results in oxygen desaturation, this is counterbalanced by improved cardiac output and total oxygen delivery. Surgical creation of a Potts shunt, an anastamosis between the left PA and the descending aorta, offers an alternative palliation strategy. Catheter-based formation of a Potts shunt is a novel technique and has been described in select patients. Both septostomy and creation of a Potts shunt are risky procedures with associated morbidity and mortality that should only be performed at experienced centers.

GENERAL MEASURES

1. Control agitation
2. Suppress fevers
3. Place filters on intravenous catheters to prevent air embolization if intracardiac shunt present
4. Deep venous thrombosis prophylaxis
5. Minimize Valsalva maneuvers (e.g., constipation)
6. Caution with colloid infusions but consider transfusion if anemic and oxygen delivery severely compromised

SUGGESTED READINGS

DeMarco T, McGlothin D. Managing right ventricular failure in PAH. *Adv Pulm Hypertens.* 2005;14(4):16–26.
  A review article with excellent flowcharts, algorithms, and detailed pathophysiology and therapeutic discussion.

Lahm T, McCaslin CA, Wozniak TC, et al. Medical and surgical treatment of acute right ventricular failure. *J Am Coll Cardiol.* 2010;56(18):1435–1446.

Excellent review of the clinical features of DRVF, including comprehensive treatment strategy.

Machuca T, de Perrot M. Interventional therapies for right ventricular failure secondary to precapillary pulmonary hypertension. *Advances in Pulmonary Hypertension.* 2015;13: 197–200.

A review of mechanical support for refractory RV failure in pulmonary hypertension.

Mebazaa A, Karpati P. Acute right ventricular failure—from pathophysiology to new treatments. *Intensive Care Med.* 2004;30(2):185–196.

A clinical case-based review.

Piazza G, Goldhaber SZ. The acutely decompensated right ventricle: pathways for diagnosis and management. *Chest.* 2005;128(3):1836–1852.

A detailed review article focusing on pathophysiology, diagnosis, and treatment of this increasingly common condition.

Taichman DB, Jeffery ME. Management of the acutely ill patient with pulmonary arterial hypertension. In: Mandel J, Taichman D, eds. *Pulmonary Vascular Disease.* Philadelphia, PA: Saunders Elsevier; 2006:254–265.

A textbook chapter which discusses issues to consider when caring for patients with PAH in the ICU.

Pulmonary Embolism

Roger D. Yusen

Intensive care unit **(ICU)** patients typically have multiple risk factors for deep vein thrombosis **(DVT)** and pulmonary embolism **(PE)** that include acute illness, comorbidities, immobilization, advanced age, hypercoagulable states, and presence of a central intravenous catheter. These risk factors make venous thromboembolism **(VTE)** a frequent diagnosis in ICU, despite the use of thromboprophylaxis. Of patients that receive care for or develop PE in the ICU, many will have **submassive PE** (i.e., signs of right ventricular [**RV**] dysfunction without arterial hypotension or cardiogenic shock), and a smaller but significant proportion will have **massive PE** (i.e., RV failure associated with arterial hypotension and cardiogenic shock).

DIAGNOSIS (Algorithm 15.1)

PE often has nonspecific **signs and symptoms** (e.g., tachycardia, tachypnea, dyspnea, pleuritic chest pain, hemoptysis, hypoxemia, presyncope, syncope, and hypotension) which frequently overlap with other conditions that occur in ICU patients. The **differential diagnosis** list for patients with signs and symptoms of PE includes sepsis, hypovolemia, acute lung injury (e.g., pneumonia, aspiration, transfusion-associated lung injury [**TRALI**]), heart failure, transfusion-associated circulatory overload (**TACO**), acute coronary syndrome, cardiac tamponade, decompensated pulmonary arterial hypertension, constrictive cardiac disease, valvular heart disease, and aortic dissection. ICU patients often have multiorgan dysfunction, and PE may occur in conjunction with illnesses such as myocardial dysfunction or sepsis. Clinicians frequently underdiagnose PE because it mimics other diseases and vice versa. Prompt diagnosis allows for appropriate treatment which will reduce mortality and recurrence rates.

Diagnostic Modalities

Since many disorders in the differential diagnosis list fall into the category of life threatening, the clinical suspicion of PE should lead to expeditious objective diagnostic testing. Pretest probability influences the diagnostic workup of patients with suspected PE, and its incorporation into the interpretation of diagnostic tests improves their accuracy. However, clinical probability scores for PE (e.g., Wells and revised Wells Prediction scores) often produce an intermediate to high pretest probability of PE in the ICU setting. Nonspecific diagnostic tests, such as **D-dimer** assay, have a low accuracy (e.g., many false positives) in the ICU setting, and waiting for the result may delay necessary additional diagnostic tests or treatments. **CXR, EKG, and ABG,** may prove useful for assisting in determining pretest probability and for evaluating

ALGORITHM 15.1 Diagnostic Evaluation for Suspected Acute Pulmonary Embolism (PE) in the Intensive Care Unit (ICU)

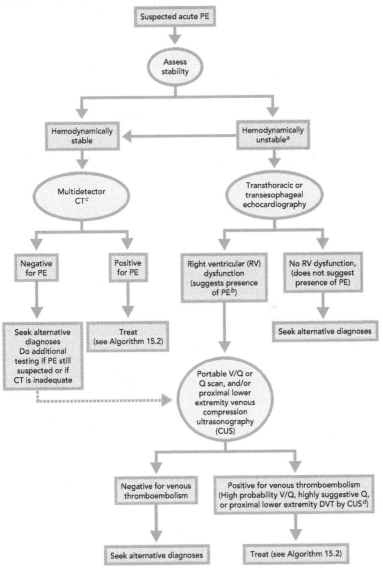

[a]Search for alternative and concomitant diagnoses.

[b]Try to confirm presence of PE with additional testing.

[c]If contraindication to intravenous (IV) contrast exist, consider V/Q scan, CUS, or MR angiography.

[d]Proximal lower extremity DVT serves as a surrogate for PE in the appropriate clinical setting.

other causes of a patient's illness, but they do not confirm or rule out the diagnosis of PE. **Cardiac biomarkers** (e.g., troponin, brain natriuretic peptide [**BNP**]) assist with prognosis, though they have low diagnostic accuracy.

Multidetector helical CT scan with contrast (PE protocol) has been the most recent gold standard test for evaluating patients for PE, and it may also help to quantify the severity of PE by showing evidence of **RV** dysfunction. CT also assists with the detection of alternative or concomitant diagnoses. The accuracy of CT for diagnosis of PE decreases with poorer scan quality and for smaller and more peripheral clots. Contraindications to PE-protocol CT include contrast allergy, severe renal dysfunction, or inability to safely travel out of the ICU. Patients who have a contraindication to CT or inadequate CT results should undergo additional testing that may include ventilation/perfusion (**V/Q**) scan, lower extremity venous compression ultrasonography (**CUS**), or echocardiography (**ECHO**).

Radionuclide scintigraphy (V/Q scan) allows for testing in the ICU because of its portability. In the setting of high clinical suspicion, a high probability (of PE) V/Q scan result rules in PE unless a mimicking diagnosis is suspected (e.g., pulmonary artery (**PA**) sarcoma, fibrosing mediastinitis). A patient who has an abnormal CXR will often have an indeterminate V/Q result, and the latter result warrants further testing. Because of the high likelihood of obtaining a nondiagnostic V/Q result, and since chest CT may reveal alternative or additional diagnoses, chest CT should remain the first-choice diagnostic test for evaluating patients in the ICU who have suspected PE.

CUS may diagnose DVT at the bedside in the ICU. Proximal lower extremity DVT may serve as a surrogate for PE in the appropriate clinical setting.

ECHO, another portable modality, may detect right-sided cardiac thrombus or signs of right heart dysfunction associated with PE (a surrogate for PE). Findings on ECHO may suggest an etiology other than PE for the signs and symptoms (e.g., cardiac tamponade, myocardial infarction, heart failure, valvular heart disease), and it may exclude these and other mimics of PE. A patient who has a possible massive PE should urgently undergo ECHO. If transthoracic ECHO does not provide good images or if other indications exist, a clinician may prefer to use transesophageal ECHO. Findings on ECHO to suggest PE include: **RV** dilatation and hypokinesis; increase in RV/ left ventricle (**LV**) diameter ratio; elevated **PA** pressure and PA dilation; tricuspid regurgitation; paradoxical septal motion; interventricular septal shift toward the left ventricle; decreased tricuspid annular plane systolic excursion (**TAPSE**); and McConnell's sign, defined by hypokinesis of the free wall of the RV with normal motion of the apex.

Stability Assessment

Cardiovascular stability helps to determine the diagnostic workup for suspected PE in an ICU setting (Algorithm 15.1). Stable patients should undergo evaluation with CT if contraindications do not exist. Unstable patients should undergo tests based on their likelihood of ruling in or ruling out diagnoses, their availability, and the ability to get rapid results. A hemodynamically unstable patient who has suspected PE should undergo rapid risk stratification to assess for RV dysfunction (i.e., ECHO and/or chest CT) and RV stress/injury (i.e., BNP and cardiac troponin). If a patient cannot transport out of the ICU for diagnostic testing due to unacceptable risk or other reasons, the patient should undergo bedside testing (e.g., ECHO, portable V/Q or Q scan, lower extremity venous CUS). For patients who have a cardiac arrest, immediate bedside ECHO might also assist with decision-making about interventions such as thrombolytic therapy.

PROGNOSIS

Hemodynamic status remains the most important acute prognostic factor for patients who have acute PE. Although treated PE in normotensive patients that do not have evidence of **RV** dysfunction has a short-term mortality rate of approximately 2%, the mortality rate increases up to 30% in patients with shock and up to 65% in patients that present with cardiac arrest. RV failure causes approximately half of the PE-associated deaths that occur during the first 30 days after diagnosis of PE. The degree of hemodynamic instability in patients with acute PE predicts in-hospital mortality. Higher severity of PE-associated cardiovascular dysfunction (i.e., ranging from the lowest severity of no cardiovascular dysfunction to higher severity categories of RV dysfunction without arterial hypotension, arterial hypotension, cardiogenic shock, and cardiopulmonary arrest) predicts mortality.

Elevated BNP and troponin in the setting of PE suggest RV stress/injury has occurred, and abnormal test results portend a poor prognosis even in the hemodynamically stable patient. Patients who have RV thrombus or RV dysfunction on ECHO or CT have a higher mortality compared to those without these findings.

Prognostic indicators may assist with decision-making regarding escalation of therapy (Tables 15.1 and 15.2). The recent European Society of Cardiology guideline has moved away from the massive/submassive/other PE classification system toward an early mortality risk–based classification system that drives treatment decisions (Table 15.1). The guideline uses four key risk assessment categories that assess for (1) hemodynamic instability (i.e., shock or hypotension present), (2) imaging-detected (echocardiogram or CT) signs of RV dysfunction, (3) elevated clinical risk score (by Pulmonary Embolism Severity Index [**PESI**] or simplified PESI [**sPESI**]; [Table 15.2]), and (4) abnormal cardiac laboratory biomarkers (i.e., troponin, BNP). **High-risk PE** patients have hemodynamic instability with imaging-detected signs of RV dysfunction, with or without an elevated clinical risk score and with or without abnormal cardiac laboratory biomarkers. **Intermediate-risk PE** patients do not have hemodynamic instability, but they have an elevated clinical risk score, and they may or may not have imaging-detected signs of RV dysfunction and/or abnormal cardiac laboratory biomarkers. **Low-risk PE** patients do not have abnormalities in any of the four key risk assessments. The PE severity classification systems do not address all important clinical events such as hypoxemia, respiratory failure requiring mechanical ventilation, or worsening cardiovascular status that might occur within a specific risk class (e.g., greater tachycardia, drop in blood pressure not meeting criteria for hypotension).

PROGNOSTIC ASSESSMENT AND SEVERITY INDICES

Indicators of poor prognosis or adverse outcomes for patients who have PE include hemodynamic instability/hypotension, signs of RV dysfunction, elevated troponin, elevated BNP, coexisting DVT, thrombus burden, and RV thrombus. Several prognostic scoring systems (e.g., the **PESI** and the **sPESI**) exist. However, the clinical prediction tools have not been specifically developed for patients in the ICU. Of note, the prognostic markers (e.g., troponin, BNP), often predict different degrees of risk in different types of patients, such as those with hypotension and those without it.

TABLE 15.1	Morality Risk Classification of Patients Who Have Acute PE			
	Risk Parameters and Scores			
Early Mortality Risk	Shock or Hypotension	PESI Class III–V or sPESI ≥1[a]	Signs of RV Dysfunction on an Imaging Test[b]	Cardiac Laboratory Biomarkers[c]
High	+	(+)[d]	+	(+)[d]
Intermediate Intermediate high	–	+	Both positive	
Intermediate low	–	+	Either one (or none) positive[e]	
Low	–	–	Assessment optional; if assessed, both negative[e]	

[a]PESI class III to V indicates moderate to very high 30-day mortality risk; sPESI ≥1 point(s) indicates high 30-day mortality risk.

[b]Echocardiographic criteria of RV dysfunction include RV dilation and/or an increased end-diastolic RV/LV diameter ratio (in most studies, the reported threshold value was 0.9 or 1.0), hypokinesia of the free RV wall, or increased velocity of the tricuspid regurgitation jet. Computed tomographic (CT) angiography (four-chamber views of the heart) criterion for RV dysfunction consists of an increased end-diastolic RV/LV diameter ratio (≥0.9 or 1.0).

[c]Markers of myocardial injury (e.g., elevated cardiac troponin I or T concentrations in plasma) or of heart failure as a result of right ventricular dysfunction (elevated natriuretic peptide concentrations in plasma).

[d]Classify shock or hypotension as high risk, despite any PESI or sPESI or cardiac biomarker score.

[e]Classify low-risk PESI (class I to II) or sPESI patients (score of 0) who have associated elevated cardiac biomarkers or signs of RV dysfunction on imaging tests into the intermediate-low-risk category.

PE, pulmonary embolism; PESI, pulmonary embolism severity index; RV, right ventricle; sPESI, simplified pulmonary embolism severity index.

Adapted from Konstantinides SV, Torbicki A, Agnelli G, et al. 2014 ESC guidelines on the diagnosis and management of acute pulmonary embolism: The Task Force for the diagnosis and management of acute pulmonary embolism of the European Society of Cardiology (ESC) endorsed by the European Respiratory Society (ERS). *Eur Heart J.* 2014;35(43):3033–3073 (Table 9).

TREATMENT (Algorithm 15.2)

General Approaches

Clinicians should make their treatment decisions for PE based on confidence in the diagnosis of PE, hemodynamic status, degree of RV dysfunction/injury, bleeding risk, prognosis, and patient preferences. For patients deemed to have a high clinical probability of PE and an acceptable bleeding risk, clinicians should initiate anticoagulation upon the initial suspicion of PE and prior to completion of any diagnostic tests. Satisfactory "exclusion" of the diagnosis of PE should lead to prompt discontinuation of anticoagulation, unless otherwise indicated, and initiation of VTE prophylaxis. Confirmation of PE should lead to continuation of or prompt initiation of anticoagulation if not contraindicated. Confirmation of PE in the setting of a contraindication to anticoagulation or the failure of therapeutic doses of anticoagulation should lead to placement of an inferior vena cava (**IVC**) filter (*see below*). **Hemodynamically unstable patients** who have PE

TABLE 15.2	Original and Simplified Pulmonary Embolism Severity Index (PESI)	
Variable	Original PESI	Simplified PESI
Age	Age, in years	1 (if >age 80 yrs)
Male sex	+10	–
History of cancer	+30	1
History of heart failure	+10	1 for either or both of these items
History of chronic lung disease	+10	
Pulse ≥110 beats/min	+20	1
Systolic blood pressure <100 mm Hg	+30	1
Respiratory rate ≥30 breaths/min	+20	–
Temperature <36°C	+20	–
Altered mental status	+60	–
Arterial oxyhemoglobin saturation (SaO_2) <90%	+20	1

30-Day Mortality Risk Strata (Based on Sum of Points)		
	Low-Risk PESI	Low-Risk sPESI
	Class I: ≤65 points (event rate 95% CI, 0–1.6%) **Class II: 66–85 points** (event rate 95% CI, 1.7–3.5%)	**0 points** (event rate 95% CI, 0–2.1%)
	High-Risk PESI	High-Risk sPESI
	Class III: 86–105 points (event rate 95% CI, 3.2–7.1%) **Class IV: 106–125 points** (event rate 95% CI, 4.0–11.4%) **Class V: >125 points** (event rate 95% CI, 10.0–24.5%)	**≥1 point** (event rate 95% CI, 8.5–13.2%)

should undergo stabilization and resuscitation (*see Chapter 4*). Resuscitation should include cautious fluid management, and supplemental oxygen and ventilatory support as deemed necessary. Vasopressors/inotropes may lead to improved stability. Prompt risk stratification will assist with further decisions regarding escalated PE treatment (i.e., thrombolytic therapy, catheter-based therapy, or surgical embolectomy). Uncommonly, a patient may need mechanical circulatory support as a bridge to escalated therapy.

Anticoagulation

Anticoagulation acts to prevent new clot formation and decrease risk for recurrent VTE. Anticoagulants that have efficacy for the initial treatment of PE include

ALGORITHM 15.2 Treatment of Confirmed Acute PE in the ICU

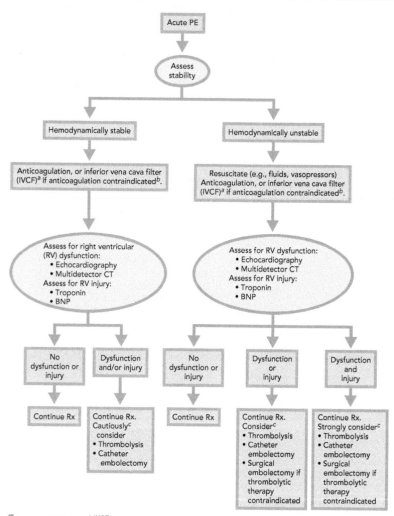

[a]Temporary or permanent IVCF.
[b]Anticoagulate after IVCF placement once contraindication to anticoagulation resolves.
[c]Assess for contraindications.

parenteral agents (i.e., unfractionated heparin [UFH], low–molecular-weight heparin [LMWH], and fondaparinux) and oral agents (i.e., rivaroxaban, apixaban, dabigatran, and edoxaban) (*see Chapter 91 for dosing, side effects, and complications*). However, most studies of anticoagulants excluded ICU patients. Since patients in the ICU often have higher than average bleeding risks, a relatively high rate of undergoing invasive procedures, and a higher chance of receiving thrombolytic therapy, IV UFH may be the preferred anticoagulant because of its bioavailability, relatively short half-life, insignificant renal clearance, and reversibility. Adjusted-dose anticoagulation (such as IV **UFH**, argatroban, or lepirudin) should undergo timely titration to therapeutic levels to lower the risk of VTE recurrence or extension. For ICU patients that have high-risk PE, and for some patients that have intermediate-risk PE, it might be prudent to check an activated partial thromboplastin time (aPTT) about 90 minutes after the UFH bolus. If the aPTT does not reach a very high value (e.g., >150 seconds) in this setting, then another UFH bolus is indicated. Guidelines suggest using drugs other than UFH for nonmassive PE. Of note, the oral agents dabigatran and edoxaban first require at least 5 days of parenteral therapy (e.g., UFH, LMWH, fondaparinux). Even though the oral agents apixaban and rivaroxaban may be used for the initial (and long-term) treatment of PE, the parenteral agents should be preferred for many ICU patients based on their short half-life, reversibility, lack of gastrointestinal absorption concerns, lower risk of drug interactions, and ability to monitor anticoagulant effect. For ICU patients who have severe renal dysfunction, or those in whom thrombolytic therapy is being considered, UFH is the anticoagulant of choice.

Thrombolytic Therapy

Thrombolytic agents convert plasminogen to plasmin and lead to rapid fibrin clot lysis. Thrombolytics may rapidly improve pulmonary perfusion, pulmonary hypertenison, RV function, and low systemic blood pressure. The high risk of death in patients who have PE and associated hypotension or shock may indicate the need for treatment more aggressive than anticoagulation (i.e., thrombolysis). Studies do not support the use of thrombolytic agents in most patients who have acute symptomatic PE. In the absence of large randomized clinical trials that demonstrate the benefit of thrombolytic therapy on mortality, the American College of Chest Physicians (**ACCP**) guidelines recommended the use of thrombolytic therapy for (1) patients with acute symptomatic PE and hypotension that do not have a high bleeding risk (evidence strength grade 2B), and (2) selected patients with acute symptomatic PE who deteriorate after starting anticoagulation and who have a low bleeding risk (evidence strength grade 2C). However, some data suggest that thrombolytic therapy followed by long-term anticoagulation, compared to sole anticoagulant therapy, has a higher risk of all-cause death among hemodynamically stable patients. More controversial indications for thrombolytic therapy for PE in normotensive patients consist of RV dysfunction, severe hypoxemia, extensive embolic burden, saddle embolism, free floating right heart thrombus, and presence of patent foramen ovale.

General contraindications to thrombolytic administration include active, recent, or high risk for bleeding (Table 15.3). Compared to UFH, thrombolytics for PE increase the major bleeding rate by 50% to 100%, from about 6% to 12% to about 9% to 22%, and they markedly increase the intracranial hemorrhage rate from <1% to about 1.5% to 3%.

Types of thrombolytics include *fibrin-specific* agents (recombinant tissue plasminogen activator [rtPA] [i.e., alteplase], recombinant plasminogen activator [rPA] [i.e., reteplase], and modified human tissue plasminogen activator [i.e., tenecteplase]). Of these, only alteplase has a U.S. Food and Drug Administration (**FDA**) indication for acute PE (i.e., massive PE). The previously used *nonselective agents* (urokinase and streptokinase) are not available for use in the United States any more. Studies have not demonstrated the superiority of one type of thrombolytic agent over another.

The standard alteplase dose for PE is 100 mg IV over 2 hours. Compared to alteplase, reteplase (rPA; Retavase) has less fibrin specificity and a longer half-life. For

| **TABLE 15.3** | Contraindications to Thrombolytic Therapy |

Absolute contraindications[a]
  Serious active bleeding
  Known major bleeding diathesis
  History of intracranial hemorrhage
  Known intracranial neoplasm, arteriovenous malformation, or aneurysm
  Recent nonhemorrhagic stroke (e.g., within the past 3 mo)
  Recent significant head trauma (e.g., within the past 3 mo)
  Recent intracranial or intraspinal surgery (e.g., within the past 3 mo)
  Suspected aortic dissection

Relative contraindications
  Recent internal bleeding (e.g., within the past 4 wks)
  Recent major surgery (see above) or organ biopsy
  Recent trauma (see above), including cardiopulmonary resuscitation (especially
    if prolonged)
  Recent blood vessel puncture at noncompressible site
  Platelet count less than 10,000/mm³
  Severe uncontrolled systemic hypertension
  Diabetic retinopathy or other hemorrhagic ophthalmic conditions
  Pregnancy
  Acute pericarditis
  Endocarditis
  Significant hemostatic defects
  Current use of long-acting anticoagulant with therapeutic dose or level
  Advanced age (e.g., greater than 75 yrs)
  Prior associated allergic reaction
  Any other condition in which bleeding would be difficult to manage

[a]Some absolute contraindications (except concurrent intracranial hemorrhage) might not be "absolute" in the most extreme circumstances. Severity of condition and judgment of clinician will determine the categorization of absolute versus relative contraindication; list not all inclusive.

PE, reteplase is typically given as 10 U IV over 2 minutes, and 30 minutes later, another 10 U is given IV over 2 minutes. Genetic engineering has produced the multiple-point mutant of rtPA, tenecteplase (TNK-tPA; TNKase). Tenecteplase's longer plasma half-life than reteplase and alteplase allows for its single intravenous bolus injection (e.g., 50 mg IV over 5 seconds) *(For dosing, side effects, and complications see PHARMACOLOGIC chapter)*. Some studies have proposed use of **low-dose lytics**, especially in those who have a relative contraindication to or a less strong indication for lytic therapy, though controversy exists around such dosing. Regarding use of **lytics during cardiac arrest**, placebo-controlled pilot studies have shown a higher rate of return of spontaneous circulation and perhaps survival after a bolus of either 50 mg of rTPA; alteplase) or 50 mg of tenecteplase.

Most guidelines recommend that clinicians discontinue anticoagulant therapy prior to initiating thrombolytic therapy. After completion of thrombolytic therapy, the clinician should reinitiate anticoagulation without a bolus to prevent recurrent VTE when the aPTT has decreased to less than twice the normal control value.

In a situation where the clinician would like to give thrombolytic therapy, but a contraindication exists, the patient should undergo assessment for **catheter or surgical embolectomy**. Though gaining in popularity, catheter embolectomy (with or without local low-dose thrombolytic therapy) lacks strong supporting data at this time, and surgical embolectomy carries a high mortality risk.

Catheter-based Therapy

For patients who have acute PE associated with hypotension and who have (i) a high bleeding risk or (ii) failed systemic thrombolysis, guidelines recommend consideration of catheter-assisted thrombus treatment if appropriate expertise and resources are available (evidence strength grade 2C). Catheter-based therapies may administer thrombolytics at low doses and may mechanically treat thrombi.

Surgical Embolectomy

Surgical embolectomy at centers that have expertise has a role in patients who have massive/high-risk PE and a contraindication to thrombolytic therapy or failed thrombolytic therapy. Surgical embolectomy for acute PE, often reserved for patients who fall within the most severe spectrum of those who have massive/high-risk PE, has had high morbidity and mortality (25%) rates. However, surgical embolectomy on cardiopulmonary bypass with the heart in arrest for rescue of patients remaining unstable despite IV thrombolytic therapy has had reasonable success, with fewer recurrent PE and a trend toward fewer deaths than those who received repeat IV thrombolysis. Patients who have a right heart thrombus that straddles the interatrial septum via a patent foramen ovale/atrial septal defect should be considered for surgical embolectomy. Embolectomy for free floating right heart thrombus remains controversial.

IVC Filters

Studies have demonstrated a decreased risk of PE and an increased risk of DVT, without a significant effect on mortality, associated with IVC filter placement. Guidelines recommend that patients should undergo (temporary or permanent) IVC filter placement if they have a contraindication to or develop VTE on therapeutic doses of anticoagulation. If and when a reversible (e.g., bleeding) contraindication to anticoagulation resolves, patients who have an IVC filter should undergo a standard course of anticoagulation and consideration of temporary filter removal. For patients who have massive PE, guidelines recommend consideration of (permanent) IVC filter placement. Patients with temporary IVC filters should have them removed, if and when deemed appropriate, according to manufacturer and treatment guidelines.

Risks of Treatment

Bleeding

In general, ICU patients have a high risk of major bleeding because of coagulopathies, liver or renal insufficiency, significant comorbidities, increased risk for stress ulcers, and invasive procedures. Concomitant use of antiplatelet agents increases the risk of bleeding (Table 15.4).

Major bleeding should lead to the immediate discontinuation of all forms of anticoagulation, appropriate monitoring, and supportive measures. Many scenarios may require blood product transfusion. Some scenarios require reversal of anticoagulant therapy (*see Chapters 63 and 91*).

TABLE 15.4	Risk Factors for Bleeding[a] With Initial Anticoagulant Therapy
Risk Factors	

Age >65 yrs
Age >75 yrs
Previous bleeding
Cancer
Metastatic cancer
Renal failure
Liver failure
Thrombocytopenia
Previous stroke
Diabetes
Anemia
Antiplatelet therapy
Poor anticoagulant control
Comorbidity and reduced functional capacity
Recent surgery
Frequent falls
Alcohol abuse

The increased bleeding risk associated with a risk factor will vary with (1) severity of the risk factor (e.g., location and extent of metastatic disease, platelet count), (2) temporal relationships (e.g., interval from surgery or a previous bleeding episode), and (3) previous effectiveness of correction of cause of bleeding (e.g., upper GI bleeding).

Compared with low-risk patients (0 risk factors), moderate-risk patients (1 risk factor) have a twofold risk, and high-risk patients (≥2 risk factors) have an eightfold risk of major bleeding.

[a]List not all inclusive.

Adapted, with permission, from Kearon C, Akl EA, Comerota AJ, et al. Antithrombotic therapy for VTE disease: antithrombotic therapy and prevention of thrombosis, 9th ed: American college of chest physicians evidence-based clinical practice guidelines. *Chest.* 2012;141(2 suppl):e432 (Table 2).

Heparin-Induced Thrombocytopenia

Clinicians should consider the possibility that heparin-induced thrombocytopenia (**HIT**) has occurred in patients who develop VTE in the setting of absolute or relative thrombocytopenia. Patients receiving UFH should undergo monitoring for HIT. Patients who have PE and suspected or confirmed HIT should not receive UFH, LMWH, or warfarin until the HIT has resolved. Such patients should undergo treatment with a direct thrombin inhibitor such as **argatroban** or **lepirudin** (*see PHARMACOLGIC chapter for indications, dosing, contraindications, and side effects*).

SUGGESTED READINGS

Chatterjee S, Chakraborty A, Weinberg I, et al. Thrombolysis for pulmonary embolism and risk of all-cause mortality, major bleeding, and intracranial hemorrhage: a meta-analysis. *JAMA.* 2014;311(23):2414–2421.
  A comprehensive review of thrombolytic therapy for patients with acute PE.

Kearon C, Akl EA, Ornelas J, et al. Antithrombotic therapy for VTE disease: CHEST guideline and expert panel report. *Chest.* 2016;149(2):315–352.

A premier guideline for antithrombotic therapy for patients who have venous thromboembolism.

Kline JA, Nordenholz KE, Courtney DM, et al. Treatment of submassive pulmonary embolism with tenecteplase or placebo: cardiopulmonary outcomes at 3 months: multicenter double-blind, placebo-controlled randomized trial (TOPCOAT). *J Thromb Haemost.* 2014;12(4): 459–468.

Konstantinides S, Geibel A, Heusel G, et al; Management Strategies and Prognosis of Pulmonary Embolism-3 Trial Investigators. Heparin plus alteplase compared with heparin alone in patients with submassive pulmonary embolism. *N Engl J Med.* 2002;347(15):1143–1150.

Konstantinides SV, Torbicki A, Agnelli G, et al. 2014 ESC guidelines on the diagnosis and management of acute pulmonary embolism: The Task Force for the diagnosis and management of acute pulmonary embolism of the European Society of Cardiology (ESC) endorsed by the European Respiratory Society (ERS). *Eur Heart J.* 2014;35(43):3033–3073.

A premier guideline for the diagnosis and management of acute PE.

Meyer G, Vicaut E, Danays T, et al; PEITHO Investigators. Fibrinolysis for patients with intermediate-risk pulmonary embolism. *N Engl J Med.* 2014;370(15):1402–1411.

Piazza G, Hohlfelder B, Jaff MR, et al; SEATTLE II Investigators. A prospective, single-arm, multicenter trial of ultrasound-facilitated, catheter-directed, low-dose fibrinolysis for acute massive and submassive pulmonary embolism: The SEATTLE II Study. *JACC Cardiovasc Interv.* 2015;8(10):1382–1392.

A recent study of ultrasound-facilitated, catheter-directed, low-dose fibrinolysis for patients with acute massive and submassive PE.

PIOPED Investigators. Value of ventilation/perfusion scan in acute pulmonary embolism: results of the prospective investigation of the pulmonary embolism diagnosis (PIOPED). *JAMA.* 1990;263(20):2753–2759.

The premier study of the diagnostic test characteristics of lung scintigraphy (ventilation/perfusion; V/Q) scan for the evaluation of patients who have suspected acute PE.

Sharifi M, Bay C, Skrocki L, et al; MOPETT Investigators. Moderate pulmonary embolism treated with thrombolysis (from the "MOPETT" Trial). *Am J Cardiol.* 2013;111(2):273–277.

Stein PD, Fowler SE, Goodman LR, et al; PIOPED II Investigators. Multidetector computed tomography for acute pulmonary embolism (PIOPED II). *N Eng J Med.* 2006;354(22): 2317–2327.

The premier study of the diagnostic test characteristics of contrast-enhanced chest CT scan for the evaluation of patients who have suspected acute PE.

16 Pleural Disorders in the Intensive Care Unit

Alexander C. Chen and Kevin Haas

Disorders of the pleura are found often in the intensive care unit (ICU). In some instances, pleural processes may be the primary cause of patients' critical illness; in most cases, pleural disorders are recognized as secondary processes related to patients' underlying illness. This chapter will review the pathophysiology of these disorders and provide guidelines for managing these conditions in the ICU.

PLEURAL EFFUSIONS

The pleural space is a potential space between the visceral pleura, which covers the outer surface of the lung, and the parietal pleura, which lines the inside of the chest wall. In this space, there is a small amount of fluid present that functions to mechanically couple the lung to the chest wall and lubricate the interface of the visceral and parietal pleura. Pleural fluid normally results from the filtration of blood through high-pressure systemic blood vessels and is drained from the pleural space through lymphatic openings in the parietal pleura which drain into parietal lymphatic vessels. In different disease states, fluid may originate from the interstitial spaces of the lungs, the intrathoracic lymphatics, the intrathoracic blood vessels, or the peritoneal cavity.

A pleural effusion is defined as an abnormal collection of fluid in the pleural space. Effusions occur when the rate of fluid formation exceeds the rate of fluid absorption. The most common causes of pleural effusions are shown in Table 16.1. Pleural effusions are commonly classified as being either exudative or transudative. An exudative pleural effusion implies that there is a disease process that is affecting the pleura directly, causing the pleura and/or its vasculature to be damaged. A transudative pleural effusion results when the pleura itself is healthy and implies that a disease process is affecting hydrostatic and/or oncotic factors that either increase the formation of pleural fluid or decrease the absorption of pleural fluid. Deciding if the pleura is injured or intact helps in formulating a concise differential diagnosis for potential causes (Table 16.2).

There are certain nonspecific signs and symptoms that may indicate the presence of a pleural effusion, but these are often difficult to ascertain in the ICU. Chest pain, particularly when sharp and made worse with breathing, can result from inflamed pleura in the presence of an effusion. Dyspnea is also common as the effusion can affect the mechanics of the diaphragm, cause a restrictive ventilatory defect, and/or cause compressive atelectasis leading to hypoxemia. The history can also help to reveal the cause of the effusion. For example, a patient with a fever and cough productive of sputum might have pneumonia causing the effusion. On physical examination, signs

TABLE 16.1	Common Causes of Pleural Effusions
CHF, 36%	
Pneumonia, 22%	
Malignancy, 14%	
Pulmonary embolism, 11%	
Other infections, 7%	
Other causes, 10%	

CHF, congestive heart failure.

that an effusion is present include dullness to percussion over the effusion, loss of fremitus, decreased breath sounds, crackles/egophony immediately above the effusion, and asymmetric diaphragmatic excursion with inspiration.

The majority of ICU patients will have their pleural effusion detected first by chest x-ray. Although a posterior–anterior (PA) and lateral chest x-ray is the preferred image, ICU patients typically have portable x-rays. Blunting of the costophrenic angle and a meniscus sign are the most common findings when an effusion is present. On the lateral chest x-ray, as little as 175 mL of fluid can be detected, while on the PA film, it takes approximately 500 mL of fluid. Portable films are less sensitive and often do not show the meniscus sign. Signs on the portable chest x-ray include loss of the diaphragm silhouette and increased basilar opacity with gradation over the entire hemithorax (more opaque at the base than the apex). Once a pleural effusion is detected radiographically, a lateral decubitus chest x-ray (where the dependent side is the side of the effusion) can quantitate the volume of fluid present and determine if the effusion is free-flowing or loculated. If the fluid is free-flowing, fluid can be detected as a straight line between the chest wall and the lower border of the lung. Measurement of the distance between the chest wall and the lower border of the lung can give an idea of how much fluid is present. It is generally accepted that if this distance is >1 cm, then the amount of fluid is significant. Diagnostic evaluation of the effusion from this point is discussed in Algorithms 16.1 and 16.2.

TABLE 16.2	Pathophysiologic Causes of Pleural Effusions	
How Pleura Are Affected	Example	Exudate/ Transudate
Pleura damaged		
• Local disease in pleural space	• Malignancy	• Exudate
• Local disease adjacent to pleural space	• Pneumonia, PE, subdiaphragmatic abscess	• Exudate
• Systemic diseases that affect the pleural surface	• Autoimmune disease (lupus, rheumatoid arthritis)	• Exudate
Pleura intact		
• Systemic disease that does not directly affect the pleural surface	• CHF, myxedema, cirrhosis	• Transudate

PE, pulmonary embolism; CHF, congestive heart failure.

ALGORITHM 16.1 Evaluation of the Unknown Effusion

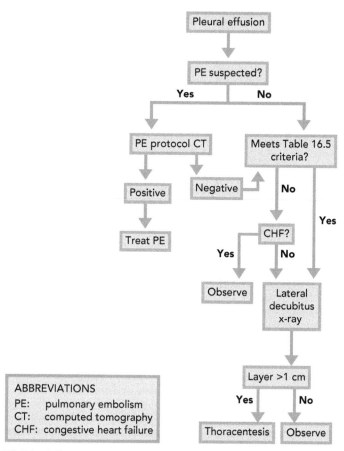

Note: 90% of pleural effusions are caused by five processes shown in Table 16.1.

Other imaging modalities can also detect, quantify, and sometimes even characterize the pleural effusion. Chest computed tomography (CT) is a useful imaging tool in assessing pleural effusions and can help the clinician diagnose not only the presence of the effusion but also delineate possible causes. Different techniques yield different information, so it is important to select the appropriate technique.

- Noncontrast CT scans can give a better idea of the amount of fluid within the pleural space, whether the fluid is loculated, and can detect abnormalities in the lungs that can be obscured by the effusion on standard chest x-ray.
- Standard contrast CT scans also assess the pleural surface for abnormalities that might suggest empyema or pleural malignancy.

ALGORITHM 16.2 Evaluation and Management of Pleural Fluid After Thoracentesis

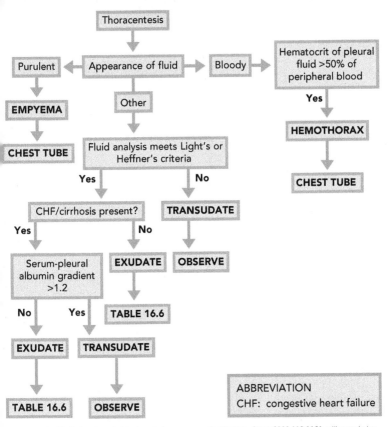

From Colice GL. Medical and surgical treatment of parapneumonic effusions. *Chest.* 2000;118:1161, with permission.

- CT scans with contrast given by pulmonary embolism protocol can detect a pulmonary embolism as the cause of the effusion but do not provide information about the pleural surface beyond that of a noncontrast CT.

CT scans cannot be done at bedside, a big disadvantage when dealing with a patient who is not stable enough to travel out of the ICU.

Ultrasound is beneficial for multiple reasons. It gives a real-time image that can be done at the bedside and used not only for diagnosis that an effusion is present but also guide diagnostic and therapeutic interventions (i.e., thoracentesis, tube thoracostomy). Ultrasound can detect whether the fluid is loculated or free-flowing and can give clues as to whether the fluid is transudative, exudative, or even whether it is an empyema.

ALGORITHM 16.3 Management of Parapneumonic Effusions

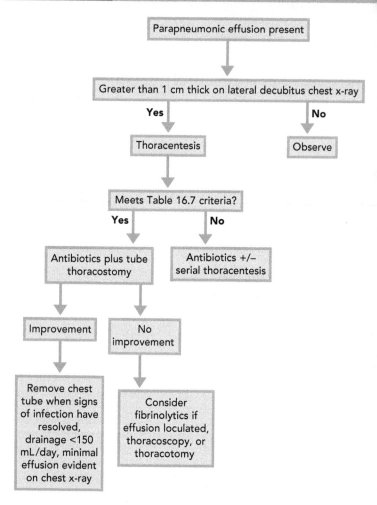

Once a pleural effusion is identified, it is important to attempt to diagnose the etiology of the effusion by obtaining a sample of the fluid for analysis. This is most often done by a thoracentesis. Thoracenteses can be safely performed as long as there is >1 cm of layered fluid on the lateral decubitus chest x-ray, even in patients receiving mechanical ventilation. One can remove a small amount of fluid for analysis or as much as 1500 mL per drainage of fluid for both diagnostic and therapeutic goals (Algorithms 16.2 to 16.4). The most common criteria used to separate exudates from transudates are Light's criteria (Table 16.3). Heffner's criteria (Table 16.4) can

TABLE 16.3	Light's Criteria

Pleural fluid to serum protein ratio >0.5
Pleural fluid to serum LDH ratio >0.6
Pleural fluid LDH >2/3 upper limit of normal for serum LDH

LDH, lactate dehydrogenase.

TABLE 16.4	Heffner's Criteria

Pleural fluid protein >2.9 g/dL
Pleural fluid LDH >0.45 upper limit of normal

LDH, lactate dehydrogenase.

ALGORITHM 16.4	Management of Recurrent Malignant Effusions

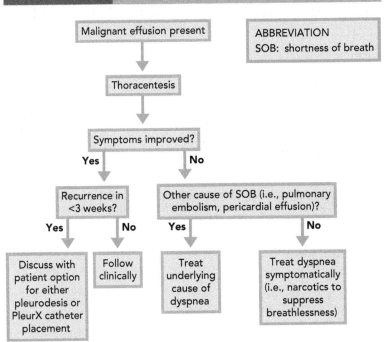

From Antunes G, Neville E, Duffy J, et al. BTS guidelines for the management of malignant pleural effusions. *Thorax.* 2003;58(suppl II):ii30, with permission.

TABLE 16.5 Indications for Thoracentesis

Pleural effusion of unknown etiology
Fever in the setting of long-standing pleural effusion
Air-fluid level in the pleural space
Rapid change in size of effusion
Concern that empyema is developing

also differentiate exudate from transudate. Heffner's criteria have a similar sensitivity (98.4%) as Light's criteria (97.9%) and do not require simultaneous blood work to be drawn.

Other specific tests (Tables 16.5 and 16.6) can help determine a specific diagnosis.

As many as 20% of pleural effusions remain undiagnosed even after extensive investigation, and it is often unclear as to what the appropriate management of these effusions is in these situations. These idiopathic effusions with no clinical or radiologic evidence of malignancy will often resolve spontaneously without further therapy. In the ICU setting, as long as the patient does not clinically deteriorate, a conservative approach may be preferred when a diagnosis cannot be made after initial evaluation. If the patient continues to deteriorate despite serial thoracenteses, thoracoscopy can be considered as the next step to assess the pleural effusion.

SPECIAL SITUATIONS

Parapneumonic Effusion

A parapneumonic effusion is defined as any pleural effusion associated with bacterial pneumonia, lung abscess, or bronchiectasis. Parapneumonic effusions progress through different stages and depending on when the patient presents, the treatment of the effusion will be different. The main distinction is whether the effusion is uncomplicated or complicated. Complicated effusions and empyemas will not resolve on their own and will require tube thoracostomy. As shown in Algorithm 16.3 and

TABLE 16.6 Diagnostic Tests to Consider in Evaluation of Pleural Effusions

Diagnostic Test	Type of Effusion
Cytology	Malignant effusion
Gram stain or culture positive	Infectious effusion (i.e., bacterial, fungal)
AFB positive; pleural fluid ADA >70 U/L	Tuberculous effusion
Rheumatoid arthritis cells	Rheumatoid effusion
Chylomicrons present; pleural fluid triglycerides >110 mg/dL	Chylothorax
Salivary amylase present in pleural fluid	Esophageal rupture
Pleural creatinine/serum creatinine >1	Urinothorax

AFB, acid-fast bacillus; ADA, adenosine deaminase

TABLE 16.7	Indication for Tube Thoracostomy in Parapneumonic Effusions

1. Radiographic
   - Pleural fluid loculation
   - Effusion filling more than half of hemithorax
   - Air-fluid level present
2. Microbiologic
   - Pus in pleural space
   - Positive Gram stain for microorganisms
   - Positive pleural fluid cultures
3. Chemical
   - Pleural fluid pH <7.2
   - Pleural fluid glucose <60

Table 16.7, radiographic, microbiologic, and chemical characteristics of the effusion will dictate whether thoracentesis with antibiotics alone will be sufficient to treat the effusion or whether a chest tube must be inserted to effectively treat the effusion. The use of intrapleural fibrinolytics and DNase twice a day for 3 days has been shown to improve pleural fluid drainage, reduce the need for surgical therapy, and decrease length of hospital stay when compared to either therapy alone. If intrapleural therapy is unsuccessful, the patient may require more invasive therapy, including thoracoscopy with breakdown of adhesions or thoracotomy with decortication.

Malignant Effusion

Malignant pleural effusions occur from a number of causes. Pleural metastases occur causing increased permeability of the pleura, and lymphatic obstruction can occur, which impairs drainage of pleural fluid through regional lymphatics. Table 16.8 shows the most common malignancies associated with pleural effusions. When these effusions occur, they are often large and lead to significant symptoms in the patient. Often, drainage of the effusion with thoracentesis alone is not sufficient as the effusion frequently recurs. Other management options include insertion of a chest tube followed by pleurodesis, which can obliterate the pleural space and prevent the effusion from recurring. Alternatively, insertion of a long-term indwelling catheter will allow the patient to drain the effusion at home and is a viable option that decreases

TABLE 16.8	Most Common Primary Tumors of Malignant Effusions
Primary Malignancy	**Rate (%)**
Lung	38
Breast	17
Lymphoma	12
Unknown primary	11
GU tract	9
GI tract	7

GU, genitourinary; GI, gastrointestinal.

TABLE 16.9	Causes of Hemothoraces
Causes	Examples
Traumatic	Penetrating trauma (gunshot wound), blunt trauma (usually with displaced rib fracture)
Nontraumatic	Metastatic malignant pleural disease, complication of anticoagulant therapy for pulmonary emboli
Iatrogenic	Perforation of a central vein from percutaneous catheter placement, following thoracentesis, following pleural biopsy

hospitalizations and increases the quality of life of the patient. Additionally, these indwelling catheters can be attached to Pleur-evac systems and used as chest tubes to support patients through their period of critical illness. Once in place, these catheters can be managed similarly to traditional tube thoracostomies. Management of this type of effusion is outlined in Algorithm 16.4.

Hemothorax

A hemothorax is the presence of blood in the pleural space such that the ratio of pleural fluid hematocrit to blood hematocrit is >0.5. This can be a serious condition and may result in ICU admission for treatment. Hemothoraces can be due to traumatic, nontraumatic, or rarely iatrogenic causes (Table 16.9). Diagnosis is made after a thoracentesis returns bloody fluid (Algorithm 16.2). It should be noted that even a small amount of blood can make pleural fluid appear bloody; therefore, the fluid's hematocrit needs to be compared with peripheral blood hematocrit to confirm the presence of a hemothorax. Initial treatment for hemothoraces of all causes is tube thoracostomy. If bleeding is voluminous and persists, transfusion and surgical intervention may be required.

Pneumothorax

A pneumothorax is the presence of air in the pleural space. When this occurs, it can be an acute emergency that requires immediate attention. A pneumothorax can be spontaneous or traumatic. Spontaneous pneumothoraces are either primary, if no other disease process is present, or secondary, if there is an underlying disease process such as chronic obstructive pulmonary disease. Traumatic pneumothoraces include iatrogenic causes that may occur following a procedure (i.e., central line placement) or barotrauma. Primary spontaneous and traumatic pneumothoraces can often be treated effectively with observation or tube thoracostomy. Secondary spontaneous pneumothoraces typically require tube thoracostomy and may also require pleurodesis for definitive treatment.

Tension pneumothorax is the most serious consequence of a pneumothorax. This occurs when a one-way valve process develops, which allows air to enter the pleural space during inspiration but not leave during expiration. As the air builds up in the pleural space, the lung and intrathoracic vasculature become compressed, leading to dyspnea, hypoxemia, and hemodynamic compromise. Physical examination may reveal absent breath sounds on the side of the pneumothorax and/or shift of the trachea to the contralateral side of the pneumothorax. Tension pneumothorax should be suspected in unstable patients with absent breath sounds over one hemithorax,

ALGORITHM 16.5 Management of Pneumothorax

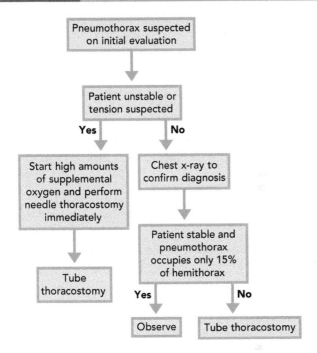

in mechanically ventilated patients who suddenly decompensate, in patients with known previously stable/improving pneumothorax who suddenly decompensate, or in patients who become unstable during or after a procedure known to cause a pneumothorax. Algorithm 16.5 gives further information on the evaluation and management of pneumothoraces. Table 16.10 covers the indications for removal of the chest tube.

Treatment of a persistent pneumothorax (air leak >72 hours) or a bronchopleural fistula is difficult, requires a multidisciplinary approach, and leads to considerable patient morbidity and mortality. The most common cause is postoperative pulmonary resection with other less common causes including necrotizing lung infections, trauma, rupture of lung bullae, or iatrogenic causes. The two main treatment options

TABLE 16.10	Indications for Removal of Chest Tube

1. Pneumothorax resolved
2. No air leak present in chest tube
3. Lung remains expanded after chest tube placed on water seal for 24 hrs

If concern remains, chest tube can be clamped for 4–8 hrs followed by chest radiograph; if lung expanded, then it is safe to remove the chest tube

are surgical repair or endoscopic management. Endoscopic options include tissue sealants, glue, silver nitrate injections, endobronchial stents, occlusion coils, and one-way valves. Success rates vary with most data limited to small sample sizes.

Chest Tube Size

The optimal size of chest tube for treating pleural disease has not been evaluated in prospective randomized trials. A clear advantage for small-bore chest tubes (≤14 French) are ease of insertion with the Seldinger technique (compared to blunt dissection with large tubes), less pain for the patient, and lower risk of procedural complications. Small-bore chest tubes are recommended for pleural drainage of fluid or air in the majority of patients. The British Thoracic Society guidelines state small-bore chest tubes (10 to 14 French) with regular flushing will be adequate for most cases of pleural infection. Hemothorax and pneumothorax due to barotrauma in the mechanically ventilated patient are likely better managed with large-bore chest tubes (≥22 French).

SUGGESTED READINGS

Abrahamian FM. Pleural effusions. http://www.emedicine.com/emerg/topic 462.htm. Accessed October 24, 2006.

Antunes G, Neville E, Duffy J, et al. BTS guidelines for the management of malignant pleural effusions. *Thorax.* 2003;58(suppl II):ii29–ii38.

Boudaya MS, Smadhi H, Zribi H, et al. Conservative management of postoperative bronchopleural fistulas. *J Thorac Cardiovasc Surg.* 2013;146:575–579.

Colice GL, Curtis A, Deslauriers J, et al. Medical and surgical treatment of parapneumonic effusions: an evidence-based guideline. *Chest.* 2000;118:1158–1171.

Davies HE, Davies RJ, Davies CW, et al. Management of pleural infection in adults: British Thoracic Society pleural disease guideline. *Thorax.* 2010;65:41–53.

Fartoukh M, Azoulay E, Galliot R, et al. Clinically documented pleural effusions in medical ICU Patients: how useful is routine thoracentesis? *Chest.* 2002;121:178–184.

Ferrer JS, Munoz XG, Orriols RM, et al. Evolution of idiopathic pleural effusion: a prospective, long-term follow-up study. *Chest.* 1996;109:1508–1513.

Heffner JE, Brown LK, Barbieri CA. Diagnostic value of tests that discriminate between exudative and transudative pleural effusions. Primary study investigators. *Chest.* 1997;111:970–980.

Lichtenstein DA, Meziere G, Lascols N, et al. Ultrasound diagnosis of occult pneumothorax. *Crit Care Med.* 2005;33:1231–1238.

Light RW. Pleural controversy: optimal chest tube size for drainage. *Respirology.* 2011;16:244–248.

Light RW. Pleural Diseases. 4th ed. Philadelphia, PA: Lippincott Willams & Wilkins; 2001.

Lin YC, Tu CY, Liang SJ, et al. Pigtail catheter for the management of pneumothorax in mechanically ventilated patients. *Am J Emerg Med.* 2010;28:466–471.

Mattison LE, Coppage L, Alderman DF, et al. Pleural effusions in the medical ICU: prevalence, causes, and clinical implications. *Chest.* 1997;111:1018–1023.

Rahman NM, Maskell NA, Davies CW, et al. The relationship between chest tube size and clinical outcome in pleural infection. *Chest.* 2010;137:536–543.

Rahman NM, Maskell NA, West A, et al. Intrapleural use of tissue plasminogen activator and DNase in pleural infection. *N Engl J Med.* 2011;365:518–526.

Travaline JM, McKenna RJ Jr, De Giacomo T, et al. Treatment of persistent pulmonary air leaks using endobronchial valves. *Chest.* 2009;136:355–360.

Tu CY, Hsu WH, Hsia TC, et al. Pleural effusions in febrile medical ICU patients: chest ultrasound study. *Chest.* 2004;126:1274–1280.

Vives M, Porcel JM, Vicente de Vera M, et al. A study of Light's criteria and possible modifications for distinguishing exudative from transudative pleural effusions. *Chest.* 1996;109:1503–1507.

17 Weaning of Mechanical Ventilation

Shweta Sood and Chad A. Witt

Intubation for airway protection and respiratory failure is common in the intensive care unit (ICU). It is estimated that 800,000 patients are intubated annually in the United States. The complications of mechanical ventilation, such as infection and airway trauma are well described. For this reason, it is important to proceed with mechanical ventilation withdrawal as quickly as the patient will tolerate. The gradual withdrawal of mechanical ventilation is termed *weaning*. Weaning can be divided into two components: (a) *liberation* refers to no longer requiring mechanical ventilatory support and (b) *extubation/decannulation* refers to the removal of the endotracheal or tracheostomy tube. The weaning of mechanical ventilation in the ICU setting for acute respiratory failure is discussed below, prolonged ventilator weaning after severe chronic illness is beyond the scope of this chapter.

There are multiple weaning strategies and spontaneous breathing trial (SBT) protocols that have been studied and utilized. Mechanical ventilation weaning is a sequential process. First, the underlying disease process causing the patient's initial respiratory failure must be significantly improved or resolved. Second, the patient must be awake, able to cooperate, hemodynamically stable, and able to cough and protect the airway. Minimal ventilator settings with positive end-expiratory pressure (PEEP) less than 8 cm H_2O and FiO_2 less than 50% are ideal. Other parameters, such as negative inspiratory force, should be assessed in selected patients including those with underlying neuromuscular disease. Patients should be on minimal or no vasopressor therapy. Third, daily spontaneous awakening trials (SATs) should begin that stop or reduce sedatives. A patient's mental status can be assessed during SATs. The patient should be cooperative, able to follow simple commands, and calm on minimal or no sedation. If an SAT is successful and the patient is on minimal ventilator settings, an SBT should be initiated. Patients who are intubated on mechanical ventilation should be evaluated for readiness to undergo an SBT on a daily basis (Algorithm 17.1). Protocols driven by nurses and respiratory therapists have been shown to improve the efficiency of the weaning process. Computer-driven protocols have also been associated with decreased duration of mechanical ventilation and ICU length of stay.

SBTs can be done using pressure support ventilation (PSV), continuous positive airway pressure (CPAP), or T-tube technique. Using PSV, a pressure support of 5 to 10 cm H_2O is delivered to help the patient overcome the resistance of the endotracheal tube, usually accompanied by a PEEP of 5 cm H_2O. During a CPAP trial, 5 cm H_2O of CPAP is provided. Lastly, the T-tube technique provides oxygen flow without any pressure support or CPAP during the trial. The duration of SBT should be 30 to 60 minutes. The head of the bed should be elevated 30 to 60 degrees to optimize diaphragmatic mechanics.

ALGORITHM 17.1 — Readiness to Liberate and Wean from Mechanical Ventilation

Is the patient ready for a spontaneous breathing trial?
- Evidence for reversal of the underlying cause of respiratory failure
- Patient is awake, alert, and cooperative
- Adequate oxygenation (e.g., PEEP ≤5 cm H_2O; PaO_2 >60 mm Hg with FiO_2 <0.50)
- Hemodynamically stable: on no vasopressor or inotropic agents or stable minimal doses of vasopressors or inotropes; no evidence of myocardial ischemia; HR <140 beats/min.
- Afebrile (T <38.0°C)
- pH and $PaCO_2$ appropriate for patient's baseline respiratory status

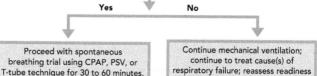

Yes → Proceed with spontaneous breathing trial using CPAP, PSV, or T-tube technique for 30 to 60 minutes.

No → Continue mechanical ventilation; continue to treat cause(s) of respiratory failure; reassess readiness for spontaneous breathing trial daily.

Is the patient tolerating the spontaneous breathing trial?
- RSBI <105 breaths/min/L
- Gas exchange acceptable (SaO_2 ≥90%; PaO_2 ≥60 mm Hg; pH ≥7.32; increase in $PaCO_2$ ≤10 mm Hg from start of trial)
- Stable respiratory rate (RR ≤30 to 35 breaths/min, change in RR <50%)
- Hemodynamically stable (HR <120 to 140, HR increase by less than 20%, SBP >90 mm Hg and <180 mm Hg, change in SBP <20%)
- No significant change in mental status, evidence of anxiety, or agitation
- No diaphoresis or signs of increased work of breathing (use of accessory muscles, paradoxical breathing)

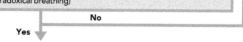

No (returns up to Continue mechanical ventilation)

Yes ↓

Is the patient ready to be extubated?
- Is the patient's airway patent?
- Can the patient protect his/her airway?
- Can the patient clear his/her secretions?

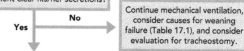

No → Continue mechanical ventilation, consider causes for weaning failure (Table 17.1), and consider evaluation for tracheostomy.

Yes ↓

Proceed with extubation

ABBREVIATIONS
PaO_2: arterial partial pressure of oxygen
FiO_2: fraction of inspired oxygen
PEEP: positive end-expiratory pressure
HR: heart rate
T: temperature
$PaCO_2$: arterial partial pressure of carbon dioxide
CPAP: continuous positive airway pressure
PSV: pressure support ventilation
RSBI: rapid shallow breathing index
SaO_2: arterial oxygen saturation
RR: respiratory rate
SBP: systolic blood pressure

TABLE 17.1	Issues to Be Considered When Weaning Efforts Fail

Weaning parameters (see Algorithm 17.1)

Endotracheal tube
  Use the largest tube possible
  Consider use of supplemental pressure support ventilation during spontaneous
    breathing trial
  Suction secretions

Arterial blood gases
  Avoid or treat metabolic alkalosis
  Maintain PaO_2 at 60–65 mm Hg to avoid increased shunt in patients with
    chronic CO_2 retention
  For patients with CO_2 retention, keep $PaCO_2$ at or above the baseline level

Nutrition
  Ensure adequate nutritional support
  Avoid electrolyte deficiencies
  Avoid excessive calories

Secretions
  Clear regularly
  Avoid excessive dehydration

Neuromuscular factors
  Avoid neuromuscular depressing drugs (neuromuscular blockers, aminoglycosides,
    clindamycin) in patients with muscle weakness
  Avoid unnecessary corticosteroids

Obstruction of airways
  Use bronchodilators when appropriate
  Exclude foreign bodies within the airway

Wakefulness
  Avoid oversedation
  Wean in morning or when patient is most awake

From Kollef MH. Critical care. In: Green GB, Harris IS, Lin GA, et al., eds. *The Washington Manual of Medical Therapeutics*. 31st ed. Philadelphia, PA: Lippincott Williams & Wilkins; 2004:192.

Determining success or failure of SBTs performed using the T-tube technique has been studied rigorously. The most useful measure is the rapid shallow breathing index, defined as the respiratory rate/tidal volume (f:Vt ratio). A rapid shallow breathing index of <105 breaths/min/L during an SBT indicates that a patient is more likely to be successfully extubated. A successful SBT is also defined by pulmonary and hemodynamic stability (respiratory rate less than 35/minute, minimal change in heart rate, blood pressure, and oxygen saturations, minimal anxiety, and no increase in work of breathing). Thus a quick physical assessment should be done before and after each SBT to assess hemodynamic parameters and overall patient comfort during the SBT.

Difficult-to-wean patients are those who do not wean from mechanical ventilation within 48 to 72 hours of resolution of their underlying disease process. In such patients, the acronym "WEANS NOW" has been developed as a set of factors to be considered in difficult-to-wean patients (Table 17.1).

A successful SAT/SBT should prompt extubation. Prior to extubation, the endotracheal tube and airways should be suctioned to clear secretions. A cuff leak test should be performed by a physician or respiratory therapist. The absence of a cuff leak in patients with prolonged intubation suggests laryngeal edema and should postpone extubation pending further evaluation and treatment if indicated. If a cuff leak is present, extubation should proceed.

After extubation, most patients can be safely transitioned to nasal cannula oxygen, although some patients may benefit from or require noninvasive positive pressure ventilation (NIPPV) after extubation. Patients should be asked to cough several times within the first few minutes of extubation to clear any secretions. It should be kept in mind that there will be extubation failures in patients who are deemed ready by all objective evaluations (reported reintubation rates 11% to 23.5%); these patients may benefit from early tracheostomy. Given this risk of recurrent respiratory failure, patients should be monitored in the ICU for a period of time in order to ensure reintubation is not required.

SUGGESTED READINGS

Calfee CS, Matthay MA. Recent advances in mechanical ventilation. *Am J Med.* 2005; 118(6):584–591.
> *Review of mechanical ventilation, including noninvasive ventilation, ventilating patients with acute respiratory distress syndrome, and weaning of mechanical ventilation.*

Ferrer M, Valencia M, Nicolas JM, et al. Early noninvasive ventilation averts extubation failure in patients at risk: a randomized trial. *Am J Respir Crit Care Med.* 2006;173(2):164–170.

Kollef MH. Critical care. In: Green GB, Harris IS, Lin GA, et al., eds. *The Washington Manual of Medical Therapeutics.* 31st ed. Philadelphia, PA: Lippincott Williams & Wilkins; 2004:192.
> *"WEANS NOW" acronym for the difficult-to-wean patient.*

Kollef MH, Shapiro SD, Silver P, et al. A randomized, controlled trial of protocol-directed versus physician-directed weaning from mechanical ventilation. *Crit Care Med.* 1997;25(4): 567–574.
> *Randomized, controlled trial showing that protocol-guided weaning of mechanical ventilation performed by nurses and respiratory therapists is effective, and resulted in earlier extubation than physician-directed weaning.*

Lellouche F, Mancebo J, Jolliet P, et al. A multicenter randomized trial of computer-driven protocolized weaning from mechanical ventilation. *Am J Respir Crit Care Med.* 2006;174(8): 894–900.
> *Randomized trial demonstrating that duration of mechanical ventilation and length of ICU stay were decreased by using a computer-driven weaning protocol versus physician-controlled weaning according to local guidelines.*

MacIntyre N. Evidence-based guidelines for weaning and discontinuing ventilatory support: a collective task force facilitated by the American College of Chest Physicians; the American Association for Respiratory Care; and the American College of Critical Care Medicine. *Chest.* 2001;120(6 suppl):375S–396S.
> *Evidence-based review and guidelines for weaning, including spontaneous breathing trials, weaning protocols, and the use of tracheostomy for failure to wean.*

Manthous CA, Schmidt GA, Hall JB. Liberation from mechanical ventilation: a decade of progress. *Chest.* 1998;114(3):886–901.
> *Review of current practices and advances in assessment of readiness for liberation, weaning strategies, and extubation.*

McConville JF, Kress JP. Weaning patients from the ventilator. *N Engl J Med.* 2012;367(23): 2233–2239.

Meade M, Guyatt G, Cook D, et al. Predicting success in weaning from mechanical ventilation. *Chest.* 2001;120(6 suppl):400–424.
Meta-analysis of 63 studies evaluating predictors of successful weaning, including the rapid shallow breathing index.

Rumbak MJ, Newton M, Truncale T, et al. A prospective, randomized, study comparing early percutaneous dilational tracheostomy to prolonged translaryngeal intubation (delayed tracheotomy) in critically ill medical patients. *Crit Care Med.* 2004;32(8):1689–1694.
Prospective, randomized trial showing the benefit of early tracheotomy over prolonged translaryngeal intubation.

Tobin MJ. Advances in mechanical ventilation. *N Engl J Med.* 2001;334(26):1986–1996.
Review of mechanical ventilation strategies, including modes of ventilation, use of positive end-expiratory pressure, and discontinuation of mechanical ventilation.

18 Noninvasive Ventilation

Britney M. Ramgopal and Adam Anderson

INTRODUCTION

Noninvasive ventilation (NIV) delivers mechanically assisted breaths using tight-fitting masks or interfaces, all with separate benefits and limitations (Table 18.1). NIV may prevent the need for endotracheal intubation, but requires optimal patient selection and frequent reevaluation. The correct NIV mode and patient-tailored settings are imperative for success.

PATIENT SELECTION

Although NIV can be used in several situations, appropriate selection is necessary for optimal outcomes. Broadly, NIV can be considered in patients with either hypoxemic or hypercarbic respiratory failure, especially if the clinical deterioration is felt to be rapidly reversible. The best evidence to support its use is with acute exacerbations of chronic obstructive pulmonary disease (AECOPD) and acute cardiogenic pulmonary edema, though the use of NIV is frequently extended to additional patients.

Equally important are contraindications to trials of NIV. Generally accepted absolute contraindications include inability to fit the NIV mask appropriately, cardiopulmonary arrest, and need for urgent intubation. There are several relative contraindications; most commonly encountered relative contraindications include encephalopathy with inability to protect ones airway, uncooperativeness, and claustrophobia. Additional relative contraindications are provided in Table 18.2.

The advantages of NIV over invasive mechanical ventilation (IMV) have resulted in its widespread implementation over a variety of clinical scenarios. Generally, patients with hypoxemia, hypercapnea, or respiratory muscle fatigue who do not have an absolute or relative contraindication warrant a trial of NIV.

Modes

Once the decision to initiate NIV is made, the optimal mode and settings must be considered. A simplified approach to understanding different NIV options is to differentiate by settings available for manipulation. Common modes of NIV are summarized in Table 18.3 with benefits and limitations emphasized.

Continuous positive airway pressure (CPAP) is the simplest mode of NIV. A constant pressure is set via the ventilator that is provided throughout the entire respiratory cycle. The correlate to an IMV setting is the positive end-expiratory pressure (PEEP). As this mode only provides a continuous pressure, CPAP is a spontaneous

TABLE 18.1	Types of Masks/Interfaces	
Interface	Advantages	Disadvantages
Nasal pillow	• Improved patient comfort • Able to speak and swallow during use	• Air leaks from the uncovered mouth • Not advised for use during acute respiratory failure
Nasal mask	• Improved patient comfort • Able to speak and swallow during use	• Air leaks from the uncovered mouth • Not advised for use during acute respiratory failure • Potential for cutaneous breakdown at nasal bridge
Full face mask (Oronasal mask)	• Better for mouth breathers • Mask of choice for initiation of NIV	• Potential for cutaneous breakdown at nasal bridge • Limited use in claustrophobic patients
Total face mask	• Better for mouth breathers • Easier use for patients with facial irregularities • No pressure applied to nasal bridge	• Limited use in claustrophobic patients
Helmet	• Better for mouth breathers • Easier use for patients with facial irregularities • More comfortable seal • Diminished leaks	• Carbon dioxide accumulates in helmet • Not approved for use by U.S. FDA

mode of ventilation that requires patient initiation and respiratory muscle effort. Therefore, no respiratory rate or minute ventilation is targeted or guaranteed. **The clinical benefit of CPAP is most evident in hypoxemic respiratory failure** as the positive airway pressure predominately augments oxygenation with the goal of recruiting alveoli, increasing functional residual capacity, and decreasing shunting. CPAP is typically less uncomfortable than other NIV modes and may improve tolerance.

Bilevel positive airway pressure (BiPAP), in contrast to CPAP, provides both an expiratory positive airway pressure (EPAP) and inspiratory positive airway pressure (IPAP). The EPAP setting is functionally synonymous with the CPAP mode providing a continuous baseline pressure throughout the respiratory cycle. The IPAP, however, is an additional inspiratory pressure that is either patient or

TABLE 18.2	Relative Contraindications to NIV	
Shock/hemodynamic instability	Facial surgery, trauma, or deformity	
Claustrophobia/anxiety	Upper airway obstruction	
Encephalopathy	Inability to protect airway	
Upper gastrointestinal bleeding	High risk for aspiration	
Unstable cardiac rhythm	Inability to clear secretions	

TABLE 18.3	Common Modes of NIV		
	CPAP	**BiPAP**	**AVAPS**
Settings	• Initiate PEEP at 5 cm H_2O • Increase by increments of 1–2 cm H_2O • Max 20 cm H_2O • FiO_2 0.21–1	• Initiate IPAP at 10 cm H_2O and EPAP at 5 cm H_2O • Increase IPAP in increments of 2–3 cm H_2O • EPAP may also need to be increased in obese patients • Max IPAP 20–25 cm H_2O • FiO_2 0.21–1	• Set goal tidal volume (6–8 mL/kg of ideal body weight) • Set EPAP at 5 cm H_2O • Set IPAP range • Min EPAP + 4 cm H_2O • Max 25 cm H_2O • FiO_2 0.21–1
Benefits	• Typically best tolerated at lower pressure requirements • Simplest titration • Widely available • Well studied	• Better tolerated than CPAP at high pressure requirements • Widely available • Well studied • Backup respiratory rate • Manipulations of IPAP/EPAP delta improve tidal volume	• Better tolerated than CPAP at high pressure requirements • Backup respiratory rate • Tidal volume guaranteed • Better approximation of goal minute ventilation
Limitations	• No respiratory rate setting • No guaranteed tidal volume/minute ventilation	• No set tidal volume/minute ventilation	• Targeted but not guaranteed minute ventilation • Newer mode of NIV • Not widely available • Less well studied

entilator triggered. The change in pressure gradient supports the muscles of respiration resulting in an improvement in tidal volume and, thus, alveolar ventilation. As the delta between IPAP and EPAP is increased on the NIV, tidal volume should also improve. Given its impact on minute ventilation, and ability to set a minimal respiratory rate, **BiPAP has utility in both hypoxemic and hypercarbic respiratory failure.**

Average volume-assured pressure support (AVAPS) is similar to BiPAP as it provides an IPAP on continuous EPAP; the inherent difference is the clinician-defined parameters. An EPAP is identically chosen as in BiPAP; however, an IPAP range is selected to target a goal tidal volume. Therefore, as patient effort varies, the NIV will either uptitrate IPAP to increase, or downtitrate to decrease to the targeted inhaled tidal volume. By setting a minimal respiratory rate and target inhaled tidal volume, a provider can more closely target a goal minute ventilation. **Thus, AVAPS also has utility in both hypoxemic and hypercarbic respiratory failure.**

Specific Clinical Scenarios

AECOPD has been the benchmark for NIV use in the intensive care unit (ICU). In these patients NIV compared to IMV reduces the risk of hospital-acquired pneumonia, shortens length of stay, decreases cost, and improves hospital mortality. Algorithm 18.1 provides a generic algorithmic approach to initiating BiPAP in a patient with AECOPD.

Asthma exacerbations, although often treated with NIV, do not have strong evidence supporting its use. Extrapolating data from AECOPD would suggest a clinical benefit. As status asthmaticus is difficult to manage with IMV, a trial of NIV is reasonable while other pharmacotherapy is administered. As with any patient, intubation and IMV should proceed if no improvement.

Acute cardiopulmonary edema treated with NIV improves gas exchange and symptomatic dyspnea better than standard oxygen therapy. CPAP is a standard therapy; however, for those with underlying lung disease, worsened lung mechanics, or hypercarbia, BiPAP may be a more appropriate choice. Use of NIV in this population results in reduced intubation rates and decreased in-hospital mortality.

Studies on patients with pneumonia treated with NIV have yielded conflicting results: some showing benefit, others demonstrating potential harm. As the pathophysiology and clinical course frequently take several days to improve, NIV may not alter the need for IMV, especially if secretions are copious and airway clearance is an issue. Practitioners should use clinical judgment while selecting these patients for a NIV trial and not hesitate to proceed to intubation if necessary. A caveat is in immunocompromised patients, supporting a different pathophysiology in the host response to pneumonia. Some trials have shown that, in immunocompromised patients with acute hypoxemic respiratory failure secondary to pneumonia, NIV showed benefit with a decrease in intubation rate, ICU duration, and ICU mortality. Other studies have been unable to demonstrate similar benefits, and showed NIV may actually increase mortality. Regardless, societal guidelines suggest a trial of NIV may be reasonable in immunocompromised patients with pneumonia.

NIV postextubation reduces the rate of reintubation and improves mortality. These benefits are most prominent in patients with COPD; however, smaller studies have shown similar outcomes in a mixed population. NIV does not prevent reintubation when applied after a recently extubated patient develops new respiratory failure and may in fact increase mortality in this population.

ALGORITHM 18.1 — Algorithm for the Initiation of BiPAP in a Patient with a COPD Exacerbation

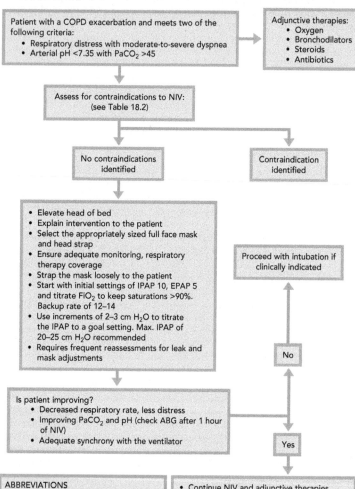

Patient with a COPD exacerbation and meets two of the following criteria:
- Respiratory distress with moderate-to-severe dyspnea
- Arterial pH <7.35 with $PaCO_2$ >45

Adjunctive therapies:
- Oxygen
- Bronchodilators
- Steroids
- Antibiotics

Assess for contraindications to NIV:
(see Table 18.2)

No contraindications identified

Contraindication identified

- Elevate head of bed
- Explain intervention to the patient
- Select the appropriately sized full face mask and head strap
- Ensure adequate monitoring, respiratory therapy coverage
- Strap the mask loosely to the patient
- Start with initial settings of IPAP 10, EPAP 5 and titrate FiO_2 to keep saturations >90%. Backup rate of 12–14
- Use increments of 2–3 cm H_2O to titrate the IPAP to a goal setting. Max. IPAP of 20–25 cm H_2O recommended
- Requires frequent reassessments for leak and mask adjustments

Proceed with intubation if clinically indicated

No

Is patient improving?
- Decreased respiratory rate, less distress
- Improving $PaCO_2$ and pH (check ABG after 1 hour of NIV)
- Adequate synchrony with the ventilator

Yes

ABBREVIATIONS
NIV: noninvasive venitlation
IPAP: inspiratory positive airway pressure
EPAP: expiratory positive airway pressure
ABG: arterial blood gas

- Continue NIV and adjunctive therapies
- Frequent reassessment of patients condition

Beyond acute indications in the ICU, chronic outpatient nocturnal NIV is common in diseases such as obstructive sleep apnea (OSA), obesity hypoventilation syndrome (OHS), and neuromuscular conditions. In this setting, benefits in sleep architecture, nocturnal oxygen, and carbon dioxide levels are evident. Patients with these comorbidities are frequently admitted to the ICU; continuation of NIV is appropriate when no contraindications exist.

MONITORING

Regardless of the interface, appropriate fit is key to assuring patient comfort and providing effective ventilatory support. Air leaks due to poorly fitting masks impair detection of inspiratory effort and end expiration. Overly tight masks can lead to pressure ulcers and skin necrosis. Careful adjustment of the ventilator settings and mask fit improves patient tolerance and compliance. Importantly, the delivered tidal volume is displayed as opposed to exhaled tidal volume as on an invasive ventilator.

Patients receiving NIV require close monitoring and frequent assessments. Most patients require admission to an intensive or respiratory care unit. Sequential assessment of mental status, respiratory rate, accessory muscle usage, chest wall movement, coordination of respiratory effort with the ventilator, and overall comfort is necessary. Periodic monitoring with arterial blood gas analysis adds objective data and evaluates response to NIV. Breaks from NIV, assuming clinically acceptable, may improve overall tolerance allowing for a longer duration if needed.

The use of NIV should never delay clinically indicated endotracheal intubation and IMV. Moreover, NIV is a supportive therapy and patients require prompt treatment of the underlying medical conditions leading to respiratory failure.

CONCLUSIONS

NIV has become a valuable tool for the management of respiratory failure. When employed appropriately, it may negate the need for endotracheal intubation and associated complications. However, mask choice, NIV settings, and close monitoring are required to optimize success.

SUGGESTED READINGS

Allison MG, Winters ME. Noninvasive ventilation for the emergency physician. *Emerg Med Clin North Am.* 2016;34(1):51–62.

Garpestad E, Brennan J, Hill NS. Noninvasive ventilation for critical care. *Chest.* 2007;132(2):711–720.

Gregoretti C, Pisani L, Cortegiani A, et al. Noninvasive ventilation in critically ill patients. *Crit Care Clin.* 2015;31(3):435–457.

Lindenauer P, Stefan M, Shieh MS, et al. Outcomes associated with invasive and noninvasive ventilation among patients hospitalized with exacerbations of chronic obstructive pulmonary disease. *JAMA Intern Med.* 2014;174(12):1982–1993.

Mas A, Masip J. Noninvasive ventilation in acute respiratory failure. *Int J Chron Obstruct Pulmon Dis.* 2014;9:837–852.

Ornico S, Lobo SM, Sanches HS, et al. Noninvasive ventilation immediately after extubation improves weaning outcome after acute respiratory failure: a randomized controlled trial. *Crit Care.* 2013;17(2):R39.

19 Acute Myocardial Infarction

Tyson Turner and Andrew M. Kates

Acute myocardial infarction (AMI) is a common diagnosis among hospitalized and critically ill patients. There are approximately 610,000 new AMIs and 310,000 recurrent AMIs diagnosed annually in the United States; three-fourths of these events will be non–ST-elevation acute coronary syndromes (NSTE-ACS). Despite improved survival during the last several decades, roughly one in five patients admitted with AMI will die within the following year.

A rapid and detailed assessment of symptoms is crucial in determining the likelihood of acute coronary syndrome (ACS) in the patient presenting with chest discomfort. Patients with ACS typically complain of moderate-to-severe chest discomfort that lasts more than 20 minutes. Atypical presentations are not uncommon in women, diabetic patients, and the elderly. An electrocardiogram (ECG) and cardiac-specific serum biomarkers (preferably troponin I or T) are needed to distinguish between ST-segment elevation ACS (STE-ACS), non–ST-segment elevation ACS (NSTE-ACS), and noncardiac chest pain. The diagnosis of *myocardial infarction* is supported by evidence of cardiac myocyte death as demonstrated by elevated cardiac-specific serum biomarkers. Patients who present with ACS and STE on ECG have actively infarcting myocardium and are termed *ST-elevation myocardial infarction* (STEMI) or STE-ACS. Previously, patients with ACS but without STEs were stratified as unstable angina (UA) in the absence of elevated serum cardiac biomarkers, or *non–ST-segment elevation myocardial infarction* (NSTEMI) in their presence. Recent guidelines emphasize the continuum between UA and NSTEMI and therefore consider these entities together under the diagnosis of NSTE-ACS. The goal of the initial evaluation for the ACS patient is prompt diagnosis of STE-ACS or NSTE-ACS with concurrent treatment of the patient's ischemia.

ST-ELEVATION ACUTE CORONARY SYNDROME

STE-ACS results from a sudden occlusion of a coronary artery, which is usually due to plaque rupture in an atherosclerotic coronary artery. Other causes, such as coronary embolism, can also precipitate an STE-ACS. The resultant cascade of events associated with plaque rupture involves platelet activation/aggregation and ultimately thrombus formation. Approximately one-third of patients presenting with STE-ACS do not survive, with nearly half of the deaths in the first hour due to ventricular arrhythmias. The extent of cardiac myocyte death worsens with ischemic time and correlates strongly with cardiac morbidity and mortality, leading to the oft-quoted phrase "time is muscle." As such, mechanical and medical therapies designed to reestablish blood flow in the shortest time possible are the mainstay of the therapy.

A management pathway which combines established benchmark goals and treatment options for the patient with STE-ACS/STEMI is essential for optimal care (Algorithm 19.1, Table 19.1). Mechanical support with an intra-aortic balloon pump (IABP) or a percutaneous ventricular assist device (such as Impella 2.5 or 5.0) in the patient with hemodynamic or rhythm instability, severe heart failure, or cardiogenic shock should be considered for mechanical support.

NON–ST-ELEVATION ACUTE CORONARY SYNDROME

The evaluation and management of patients with NSTE-ACS is outlined in Algorithm 19.2. Patients who present with NSTE-ACS should undergo evaluation to assess for risk of major adverse cardiac events (MACE), defined as death, nonfatal myocardial infarction, and stroke. A useful and well-validated method for risk stratification is the Thrombolysis in Myocardial Infarction (TIMI) risk score. Patients with a higher score are more likely to suffer from MACE than those with a lower score. All patients should receive medical management appropriate to their level of risk and, importantly, should be considered for diagnostic angiography with intent to perform percutaneous coronary intervention (PCI). High-risk patients benefit from early revascularization therapies.

HOSPITAL CARE OF THE ACS PATIENT

Patients with ACS are at an increased risk for recurrent MI and death during both hospitalization and after discharge. Hospitalization and subsequent office visits provide venues with which to work with patients to reduce the risk of further events. The mnemonic "ABCDE" is a thoughtful way to organize the various in-hospital and postdischarge treatments (Table 19.2). These items can be considered an acute treatment guide as well as a discharge checklist for any patient admitted with ACS.

Classifying Myocardial Infarctions

Classification of different types of myocardial infarctions is important as their management may differ from the recommendations for STE and NSTE-ACS (Table 19.3). A type 1 MI is due to ischemia from an unstable coronary plaque and leads to thrombus formation, which may (as in STE-ACS) or may not (as in NSTE-ACS) completely occlude blood flow. A type 2 MI occurs with an increased demand or a decreased supply of myocardial oxygen. Typically, patients with type 2 MIs have fixed coronary artery atheromas that do not cause ischemia at rest but can induce ischemia at times of increased oxygen utilization (e.g., tachycardia, surgery, severe hypertension) or decreased oxygen delivery (e.g., anemia, hypoxia, hypotension, sepsis). Intraoperative MIs are most commonly due to myocardial oxygen supply–demand mismatch and often manifest postoperatively as elevated cardiac biomarkers. Our recommended algorithm for the treatment of type 2 MI is shown in Algorithm 19.3.

Two unique forms of type 2 MIs are stress-induced ("Takotsubo") and sepsis-induced cardiomyopathies. Both syndromes are driven by an excess of catecholamines and can be difficult to differentiate from ACS. Patients with these syndromes manifest ischemic ECG changes, echocardiographic abnormalities including focal wall motion abnormalities and depressed left ventricular (LV) systolic function, and elevated cardiac biomarkers. Patients with suspected stress-induced cardiomyopathy

ALGORITHM 19.1 Goals and Treatment of ST-Segment Elevation Myocardial Infarction/ST-Segment Elevation Acute Coronary Syndrome

PATIENT
GOAL: Time of symptom onset to calling EMS ≤5 minutes[a]

↓

TRANSPORT
GOAL: EMS on the scene ≤8 minutes
Consider prehospital fibrinolysis (if available).

↓

MEDICAL FACILITY-3D'S-DATA, DECISION, DRUGS
DATA—Focused history and physical exam.
GOAL: ECG ≤10 minutes
STEMI = ischemic symptoms <u>with:</u>
    1) ≥1-mm ST elevation in two contiguous leads **OR**
    2) New LBBB

- If inferior MI (leads II, III, avF)→ <u>right-sided ECG</u> (rV4) for right ventricular MI
- If ST depression in precordial leads→ <u>posterior ECG</u> (V7, V8, V9) for posterior MI

↓

DECISION—PRIMARY PCI

GOAL: Medical contact-to-balloon time ≤90 minutes

<u>Preferred over fibrinolytics if available</u>

Also preferred when:
- Severe congestive heart failure
- Cardiogenic shock
- Unstable ventricular arrhythmias
- Contraindication to fibrinolytic therapy
- Late presentation (>3 hours of symptoms)
- The diagnosis of STEMI is in doubt

DECISION—FIBRINOLYTIC THERAPY

GOAL: Medical contact-to-needle time ≤30 minutes

Preferred when:
- Lack of available PCI facility
- Delay in transport to PCI facility
- Contraindication to PCI

<u>Absolute</u> contraindications to fibrinolytics:
  History of any intracranial hemorrhage
  Ischemic stroke <3 months
  Known intracranial malignant neoplasm
  Known cerebral vascular lesion
  Active bleeding or bleeding diathesis
  Known or suspected aortic dissection
  Closed head or facial trauma <3 months

<u>Relative</u> contraindications to fibrinolytics:
  BP >190/110
  CPR >10 minutes
  Ischemic stroke >3 months
  INR >2.0
  Recent internal bleeding within 2–4 weeks
  Noncompressible vascular puncture
  Pregnancy
  Recent major surgery

DECISION—PCI AFTER FIBRINOLYSIS

If a patient has received fibrinolytics at a non–PCI-capable facility and is a high-risk STEMI, then immediate transfer to a PCI-capable facility should be arranged

Continued on next page

Continued on next page

ALGORITHM 19.1 Goals and Treatment of ST-Segment Elevation Myocardial Infarction/ST-Segment Elevation Acute Coronary Syndrome (*Continued*)

DRUGS—Unless contraindicated, all patients receive:
- Aspirin 162–325 mg chewed
- Metoprolol 5 mg IV every 5 minutes × 3 doses unless patient has any contraindications[b]
- IV nitroglycerin, started at 10 mcg/min and titrated for symptoms[c]
- Consider morphine sulfate 2–4 mg IV for chest pain unresponsive to nitrates
- Options for anticoagulant therapy in patients treated with **primary PCI:**
  - Unfractionated heparin (UFH): 50–70 U/kg IV bolus, max 4000–5000 U; then 12 U/kg/hr, max 1000 U/hr
  - Bivalirudin: 0.75 mg/kg IV bolus; then 1.75 mg/kg/hr IV infusion until PCI
- Options for anticoagulant therapy in patients treated with **fibrinolysis:**
  - Enoxaparin (Lovenox): If <75 years, 30 mg IV bolus followed by 1 mg/kg SQ Q12H (first SQ dose should be given with IV bolus, max of 100 mg for first two SQ doses); if >75 years, then omit IV bolus and inject 0.75 mg/kg SQ Q12H; avoid if Cr >2.0
  - UFH: 60–100 U/kg IV bolus, max 4000 units, then 12 U/kg/hr (max 1000 U/hr) to goal aPTT 50–70 seconds
  - Fondaparinux: 2.5 mg IV, then 2.5 mg SQ Q24H; avoid in CrCl <30 mL/min
- Options for antiplatelet therapy:
  Note: If there is a high suspicion for CAD that may require CABG (i.e., diabetes or known multivessel CAD), consider withholding a loading dose until the anatomy is defined:
  - Clopidogrel (Plavix) 300–600 mg PO loading dose
  - Ticagrelor (Brilinta) 180 mg loading dose
  - Prasugrel (Effient) 60 mg PO loading dose for patients at the time of PCI only; avoid use if body weight <60 kg, history of stroke/TIA, age ≥75 years, or increased risk of bleeding

DRUGS—PRIMARY PCI
Use and selection of a GP-IIb/IIIa inhibitor should be determined at the time of PCI by the interventional cardiologist

REPERFUSION—PRIMARY PCI
GOAL: Restoration of TIMI 3 flow (i.e., complete perfusion)
Advantages of PCI over fibrinolytics:
1) Superior restoration of coronary flow
2) Defines anatomy
3) Fewer complications
4) Treatment of thrombus AND plaque

DRUGS—FIBRINOLYTIC
Regimens include:
Alteplase + UFH
    Alteplase 15 mg bolus, then 0.75 mg/kg (max 50 mg) over 30 minutes, then 0.5 mg/kg (max 35 mg) over next 60 minutes
    UFH IV as detailed above

Reteplase (Retavase) + UFH
    Reteplase 10 U IV bolus over 2 minutes and repeat 10 U IV bolus 30 minutes later
    UFH IV as detailed above

Tenecteplase (TNKase) + UFH
    TNKase dose is based on weight (see **Table 19.1**)
    UFH IV as detailed above

REPERFUSION—THROMBOLYSIS
Considered successful if:
1) Complete resolution of chest pain
2) ST-segment elevation improvement >50%

If unsuccessful or the development of hemodynamic or electrical instability, consider transfer to center capable of rescue PCI

ABBREVIATIONS
aPPT:	activated partial thromboplastin time
BP:	blood pressure
CABG:	coronary artery bypass grafting
CAD:	coronary artery disease
CPR:	cardiopulmonary resuscitation
Cr:	creatinine
ECG:	electrocardiogram
EMS:	emergency medical services
GP:	glycoprotein
INR:	international normalized ratio
IV:	intravenous
LBBB:	left bundle branch block
MI:	myocardial infarction
PCI:	percutaneous coronary intervention
PO:	by mouth
Q12H:	every 12 hours
Q2H4:	every 24 hours
SQ:	subcutaneous
STEMI:	ST-elevation myocardial infarction
TIA:	transient ischemic attack
TIMI:	thrombolysis in myocardial infarction
UFH:	unfractionated heparin

TABLE 19.1	TNKase Dosing
Weight (kg)	**TNKase (mg)**
<60	30
60–69	35
70–79	40
80–89	45
≥90	50

[a]Patients who have taken SL nitroglycerin should call 911 if symptoms do not improve or worsen within 5 minutes of taking one SL nitroglycerin.

[b]Signs of heart failure; evidence of a low cardiac output; increased risk of cardiogenic shock (age >70 years, SBP <120 mm Hg, HR <60 bpm, or sinus tachycardia >120 bpm, and increased time since onset of symptoms); or relative contraindications to beta blockers (PR interval >0.24 seconds, second- or third-degree heart block, active asthma or reactive airway disease).

[c]Caution if suspected inferior MI, SBP <90 mm Hg, HR <50 bpm or >100 bpm, or phosphodiesterase inhibitors for erectile dysfunction in past 24 to 48 hours.

ALGORITHM 19.2 Risk Stratification and Treatment Algorithm for Non–ST-Segment Elevation Myocardial Infarction

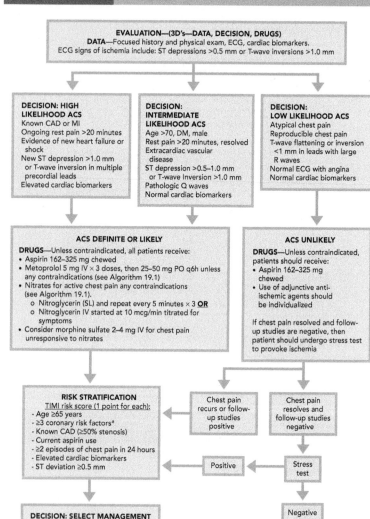

EVALUATION—(3D's—DATA, DECISION, DRUGS)
DATA—Focused history and physical exam, ECG, cardiac biomarkers.
ECG signs of ischemia include: ST depressions >0.5 mm or T-wave inversions >1.0 mm

DECISION: HIGH LIKELIHOOD ACS
Known CAD or MI
Ongoing rest pain >20 minutes
Evidence of new heart failure or shock
New ST depression >1.0 mm or T-wave inversion in multiple precordial leads
Elevated cardiac biomarkers

DECISION: INTERMEDIATE LIKELIHOOD ACS
Age >70, DM, male
Rest pain >20 minutes, resolved
Extracardiac vascular disease
ST depression >0.5–1.0 mm or T-wave Inversion >1.0 mm
Pathologic Q waves
Normal cardiac biomarkers

DECISION: LOW LIKELIHOOD ACS
Atypical chest pain
Reproducible chest pain
T-wave flattening or inversion <1 mm in leads with large R waves
Normal ECG with angina
Normal cardiac biomarkers

ACS DEFINITE OR LIKELY
DRUGS—Unless contraindicated, all patients receive:
- Aspirin 162–325 mg chewed
- Metoprolol 5 mg IV × 3 doses, then 25–50 mg PO q6h unless any contraindications (see Algorithm 19.1)
- Nitrates for active chest pain any contraindications (see Algorithm 19.1).
  o Nitroglycerin (SL) and repeat every 5 minutes × 3 **OR**
  o Nitroglycerin IV started at 10 mcg/min titrated for symptoms
- Consider morphine sulfate 2–4 mg IV for chest pain unresponsive to nitrates

ACS UNLIKELY
DRUGS—Unless contraindicated, patients should receive:
- Aspirin 162–325 mg chewed
- Use of adjunctive anti-ischemic agents should be individualized

If chest pain resolved and follow-up studies are negative, then patient should undergo stress test to provoke ischemia

RISK STRATIFICATION
TIMI risk score (1 point for each):
- Age ≥65 years
- ≥3 coronary risk factors[a]
- Known CAD (≥50% stenosis)
- Current aspirin use
- ≥2 episodes of chest pain in 24 hours
- Elevated cardiac biomarkers
- ST deviation ≥0.5 mm

Chest pain recurs or follow-up studies positive

Chest pain resolves and follow-up studies negative

Positive

Stress test

DECISION: SELECT MANAGEMENT STRATEGY

Negative

Continued on next page

Diagnosis: Likely noncardiac chest discomfort

Arrange for outpatient follow-up

Discharge medications based on risk factors for cardiovascular disease

ALGORITHM 19.2 **Risk Stratification and Treatment Algorithm for Non–ST-Segment Elevation Myocardial Infarction (*Continued*)**

DECISION: SELECT MANAGEMENT STRATEGY

Favors Invasive Strategy:
Recurrent chest pain despite maximal medical therapy
Elevated cardiac biomarkers
New ST-segment depression
Signs of heart failure
New or worsening mitral regurgitation
Hemodynamic instability
Sustained ventricular tachycardia
Prior CABG
High-risk score (e.g., TIMI 5–7)
PCI within 6 months
Reduced LV ejection fraction

Favors Conservative Strategy:
Low-risk score (e.g., TIMI 0–2)
Patient or physician preference
Risk of revascularization outweighs benefits

Calculated TIMI Score	14-day Risk of MACE
0 or 1	5%
2	8%
3	13%
4	20%
5	26%
6 or 7	41%

INVASIVE STRATEGY
(i.e., Diagnostic catheterization with intent to perform PCI)

Early invasive strategy (i.e., requiring immediate catheterization) should be considered in patients with:
- Refractory chest discomfort despite vigorous medical therapy
- Hemodynamic or rhythm instability

CONSERVATIVE STRATEGY

DRUGS—Unless contraindicated, all patients should receive the following regardless of the strategy:
- Options for anticoagulant therapy:
  - Unfractionated heparin, **preferred in early invasive approach**: 60–70 U/kg IV bolus, max 4000–5000 U; then 12 U/kg/hr (max 1000 U/hr), adjusted to achieve goal aPTT of 50–70 seconds
  - Bivalirudin (Angiomax), **preferred in early invasive approach**: 0.1 mg/kg IV bolus; then 0.25 mg/kg/hr until angiography performed
  - Enoxaparin (Lovenox), **preferred in noninvasive strategy**: If NSTE-ACS and not undergoing early invasive approach, no loading dose necessary. Dosing is 1 mg/kg SQ q12h. If CrCl <30 mL/min, dose is 1 mg/kg q24h
  - Fondaparinux (Arixtra), **preferred in noninvasive strategy**: 2.5 mg SQ q24h, avoid if CrCl <30 mL/min
- Options for dual antiplatelet therapy:
  - *For the invasive strategy, if there is a high suspicion for CAD that may require CABG (e.g., diabetes or known multivessel CAD), then consider with holding therapy and starting a GP IIb/IIIa inhibitor until the anatomy is defined:*
  - Clopidogrel (Plavix) 300–600 mg PO loading dose then 75 mg daily
  - Ticagrelor 180 mg loading dose
    Note: for patients undergoing PCI, can consider Prasugrel 60 mg PO loading dose at the time of PCI then 10 mg daily (see Algorithm 19.1 for contraindications)

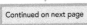

Continued on next page

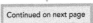

Continued on next page

ALGORITHM 19.2 Risk Stratification and Treatment Algorithm for Non–ST-Segment Elevation Myocardial Infarction (*Continued*)

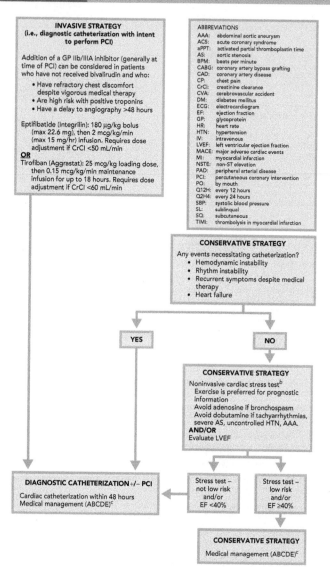

INVASIVE STRATEGY
(i.e., diagnostic catheterization with intent to perform PCI)

Addition of a GP IIb/IIIa inhibitor (generally at time of PCI) can be considered in patients who have not received bivalirudin and who:

- Have refractory chest discomfort despite vigorous medical therapy
- Are high risk with positive troponins
- Have a delay to angiography >48 hours

Eptifibatide (Integrilin): 180 µg/kg bolus (max 22.6 mg), then 2 mcg/kg/min (max 15 mg/hr) infusion. Requires dose adjustment if CrCl <50 mL/min
OR
Tirofiban (Aggrastat): 25 mcg/kg loading dose, then 0.15 mcg/kg/min maintenance infusion for up to 18 hours. Requires dose adjustment if CrCl <60 mL/min

ABBREVIATIONS

AAA: abdominal aortic aneurysm
ACS: acute coronary syndrome
aPPT: activated partial thromboplastin time
AS: aortic stenosis
BPM: beats per minute
CABG: coronary artery bypass grafting
CAD: coronary artery disease
CP: chest pain
CrCl: creatinine clearance
CVA: cerebrovascular accident
DM: diabetes mellitus
ECG: electrocardiogram
EF: ejection fraction
GP: glycoprotein
HR: heart rate
HTN: hypertension
IV: intravenous
LVEF: left ventricular ejection fraction
MACE: major adverse cardiac events
MI: myocardial infarction
NSTE: non-ST elevation
PAD: peripheral arterial disease
PCI: percutaneous coronary intervention
PO: by mouth
Q12H: every 12 hours
Q2H4: every 24 hours
SBP: systolic blood pressure
SL: sublingual
SQ: subcutaneous
TIMI: thrombolysis in myocardial infarction

CONSERVATIVE STRATEGY

Any events necessitating catheterization?
- Hemodynamic instability
- Rhythm instability
- Recurrent symptoms despite medical therapy
- Heart failure

YES   **NO**

CONSERVATIVE STRATEGY

Noninvasive cardiac stress test[b]
Exercise is preferred for prognostic information
Avoid adenosine if bronchospasm
Avoid dobutamine if tachyarrhythmias, severe AS, uncontrolled HTN, AAA.
AND/OR
Evaluate LVEF

DIAGNOSTIC CATHETERIZATION +/– PCI

Cardiac catheterization within 48 hours
Medical management (ABCDE)[c]

Stress test – not low risk and/or EF <40%

Stress test – low risk and/or EF ≥40%

CONSERVATIVE STRATEGY

Medical management (ABCDE)[c]

[a]Coronary risk factors include diabetes mellitus, cigarette smoking, hypertension (>140/90 mm Hg or on antihypertensive medication), low HDL cholesterol (<40 mg/dL), family history of premature CAD (male first-degree relative ≤55 years old or female first-degree relative ≤65 years old), and age (men ≥45 years old; women ≥55 years old).
[b]Diagnostic accuracy of various stress tests is: Exercise treadmill: men—68% sensitive, 77% specific, women—61% sensitive, 70% specific; Exercise, adenosine thallium—88% sensitive, 77% specific; Exercise or dobutamine echo—76% sensitive, 88% specific.
[c]See Table 19.2.

TABLE 19.2		ABCDEs as an Inpatient Treatment Guide and Discharge Checklist for Patients With ACS
A	Antiplatelet	Aspirin indefinitely
		Clopidogrel (or other antiplatelet agent) for at least 1 yr
		Consider PPI prophylaxis in patients with risk factors for or history of PUD/GI bleeding
	Anticoagulation	Heparin or enoxaparin during hospitalization
	ACE inhibitor (ACE-I)	Consider if EF (≤40%), heart failure with preserved EF, DM, CRI, or HTN
	Angiotensin receptor blocker	For ACE-I intolerant patients
	Aldosterone receptor blocker	For patients with EF <40% with DM or HF who are already on an ACE-I and beta blocker; caution in patients with hyperkalemia or CRI
B	Beta blocker	All patients unless contraindicated
	Blood pressure	Goal <140/90; for CRI or DM, goal is <130/80 (maximize therapy with beta blocker and ACE-I before adding additional anti-HTN medications)
C	Cigarette cessation	Complete cessation. Nicotine replacement, oral medications, counseling
	Cholesterol	High-intensity statin therapy regardless of LDL
D	Diet	If BMI >25, initial goal is to reduce weight by 10%
	Diabetes	Goal Hgb A1c <7.0%
E	Exercise	30 min of aerobic activity a minimum of 5 days/wk
		Referral for cardiac rehabilitation
	Ejection fraction	Measurement of ejection fraction prior to discharge

ACE, angiotensin converting anzyme; BMI, body mass index; CRI, chronic renal insufficiency; DM, diabetes mellitus; EF, ejection fraction; HF, heart failure; GI, gastrointestinal; Hgb, hemoglobin; HTN, hypertension; LDL, low-density lipoprotein; PPI, proton pump inhibitor; PUD, peptic ulcer disease.

TABLE 19.3	Classification of Different Types of Myocardial Infarction
	Clinical Scenario
Type 1	Spontaneous MI secondary to a primary coronary event due to plaque instability
Type 2	MI secondary to myocardial oxygen supply–demand mismatch
Type 3	Sudden cardiac death
Type 4a	MI secondary to PCI
	(Note: cTn values must be >5 × 99th percentile URL)
Type 4b	MI secondary to stent thrombosis
Type 5	MI associated with CABG
	(Note: cTn values must be >10 × 99th percentile URL)

CABG, coronary artery bypass grafting; MI, myocardial infarction; PCI, percutaneous coronary intervention; cTn, cardiac troponin; URL, upper reference limit.

ALGORITHM 19.3 Management Algorithm for Type 2 Myocardial Infarction

EVALUATION—(3D's—DATA, DECISION, DRUGS)

DATA—Focused history and physical exam, assess cardiac risk factors, ECG, cardiac biomarkers
ECHO recommended to assess focal wall motion abnormalities or new cardiomyopathy (e.g., myocarditis)

DECISION—Risk stratify patient based on above
Trend cardiac biomarkers every 6 hours until downtrending
IMPORTANT: Treat and correct the underlying cause for oxygen mismatch

DRUGS—Unless contraindicated, all patients receive:
- Aspirin 162–325 mg chewed
- Metoprolol 5 mg IV × 3 doses, then 25–50 mg PO q6h unless any contraindications (see STEMI/STE-ACS algorithm)
- Nitrates for active chest pain if no contraindications (see STEMI/STE-ACS algorithm)
  - o Nitroglycerin (SL) and repeat every 5 minutes × 3 **OR**
  - o Nitroglycerin IV started at 10 mcg/min titrated for symptoms
- Consider morphine sulfate 2–4 mg IV for chest pain unresponsive to nitrates

For certain higher-risk patients, consider:
- Anticoagulant therapy:
  Unfractionated heparin: 60–70 U/kg IV bolus (max 4000 U); then 12 U/kg/hr (max 1000 U/hr), adjusted to achieve goal aPTT of 50–70 seconds
  OR,
  Enoxaparin (Lovenox): 1 mg/kg SQ q12h (caution if CrCl <30)

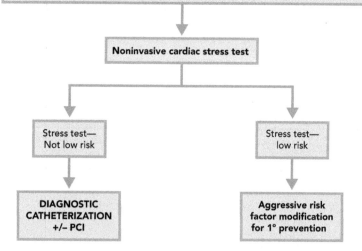

Noninvasive cardiac stress test

Stress test—Not low risk

Stress test—low risk

DIAGNOSTIC CATHETERIZATION +/− PCI

Aggressive risk factor modification for 1° prevention

should undergo diagnostic angiography. This may be normal or show only mild CAD. They should, likewise, undergo evaluation by transthoracic echocardiogram or cardiac MRI to evaluate for possible LV dysfunction and LV outflow tract obstruction. Management includes adrenergic-blocking agent (i.e., nonselective beta blockers with alpha-blocking activity), afterload reduction with ACE inhibitors, diuretics as needed, and serial transthoracic echocardiograms to monitor for persistence of ventricular dysfunction. Patients with a severely depressed LV ejection fraction (LVEF) or LV thrombus should be considered for short-term oral anticoagulation. The majority of patients who overcome the inciting event or medical illness will fully recover.

COMPLICATIONS AFTER MYOCARDIAL INFARCTION

Postinfarction complication rates have fallen dramatically since the advent of early reperfusion strategies. Nevertheless, many patients, including those with large infarction, silent infarction, late presentation, and delayed or incomplete reperfusion, remain at high risk for complications. The mnemonic FEAR AMI is a helpful way to remember these potential life-threatening complications. The following sections discuss the individual letters of this mnemonic.

Failure

LV dysfunction is the most powerful predictor of survival following MI. Clinical symptoms of LV dysfunction range from mild heart failure (e.g., rales or S3) to cardiogenic shock. The severity of LV dysfunction correlates with the size of the infarct, advanced age, and other clinical risk factors such as diabetes. Treatment for post-MI LV dysfunction is determined by its severity and includes supplemental oxygen, afterload reduction with vasodilators (e.g., nitroglycerin or nitroprusside) and inhibition of the renin–angiotensin system, and diuretic therapy. Patients who develop cardiogenic shock warrant insertion of a pulmonary artery catheter (PAC) and may require beta agonists (e.g., dobutamine and dopamine), a phosphodiesterase inhibitor (e.g., milrinone), and/or vasopressor therapy. Consideration of early use of an IABP or percutaneous ventricular assist device is essential.

Right ventricular (RV) dysfunction occurs in about 10% of patients with inferior or posterior MIs. It should be suspected in those patients who develop hypotension with standard medical therapy for MI and who have an elevated jugular venous pulse in the absence of pulmonary edema. In these patients, PAC will reveal a high central venous pressure and low pulmonary capillary wedge pressure (PCWP). Management includes judicious intravenous fluids for preload and the use of dobutamine to maintain adequate cardiac output.

Embolism and Effusions/Pericarditis

Up to 20% of all patients and 60% of patients suffering a large anterior wall MI will develop a mural thrombus. Echocardiography should be performed in all patients with an MI to determine the presence of either a mural thrombus or akinetic segments that predispose to thrombus formation. If found, these should prompt a discussion between provider and patient regarding the risk of embolization versus the risk of bleeding with anticoagulation therapy. This is of particular concern when anticoagulation is in addition to aspirin and a P2Y$_{12}$ receptor inhibitor after PCI. If anticoagulation is desired, systemic heparin followed by approximately 3 to 6 months of oral vitamin K antagonist therapy can be initiated.

Post-MI pericardial effusions are rarely life-threatening. However, when tamponade physiology is present in a post-MI patient, a hemorrhagic effusion from a ventricular rupture must be considered. In the presence of an effusion on echocardiogram, anticoagulation should be withheld in the post-MI period to avoid possible hemopericardium. If anticoagulation cannot be stopped, heightened vigilance for this complication is warranted.

Post-MI pericarditis can present at any point from the first days after MI up to 6 weeks following infarct. This complication is due to local pericardial irritation, usually by a transmural infarct. Pericarditis must be distinguished from recurrent ischemia. Pain secondary to pericarditis is classically worse with deep inspiration, improves with sitting forward, radiates to the scapulae, and can be associated with characteristic ECG findings. This is treated with high-dose aspirin 650 mg every 8 hours plus colchicine 0.5 to 0.6 mg twice daily, especially in early pericarditis.

Dressler syndrome is a type of postinfarction pericarditis that occurs 1 to 8 weeks after the infarct. It is thought to be immune mediated and is best treated with high-dose aspirin. Glucocorticosteroids and other nonsteroidal anti-inflammatory agents are avoided in the first month after infarction because of the potential to impair ventricular healing and increase rates of ventricular rupture.

Arrhythmia

The management of many common arrhythmias is discussed elsewhere (see Chapter 20). Several infarction-specific arrhythmias are presented here.

Various ventricular arrhythmias have been previously associated with infarction and subsequent reperfusion. The best evidence for a "reperfusion rhythm" is accelerated idioventricular rhythm (AIVR), as it is often seen immediately following successful reperfusion. Despite this, AIVR is neither very sensitive nor specific for a successful reperfusion and, if seen in the setting of reperfusion, does not require any specific intervention. More common ECG changes following successful reperfusion involve ST-T changes, such as resolution of prior ST elevation.

Ventricular tachycardia (VT) is often the terminal rhythm in the peri-infarct period and is associated with increased mortality when occurring in the first 48 hours of hospitalization. VT can be stratified into *monomorphic* VT, in which all ventricular beats have a similar morphology as is seen when the VT originates from a single focus or circuit, and *polymorphic* VT, which has a changing morphology in its ventricular beats. In each case, aggressive restoration of sinus rhythm is achieved through the use of antiarrhythmic medications (e.g., amiodarone, lidocaine) and/or synchronized direct current cardioversion as per Advanced Cardiac Life Support (ACLS) guidelines. Because hypokalemia and hypomagnesemia have been associated with development of sustained VT, it is important to correct potassium (K) and magnesium (Mg) levels in the setting of an infarction (K >4 mEq/L and Mg >2 mEq/L). In contrast, nonsustained VT (NSVT) is not associated with an increased risk of death during the index hospitalization or during the first year after infarction and suppressive treatment of asymptomatic NSVT is not routinely recommended in the post-MI patient.

Infarction can cause block at any level of the conduction system. The location of the infarct has an important influence on the patient's prognosis and treatment of conduction disease. In general, right coronary artery infarct is associated with proximal (atrioventricular [AV] nodal) conduction disease. This AV block is usually transient and, in the absence of symptoms, typically does not warrant transvenous pacemaker placement. One exception is symptomatic AV block in the setting of RV infarction,

TABLE 19.4	Features of Ischemia-Related Atrioventricular Conduction Disease	
	Proximal Conduction Disease	**Distal Conduction Disease**
Compromised artery	Right coronary/posterior descending (90%)	Septal perforators of left anterior descending
Site of block	Intranodal	Infranodal
Site of infarction	Inferoposterior	Anteroseptal
Type of AV block	First degree or Mobitz I	Mobitz II or third degree
Duration of AV block	Transient (2–3 days)	Variable
Mortality rate	Low, unless CHF or hypotension	High, because of extensive infarct
Temporary pacemaker	Rare	Early consideration, especially for anterior infarct and bifascicular block
Permanent pacemaker	Almost never	Indicated if high-grade block in His–Purkinje system or associated bundle branch block

CHF: congestive heart failure.

as restoration of AV synchrony can improve RV filling and thus cardiac output. Left anterior descending/septal infarct is associated with distal (infranodal) conduction disease and is potentially life-threatening. Immediate pacing efforts should be pursued. Additional features of AV conduction disease are shown in Table 19.4. Acute treatment is discussed in Chapter 20.

Rupture and Regurgitation

The clinical presentation of a ventricular rupture is often striking and usually life-threatening. The rupture can be in the ventricular free wall, ventricular septum, or papillary muscle (Table 19.5).

Ventricular free wall rupture presents with hypotension and signs of cardiac tamponade. Any clinical suspicion warrants immediate use of echocardiography as well as PAC for prompt diagnosis. Emergent surgery is usually the only chance for survival.

Ventricular septal rupture (VSR) should be suspected in patients with a new pansystolic murmur or palpable thrill with signs of worsening biventricular failure. Echocardiography is needed to detect and localize the VSR. PAC is useful to assess for an increase in the oxygen saturation in the right ventricle ("step-up"), which is characteristic of a VSR. PAC can also be used to calculate a shunt fraction. All patients with a VSR should be considered for early surgical therapy. IABP and/or the use of nitroprusside can be used to bridge patients to surgery by reducing the shunt.

Mitral regurgitation (MR) is a common complication of MI, occurring in almost half of all patients. Ischemic MR may be caused by mitral annular dilatation in LV dysfunction, papillary muscle dysfunction, or papillary muscle rupture. Typically, MR is transient and asymptomatic and does not warrant further intervention. However, MR secondary to papillary muscle rupture may be severe and should be suspected in patients with a new pansystolic murmur in the setting of heart failure

TABLE 19.5	Clinical Profile of Mechanical Complications of Myocardial Infarction		
	Ventricular Septal Defect	Free Wall Rupture	Papillary Muscle Rupture
Days post-MI	1–5	1–7	3–5
Anterior MI	66%	50%	25%
New murmur	90%	25%	50%
Palpable thrill	Yes	No	Rare
2D Echo findings	Visualize defect	May have pericardial effusion	Flail or prolapsing leaflet
Doppler Echo findings	Detect shunt		Regurgitant jet in LA
PA catheterization	Oxygen step-up in RV	Equalization of diastolic pressure	Prominent *c-v* wave in PCW tracing
Medical mortality	90%	90%	90%
Surgical mortality	50%	Case reports	40–90%

MI, myocardial infarction; LA, left atrium; PA, pulmonary artery; RV, right ventricle; PCW, pulmonary capillary wedge.
Modified from Labovitz AJ, et al. Mechanical complications of acute myocardial infarction. *Cardiovasc Rev Rep.* 1984;5:948.

or hemodynamic compromise. Notably, some patients with severe MR in this setting may not have a prominent murmur. Echocardiography (TTE and TEE) is essential to the diagnosis and determining the etiology of MR. PAC reveals large V waves on the PCWP tracing. For patients with suspected papillary muscle rupture, immediate surgery is indicated with the use of nitroprusside or IABP in the setting of hypotension to stabilize the patient until surgery.

Aneurysm

True LV aneurysms complicate <5% of acute infarctions. They are thought to be a consequence of a complete occlusion of the supplying coronary artery without significant collateral blood flow. As such, anteroapical aneurysms (due to left anterior descending artery occlusion) are four times more common than inferoposterior aneurysms.

LV aneurysms are associated with a sixfold increase in mortality, mainly resulting from ventricular arrhythmias. LV aneurysms are often supported by fibrous tissue and thus rarely rupture. The characteristic ECG findings of LV aneurysms are Q waves with persistent ST elevations, although the diagnosis is best made by a noninvasive imaging study. Because of the risk of mural thrombus formation and systemic embolization, patients with an LV aneurysm are often treated with long-term anticoagulation with warfarin, particularly if there is evidence of significant LV dysfunction or suspected thrombus. Additionally, as ST segments may remain elevated for some time after successful reperfusion, persistent ST elevations (>4 weeks after AMI) are generally required for the ECG diagnosis of LV aneurysm. Acute aneurysms lead to decompensated heart failure and cardiogenic shock and are managed with vasodilators and an IABP. ACE inhibitors can reduce progression of the aneurysm and

ould be initiated in the absence of hypotension. Chronic aneurysms lead to heart
ailure or arrhythmias and should be treated accordingly. For patients with refractory
ymptoms, surgery may be considered to repair a chronic aneurysm.

Distinct from an aneurysm is a pseudoaneurysm. Rather than involving layers of
muscle, the myocardium perforates, allowing this clinical entity to be thought of as
"contained rupture." It is most often seen with inferior infarctions, and treatment
f choice is surgery. Both surgical and medical treatments carry a very high mortality
ue to the risk for spontaneous rupture.

Recurrent Myocardial Infarction

The complaint of chest pain after an MI may represent recurrent ischemia from
ncomplete revascularization, infarct extension, reinfarction, or postinfarction angina.
schemia recurs in 20% to 30% of patients receiving thrombolytic therapy and up
o 10% of patients after percutaneous revascularization. Serial cardiac biomarkers
nd ECGs can help identify at-risk patients. Troponins may not be useful given their
ersistent elevation beyond 1 week after an MI. Increases in CK-MB isoenzymes after
owntrending may be a more diagnostic marker of reinfarction. Aggressive medical
herapy with anti-ischemic medications (e.g., aspirin, heparin, nitrates, beta blockers)
s important to control symptoms. Revascularization should be considered in patients
whose symptoms are refractory to medical therapy.

New postinfarct ST elevations can be caused by reinfarction, pericarditis, or
dyskinetic/aneurysmal ventricular segments. Reinfarction due to stent thrombosis
usually has a dramatic presentation with severe anginal pain refractory to medical
herapy and evolving ST elevations on ECG. These findings warrant immediate
evascularization efforts.

SUGGESTED READINGS

Amsterdam EA, Wenger NK, Brindis RG, et al. 2014 AHA/ACC guideline for the management
of patients with non-ST-elevation acute coronary syndromes: a report of the American
College of Cardiology/American Heart Association Task Force on Practice Guidelines.
Circulation. 2014;130(25):e344–e426.
Equally invaluable consensus guidelines for patients with NSTE-ACS.

Antman EM, Cohen M, Bernink PJ, et al. The TIMI risk score for unstable angina/non-ST
elevation MI: a method for prognostication and therapeutic decision making. *JAMA.*
2000;284(7):835–842.
One of several validations of the popular TIMI risk score for NSTE-ACS.

Bybee KA, Prasad A. Stress-related cardiomyopathy syndromes. *Circulation.* 2008;118(4):397–409.
*Nice review on various types of stress-induced cardiomyopathies including their mechanism,
diagnosis, and suggested management.*

O'Gara PT, Kushner FG, Ascheim DD, et al. 2013 ACCF/AHA guideline for the management
of ST-elevation myocardial infarction: a report of the American College of Cardiology
Foundation/American Heart Association Task Force on Practice Guidelines. *Circulation.*
2013;127(4):e362–e425.
*Invaluable consensus guidelines detailing the state of the art for management of patients with
STEMI.*

Thygesen K, Alpert JS, Jaffe AS, et al. Third universal definition of myocardial infarction.
Circulation. 2012;126(16):2020–2035.
Updated definitions for diagnosing myocardial infarction in different clinical settings.

20 Cardiac Arrhythmias and Conduction Abnormalities

Sandeep S. Sodhi and Daniel H. Cooper

This chapter addresses the causes, recognition, and treatment of cardiac arrhythmias occurring in hospitalized and critically ill patients. Cardiac arrhythmias can disrupt cardiac output (CO) by impairing the heart rate (HR) and/or stroke volume (SV)—evidenced by the equation $CO = HR \times SV$. The clinical presentation of cardiac arrhythmias varies widely, and may include: (a) asymptomatic findings on an electrocardiogram (ECG) or telemetry, (b) symptoms without hemodynamic instability (e.g., palpitations, shortness of breath, syncope, or chest pain), (c) hemodynamic instability in conscious patients, or (d) cardiac arrest. Initial evaluation in hospitalized patients includes ensuring: (a) adequate airway and breathing support; (b) continuous monitoring of cardiac rhythm, blood pressure, and oxyhemoglobin saturation; (c) adequate intravenous (IV) access; and, (d) adequate support personnel. The cardiac rhythm should be analyzed by 12-lead ECG when possible, but initial treatment may be based on the rhythm seen on the intensive care unit bedside monitor or external defibrillator. If time permits, the specific underlying rhythm should be identified, the cause sought, and therapy tailored accordingly. However, *cardiac arrest and severely symptomatic tachycardia and bradycardia require immediate treatment based on the advanced cardiac life support (ACLS) algorithms* shown later in this chapter in Algorithms 20.1, 20.2, and 20.3.

TACHYARRHYTHMIAS

Tachycardia, defined as an HR >100 beats/min, can be separated into (a) those with origins above the ventricles, termed **supraventricular tachycardias**, and (b) those that arise within the ventricles, termed **ventricular tachycardias (VTs)**. Tachycardia can generally be distinguished on the basis of the HR, the width and morphology of the QRS complex, and the length of the PR interval. The approach to differentiating narrow and wide QRS complex tachycardias is outlined in Algorithms 20.4 and 20.5, respectively.

Supraventricular Tachycardias

Sinus tachycardia originates from the sinus node, and is not considered a primary arrhythmia. The ECG shows a normal P wave preceding each QRS complex, with upright morphology in lead II and a downward morphology in lead aVL. Sinus tachycardia in the intensive care unit can be a physiologic response to volume depletion, fever, pain, anxiety, shock, hypoxia, or in patients on vasopressor or inotropic support. Maximum heart rate (MHR) is age dependent and roughly limited to 220—age in years (e.g., in a 70-year-old man, MHR = 220 − 70 = 150).

ALGORITHM 20.1   Advanced Cardiac Life Support Tachycardia Treatment Algorithm

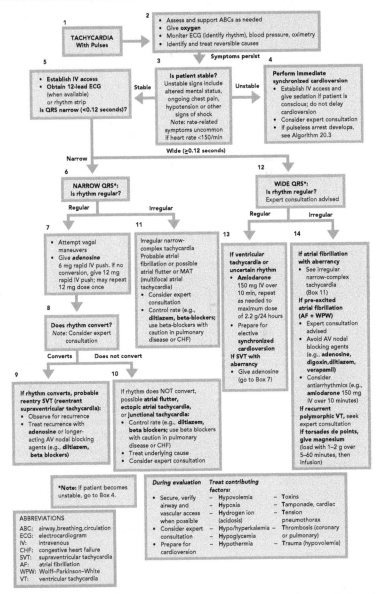

From 2005 American Heart Association Guidelines for Cardiopulmonary Resuscitation and Emergency Cardiovascular Care. Part 7.3: Management of symptomatic bradycardia and tachycardia. *Circulation.* 2005;112(suppl IV):IV-70, with permission.

ALGORITHM 20.2 Advanced Cardiac Life Support Bradycardia Treatment Algorithm

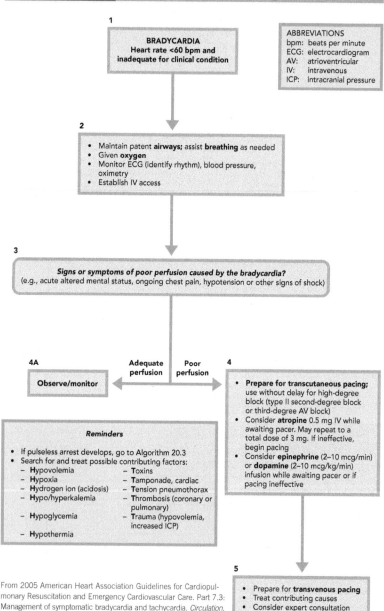

1

BRADYCARDIA
Heart rate <60 bpm and
inadequate for clinical condition

ABBREVIATIONS
bpm: beats per minute
ECG: electrocardiogram
AV: atrioventricular
IV: intravenous
ICP: intracranial pressure

2

- Maintain patent **airways**; assist **breathing** as needed
- Given **oxygen**
- Monitor ECG (identify rhythm), blood pressure, oximetry
- Establish IV access

3

Signs or symptoms of poor perfusion caused by the bradycardia?
(e.g., acute altered mental status, ongoing chest pain, hypotension or other signs of shock)

4A   Adequate   Poor   **4**
    perfusion   perfusion

Observe/monitor

- **Prepare for transcutaneous pacing;**
  use without delay for high-degree
  block (type II second-degree block
  or third-degree AV block)
- Consider **atropine** 0.5 mg IV while
  awaiting pacer. May repeat to a
  total dose of 3 mg. If ineffective,
  begin pacing
- Consider **epinephrine** (2–10 mcg/min)
  or **dopamine** (2–10 mcg/kg/min)
  infusion while awaiting pacer or if
  pacing ineffective

Reminders

- If pulseless arrest develops, go to Algorithm 20.3
- Search for and treat possible contributing factors:
  - Hypovolemia
  - Hypoxia
  - Hydrogen ion (acidosis)
  - Hypo/hyperkalemia
  - Hypoglycemia
  - Hypothermia
  - Toxins
  - Tamponade, cardiac
  - Tension pneumothorax
  - Thrombosis (coronary or pulmonary)
  - Trauma (hypovolemia, increased ICP)

5

- Prepare for **transvenous pacing**
- Treat contributing causes
- Consider expert consultation

From 2005 American Heart Association Guidelines for Cardiopulmonary Resuscitation and Emergency Cardiovascular Care. Part 7.3: Management of symptomatic bradycardia and tachycardia. *Circulation.* 2005;112(suppl IV):IV-68, with permission.

ALGORITHM 20.3 **Advanced Cardiac Life Support Pulseless Arrest Algorithm**

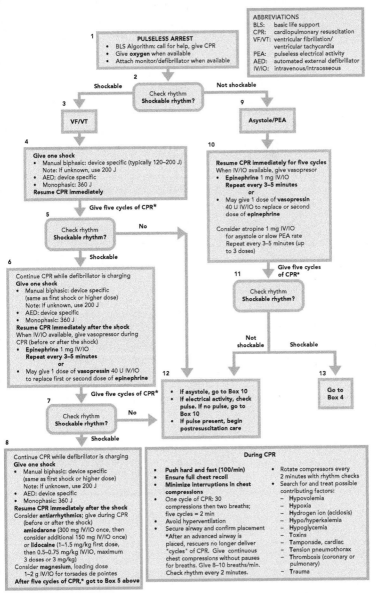

ABBREVIATIONS
BLS: basic life support
CPR: cardiopulmonary resuscitation
VF/VT: ventricular fibrillation/ventricular tachycardia
PEA: pulseless electrical activity
AED: automated external defibrillator
IV/IO: intravenous/intraosseous

1 PULSELESS ARREST
- BLS Algorithm: call for help, give CPR
- Give **oxygen** when available
- Attach monitor/defibrillator when available

2 Check rhythm
Shockable rhythm?
Shockable → **3 VF/VT**
Not shockable → **9 Asystole/PEA**

4 Give one shock
- Manual biphasic: device specific (typically 120–200 J)
  Note: If unknown, use 200 J
- AED: device specific
- Monophasic: 360 J
Resume CPR immediately

Give five cycles of CPR*

5 Check rhythm
Shockable rhythm?
No →
Shockable ↓

6
Continue CPR while defibrillator is charging
Give one shock
- Manual biphasic: device specific (same as first shock or higher dose)
  Note: If unknown, use 200 J
- AED: device specific
- Monophasic: 360 J
Resume CPR immediately after the shock
When IV/IO available, give vasopressor during CPR (before or after the shock)
- **Epinephrine** 1 mg IV/IO
  Repeat every 3–5 minutes
  or
- May give 1 dose of **vasopressin** 40 U IV/IO to replace first or second dose of **epinephrine**

Give five cycles of CPR*

7 Check rhythm
Shockable rhythm?
No →
Shockable ↓

8
Continue CPR while defibrillator is charging
Give one shock
- Manual biphasic: device specific (same as first shock or higher dose)
  Note: If unknown, use 200 J
- AED: device specific
- Monophasic: 360 J
Resume CPR immediately after the shock
Consider **antiarrhythmics**; give during CPR (before or after the shock)
  amiodarone (300 mg IV/IO once, then consider additional 150 mg IV/IO once) or **lidocaine** (1–1.5 mg/kg first dose, then 0.5–0.75 mg/kg IV/IO, maximum 3 doses or 3 mg/kg)
Consider **magnesium**, loading dose 1–2 g IV/IO for torsades de pointes
After five cycles of CPR,* got to Box 5 above

10
Resume CPR immediately for five cycles
When IV/IO available, give vasopressor
- **Epinephrine** 1 mg IV/IO
  Repeat every 3–5 minutes
  or
- May give 1 dose of **vasopressin** 40 U IV/IO to replace or second dose of **epinephrine**

Consider atropine 1 mg IV/IO for asystole or slow PEA rate
Repeat every 3–5 minutes (up to 3 doses)

Give five cycles of CPR*

11 Check rhythm
Shockable rhythm?
Not shockable → **12**
Shockable → **13**

12
- If asystole, go to Box 10
- If electrical activity, check pulse. If no pulse, go to Box 10
- If pulse present, begin postresuscitation care

13
Go to Box 4

During CPR
- **Push hard and fast (100/min)**
- **Ensure full chest recoil**
- **Minimize interruptions in chest compressions**
- One cycle of CPR: 30 compressions then two breaths; five cycles = 2 min
- Avoid hyperventilation
- Secure airway and confirm placement
- *After an advanced airway is placed, rescuers no longer deliver "cycles" of CPR. Give continuous chest compressions without pauses for breaths. Give 8–10 breaths/min. Check rhythm every 2 minutes.

- Rotate compressors every 2 minutes with rhythm checks
- Search for and treat possible contributing factors:
  - Hypovolemia
  - Hypoxia
  - Hydrogen ion (acidosis)
  - Hypo/hyperkalemia
  - Hypoglycemia
  - Toxins
  - Tamponade, cardiac
  - Tension pneumothorax
  - Thrombosis (coronary or pulmonary)
  - Trauma

From 2005 American Heart Association Guidelines for Cardiopulmonary Resuscitation and Emergency Cardiovascular Care. Part 7.2: Management of cardiac arrest. *Circulation.* 2005;112(suppl IV):IV-59, with permission.

ALGORITHM 20.4 Approach to Differentiating Narrow QRS Complex Tachycardias

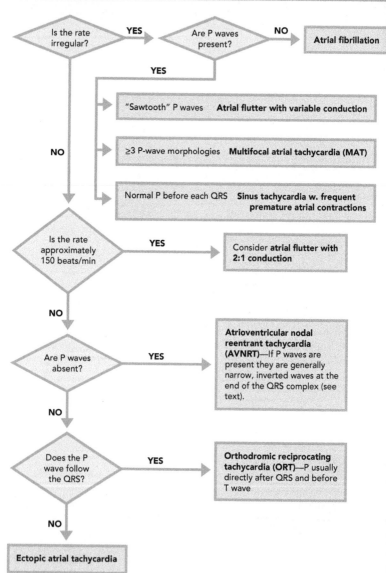

ALGORITHM 20.5 Approach to Differentiating Wide QRS Complex Tachycardias

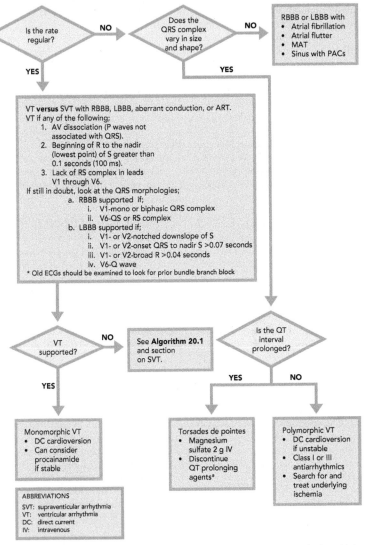

Wide complex tachycardias (except clear sinus tachycardia with aberrancy) should initially be assumed to be ventricular tachycardia (VT) and treatment urgency based on assessment of patient condition and hemodynamics (see text for details).

Treatment of sinus tachycardia is directed at remedying the underlying cause, which includes treating infections and fever, repleting volume, administering anxiolytics as needed, and controlling pain. Rate-controlling agents are generally not indicated unless the tachycardia causes symptoms of low CO. Reflex sinus tachycardia may be important to maintain adequate CO. Direct treatment of the tachycardia without treatment of the underlying cause may be deleterious.

Atrial fibrillation is a chaotic rhythm within the atria of 350 to 600 beats/min without an appreciable P wave on ECG. All atrial beats are not conducted because of the refractory period in the atrioventricular (AV) node, and conduction is variably timed, resulting in an irregular ventricular rate. If the ventricular rate is greater than 100 beats/min, a rapid ventricular response is said to be present. The associated rapid HR and the lack of atrial contribution to pumping blood can compromise CO (primarily in patients with reduced cardiac function at baseline), requiring immediate treatment. Loss of organized atrial contraction creates stasis of the blood pool within the atria, which predisposes intracardiac thrombus formation and thromboembolism.

Atrial fibrillation is seen in association with chronic cardiopulmonary disease. It can also be the presenting finding of the elderly with conduction disturbances; patients with thyrotoxicosis, infection, pulmonary embolization, acute alcohol intoxication, pericarditis, and stress; and is common postoperatively. It is a rare presentation of acute myocardial infarction.

Typical *atrial flutter* is caused by a reentrant rhythm localized to the right atrium, which generates impulses at a rate of approximately 300 beats/min. The ventricular rate is frequently 150 beats/min (half the atrial rate) due to 2:1 block within the AV node. In 3:1 block, every third beat is conducted, and the ventricular rate is approximately 100 beats/min. A large portion of the atria is depolarized at once, causing a classic "sawtooth" appearance on the baseline of the ECG, with fairly narrow, negative flutter waves in the inferior leads (II, III, aVF). The ventricular rate may be regular, but can be irregular if conduction is variable (i.e., 2:1 alternating with 3:1). It is seen in patients with underlying heart disease and is also commonly seen in patients after cardiac surgery. If left untreated, atrial flutter may degrade to atrial fibrillation.

Initial management of atrial fibrillation and atrial flutter is outlined in Algorithm 20.6. Precipitating factors should be sought and treated. Preoperative beta blockers can reduce the incidence of postoperative atrial fibrillation/flutter. For atrial fibrillation or flutter that persists despite electrical cardioversion and/or pharmacotherapy, consider electrophysiology consultation for evaluation of ablation procedures.

Thromboembolic risk management typically involves anticoagulation with IV heparin overlapping with warfarin until the international normalized ratio (INR) is >2. Long-term anticoagulation can be achieved with warfarin alone. Alternatively, novel oral anticoagulants (NOACs) such as apixaban, rivaroxaban, dabigatran, or edoxaban may be used for stroke prevention in patients with nonvalvular atrial fibrillation or flutter. Risk factors such as age, hypertension, heart failure, diabetes, prior stroke, female gender, and vascular disease portend atrial thrombus formation and increase the risk of subsequent cerebrovascular accident (CVA) related to atrial fibrillation or flutter.

Paroxysmal supraventricular tachycardias (PSVT) are characterized by sudden onset and termination. The most common PSVT in adults is *AV nodal reentrant tachycardia* (AVNRT). It is caused by a reentrant electrical loop within the AV node. The rate generally varies from 120 to 250 beats/min and is associated with a narrow QRS complex in the absence of aberrancy or an underlying bundle

ALGORITHM 20.6 Treatment of Atrial Fibrillation and Atrial Flutter (See Chapter 91 Common Drug Dosages and Side Effects)

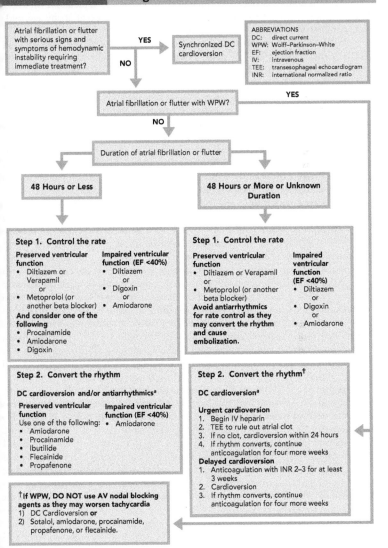

ABBREVIATIONS
DC: direct current
WPW: Wolff–Parkinson–White
EF: ejection fraction
IV: intravenous
TEE: transesophageal echocardiogram
INR: international normalized ratio

Atrial fibrillation or flutter with serious signs and symptoms of hemodynamic instability requiring immediate treatment? **YES** → Synchronized DC cardioversion

NO

Atrial fibrillation or flutter with WPW? **YES**

NO

Duration of atrial fibrillation or flutter

48 Hours or Less

48 Hours or More or Unknown Duration

48 Hours or Less

Step 1. Control the rate

Preserved ventricular function	Impaired ventricular function (EF <40%)
• Diltiazem or Verapamil or • Metoprolol (or another beta blocker)	• Diltiazem or • Digoxin or • Amiodarone

And consider one of the following
• Procainamide
• Amiodarone
• Digoxin

Step 2. Convert the rhythm

DC cardioversion and/or antiarrhythmics[a]

Preserved ventricular function	Impaired ventricular function (EF <40%)
Use one of the following: • Amiodarone • Procainamide • Ibutilide • Flecainide • Propafenone	• Amiodarone

[†]**If WPW, DO NOT use AV nodal blocking agents as they may worsen tachycardia**
1) DC Cardioversion or
2) Sotalol, amiodarone, procainamide, propafenone, or flecainide.

48 Hours or More or Unknown Duration

Step 1. Control the rate

Preserved ventricular function	Impaired ventricular function (EF <40%)
• Diltiazem or Verapamil or • Metoprolol (or another beta blocker) **Avoid antiarrhythmics for rate control as they may convert the rhythm and cause embolization.**	• Diltiazem or • Digoxin or • Amiodarone

Step 2. Convert the rhythm[†]

DC cardioversion[a]

Urgent cardioversion
1. Begin IV heparin
2. TEE to rule out atrial clot
3. If no clot, cardioversion within 24 hours
4. If rhythm converts, continue anticoagulation for four more weeks

Delayed cardioversion
1. Anticoagulation with INR 2–3 for at least 3 weeks
2. Cardioversion
3. If rhythm converts, continue anticoagulation for four more weeks

[a]Premedicate when possible with a sedative (e.g., diazepam, midazolam, ketamine, etomidate) and analgesic (e.g., fentanyl, morphine). Perform synchronized cardioversion with 100 J, 200 J, 300 J, 360 J, biphasic energy or monophasic equivalent, starting with lowest energy level and increasing if needed. Perform asynchronous cardioversion if delays in synchronized cardioversion with worsening clinical status. DC, direct current; WPW, Wolff–Parkinson–White; EF, ejection fraction; IV, intravenous; TEE, transesophageal echocardiogram; INR, international normalized ratio.

branch block. The atria and ventricles typically depolarize at virtually the same tim
thus, the P waves are frequently not visible, obscured by the QRS complexes.
visible, they generally present as narrow inverted P waves at the end of the QR
complex, commonly described as a "pseudo R" in V1 and/or "a pseudo S" in lead I
AVNRT is not typically associated with specific diseases, can occur at any age, and
more common in women.

PSVT may also be mediated by an accessory pathway between the atria an
ventricles that bypasses the AV node. *Manifest* accessory pathways are seen on th
sinus rhythm ECG as a "delta wave" of pre-excitation. The pre-excitation also cause
a short PR interval because the accessory pathway does not have the delayed conduc
tion of the AV node. Accessory pathways may conduct antegrade (forming the delt
wave) or retrograde. *Concealed* accessory AV pathways only conduct retrograde, an
are invisible in sinus rhythm. Either of these pathways may mediate an ***orthodrom***
reentrant tachycardia (ORT) in which the electrical impulse propagates antegrad
through the AV node and retrograde (from ventricle to atrium) through the accessor
pathway. The result is a narrow QRS complex tachycardia, typically with inverted
retrograde P waves between the QRS and T wave (although the QRS may be wid
because of aberrancy, e.g., bundle branch block or fascicular block).

The patient with visible pre-excitation (delta wave and short PR interval) i
sinus rhythm and with palpitations (usually from paroxysmal ORT) is said to hav
Wolff–Parkinson–White syndrome (WPW). Patients with WPW are also prone t
arrhythmias with antegrade conduction through the accessory pathway. These includ
antidromic reentrant tachycardia, in which the excitation propagates antegrad
through the accessory pathway and retrograde through the AV node. Atrial arrhyth
mias (including atrial fibrillation) may also conduct antegrade through the accessor
pathway. The short refractory period of the accessory pathway may allow very rapi
conduction of impulses to the ventricles, resulting in rapid "pre-excited atrial fibril
lation" with ventricular rates up to 300 beats/min, often resulting in hemodynami
instability requiring urgent intervention. Rapid conduction of atrial fibrillatio
through an accessory pathway may also induce ventricular fibrillation (VF). Thi
is thought to be the pathogenesis of the rare sudden death that is associated wit
WPW.

Treatment of PSVT aims at aborting the reentrant rhythm by blocking conduc
tion through the AV node with vagal maneuvers (valsalva, carotid massage, and fac
immersion in cold water [diving reflex]) or adenosine given as a 6 mg IV bolus ($t_{1/}$
approximately 10 seconds). A second 12-mg dose can be given after 1 to 2 minute
if the first was ineffective, and a third dose of 12 or 18 mg can be given if needed. I
these treatments fail, AV nodal blocking agents, calcium channel blockers, or digoxi
should be used. Patients with WPW and pre-excited atrial fibrillation or flutter mus
be rapidly treated with direct current cardioversion or class IA, IC, or III drugs (e.g.
procainamide, flecainide, and amiodarone), which slow myocardial conduction and
prolong the refractory period. AV nodal blocking agents are not to be used espe
cially when the accessory pathway has a short antegrade refractory period capable of
rapid ventricular conduction (Algorithm 20.6). Advanced management of PSVT
includes evaluation by electrophysiology for potential ablative therapy targeting the
mechanism of arrhythmia.

Ectopic atrial tachycardia occurs when there is automaticity at a single focus
outside the sinoatrial (SA) node. A P wave precedes each QRS as in sinus tachycardia, but the P-wave axis and morphology are typically altered. When increased

automaticity occurs at three or more different atrial sites, which may include the SA node, it is termed **multifocal atrial tachycardia**, with the alternating foci causing at least three P-wave morphologies on ECG. Both can be seen in cases of digitalis toxicity (which causes increased automaticity), severe cardiopulmonary disease, hypokalemia, hyperadrenergic states, and as a side effect of theophylline. Treatment includes AV nodal blocking agents and removal of inciting agents/factors (i.e., chronic obstructive pulmonary disease exacerbations, infections, stimulants).

Ventricular Tachycardias

The two main tachyarrhythmias arising from the ventricles are **ventricular tachycardia** (VT) and **ventricular fibrillation** (VF). VT may be monomorphic, if the QRS morphology is fixed, or polymorphic, if the QRS complex is variable. Polymorphic VT results in chaotic ventricular activation, often with hemodynamic instability, possibly leading to cardiac arrest and sudden death. It is more likely to occur in the setting of acute ischemia, infarct, or acute heart failure.

Monomorphic VT results from reentrant electrical impulses within the ventricles or from a focal site with frequent spontaneous action potentials that propagate to the remainder of the ventricles. VT is characterized on ECG by a wide QRS complex (>0.12 seconds), and a rate usually between 100 and 200 beats/min (although it may be higher). VT lasting <30 seconds is termed *nonsustained VT* (NSVT), while sustained VT lasts >30 seconds. The most common substrates for monomorphic VT are healed myocardial infarction or significant cardiomyopathy. It occurs less commonly in acute ischemia or active infarction. Importantly, monomorphic VT may occur in the absence of structural heart disease. These "idiopathic VTs" do not have a poor prognosis and may not cause hemodynamic instability, emphasizing the need to assess and treat the patient's condition, and not solely the ECG.

An important type of polymorphic VT is **torsades de pointes**, characterized by polymorphic VT associated with prolongation of the QT interval (in sinus rhythm) from numerous causes, including (a) drugs (especially tricyclic antidepressants, antipsychotics, certain antiarrhythmics, macrolides, and fluoroquinolones), (b) electrolyte abnormalities (hypokalemia, hypomagnesemia, and hypocalcemia), and (c) congenital long QT syndromes. Torsades de pointes appears on ECG as a characteristic pattern of oscillating amplitude of the QRS, or "twisting," around the baseline. Torsades de pointes is generally symptomatic but may be nonsustained. If prolonged, hemodynamic instability, syncope, and/or sudden death may result.

Wide complex tachycardias (except clear sinus tachycardia with aberrancy) should initially be assumed to be VT and the urgency of treatment should depend on assessment of the patient and the hemodynamic situation. Distinguishing VT from SVT with a wide QRS is therefore of secondary importance. Mistaken diagnosis of "SVT with aberrancy" can result in mistreatment. The differential diagnosis of wide complex tachycardia is threefold: (a) VT, (b) SVT with aberrancy (typical bundle branch or fascicular blocks or atypical aberrancy), and (c) pre-excited supraventricular rhythm (including atrial fibrillation)—in which case the ECG in sinus rhythm will typically feature a delta wave.

Algorithm 20.5 reviews the ECG criteria that favor VT. Also, old ECGs should be examined for bundle branch blocks or ventricular pre-excitation syndromes. As previously mentioned, if the diagnosis of the wide complex rhythm is uncertain, it should be assumed to be VT, and treatment should proceed according to the patient's condition.

NSVT may be idiopathic or occur in the setting of acute ischemia or heart failure, and evaluation and treatment should be focused on the underlying etiology if one is present. Direct pharmacologic treatment (e.g., lidocaine, amiodarone) of NSVT in ischemia/infarct is not advisable. If the patient is not suffering from ischemia, NSVT can frequently be asymptomatic and has little prognostic utility for malignant arrhythmia, especially in the absence of structural heart disease and ventricular dysfunction. Symptomatic NSVT may be treated pharmacologically with beta blockers, primarily to relieve symptoms.

Sustained VT generally causes symptoms by impairing CO, resulting in hypotension, loss of consciousness, and possibly cardiac arrest. It may also deteriorate into VF.

Treatment of symptomatic VT with a detectable pulse is *synchronous* direct current cardioversion (with sedation or anesthesia in the awake patient) or, if the VT is hemodynamically tolerated by the patient, with an antiarrhythmic drug (such as amiodarone or lidocaine). Patients with hemodynamically compromising, pulseless monomorphic or polymorphic VT usually require immediate treatment with asynchronous defibrillation (see section "Cardiac Arrest"), followed by antiarrhythmic drugs if necessary. Once the patient is stable, consideration should be given to VT ablation in addition to antiarrhythmic medications for long-term management of VT and to prevent further defibrillation therapy.

Sustained torsades de pointes with hemodynamic collapse also requires asynchronous cardioversion. Treatment of torsades de pointes aims at correcting any underlying electrolyte abnormalities (i.e., magnesium, potassium) and stopping any drugs known to prolong the QT interval. Torsades de pointes is likely to recur if the inciting factors cannot be eliminated immediately. Lidocaine or phenytoin may also be suppressive. Torsades de pointes is frequently *bradycardia dependent*, and temporary pacing or isoproterenol infusion may be used to increase the HR and prevent recurrences.

VF is the result of chaotic electrical currents within the ventricles, preventing coordinated contractions. VF on ECG has a chaotic appearance without any discernable QRS complex. Untreated VF rapidly results in death. VF may be preceded by VT and is most commonly seen in patients with acute myocardial infarction or profound heart failure.

Treatment is immediate asynchronous electrical defibrillation, followed by antiarrhythmic drugs when a stable rhythm returns (see "Cardiac Arrest"). Treatment Algorithm 20.3 outlines the management of VF in the setting of cardiac arrest. Increasingly, ablation procedures are being employed for management of VF. VF triggered by PVCs, in particular, can be targeted for ablation once the patient has been stabilized. Patients who survive cardiac arrest caused by any ventricular arrhythmia should be evaluated for secondary prevention implantable cardioverter-defibrillator (ICD) prior to hospital discharge.

BRADYARRHYTHMIAS

Bradycardia, defined as an HR of less than 60 beats/min, occurs from (a) SA node dysfunction or (b) disturbances of the AV conduction system. Clinically significant bradycardia occurs when there is inadequate CO, generally associated with hypotension, and which may manifest as presyncope, syncope, fatigue, confusion, depressed level of consciousness, chest pain, shock, and/or congestive heart failure. Appropriate management entails identifying the underlying rhythm and cause of the bradycardia. Acute treatment aims at restoring adequate CO and its cause.

SA node dysfunction occurs in a number of pathophysiologic states seen in the intensive care unit including increased intracranial pressure, prolonged apneic periods in patients with the obstructive sleep apnea/hypopnea syndrome, myocardial infarction, advanced liver disease, hypothyroidism, hypothermia, hypercapnia, acidemia, hypervagotonia, and certain infections. It may also be due to depression of the sinus node by drugs, including sympatholytics such as beta blockers and clonidine, the cardioselective calcium channel blockers verapamil and diltiazem, parasympathomimetics, and antiarrhythmic drugs such as amiodarone. Sick sinus syndrome refers to intrinsic sinus node dysfunction with any of the previously mentioned clinical symptoms resulting in decreased CO. An important variant of sick sinus syndrome is associated with sinus bradycardia or prolonged sinus pause occurring after termination of atrial fibrillation or other atrial arrhythmias due to depression of SA node automaticity during the tachyarrhythmia, which may be slow to recover. Syncope or near-syncope is a common presentation of this variant, termed the *tachy-brady syndrome.*

Disturbances of the AV conduction system can occur in the atria, AV node, or His–Purkinje system. When there is complete block in any part of the AV conduction system (termed *third-degree AV block*) an escape pacemaker generally develops. When complete blockage occurs in the AV node, the His bundle escape pacemaker generally takes over at a rate of 40 to 60 beats/min, and is associated with a narrow QRS complex (in the absence of an underlying bundle branch block or other aberrant conduction). Complete heart block distal to the AV node often results in an escape pacemaker originating from the more distal conduction system, usually with a rate between 25 and 45 beats/min. These fascicular escape rhythms generate a QRS complex consistent with their origin (e.g., if the origin is in the right bundle, the QRS has a left bundle branch block pattern). If the conduction system fails, a rhythm from the ventricular myocardium may generate a heartbeat, with a wide complex of ventricular origin. Thus, in general, the more distal the escape rhythm, the slower and less reliable it tends to be. Heart block with irregular fascicular escapes may require urgent temporary pacing. The ECG shows AV dissociation with nonconducted P waves that "march" out independently of the ventricular escape rhythm. There are many causes of third-degree heart block including acute myocardial infarction, idiopathic fibrosis, drug toxicity (e.g., digitalis, beta blockers, cardioselective calcium channel blockers), chronic cardiopulmonary disease, congenital heart disease, infiltrative diseases (sarcoidosis), infections/inflammatory diseases, collagen vascular diseases, trauma, and tumors.

First-degree AV block is not truly heart *block,* but rather represents a delay in normal cardiac conduction. It is defined by a PR interval >200 ms. First-degree AV block is generally benign, but may result in symptoms if the degree of AV dyssynchrony is severe.

Second-degree AV block occurs when some atrial impulses fail to conduct to the ventricles. **Mobitz type I second-degree AV block** (Wenckebach block) is characterized on ECG by a variable (usually progressively prolonging) PR interval culminating in a nonconducted atrial beat. Mobitz I uncommonly progresses to complete heart block. When it does, the escape pacemaker of 40 to 60 beats/min in the His bundle usually provides an adequate backup rate to maintain CO. Mobitz I block can be caused by drugs such as digoxin, beta blockers, certain calcium channel blockers, or by ischemia (especially of the inferior wall) or hypervagotonia in otherwise healthy individuals.

Mobitz type II second-degree AV block generally is due to disease in the His–Purkinje system and is characterized on ECG by a fixed PR interval with one or more nonconducting atrial impulses. It is more likely to progress, sometimes precipitously, to complete heart block than Mobitz I. The typical escape pacemaker rate of 25 to 45 arises in the more distal His–Purkinje system and has a wide QRS. The escape rhythm may not be sufficient to maintain CO and can progress rapidly to cardiac arrest and death. Mobitz II heart block can occur from ischemia (especially anteroseptal infarcts), endocarditis, valvular or congenital heart disease, drugs (such as procainamide, disopyramide, and quinidine), or idiopathic progressive cardiac conduction system diseases.

Treatment of clinically significant bradycardia follows the ACLS algorithm outlined in Algorithm 20.2, and aims at maintaining adequate CO. Reversible causes should be identified. Atropine is a first-line transient pharmacologic therapy, and is more successful in patients with sinus bradycardia or block within the AV node, rather than block in the more distal His–Purkinje system. Patients who remain clinically unstable require immediate transcutaneous or transvenous pacing. In patients with sinus node dysfunction in which the cause is not reversible, permanent pacing can relieve symptoms. Permanent pacing is typically indicated in Mobitz II or third-degree AV block. If symptoms of bradycardia are present in Mobitz I AV block, permanent pacing is indicated.

CARDIAC ARREST

Cardiac arrest refers to the cessation of a detectable noninvasive blood pressure and pulse. Cardiac arrest can be separated into three main types: (a) pulseless electrical activity (PEA), (b) VT and VF, and (c) asystole. All three fall under the overall heading of pulseless arrest outlined in Algorithm 20.3. Treatment of PEA and asystole are similar and center on identifying reversible causes and employing pharmacologic intervention. VT and VF are treated with immediate electrical defibrillation. The most important aspect of resuscitation remains adequate cardiopulmonary resuscitation (CPR).

Treatment of cardiac arrest in an intensive care unit setting requires a team of nurses and physicians trained in ACLS. Ideally there should be an established and easily identifiable team leader responsible for continuously evaluating the patient's condition and cardiac rhythm, assimilating incoming data, and giving all orders. In addition, there should be a scribe, recording changes in condition, diagnostic and laboratory data, and therapies delivered. Initial patient evaluation follows the ABCs of cardiac arrest in a coordinated and overlapping fashion, ensuring adequate airway control, breathing (i.e., ventilation), and circulation. In nonintubated patients, an oral airway device should be placed and a bag-valve-mask should be used to deliver breaths. Intubation is performed when possible. CPR should begin immediately with chest compressions given at a rate of 100 compressions/min at 1.5 to 2 in depth, allowing full chest recoil between compressions. Patients should also be immediately connected to an automated external defibrillator (AED), or a manual defibrillator if an AED is not available. The defibrillator is connected to two pads or paddles placed on the chest wall, with one to the right of the sternum centered on the second intercostal space, and one on the left chest wall centered in the midaxillary line at the fifth intercostal space. IV access should be ensured for delivery of medications and fluids. Peripheral IV access is initially adequate. However, central IV access should be obtained as soon as possible via the femoral vein, subclavian vein, or internal jugular vein. Endotracheal intubation or central IV access should not interfere with CPR. Pulses are best monitored in the femoral artery, but the carotid arteries may be used. Once airway control is established and the patient is connected to an external defibrillator, the cardiac rhythm should be rapidly analyzed (Table 20.1).

Pulseless VT and VF

Confirmed VT and VF with hemodynamic collapse should be treated with *immediate* asynchronous defibrillation. Automated AED devices typically deliver escalating biphasic shocks at 200, 300, and 360 J. Manual devices may generate monophasic or biphasic waveforms. If a manual biphasic device is used and the device recommended dose scale is unknown, an initial dose of 200 J should be used, with subsequent shocks at the same or higher doses. If a monophasic device is used, the dose should be 360 J for all shocks. The patient's rhythm, blood pressure, and responsiveness must be continuously monitored with appropriate adjustment of therapy (e.g., continuation/discontinuation of CPR, infusion of new medications). If VT/VF persists or recurs after initial treatment, CPR should be resumed immediately after the first shock is given and continued for 2 minutes along with continuous ventilation via a mask airway or endotracheal tube. The rhythm and pulse should be reassessed 2 minutes after the shock is given. Shocks should be repeated if patients remain in pulseless VT/VF and the CPR cycle repeated. When IV access is established, patients should be concomitantly treated with 1 mg IV epinephrine every 3 to 5 minutes. After the third shock is given, patients who remain in VF/VT should be considered for amiodarone or lidocaine at the doses shown in Algorithm 20.3. Careful evaluation for a treatable cause should be sought. If a pulse becomes present at any point in treatment, the rhythm should be identified and appropriately treated according to Algorithms 20.4 and 20.5.

PEA and Asystole

PEA includes numerous pulseless rhythms such as bradyasystolic rhythms, idioventricular rhythms, and ventricular escape rhythms. PEA and asystole are not treated with electrical defibrillation. Treatment centers on well-delivered CPR and pharmacologic intervention as illustrated in Algorithm 20.3. Epinephrine should be given at 1 mg IV every 3 to 5 minutes. If a slow rhythm is seen on the monitor, consider giving atropine 1 mg IV. If IV access is not available, the drugs may be given endotracheally, in which case the dose is generally doubled.

The five H's and five T's listed in Algorithm 20.1 are common conditions that may contribute to cardiac arrest. Airway control and ventilation can correct *hypoxemia*. IV fluids should be given at a wide open rate or via a rapid infuser to correct *hypovolemia*. If *hypoglycemia* is suspected, give 1 ampule (amp) of 50% dextrose, or 1 mg of intramuscular glucagon if IV access is not available. If *hypokalemia* or acidosis (*hydrogen ion*) is suspected, give 1 amp of sodium bicarbonate (50 mEq NaHCO$_3$). *Hypothermia* should be treated as outlined in Chapter 32. Cases of suspected cardiac *tamponade* should be treated with immediate pericardiocentesis (see Chapter 79). Suspected *tension* pneumothorax should be treated with rapid decompression by inserting a large-bore catheter (14 or 16 gauge) into the second intercostal space in the midclavicular line, or unilateral or bilaterally inserted thoracostomy tubes. Ischemia from coronary *thrombosis* should be rapidly identified and treated when patients are stabilized (see Chapter 15). If pulmonary thrombosis is suspected, fibrinolytics may be beneficial but are not recommended for routine use.

TABLE 20.1	ACLS Pharmacotherapies: Dosing and Side Effects	
Medications	IV Dosing	Side Effects
Metoprolol	SVT: 2.5–5 mg IV q5min (max dose 15 mg over 15 min)	Hypotension, bradycardia, bronchoconstriction, CHF
Diltiazem	SVT: 0.25 mg/kg IV over 2 min, repeat bolus (after 15 min if response inadequate) 0.35 mg/kg IV over 2 min	Hypotension, bradycardia, CHF
Adenosine	SVT: initial dose: 6 mg IV rapid push Repeat bolus (after 2 min if response inadequate) 12 mg IV rapid push (always flush with saline)	Flushing, headache, AV block, asystole
Digoxin	SVT: initial loading dose: 0.25–0.5 mg IV slow push (reduce dose by 50% in renal failure), up to 1.5 mg in 24 hrs	Atrial tachycardia with or without AV block, nausea, blurred vision
Epinephrine (1:10,000)	PEA/asystole: 1 mg IV q3–5min × 3 doses (higher doses or continuous infusions can be used to treat specific problems)	Tachyarrhythmias, chest pain, hypertension
Vasopressin	PEA/asystole: 40 units IV may replace first or second dose of epinephrine	Tachyarrhythmias, asystole, chest pain, hypertension
Atropine	Slow PEA/asystole: 1 mg IV q3–5min × 3 doses Bradycardia: 0.5–1 mg IV q3–5min, up to 0.04 mg/kg in 24-hr period	Anticholinergic side effects, tachyarrhythmias, hypotension
Dopamine	Hemodynamic support: 1–5 mcg/kg/min, max dose 50 mcg/kg/min	Vasoconstriction, arrhythmias, hypotension (at lower doses), chest pain
Norepinephrine	Hemodynamic support: 0.5–1 mcg/min, max dose titrate to response	Vasoconstriction, arrhythmias, chest pain
Amiodarone	300 mg IV push, can redose if inadequate response 150 mg IV push	Hypotension, prolonged QT interval, bradycardia arrhythmias
Lidocaine	1–1.5 mg/kg IV over 2–3 min, may repeat 0.5–0.75 mg/kg IV q10min for total of 3 doses	Tachyarrhythmias, bradycardia, hypotension, AV block
Procainamide	20–50 mg/min until arrythmia controlled	Hypotension, lupus-like syndrome, QRS widening
Magnesium	Torsades de pointes: 1–2 mg IV push over 5–20 min	Flushing, hypotension

ACLS, advanced cardiac life support; IV, intravenous; SVT, supraventricular arrhythmia.

Cycles of CPR should continue until patients have palpable pulses and a detectable blood pressure or until resuscitation efforts have failed. There is no set period for when to stop resuscitation efforts. The decision to stop CPR is made by the medical team once a full trial at resuscitation has failed and the patient's chances of regaining a pulse and neurologic function are negligible. If patients do regain a pulse, the rhythm on the monitor should be identified and the patient treated accordingly. Blood pressure should be checked and hypotension should be treated with IV vasopressors and IV fluids. An arterial blood gas and other laboratory tests should be checked and abnormalities treated. Consideration of inotropic support or other advanced heart failure therapies should also be made once the patient has been stabilized if cardiogenic shock is associated with the arrest.

Postresuscitation hypothermia often occurs naturally after cardiac arrest. Active induction of hypothermia has also been evaluated in numerous randomized trials of patients with VF arrest and PEA/asystolic arrest occurring both in and out of the hospital. Patients were generally hemodynamically stable but comatose. They were cooled within minutes to hours to between approximately 32°C and 34°C, generally with cooling blankets. There were improved outcomes and metabolic endpoints in patients who were actively cooled. Thus, it is a current American Heart Association class IIb recommendation for in-hospital cardiac arrest and non-VF arrest, and class IIa for out-of-hospital VF arrest to cool hemodynamically stable but unconscious patients to between 32°C and 34°C for 12 to 24 hours after cardiac arrest. Patients with spontaneous hypothermia should not be actively rewarmed. Complications of cooling include coagulopathies and arrhythmias.

SUGGESTED READINGS

2015 American Heart Association Guidelines Update for Cardiopulmonary Resuscitation and Emergency Cardiovascular Care. Part 4: systems of care and continuous quality improvement, part 5: adult basic life support and cardiopulmonary recuscitation quality, part 6: alternative techniques and ancillary devices for cardiopulmonary recuscitation, part 7: adult advanced cardiovascular life support, part 8: post-cardiac arrest care. *Circulation*. 2015;132(18 suppl 2):S397–S482.

Current recommendations from the AHA based on evaluation of current treatment evidence reviewed at the 2015 International Consensus Conference on Cardiopulmonary Resuscitation and Emergency Cardiovascular Care, and published in the supplement to Circulation.

Hypothermia After Cardiac Arrest Study Group. Mild therapeutic hypothermia to improve the neurologic outcome after cardiac arrest. *N Engl J Med.* 2002;346(8):549–556.

Multicenter trial of patients resuscitated after cardiac arrest due to ventricular fibrillation who were randomly assigned to undergo therapeutic hypothermia or standard treatment with normothermia. The primary endpoint was a favorable neurologic outcome within 6 months after cardiac arrest, which was achieved by 55% of patients in the hypothermia group compared to 39% in the normothermia group. Mortality was 41% versus 55%, favoring the hypothermia group.

Stevenson WG, Wilber DJ, Natale A, et al; Multicenter Thermocool Ventricular Tachycardia Ablation Trial. Irrigated radiofrequency catheter ablation guided by electroanatomic mapping for recurrent ventricular tachycardia after myocardial infarction: the multicenter thermocool ventricular tachycardia ablation trial. *Circulation.* 2008;118(25):2773–2782.

Multicenter trial of patients with sustained, recurrent, monomorphic VT after myocardial infarction targeted for ablation. Primary endpoint was freedom from recurrent incessant or intermittent VT after 6 months. Fifty-three percent of patients achieved the primary endpoint with statistical significance.

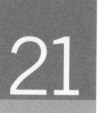

21 Aortic Dissection

Matthew J. Chung and Alan C. Braverman

Aortic dissection is a life-threatening condition that accounts for a small, but sig nificant proportion of cardiovascular disease, with an incidence of approximatel 3 to 6 per 100,000 people per year. It carries substantial morbidity and mortalit with a mortality rate up to 1% per hour within the first several hours. An algorithr for the immediate approach to the patient with aortic dissection is presented i Algorithms 21.1 and 21.2.

"Classic" aortic dissection results from a tear in the intimal layer of the aort allowing blood to enter the media and propagate in an anterograde or retrograd direction, resulting in a second or "false" lumen (Fig. 21.1A). Additional intim tears may occur and allow reconnection with the true lumen. Variants of aortic di section include aortic intramural hematoma (IMH) and penetrating atherosclerot ulcer (PAU), which together account for 10% to 20% of acute aortic syndrome (Fig. 21.1B,C). In aortic IMH, rupture of the vasa vasorum leads to hemorrhag in the medial layer without a visible intimal tear or communication with the aort lumen. IMH of the aorta is generally treated in a similar fashion as aortic dissectior with emergency surgery for type A IMH and medical therapy for type B IMH. PAl arises when an atherosclerotic lesion of the aorta develops ulceration that penetrate the intimal and medial layers, which may lead to a false aneurysm that can dissect o rupture. Between these two variants of acute aortic syndromes, IMH is more likel to progress to classic aortic dissection, and PAU, more common in the descendin aorta, may be more likely to rupture. Once aortic dissection occurs, shear stres stemming from the rate of change in pressure (dP/dt) and mean arterial blood pres sure contribute to spread of the tear.

Several conditions predispose the aorta to dissection, either due to abnor malities in the aortic wall composition or due to excess shear stress (Table 21.1) Approximately 75% of patients with aortic dissection have hypertension. Patient with genetically triggered aortic disorders, such as bicuspid aortic valve, Marfar syndrome, Loeys–Dietz syndrome, vascular Ehlers–Danlos syndrome, Turner syn drome, and Familial Thoracic Aortic Aneurysm/Dissection syndrome, are particu larly prone to aortic dilation and dissection. Cocaine- or methamphetamine-induced hypertension, inflammatory conditions such as giant cell arteritis, and direct traum from catheterization or aortic surgery can disrupt the aortic wall. Once the intim becomes injured, it is vulnerable to shear stress and may progress to dissection o rupture.

There are several anatomic classification systems of aortic dissection, and involvement of the ascending aorta is the defining characteristic (Fig. 21.2). DeBake

ALGORITHM 21.1   Evaluation of Aortic Dissection

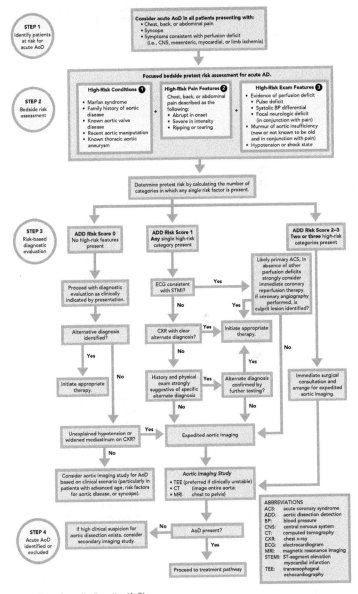

Evaluation pathway for aortic dissection (AoD).

Reproduced with permission from Rogers AM, Hermann LK, Booher AM, et al. Sensitivity of the aortic dissection detection risk score, a novel guideline-based tool for identification of acute aortic dissection at initial presentation: results from the International Registry of Acute Aortic Dissection. *Circulation.* 2011;123(20):2213–2218.

ALGORITHM 21.2 Management of Aortic Dissection

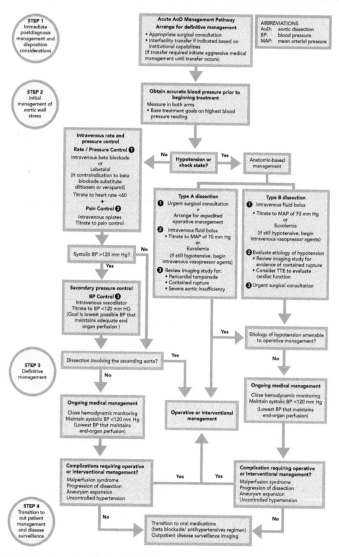

Management pathway for acute aortic dissection (AoD).

Reproduced with permission from Hiratzka LF, Bakris GL, Beckman JA, et al. 2010 ACCF/AHA/AATS/ACR/ASA/SCA/SCAI/SIR/STS/SVM guidelines for the diagnosis and management of patients with thoracic aortic disease: a report of the American College of Cardiology Foundation/American Heart Association Task Force on Practice Guidelines, American Association for Thoracic Surgery, American College of Radiology, American Stroke Association, Society of Cardiovascular Anesthesiologists, Society for Cardiovascular Angiography and Interventions, Society of Interventional Radiology, Society of Thoracic Surgeons, and Society for Vascular Medicine. *J Am Coll Cardiol*. 2010; 55(14):e27–e129.

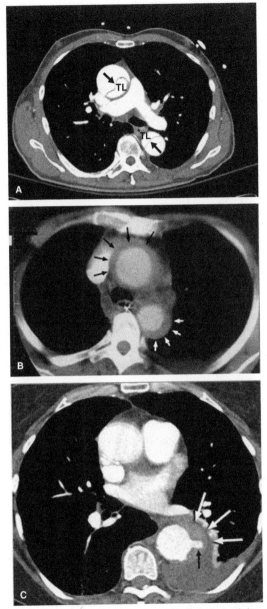

Figure 21.1. Types of acute aortic syndromes. **A:** "Classic" type A aortic dissection. *Black arrows* indicate intimal flaps. The true lumen (TL) is usually the smaller lumen. **B:** Type A intramural hematoma (IMH) of the aorta. *Black arrows* indicate circumferential IMH in the ascending aorta and *white arrows* denote crescentic IMH in descending aorta. **C:** Penetrating atherosclerotic ulcer (PAU) of the aorta (*black arrow*). *White arrows* point to associated intramural hematoma. (Reproduced with permission from Braverman AC. Diseases of the aorta. In: Bonow RO, Mann DL, Zipes DP, et al., eds. *Braunwald's Heart Disease.* 10th ed. Philadelphia, PA: Elsevier; 2015:1277–1311.)

TABLE 21.1 Risk Factors for Aortic Dissection

- Hypertension
- Hereditary aortic diseases[a] (gene responsible)
  - Marfan syndrome (*FBN1*)
  - Loeys–Dietz syndrome (*TGFBR1* and *TGFBR2*)
  - Familial thoracic aortic aneurysm/ dissection syndromes (*TGFBR1, TGFBR2, SMAD3, TGFB2, TGFB3, MYH11, ACTA2, MYLK*, others)
  - Vascular Ehlers–Danlos syndrome (*COL3A1*)
- Congenital conditions
  - Bicuspid aortic valve[a]
  - Turner syndrome
  - Aortic coarctation
- Cocaine/methamphetamine use
- Pheochromocytoma
- Atherosclerosis/penetrating aortic ulcer
- Trauma—blunt or iatrogenic
  - Catheter-induced
  - Aortic valve surgery/transcatheter aortic valve replacement (TAVR)
  - Coronary artery bypass grafting
  - Deceleration injury (e.g., motor vehicle accident)
- Inflammatory conditions
  - Giant cell arteritis
  - Takayasu's arteritis
  - Behçet's disease
  - Syphilitic aortitis
- Pregnancy[b]
- Weightlifting[b]

[a]First-degree relatives of patients with these conditions should be screened for aortic disease.
[b]With concomitant aortopathy.
Reproduced with permission from Braverman AC. Diseases of the aorta. In: Bonow RO, Mann DL, Zipes DP, et al., eds. *Braunwald's Heart Disease.* 10th ed. Philadelphia, PA: Elsevier; 2015: 1277–1311.

types I and II, and Stanford type A dissections involve the ascending aorta. DeBakey type III or Stanford type B dissections do not involve the ascending aorta. Classification of the anatomy is important because the decision regarding surgical or medical management is dependent on the location of the dissection. Broadly, dissections of the ascending aorta (types I, II, and A) require immediate surgical repair, while uncomplicated dissections involving the descending aorta (types III and B) are initially treated medically. Aortic dissection involves the ascending aorta nearly twice as frequently as the descending aorta. The chronicity of aortic dissection is defined by the duration of symptoms at the time of presentation, with less than 2 weeks considered acute and greater than 2 weeks considered chronic. Importantly, potentially fatal complications such as aortic rupture and branch vessel occlusion are more likely to occur in the acute phase compared with the chronic phase. A recent classification system from the International Registry of Acute Aortic Dissection (IRAD) stratifies aortic dissection into four temporal groups based on the risk of mortality during each time period and includes hyperacute (0 to 24 hours), acute (2 to 7 days), subacute (8 to 30 days), and chronic (>30 days). The IRAD classification scheme highlights the marked increase in risk of mortality in the immediate period (hyperacute) after developing symptoms of aortic dissection with lower risks of mortality during each subsequent time period (Fig. 21.3).

The clinical presentation of aortic dissection may be quite variable, and one must maintain a high index of suspicion for the diagnosis. In contrast to the crescendo discomfort of angina pectoris, the pain of acute dissection is maximal at its onset, usually

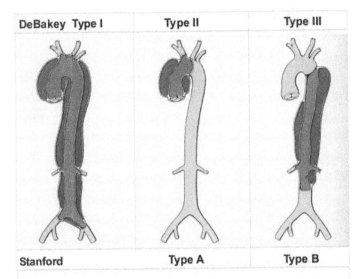

DeBakey

Type I   Originates in the ascending aorta, propagates at least to the aortic arch and often beyond it distally

Type II   Originates in and is confined to the ascending aorta

Type III Originates in the descending aorta and extends distally down the aorta or, rarely, retrograde into the aortic arch and ascending aorta

Stanford

Type A   All dissections involving the ascending aorta, regardless of the site of origin

Type B   All dissections not involving the ascending aorta

Figure 21.2. Classification systems of aortic dissection: DeBakey and Stanford. (Reproduced with permission from Nienaber CA, Eagle KA. Aortic dissection: new frontiers in diagnosis and management. Part I: from etiology to diagnostic strategies. *Circulation.* 2003;108(5):628–635.)

sudden, sharp, and severe, located in the chest or back. Syncope may accompany type A dissection, usually heralding cardiac tamponade, aortic rupture, or cerebral involvement. In addition to the dissection itself, presenting symptoms may also be related to malperfusion or complications involving various organ systems. Physical examination should include a complete pulse exam and blood pressure in both arms and legs, as there may be pulse or blood pressure deficits. Cardiac auscultation may reveal an aortic regurgitation murmur. However, pulse deficits are present in only ~25% of patients and an aortic regurgitation murmur in less than half. Thus, absence of these features on physical examination is not sufficient to rule out aortic dissection.

Significant morbidity and mortality from dissection is attributed to malperfusion with end-organ damage and aortic rupture (Table 21.2). Organ systems may become compromised by compression of branch vessels due to an expanding false lumen or direct extension of a dissection into the vessel. Cardiovascular and neurologic manifestations are two particularly devastating complications of aortic

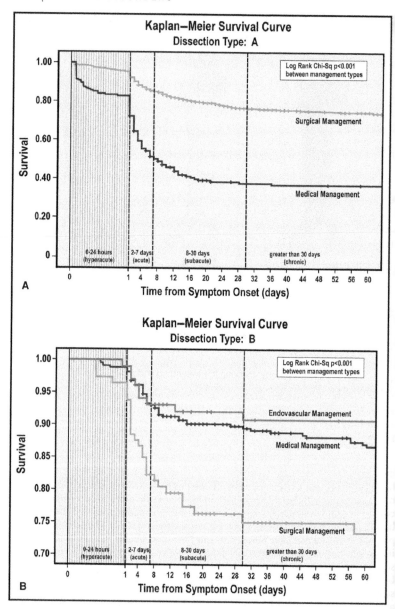

Figure 21.3. Survival curves for acute aortic dissection by type and management. **A:** Kaplan–Meier survival curve for type A dissection stratified by treatment type. **B:** Kaplan–Meier survival curve for type B dissection stratified by treatment type. (Reproduced with permission from Booher AM, Isselbacher EM, Nienaber CA, et al. The IRAD classification system for characterizing survival after aortic dissection. *Am J Med.* 2013; 126(8):730.e19–e24.)

TABLE 21.2	Complications of Aortic Dissection
Cardiovascular	Cardiac arrest Syncope Aortic regurgitation Congestive heart failure Myocardial ischemia or infarction Cardiac tamponade Pericarditis Upper or lower extremity limb ischemia
Pulmonary	Pleural effusion Hemothorax Hemoptysis
Renal	Acute renal failure Renovascular hypertension Renal ischemia or infarction
Neurologic	Transient ischemic attack or stroke Paraparesis or paraplegia Encephalopathy or coma Spinal cord syndrome Ischemic neuropathy
Gastrointestinal	Mesenteric ischemia or infarction Pancreatitis Ischemic hepatitis Nausea and vomiting Hematemesis
Systemic	Fever

Reproduced with permission from Braverman AC. Diseases of the aorta. In: Bonow RO, Mann DL, Zipes DP, et al., eds. *Braunwald's Heart Disease*. 10th ed. Philadelphia, PA: Elsevier; 2015: 1277–1311.

dissection. In type A dissection, cardiac tamponade, aortic regurgitation leading to heart failure, aortic rupture, or myocardial infarction from coronary artery involvement may lead rapidly to hemodynamic shock and death. When cardiac tamponade complicates type A dissection, emergency surgery is recommended. Poor outcomes have been reported with pericardiocentesis owing to lowering of the intrapericardial pressure, which may cause further bleeding and hemodynamic collapse. However, if emergency surgery cannot be performed expediently in the setting of refractory shock, limited pericardiocentesis to remove just enough pericardial blood to allow for better diastolic filling can improve the blood pressure and be lifesaving. Neurologic sequelae may result from acute dissection involving the carotid or vertebral arteries, as cerebral hypoperfusion may lead to syncope, altered mental status, and stroke. Transverse myelitis, myelopathy, paraplegia, or quadriplegia may result from spinal malperfusion. Mesenteric, limb, or renal ischemia may occur due to branch vessel occlusion. Hence, the clinician must remain vigilant in monitoring for evidence of end-organ malperfusion in the patient with known aortic dissection.

TABLE 21.3 Comparison of Diagnostic Imaging Modalities

Test	Sensitivity (%)	Specificity (%)	Advantages	Disadvantages
TTE[a]	77–80	93–96	Rapidly available, can be done at bedside	Poor sensitivity for type B aortic dissection, may be limited by poor acoustic windows
TEE	98–99	94–97	Excellent evaluation of aortic root, descending thoracic aorta, aortic valve, and pericardium, can be done at the bedside	Requires esophageal intubation which may affect hemodynamics, limited to thoracic aorta
CT[b]	96–100	96–100	Widely and rapidly available, superior imaging of entire aorta, heart, branch vessels, and complications such as rupture and hemopericardium	Ionizing radiation and nephrotoxic iodinated contrast required
MRI[c]	>98	>98	Superior accuracy, sensitivity, and specificity for all types of dissection	Limited availability, time-consuming procedure, more difficult to monitor patient during test

[a]Sensitivity and specificity for the use of TTE in identifying type A dissection; the ability of TTE to identify type B aortic dissection is much lower.
[b]With iodinated contrast.
[c]With gadolinium-based contrast.
TTE, transthoracic echocardiogram; TEE, transesophageal echocardiogram; CT, computed tomography; MRI, magnetic resonance imaging.

Standard imaging and laboratory tests may assist in the evaluation of aortic dissection. The chest x-ray (CXR) may demonstrate a widened mediastinum or abnormal aortic contour. Pleural effusion may represent hemothorax, and separation of the intimal calcification from the outer aortic soft tissue border by more than 10 mm, the radiologic "calcium sign," may indicate an intimal flap. However, since up to 20% of CXRs do not demonstrate abnormal findings, a normal CXR cannot exclude an aortic dissection. The electrocardiogram (ECG) is often nonspecific, although evidence of coronary ischemia or injury may be present when the dissection involves a coronary artery. The D-dimer, a degradation product of cross-linked fibrin, may be of assistance in suspecting the diagnosis; it is usually markedly elevated in acute aortic dissection, and when <500 ng/mL has a negative predictive value of 95% in the first 24 hours from symptom onset. Importantly, in IMH or PAU, the D-dimer may not be elevated, and in the setting of a high clinical index of suspicion a normal D-dimer does not rule out an acute aortic syndrome. Given these limitations, a clear role for the D-dimer in the evaluation of aortic dissection has not been established. Other laboratory tests important to obtain to evaluate for complications of aortic dissection include complete blood count, comprehensive metabolic profile, lactic acid, troponin, lactate dehydrogenase, and creatine kinase levels.

Due to the critical nature of aortic dissection, immediate diagnostic confirmation and definition of the extent of the dissection is imperative once it is suspected. The choice of imaging should be made on the basis of patient hemodynamic stability and operator availability. The sensitivity and specificity of the most commonly used imaging modalities and their relative advantages and disadvantages are shown in Table 21.3. If the patient presents with hemodynamic instability, rapid evaluation by transthoracic echocardiogram (TTE), transesophageal echocardiogram (TEE), or computed tomography (CT) scan should be performed to assess for complications of dissection, including pericardial effusion, aortic regurgitation, or aortic rupture. Given the lower sensitivity of TTE, a normal TTE cannot exclude dissection. CT is widely and rapidly available and the most commonly used initial diagnostic test. Though CT scans require intravenous contrast dye, they offer superior imaging of the entire aorta,

---

TABLE 21.4 | Pharmacologic Therapy for Acute Aortic Syndromes[a]

1. Intravenous β-blocker (preferred initial therapy)[b]
   - **Esmolol:** Give 1 mg/kg over 30 s, then continuous IV infusion at 150–300 mcg/kg/min, titrated to effect. Short half-life allows rapid titration.
   - **Labetalol:** As bolus, give 20 mg IV over 2 min, then 40–80 mg IV every 10 min until adequate response (maximum dose 300 mg); as infusion start at 2 mg/min and titrate to response up to 300 mg total cumulative dose (prolonged continuous infusions >300 mg/day may be required, however, there are limited data to guide this use).
2. Intravenous vasodilator (use only after initiation of β-blocker therapy)
   - **Sodium nitroprusside:** Start continuous infusion at 0.3–0.5 mcg/kg/min, titrate by 0.5 mcg/kg/min every few minutes to desired effect; maximum dose of 10 mcg/kg/min (to avoid toxicity, some recommend a maximum dose of 2 mcg/kg/min).
     - *Caution: thiocyanate toxicity may occur with prolonged infusions or in patients with renal impairment.*
   - **Nicardipine:** Start continuous infusion at 5 mg/hr, then increase by 2.5 mg/hr every 5 min (for rapid titration) to every 15 min (for gradual titration) up to a maximum of 15 mg/hr; for rapidly titrated patients, consider reduction to 3 mg/hr after response is achieved.
   - **Enalaprilat:** Give 0.625–1.25 mg/dose IV over 5 min, then increase by 0.625–1.25 mg/dose every 6 hrs to a maximum of 5 mg/dose every 6 hrs, titrated to effect.

[a]Goal of therapy is HR less than 60 beats/min and systolic blood pressure as low as possible without compromising end-organ perfusion.
[b]If β-blockers are contraindicated, use diltiazem: 0.25 mg/kg IV over 2 minutes, then continuous IV infusion at 5–15 mg/hr, titrated to effect.

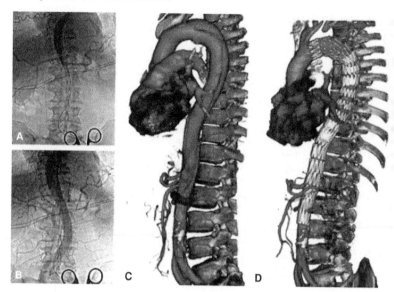

Figure 21.4. Thoracic endovascular repair (TEVAR) for complicated type B aortic dissection with aortic malperfusion above the renal arteries before and after emergency stent-graft implantation. **A:** Aortogram with no flow to the abdominal aorta. **B:** Aortogram demonstrating markedly improved distal flow after stent-graft placement. **C:** Three-dimensional reconstruction of the complicated type B dissection before TEVAR. **D:** After stent-graft placement. (Reproduced with permission from Akin I, Kische S, Tehders TC, et al. TEVAR, the solution to all aortic problems? *Herz.* 2011;36(6):539–547.)

aortic arch, and branch vessels and provide the ability to create three-dimensional CT reconstructions that can aid in treatment planning. TEE requires an experienced operator and esophageal intubation to perform the procedure; however, it can be performed at the bedside, does not require contrast dye, and visualizes the aortic valve, aortic root, and pericardium well. Although associated with a very high sensitivity and specificity for diagnosis, MRI is not typically the test of first choice in acute dissection, due to the longer image acquisition time and lesser availability on an emergency basis.

When aortic dissection is suspected, immediate initiation of β-blocker therapy to reduce shear stress is paramount, while simultaneously pursuing confirmation of the diagnosis (Table 21.4). Intravenous β-blocker therapy is recommended to achieve a target heart rate below 60 beats/min and systolic blood pressure below 120 mm Hg. Systolic blood pressure should be lowered as much as possible without compromising end-organ perfusion. Nondihydropyridine calcium channel blockers (e.g., diltiazem, verapamil) may be used if β-blocker therapy is contraindicated. If, after β-blocker therapy, the systolic blood pressure remains elevated, vasodilators, such as intravenous sodium nitroprusside, nicardipine, or angiotensin-converting enzyme (ACE) inhibitors should be added. Importantly, vasodilator therapy should not be initiated prior to starting β-blocker therapy, as vasodilators may induce reflex tachycardia, thereby increasing dP/dt, which may extend the dissection. Intravenous opiates for pain control are an important adjunct to aid in achieving target heart rate and blood pressure goals. Once the patient is stabilized, without complications, and heart rate nd blood pressure goals are met, the patient can be transitioned to oral β-blocker nd other antihypertensive therapy.

Emergent surgery is indicated in patients with type A dissection because medical herapy alone is associated with a high risk of morbidity and mortality (Fig. 21.3). Thoracic endovascular repair (TEVAR) is recommended for complicated type B dissection with typical indications being malperfusion syndromes, refractory pain, uncontrolled hypertension, rapidly expanding aortic enlargement, and rupture (Fig. 21.4). Endovascular stent grafting covers the intimal tear, decompresses the false channel, and improves perfusion to the true lumen and its branches. Open surgery for complicated type B dissection carries high risk and is reserved for complications that are unable to be managed by TEVAR. Trials are underway for TEVAR in uncomplicated type B dissection, but at present, uncomplicated patients are treated medically.

SUGGESTED READINGS

Booher AM, Isselbacher EM, Nienaber CA, et al. The IRAD classification system for characterizing survival after aortic dissection. *Am J Med*. 2013;126(8):730.e19–e24.
  Newer classification scheme for chronicity of aortic dissection based on risk of mortality.
Braverman AC. Acute aortic dissection: clinician update. *Circulation*. 2010;122(2):184–188.
  Overview of acute aortic dissection and clinical features.
Braverman AC. Aortic dissection: prompt diagnosis and emergency treatment are critical. *Cleve Clin J Med*. 2011;78(10):685–696.
  Review of aortic dissection.
Braverman AC. Diseases of the aorta. In: Mann DL, Zipes DP, Libby P, et al., eds. *Braunwald's Heart Disease*. 10th ed. Philadelphia, PA: Elsevier; 2015.
  Comprehensive overview of entire spectrum of aortic disease.
Erbel R, Aboyans V, Boileau C, et al. 2014 ESC guidelines on the diagnosis and treatment of aortic diseases: document covering acute and chronic aortic diseases of the thoracic and abdominal aorta of the adult. The Task Force for the Diagnosis and Treatment of Aortic Diseases of the European Society of Cardiology (ESC). *Eur Heart J*. 2014;35(41): 2873–2926.
  Comprehensive guideline on aortic diseases from the European Society of Cardiology.
Estrera A, Miller C, Lee T, et al. Acute type A intramural hematoma: analysis of current management strategy. *Circulation*. 2009;120(11 suppl):S287–S291.
  Nice review of management of type A IMH.
Evangelista A, Czerny M, Nienaber C, et al. Interdisciplinary expert consensus on management of type B intramural haematoma and penetrating aortic ulcer. *Eur J Cardiothorac Surg*. 2015;47(2):209–217.
  Comprehensive overview of the management of type B IMH and PAU.
Hiratzka LF, Bakris GL, Beckman JA, et al. 2010 ACCF/AHA/AATS/ACR/ASA/SCA/SCAI/ SIR/STS/SVM guidelines for the diagnosis and management of patients with thoracic aortic disease: a report of the American College of Cardiology Foundation/American Heart Association Task Force on Practice Guidelines, American Association for Thoracic Surgery, American College of Radiology, American Stroke Association, Society of Cardiovascular Anesthesiologists, Society for Cardiovascular Angiography and Interventions, Society of Interventional Radiology, Society of Thoracic Surgeons, and Society for Vascular Medicine. *J Am Coll Cardiol*. 2010;55(14):e27–e129.
  Comprehensive joint American guideline on thoracic aortic diseases.
Mehta RH, Suzuki T, Hagan PG, et al. Predicting death in patients with acute type A aortic dissection. *Circulation*. 2002;105(2):200–206.
  IRAD study of 547 patients which develops a risk prediction tool in patients with acute type A aortic dissection.

Nienaber CA, Clough RE. Management of aortic dissection. *Lancet.* 2015;385(9970):800–811
  Excellent comprehensive update on the diagnosis and management of aortic dissection.

Nienaber CA, Kische S, Rousseau H, et al. Endovascular repair of type B aortic dissection:
  long-term results of the randomized investigation of stent grafts in aortic dissection trial.
  Circ Cardiovasc Interv. 2013;6:407–416.
  *Results of the INSTEAD-XL trial, suggesting that TEVAR in addition to optimal medical
    treatment may improve outcomes in stable type B aortic dissection.*

Pape LA, Awais M, Woznicki EM, et al. Presentation, diagnosis, and outcomes of acute aortic
  dissection. 17-year trends from the international registry of acute aortic dissection. *J Am
  Coll Cardiol.* 2015;66(4):350–358.
  *Most recent update on trends in the diagnosis and management of aortic dissection from the
    IRAD.*

Rogers AM, Hermann LK, Booher AM, et al. Sensitivity of the aortic dissection detection risk
  score, a novel guideline-based tool for identification of acute aortic dissection at initial
  presentation: results from the international registry of acute aortic dissection. *Circulation.*
  2011;123(20):2213–2218.
  *Study that found the AHA/ACC aortic dissection detection (ADD) risk score to be highly
    sensitive.*

Tsai TT, Nienaber CA, Eagle KA. Acute aortic syndromes. *Circulation.* 2005;112(24):
  3802–3813.
  *Outstanding review of the three different acute aortic syndromes, and key points for diagnosis,
    imaging, and management.*

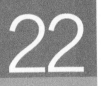

22 Acute Decompensated Heart Failure

Luigi Adamo, Shane J. LaRue, and Gregory A. Ewald

The combination of an increasing elderly population and successful reperfusion strategies for acute myocardial infarction (MI) has led to an epidemic in the number of patients with left ventricular dysfunction and heart failure (HF). It is estimated that there are nearly 6 million Americans living with HF, and 900,000 new cases occurring each year. In fact, HF is the leading cause of hospitalization for patients aged 65 or over and costs nearly 40 billion dollars per year in the United States and is an estimated 1% to 2% of the entire health care budget in Europe. The 1-year mortality from this condition approaches 50% for patients with advanced HF, resulting in 300,000 deaths annually in the United States.

The management of chronic HF has improved substantially during the past decade. Successful approaches validated by clinical trials have become well established and are documented in numerous evidence-based guidelines. These approaches will not be detailed here but involve (a) modulation of neurohormonal activation, specifically the renin–angiotensin–aldosterone system (via angiotensin-converting enzyme inhibitors [ACEIs], angiotensin receptor blockers [ARBs], ARB/neprilysin inhibitors [ARNIs], and aldosterone antagonists) and sympathetic nervous system (via beta blockers); (b) fluid management (via diuretics and sodium/water restriction); (c) reducing cardiac work and improving cardiac output (via hydralazine, nitrates, and digoxin); and (d) attempting to restore synchronized ventricular contraction and preventing sudden cardiac death (via implantation of biventricular pacemakers and cardiac defibrillators).

In contrast to chronic HF, the management of acute decompensated HF (ADHF) is not as well studied in randomized controlled trials, and evidence-based guidelines have only recently been developed. There are now three sets of guidelines that provide the clinician with recommendations for treating ADHF, one from the European Society of Cardiology, one from the American College of Cardiology/American Heart Association, and another from the Heart Failure Society of America. Our approach to HF in the critical care setting is consistent with these guidelines and is summarized in this chapter.

ADHF refers to a rapid onset or significant worsening of symptoms and signs of HF. Recognizing these signs is an important first step, as pre-existing HF may not have been diagnosed yet or acute HF may present in the setting of MI or acute cardiomyopathy. The patients presenting with ADHF are nearly equally split between those having reduced left ventricular ejection fraction and those with preserved ejection fraction. Typically, ADHF patients are elderly, have a history of hypertension, coronary artery disease, MI, or HF with subjective complaints of paroxysmal nocturnal dyspnea, orthopnea, and dyspnea on exertion. Physical findings that correlate with HF include a third heart sound (S3) and signs of volume overload, including jugular venous distention, hepatojugular reflux, pulmonary rales, and lower extremity edema. Chest radiography may show cardiomegaly or pulmonary venous congestion but up to 20% of patients with ADHF have none of these findings. Electrocardiographic findings are not specific but may show atrial fibrillation, ventricular hypertrophy, or evidence of prior MI. A completely normal EKG has a high negative predictive value for ADHF.

It is important to remember that although HF is a clinical diagnosis, echocardiography, angiography, and invasive hemodynamic monitoring are useful to document systolic or diastolic dysfunction. The role of blood testing is limited in the diagnosis of HF, however, B-type natriuretic peptide (BNP) levels can be helpful if the diagnosis is uncertain. Specifically, patients with serum BNP <100 pg/mL or NT-proBNP <300 pg/mL are very unlikely to have decompensated HF. It is important to note, however, that elevated plasma levels of the natriuretic peptides do not confirm a diagnosis of ADHF because they can be associated with a variety of other conditions including severely reduced glomerular filtration rate (<60 mL/min), ischemic stroke, liver dysfunction, severe infection, severe burns, and severe metabolic abnormalities. Once the diagnosis of ADHF is confirmed, it is critical to make an accurate assessment regarding the precipitating events for the patient's decompensated state and to make an estimation of the mortality risk of the patient. Common precipitants of ADHF include myocardial ischemia/infarction, mechanical complications of MI, hypertensive crisis, arrhythmias, sepsis, anemia, and decompensation of pre-existing HF secondary to medical or dietary nonadherence. Less common precipitating factors include acute myocarditis, peripartum cardiomyopathy, valvular heart disease (including infective endocarditis), pulmonary embolism, cardiac tamponade, drugs (e.g., non steroidal anti inflammatory drugs (NSAIDs), negative inotropic agents), and thyrotoxicosis (Table 22.1). Useful laboratory tests to evaluate patients presenting with ADHF are creatinine, blood urea nitrogen, liver function tests (often altered in patients with hypoperfusion or severe congestion), and basic electrolytes. Of note, mildly elevated cardiac troponin levels are detected in many patients with ADHF and should not be mistakenly interpreted as evidence of an acute coronary syndrome.

Approximately 4% of patients admitted with ADHF die in the hospital and it is therefore critical to identify the patients at highest risk of adverse outcomes. The need for hospital admission is determined with clinical judgment but admission is always warranted in the presence of dyspnea at rest (typically represented by resting tachypnea or oxygen saturation <90%), hemodynamically significant arrhythmias, worsening renal function, worsening pulmonary congestion, major electrolyte disturbances,

TABLE 22.1	Precipitants of Acute Decompensated Heart Failure
Common	Less Common
Medical/dietary noncompliance	Peripartum cardiomyopathy
Acute myocardial infarction	Acute myocarditis
Hypertensive crisis	Infective endocarditis
Arrhythmias	Valvular heart disease
Sepsis	Cardiac tamponade
Anemia	Thyrotoxicosis

r new-onset HF. In most cases, patients with ADHF present with either preserved r elevated blood pressure. Only 5% to 8% of patients present with systolic blood pressure <90 mm Hg. These patients have a poor prognosis with an inpatient mortality of more than 16% in the presence of serum creatinine >2 mg/dL. These patients nd those with evidence of hypoperfusion should be considered for admission to n intensive care unit. An initial algorithmic approach should focus on stabilizing he patient and performing noninvasive assessments of heart rhythm, oxygenation, emodynamics, and volume status (Algorithm 22.1). This will guide therapies such s amiodarone or cardioversion for atrial fibrillation with rapid ventricular response, asodilators to reduce afterload and the work of the failing heart, or inotropes for the atient with low cardiac output and inadequate end-organ perfusion. The Forrester lassification is useful with either noninvasive data (clinical perfusion status and evidence of pulmonary congestion) or invasive hemodynamic data (Algorithm 22.2). When an accurate clinical assessment of hemodynamic and volume status cannot be nade or in the presence of shock, a pulmonary artery catheter (Swan–Ganz) can be useful to measure the cardiac index, pulmonary capillary wedge pressure (PCWP), and systemic vascular resistance (SVR), with the additional benefit of monitoring the esponse to therapy. However, the placement of a pulmonary artery catheter is not without risks and thus should be reserved for selected cases and only performed by an experienced operator (see Chapter 82).

TREATMENT

General Measures

Oxygen supplementation should not be routinely used in nonhypoxic patients as oxygen causes vasoconstriction and may decrease cardiac output. Morphine should be used cautiously. While it can relieve dyspnea and reduce pulmonary vascular resistance, it can also exacerbate hypotension. If sedation is needed, cardiodepressive drugs like propofol should be avoided. Midazolam is considered a safer option in patients with ADHF. Patients with HF are hypercoagulable and therefore deep venous thrombosis (DVT) prophylaxis should be implemented in all patients who are not therapeutically anticoagulated.

Management of Chronic HF Medications in ADHF

ACEIs and ARBs have an important role in the management of chronic HF, but their role in the setting of ADHF is less clear. Chronic ACEI or ARB therapy promotes afterload reduction, but may require dosage reduction or discontinuation in patients with ADHF to facilitate diuresis without impairment of renal function. Cautious initiation of ACEI or ARB therapy in the intensive care unit setting may be helpful with careful monitoring of renal function and electrolytes. The short-acting ACEI, captopril at a starting dose of 6.25 to 12.5 mg every 6 to 8 hours, may be carefully titrated with each dose until a prespecified goal is met (e.g., systolic blood pressure <100 mm Hg, reduced SVR, or 300 mg daily dose). For patients with chronic HF, ACEIs or ARBs should be initiated approximately 48 hours after stabilization of an ADHF episode, most likely after transfer out of the critical care setting (class I recommendation, Level of Evidence A). Fluid restriction (<2 L/day) is recommended in patients with moderate hyponatremia and is advisable in all patients with fluid overload. In patients with severe hyponatremia, vasopressin receptor antagonists ("vaptans") can be carefully considered. Fluid restriction should be relaxed during treatment with these agents.

ALGORITHM 22.1 Algorithmic Approach to Acute Decompensated Heart Failure

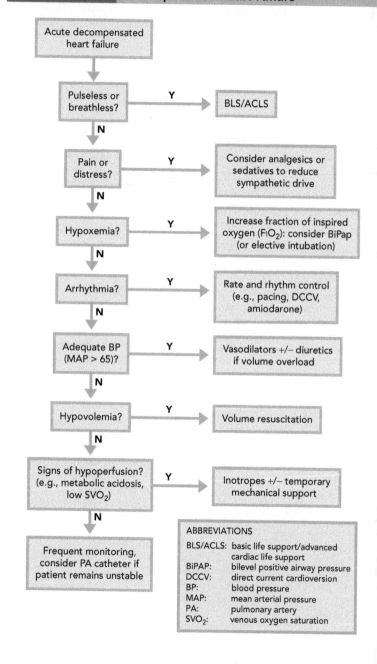

Acute decompensated heart failure

Pulseless or breathless? — **Y** → BLS/ACLS

N

Pain or distress? — **Y** → Consider analgesics or sedatives to reduce sympathetic drive

N

Hypoxemia? — **Y** → Increase fraction of inspired oxygen (FiO₂): consider BiPap (or elective intubation)

N

Arrhythmia? — **Y** → Rate and rhythm control (e.g., pacing, DCCV, amiodarone)

N

Adequate BP (MAP > 65)? — **Y** → Vasodilators +/− diuretics if volume overload

N

Hypovolemia? — **Y** → Volume resuscitation

N

Signs of hypoperfusion? (e.g., metabolic acidosis, low SVO₂) — **Y** → Inotropes +/− temporary mechanical support

N

Frequent monitoring, consider PA catheter if patient remains unstable

ABBREVIATIONS

BLS/ACLS: basic life support/advanced cardiac life support
BiPAP: bilevel positive airway pressure
DCCV: direct current cardioversion
BP: blood pressure
MAP: mean arterial pressure
PA: pulmonary artery
SVO₂: venous oxygen saturation

ALGORITHM 22.2 **Acute Decompensated Heart Failure Therapies by Clinical Presentation (Forrester Classification)**

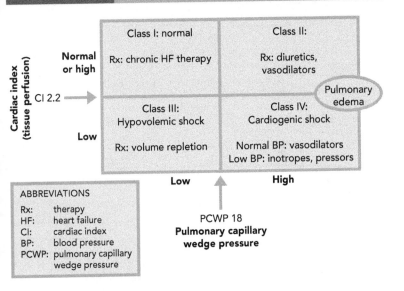

Other medical therapies such as beta blockers and calcium channel blockers have a limited role in the management of patients with ADHF. Beta blockade is a mainstay of treatment for acute MI as well as for chronic HF, but patients presenting with MI and ADHF involving hypotension or more than mild-to-moderate pulmonary congestion have not been included in most of the relevant clinical trials. As such, IV metoprolol and other agents should be used with caution in this setting. Patients receiving chronic beta-blocker therapy may require a dose reduction, but beta blockers should not be abruptly discontinued in the absence of hypoperfusion to avoid adverse events related to elevated catecholamine levels. Milrinone should be considered for these patients if they require inotropic support as it acts downstream from the beta-adrenergic receptor. Calcium channel blockers (including diltiazem, verapamil, and amlodipine) are contra-indicated in patients with ADHF, secondary to their negative inotropic effects.

Diuresis

Most patients with ADHF present with volume overload and pulmonary congestion. The mainstays of therapy are diuretics and vasodilators, reserved for those patients with adequate cardiac output to maintain sufficient systolic blood pressure (>85 to 90 mm Hg) and end-organ perfusion (Algorithm 22.2, Forrester class II) prior to their initiation. These therapies are considered class I recommendations and reduce the work that must be performed by the failing heart by reducing both preload and afterload while providing symptomatic relief. Initial therapy with intravenous (IV) diuretics (2 to 2.5 times usual daily oral dose) has a relatively rapid effect, with reductions in right atrial pressure, PCWP, and PVR within 5 to 30 minutes. For patients

TABLE 22.2 Diuretics for Acute Decompensated Heart Failure

Severity of Volume Overload	Diuretic	Dose	Comments
Mild to moderate	Furosemide	20–80 mg PO or IV	Follow Na^+ and K^+
Severe	Furosemide	40–120 mg IV, or IV drip at 2–20 mg/hr	Up to every 6 hrs for bolus dosing
Refractory to loop diuretics	Add metolazone or chlorothiazide 30 min prior to each furosemide dose	2.5–5 mg PO 250–500 mg IV	Most helpful when CrCl <30 mL/min
Refractory to combination of loop and thiazide diuretics	Consider inotrope (dobutamine) if renal perfusion is inadequate Consider renal replacement therapy if renal failure (HD or CVVHDF)		

PO, by mouth; IV, intravenously; CrCl, creatinine clearance; HD, hemodialysis; CVVHDF, continuous venovenous hemodiafiltration.

requiring high doses of furosemide, a continuous drip may be more practical than boluses >1 mg/kg. Guidelines for practical diuretic use are shown in Table 22.2, and include adding thiazide diuretics for refractory cases. Patients with significant renal dysfunction and evidence of fluid retention should still be treated with IV diuretics as renal dysfunction often improves with diuresis and decongestion.

Afterload Reduction

In selected patients with ADHF (such as MI with pulmonary edema), vasodilator therapy with IV nitroglycerin should be considered the first-line agent (Table 22.3). IV nitroglycerin is a balanced arterial and venous vasodilator when given in appropriate doses, effectively reducing both preload and afterload without impairing tissue perfusion. At low doses, IV nitroglycerin induces venodilation (without significant coronary artery dilation), and may not effectively unload the failing heart. Therefore, IV nitroglycerin should be titrated aggressively (with careful blood pressure monitoring) in patients suffering from ADHF in the setting of myocardial ischemia. In other patients with pulmonary congestion in the setting of ADHF, the combination of IV nitroglycerin and IV loop diuretics provides rapid symptomatic relief and has been found to be more effective than high-dose diuretics alone.

TABLE 22.3 Vasodilators (All Have Potential for Causing Hypotension)

Indication	Vasodilator	Dose (mcg/min)	Comments
ADHF	Nitroglycerin	10–200	Headache, tachyphylaxis
ADHF	Nesiritide	0.01–0.03	Use bolus dosing with caution
Hypertensive crisis	Nitroprusside	0.5–5	Isocyanate toxicity

ADHF, acute decompensated heart failure.

Nesiritide is a recombinant BNP that, like nitroglycerin, is a balanced arterial and venous vasodilator, but also promotes natriuresis in combination with loop diuretics. Nesiritide decreases PCWP promptly, improves dyspnea in patients with ADHF, and can be initiated most safely without a bolus at 0.01 mcg/kg/min, with titration to a maximum dose of 0.03 mcg/kg/min.

Inotropes and Vasopressors

For patients in cardiogenic shock with hypotension and evidence of inadequate tissue perfusion (Algorithm 22.2, Forrester group IV) dobutamine and milrinone are the inotropic agents of choice. Dobutamine is predominantly a beta-1 and beta-2 adrenergic receptor agonist, which augments both inotropy and chronotropy. There is frequently a reflex decrease in sympathetic tone that leads to lowered SVR, further augmenting cardiac output. In patients receiving chronic beta-blocker therapy or in patients in whom tachycardia is problematic, milrinone is an effective alternative to dobutamine. Milrinone is a type III phosphodiesterase inhibitor with characteristics of both an inotrope and peripheral vasodilator. It has the disadvantage of renal clearance, and must be used with caution in patients with acute or chronic renal failure. The peripheral vasodilation of milrinone may also cause hypotension, particularly if it is given inappropriately in the setting of volume depletion (Algorithm 22.2, Forrester class III). Dobutamine and milrinone increase myocardial oxygen demand and should be reserved for cases of documented or suspected cardiogenic shock and systemic hypoperfusion. They do not have a role for mild episodes of ADHF. The use of vasopressors (e.g., dopamine or norepinephrine) may also be necessary in urgent situations to maintain blood pressure while the patient is being stabilized, but they should be weaned quickly as they increase afterload, and may further reduce end-organ perfusion. Table 22.4 shows typical dosing of inotropic agents and vasopressors.

Mechanical Support

For patients who cannot be stabilized with medical therapy, consideration should be given to mechanical circulatory support, particularly if the patient is a candidate for advanced HF therapies such as cardiac transplantation or a left ventricular assist device (LVAD). Acute dialysis, especially continuous venovenous hemodialysis, can be used for volume control of selected diuretic refractory patients with renal failure. Intra-aortic balloon pump placement can provide mechanical afterload reduction, and augmented diastolic pressure to improve coronary artery filling in low-output states. Several temporary VADs have recently become available to provide less invasive

TABLE 22.4	Inotropic Agents and Vasopressors		
Drug	Class	Dose (mcg/kg/min)	Comments
Dobutamine	Inotrope	2.5–10	First line for ADHF
Milrinone	Inotrope/vasodilator	0.25–0.75	Useful with beta blockade
Dopamine	Inotrope/vasopressor	5–50	Relatively weak agonist
Epinephrine	Inotrope/vasopressor	0.05–0.5	If refractory to dobutamine
Norepinephrine	Vasopressor	0.05–1	More appropriate for sepsis

ADHF, acute decompensated heart failure.

short-term mechanical circulatory support. The TandemHeart is a left atrial to femoral artery bypass system capable of providing up to 4 L/min of flow. It consists of an inflow cannula placed into the left atrium from the femoral vein via transseptal puncture, a continuous flow centrifugal (extracorporeal) pump, and an outflow cannula to the femoral artery. The Impella is an all-arterial percutaneous LVAD which utilizes a contained microaxial pump placed retrograde across the aortic valve via the femoral artery. The catheter removes blood from the left ventricular cavity and pumps it into the ascending aorta. Three different sizes are available, capable of providing 2.5, 3.5 and 5 L/min of flow, respectively. Finally, surgically implanted, extracorporeal temporary VADs (CentriMag, Rotaflow) can be used to bridge severely decompensated HF patients to definitive therapy with LVAD or heart transplant. Pursuing more advanced mechanical therapy (e.g., LVAD support) or cardiac transplantation is an increasingly viable option for patients without irreversible end-organ damage who are at centers with the appropriate resources, thus early involvement of HF cardiologist and cardiac surgery specialists should be considered in such patients to facilitate institution of appropriate advanced therapy.

SUGGESTED READINGS

Abraham WT, Fonarow GC, Albert NM, et al; OPTIMIZE-HF Investigators and Coordinators. Predictors of in-hospital mortality in patients hospitalized for heart failure: insights from the Organized Program to Initiate Lifesaving Treatment in Hospitalized Patients with Heart Failure (OPTIMIZE-HF). *J Am Coll Cardiol.* 2008;52(5):347–356.

Cuffe MS, Califf RM, Adams KF Jr, et al. Short-term intravenous milrinone for acute exacerbation of chronic heart failure: a randomized controlled trial. *JAMA.* 2002;287(12):1541–1547.
This RCT highlights the dangers of routine inotrope use in ADHF and demonstrates that inotropic agents should be reserved for those patients with evidence of clinically significant hypoperfusion.

Heart Failure Society of America. Executive summary: HFSA (Heart Failure Society of America) 2010 comprehensive heart failure practice guideline. *J Card Fail.* 2010;16(6):475–539.
While the ESC guidelines are dedicated specifically to ADHF, the 2010 HFSA guidelines represent a consensus-driven approach to establish best practices for diagnosis and treatment of HF in general, including ADHF.

Lloyd-Jones D, Adams RJ, Brown TM, et al; American Heart Association Statistics Committee and Stroke Statistics Subcommittee. Heart disease and stroke statistics–2010 update: a report from the American Heart Association. *Circulation.* 2010;121(7):e46–e215.
This AHA update details the extensive cardiovascular disease burden in the United States.

McCullough PA, Nowak RM, McCord J, et al. B-type natriuretic peptide and clinical judgment in emergency diagnosis of heart failure: analysis from Breathing Not Properly (BNP) Multinational Study. *Circulation.* 2002;106(4):416–422.
This study is the most widely recognized trial validating the utility of serum BNP measurement for differentiating heart failure from other entities with similar presentations.

Ponikowski P, Voors AA, Anker SD, et al; Authors/Task Force Members; Document Reviewers. 2016 ESC Guidelines for the diagnosis and treatment of acute and chronic heart failure: The Task Force for the diagnosis and treatment of acute and chronic heart failure of the European Society of Cardiology (ESC). Developed with the special contribution of the Heart Failure Association (HFA) of the ESC. *Eur J Heart Fail.* 2016;18(8):891–975.

Publication Committee for the VMAC Investigators (Vasodilatation in the Management of Acute CHF). Intravenous nesiritide vs nitroglycerin for treatment of decompensated congestive heart failure: a randomized controlled trial. *JAMA.* 2002;287(12):1531–1540.
This trial demonstrates the utility of nesiritide for improving the hemodynamics of patients with ADHF.

Sarkar K, Kini AS. Percutaneous left ventricular support devices. *Cardiol Clin.* 2010;28(1):169–184. *This review describes available percutaneous mechanical support devices. The authors also provide details of placement technique, complications, contraindications, and hemodynamics of each device.*

Yancy CW, Jessup M, Bozkurt B, et al; American College of Cardiology Foundation; American Heart Association Task Force on Practice Guidelines. 2013 ACCF/AHA guideline for the management of heart failure: a report of the American College of Cardiology Foundation/ American Heart Association Task Force on Practice Guidelines. *J Am Coll Cardiol.* 2013; 62(16):e147–e239.

23 Approach to Hypertensive Emergencies

Paul Juang and Mollie Gowan

Hypertensive emergencies have become a less frequent cause for admission to the intensive care unit (ICU) with the widespread availability of antihypertensive medications in the current medical era. Only 1% of patients with hypertension will present with a hypertensive emergency during their lifetime. Unfortunately, severe hypertension is still very common, so distinguishing a true hypertensive emergency from hypertensive urgency is key to guiding therapy. Therefore, the following terms are worth defining.

- **Hypertensive crisis:** A generic term for severe elevations in blood pressure (BP) that have the potential to cause target organ (heart, vasculature, kidneys, eyes, and brain) damage. This includes both *hypertensive emergency* and *hypertensive urgency.*
- **Hypertensive urgency:** A severe elevation in BP *without* evidence of acute and ongoing target organ damage (TOD).
- **Hypertensive emergency:** A severe elevation in BP *with* evidence of acute, ongoing TOD.
  - *Hypertensive encephalopathy:* A specific hypertensive emergency characterized by irritability, headaches, and mental status changes caused by significant and often, rapid elevations in BP.
  - *Accelerated malignant hypertension:* A specific hypertensive emergency characterized by fundoscopic findings of papilledema and/or acute retinal hemorrhages and exudates. See Figure 23.1.

Timely differentiation between hypertensive emergencies and urgencies is imperative so that patients with severely elevated BP can be triaged to the appropriate level of care and monitoring (i.e., outpatient follow-up vs. inpatient ward vs. ICU) with the appropriate antihypertensive agents initiated (parenteral vs. oral) and the establishment of BP-lowering goals at the appropriate time interval (minutes to hours vs. days to weeks). In the absence of acute, progressive end-organ damage, elevated BP alone does not require immediate, emergent therapy. The above definitions intentionally are devoid of any absolute BP numbers because the level at which individuals develop TOD can vary depending on clinical substrate and the rapidity with which the BP rises. For example, a patient with long-standing poorly controlled hypertension may tolerate a BP in excess of 230/120 mm Hg without evidence of acute end-organ damage while the young healthy patient who acutely develops glomerulonephritis may become encephalopathic from hypertension at much lower pressures.

The approach to severely elevated BP is outlined in Algorithm 23.1. It should be emphasized that when presented with these patients one should perform a truncated

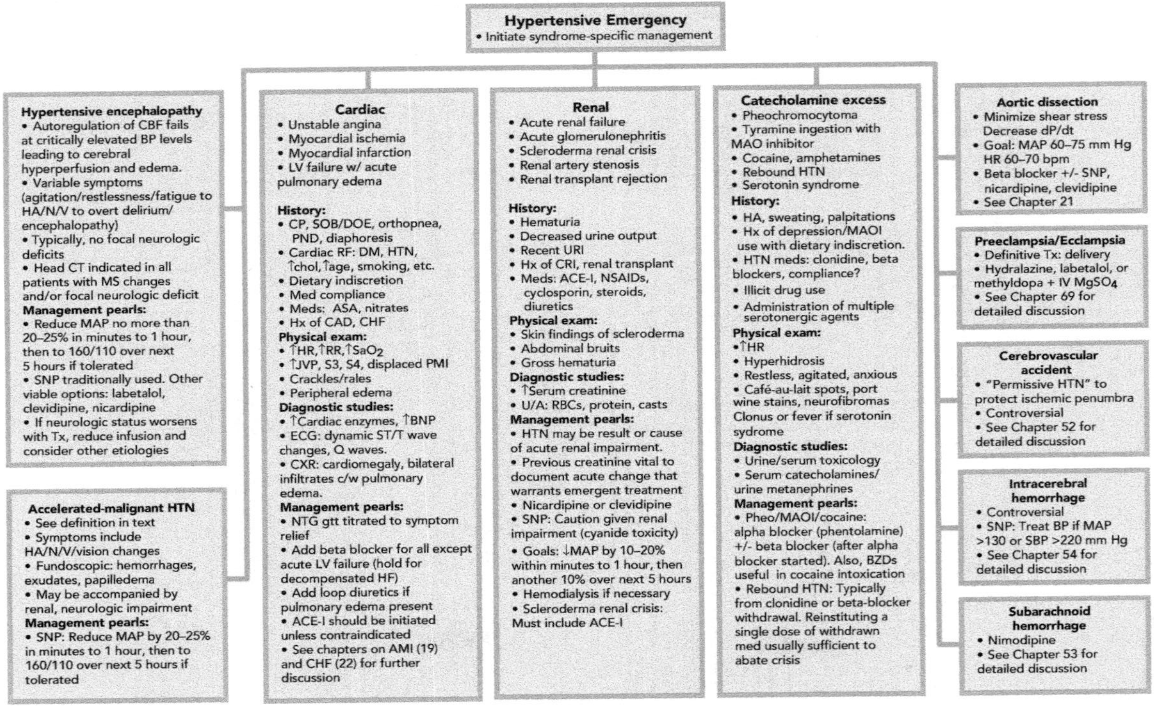

Hypertensive Emergency
- Initiate syndrome-specific management

Hypertensive encephalopathy
- Autoregulation of CBF fails at critically elevated BP levels leading to cerebral hyperperfusion and edema.
- Variable symptoms (agitation/restlessness/fatigue to HA/N/V to overt delirium/encephalopathy)
- Typically, no focal neurologic deficits

Management pearls:
- Head CT indicated in all patients with MS changes and/or focal neurologic deficit
- Reduce MAP no more than 20–25% in minutes to 1 hour, then to 160/110 over next 5 hours if tolerated
- SNP traditionally used. Other viable options: labetalol, clevidipine, nicardipine
- If neurologic status worsens with Tx, reduce infusion and consider other etiologies

Accelerated-malignant HTN
- See definition in text
- Symptoms insidue
- HA/N/V/vision changes
- Fundoscopic: hemorrhages, exudates, papilledema
- May be accompanied by renal, neurologic impairment

Management pearls:
- SNP: Reduce MAP by 20–25% in minutes to 1 hour, then to 160/110 over next 5 hours if tolerated

Cardiac
- Unstable angina
- Myocardial ischemia
- Myocardial infarction
- LV failure w/ acute pulmonary edema

History:
- CP, SOB/DOE, orthopnea, PND, diaphoresis
- Cardiac RF: DM, HTN, 'chol, 'age, smoking, etc.
- Dietary indiscretion
- Med compliance
- Meds: ASA, nitrates
- Hx of CAD, CHF

Physical exam:
- ↑HR, ↑RR, ↑SaO₂
- ↑JVP, S3, S4, displaced PMI
- Crackles/rales
- Peripheral edema

Diagnostic studies:
- ↑Cardiac enzymes, ↑BNP
- ECG: dynamic ST/T wave changes, Q waves.
- CXR: cardiomegaly, bilateral infiltrates c/w pulmonary edema.

Management pearls:
- NTG gtt titrated to symptom relief
- Add beta blocker for all except acute LV failure (hold for decompensated HF)
- Add loop diuretics if pulmonary edema present
- ACE-I should be initiated unless contraindicated
- See chapters on AMI (19) and CHF (22) for further discussion

Renal
- Acute renal failure
- Acute glomerulonephritis
- Scleroderma renal crisis
- Renal artery stenosis
- Renal transplant rejection

History:
- Hematuria
- Decreased urine output
- Recent URI
- Hx of CRI, renal transplant
- Meds: ACE-I, NSAIDs, cyclosporin, steroids, diuretics

Physical exam:
- Skin findings of scleroderma

Diagnostic studies:
- ↑Serum creatinine
- U/A: RBCs, protein, casts

Management pearls:
- HTN may be result or cause of acute renal impairment.
- Previous creatinine vital to document acute change that warrants emergent treatment
- Nicardipine or clevidipine
- SNP: Caution given renal impairment (cyanide toxicity)
- Goals: ↓MAP by 10–20% within minutes to 1 hour, then another 10% over next 5 hours
- Hemodialysis if necessary
- Scleroderma renal crisis: Must include ACE-I

Catecholamine excess
- Pheochromocytoma
- Tyramine ingestion with MAO inhibitor
- Cocaine, amphetamines
- Rebound HTN
- Serotonin syndrome

History:
- HA, sweating, palpitations
- Hx of depression/MAOI use with dietary indiscretion.
- HTN meds: clonidine, beta blockers, compliance?
- Illicit drug use
- Administration of multiple serotonergic agents

Physical exam:
- ↑HR
- Hyperhidrosis
- Restless, agitated, anxious
- Café-au-lait spots, port wine stains, neurofibromas
- Clonus or fever if serotonin syndrome

Diagnostic studies:
- Urine/serum toxicology
- Serum catecholamines/ urine metanephrines

Management pearls:
- Pheo/MAOI/cocaine: alpha blocker (phentolamine) +/- beta blocker (after alpha blocker started). Also, BZDs useful in cocaine intoxication
- Rebound HTN: Typically from clonidine or beta-blocker withdrawal. Reinstituting a single dose of withdrawn med usually sufficient to abate crisis

Aortic dissection
- Minimize shear stress
- Decrease dP/dt
- Goal: MAP 60–75 mm Hg HR 60–70 bpm
- Beta blocker +/- SNP, nicardipine, clevidipine
- See Chapter 21

Preeclampsia/Eclampsia
- Definitive Tx: delivery
- Hydralazine, labetalol, or methyldopa + IV MgSO₄
- See Chapter 69 for detailed discussion

Cerebrovascular accident
- "Permissive HTN" to protect ischemic penumbra
- Controversial
- See Chapter 52 for detailed discussion

Intracerebral hemorrhage
- Controversial
- SNP: Treat BP if MAP >130 or SBP >220 mm Hg
- See Chapter 54 for detailed discussion

Subarachnoid hemorrhage
- Nimodipine
- See Chapter 53 for detailed discussion

Figure 23.1. Management of specific hypertensive emergencies.

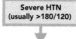

ALGORITHM 23.1 | General Approach to Hypertensive Emergencies

```
┌─────────────────────┐
│ Severe HTN          │
│ (usually >180/120)  │
└─────────────────────┘
```

Goals: Perform targeted, brief, and, often, simultaneous history and physical exam:
1) Identify patient characteristics that increase risk for HTN emergency.
2) Identify signs and symptoms of target organ damage (TOD).

History:
- **HPI:**
  Symptoms of TOD?
    - CNS: - Cardiac: - Renal:
      MS changes   Chest pain   Hematuria
      HA   SOB/DOE   ↓ Urine output
      Weakness   Orthopnea
      Vision change
- **PMH:**
    - Hx of HTN
    - Hx of CNS, cardiac/aortic, or renal disease
    - Ob/Gyn Hx
- **Medications:**
    - Anti-HTN meds: dose changes, compliance
    - MAO inhibitors, OTCs, herbal remedies
- **Social/Family history:**
    - Cocaine/amphetamine use
    - Hx of cardiac/aortic disease in family

Physical exam:
- **Vitals:**
    - BP in both arms and legs, ↑HR, ↓SaO₂
- **General:**
    - Agitation, anxiety, restlessness
- **Fundoscopic:**
    - Hemorrhages, exudates, papilledema
- **CV:**
    - S3, S4, diastolic murmur of AI,
      elevated JVP, peripheral edema
    - Arterial bruits, pulse deficits
- **Pulm:**
    - Crackles/rales
- **Neuro:**
    - Mental status changes, "AAO <4"
    - Focal neurologic deficits

Diagnostic studies:
- CBC
- Electrolytes
- BUN/Creatinine
- Glucose
- U/A(RBCs, casts)
- Cardiac enzymes
- CXR (wide mediastinum, pulmonary edema)
- ECG (ST/T wave changes, Q waves, LVH)

Note: When available, obtain previous ECG/CXR/ labs to establish baseline and confirm dynamic changes.

```
┌──────────────────────────────┐
│ Evidence of acute, ongoing TOD? │
└──────────────────────────────┘
```

Yes   No

Hypertensive emergency
General goals:
- Stop progression of TOD.
- Avoid organ hypoperfusion during treatment.

Points of emphasis:
- Parenteral therapy should be initiated immediately. Further diagnostic testing should not delay treatment.
- ICU admission with intra-arterial BP monitoring is preferred.
- In general, one should aim to lower the MAP by no more than 20% within minutes to an hour. Over the next 2–6 hours, one should aim for a goal BP of approximately 160/110 mm Hg if initial reduction was well tolerated.
- The parenteral agents used should be chosen based on the specific hypertensive syndrome being managed as outlined in Figure 2.
- Begin to plan oral regimen based on medical comorbidities and home meds so that one may transition once crisis is resolved.
- One can typically start weaning parenteral agents and institute appropriate oral therapy once BP is controlled for 12–24 hours and autoregulation is reestablished.
- After acute treatment has begun, consider initiating workup of secondary causes of hypertension in appropriate patients.

Hypertensive urgency
- Intitiate oral hypertensive therapy based on medical comorbities and home meds.
- Determine level of monitoring required based on clinical substrate and availability of close outpatient follow-up.
- Most patients can be managed as outpatients with goal of lowering MAP by 20% in 1–2 days with further reduction to goal ambulatory levels in weeks to months.
- Outpatient follow-up should be arranged within 48–72 hours to ensure compliance and to emphasize need for long term BP control to lower CV risk.

```
┌──────────────────────────────┐
│ Proceed to Figure 23.1 for   │
│ syndrome-specific            │
│ management goals             │
└──────────────────────────────┘
```

ABBREVIATIONS

AI:	aortic insufficiency
JVP:	jugular venous pressure
LVH:	left ventricular hypertrophy
CV:	cardiovascular
HTN:	hypertension
TOD:	target organ damage
CNS:	central nervous system
MS:	mental status
HA:	headache
SOB:	shortness of breath
DOE:	dyspnea on exertion
MAO:	monoamine oxidase
OTC:	over the counter
HR:	heart rate
SaO₂:	arterial oxygen saturation

TABLE 23.1 Parenteral Agents Used in Hypertensive Emergencies

Drug	Dose	Onset/Duration	Adverse Effects[a]	Points of Emphasis
Sodium nitroprusside (SNP)	Initial: 0.25–0.50 mcg/kg/min continuous infusion Maint: titrate to goal BP up to 8–10 mcg/kg/min continuous infusion	Onset: Seconds Duration: 2–3 min after infusion is stopped	Thiocyanate and cyanide poisoning, nausea, vomiting, ↓BP	• Potent arterial and venous dilator with rapid onset and offset of effect. • Use with beta blocker if used in aortic dissection. • Administer via continuous infusion in ICU, guided by intra-arterial BP monitoring. • Caution in renal or hepatic impairment due to thiocyanate/cyanide accumulation. Signs of toxicity include metabolic acidosis, tremors, seizures, nausea, and vomiting. Thiocyanate levels >10 mg/dL should be avoided. Max level infusions should be used for no more than 10 min to limit toxicity. • Avoid prolonged use (>24–48 hrs) in all patients. • Increases intracranial pressure but the simultaneous fall in SVR offsets this effect. Therefore, it is still recommended in hypertensive encephalopathy.
Labetalol	Bolus: 20 mg × 1, then 20–80 mg q10min to total dose 300 mg or Infusion: 0.5–2 mg/min	Onset: 5–10 min Duration: 3–6 hrs	↓HR, HB, HF, bronchospasm, nausea, vomiting, flushing	• Combined alpha- and beta-adrenergic blocker. • Can be given as IV bolus or IV infusion. Excessive BP drops are unusual. • Useful in most hypertensive emergencies but avoid in CHF and severe asthma. • Commonly used agent (along with hydralazine) in HTN in pregnancy.

(continued)

TABLE 23.1 Parenteral Agents Used in Hypertensive Emergencies (Continued)

Drug	Dose	Onset/Duration	Adverse Effects[a]	Points of Emphasis
Nitroglycerin	Initial: 5 mcg/min Maint: titrate q3–5min up to 100 mcg/min	Onset: 2–5 min Duration: 5–15 min	Tolerance, HA, ↓BP, nausea, methemoglobinemia	• Similar to SNP, but causes mostly venodilation with only modest arteriolar dilation effects at higher doses. • Most useful in emergencies complicated by cardiac compromise (i.e., myocardial ischemia/infarct, LV failure/pulmonary edema). • Also indicated in management of postoperative HTN following CABG. • Avoid use with phosphodiesterase-5 inhibitors. • Tolerance will develop with prolonged use.
Hydralazine	Bolus: 10–20 mg q30min until goal BP	Onset: 10–30 min Duration: 2–4 hrs	↓BP, ↑HR, flushing	• Direct arteriolar vasodilator with no significant venous effects. • Caution in patients with CAD or aortic dissection given reflex sympathetic stimulation. Must use with beta blocker in these patients. • Avoid in patients with increased ICP. • BP lowering response is less predictable than with above agents and, therefore, use should be limited to HTN in pregnancy if possible.
Enalaprilat	Initial: 1.25 mg × 1, then 1.25–5 mg q6hr	Onset: 15–30 min Duration: 6–12 hrs	↓BP, renal failure, hyperkalemia	• The only available IV ACE inhibitor. • Response to agent is unpredictable and depends on plasma renin activity and volume status of patient. • Most useful as an adjunctive agent in patients with CHF or scleroderma renal crisis. • Contraindicated in pregnancy and in renal artery stenosis.

Nicardipine	Initial: 5 mg/hr, increase by 2.5 mg/hr q20min up to max dose, 15 mg/hr (0.2–1 mcg/kg/min, increase by 0.5 mcg/kg/min up to 1.5 mcg/kg/min)	Onset: 10–30 min Duration: 1–4 hrs	↓BP, ↑THR, HF, HA nausea, flushing	• Dihydropyridine calcium channel blocker. • Can be used effectively in most emergencies, but should be avoided in acute heart failure. • Reflex tachycardia may be avoided with addition of beta blocker.
Clevidipine	Initial: 1–2 mg/hr, double dose q90s up to max dose, 32 mg/hr	Onset: 2–4 min Duration: 30 min	↓BP, ↑THR, HF, HA nausea	• Dihydropyridine calcium channel blocker. • Can be used effectively in most emergencies, but should be avoided in acute heart failure. • Reflex tachycardia may be avoided with addition of beta blocker. • Formulated in 20% lipid emulsion.
Esmolol	Bolus: 500 mcg/kg, repeat after 5 min Infusion: 50–100 mcg/kg/min, up to 300 mcg/kg/min	Onset: 1–5 min Duration: 15–30 min	↓HR, HB, HF, bronchospasm, nausea, vomiting, flushing	• Short-acting, cardioselective beta-adrenergic blocker. • Useful in ICU patients with variable hemodynamics because of short half-life.
Phentolamine	Bolus: 5–10 mg, repeat q5–15min Infusion: 0.2–5.0 mg/min	Onset: 1–2 min Duration: 10–20 min	↑THR, HA, nausea	• Alpha-adrenergic blocker, used primarily in syndromes associated with excess catecholamines (i.e., pheochromocytoma, tyramine ingestion while on MAOI).

[a]Either common or life-threatening adverse effects of these medications are listed. This does not represent a comprehensive list of all possible adverse effects. ↓BP, hypotension; ↓HR, bradycardia; ↑HR, tachycardia; HB, heart block; HF, heart failure; CHF, congestive heart failure; HA, headache; Maint, maintenance dose; SNP, Sodium nitroprusside, LV, left ventricle; HTN, hypertension; CAD, coronary artery disease; ICP, intracranial pressure; ACE, angiotensin converting enzyme; SVR, systemic vascular resistance; CABG, coronary artery bypass grafting; IV, intravenous; MAOI, monoamine oxidase inhibitor.

history and physical exam that, (1) quickly identifies patient characteristics that place the patient at risk for hypertensive emergencies, and, (2) searches for signs and/or symptoms of underlying TOD. If this rapid assessment reveals evidence for a true hypertensive emergency then treatment should be initiated immediately, preferably in an ICU setting.

The goal of treating hypertensive emergency is to sufficiently lower arterial pressure to stop the progression of TOD without overcorrecting and causing organ hypoperfusion. This careful balance is best achieved with parenteral agents that have a rapid onset and short half-life, administered under the guidance of intra-arterial BP monitoring in an ICU setting. Oral and sublingual agents should not be used as initial treatment for hypertensive emergency due to their variable effects with slower onset and longer half-life. Sodium nitroprusside can be rapidly titrated and is the preferred agent in most hypertensive emergencies. (Table 23.1 has details for agents used in hypertensive emergencies.) One must tailor therapy with syndrome-specific management, as outlined in Figure 23.1.

SUGGESTED READINGS

Calhoun DA, Oparil S. Treatment of hypertensive crisis. *N Engl J Med.* 1990;323(17):1177–1183.
  A review of treatment options for the hypertensive crisis.
Chobanian AV, Bakris GL, Black HR, et al; Joint National Committee on Prevention, Detection, Evaluation, and Treatment of High Blood Pressure; National Heart, Lung, and Blood Institute; National High Blood Pressure Education Program Coordinating Committee. Seventh report of the joint national committee on prevention, detection, evaluation and treatment of high blood pressure. *Hypertension.* 2003;42(6):1206–1252.
  JNC VII, a comprehensive expert review of hypertension, including sections dedicated to addressing approach to hypertensive emergencies.
Elliot WJ. Clinical features in the management of selected hypertensive emergencies. *Prog Cardiovasc Dis.* 2006;48(5):316–325.
  Concise review of definitions, epidemiology, pathophysiology, and syndrome-specific treatment options.
Gifford RW Jr. Management of hypertensive crises. *JAMA.* 1991;266(6):829–835.
  A review of treatment options for the hypertensive crisis.
Kaplan NM, Victor RG. Hypertensive crisis. *Kaplan's Clinical Hypertension.* 11th ed. Philadelphia, PA: Lippincott, Williams, and Wilkins; 2015:263.
  A leader in hypertension provides his approach to management of hypertensive crises. Also embedded elsewhere in text are chapters that address HTN in pregnancy, catecholamine excess states, renal failure, etc. in greater detail.
Marik PE, Rivera R. Hypertensive emergencies: an update. *Curr Opin Crit Care.* 2011;17(6): 569–580.
  An updated review of treatment options for the hypertensive crisis. Rehman SU, Basile JN.
Rehman SU, Basile JN, Vidt DG. Hypertensive emergencies and urgencies. In: Black HR, Elliot WJ, eds. *Hypertension: A Companion to Braunwald's Heart Disease.* Philadelphia, PA: Saunders-Elsevier; 2007:517–524.
  A current review of approach to hypertensive urgencies and emergencies in a comprehensive text dedicated to addressing all aspects of hypertension, written by leaders in the field.

24

Electrolyte Abnormalities

Usman Younus and Seth Goldberg

DISORDERS OF WATER BALANCE

Hyponatremia and hypernatremia are primarily disorders of *water* balance (osmoregulation) or *water* distribution across the various fluid compartments in the body. The countercurrent mechanisms of the kidneys in concert with the hypothalamic osmoreceptors via antidiuretic hormone (ADH) secretion maintain a very finely tuned balance of water. When the serum osmolality becomes too dilute (<280 mOsm/kg), excess water is excreted by the kidneys as dilute urine. Conversely, when the serum osmolality becomes too concentrated (>290 mOsm/kg), ADH release and thirst result in water retention to bring the system back into balance. Defects in such handling of water present as hyponatremia or hypernatremia (Fig. 24.1).

An important concept in distinguishing water (osmotic) balance from volume homeostasis is that Na^+ *concentration* is not affected by the *total* Na^+ balance. These are regulated independently; osmoregulation is mediated by ADH and thirst, and volume regulation is driven by the renin–angiotensin–aldosterone system, atrial natriuretic peptide, and the sympathetic nervous system (Fig. 24.2). ADH does play a small overlapping role in volume regulation, where it can maintain volume, but at the expense of osmolality.

The incidence of hyponatremia and hypernatremia in the intensive care unit (ICU) may each be 15% to 30%. Their significance lies not only in their direct clinical effects in the individual patient but also through their ability to predict mortality. The in-hospital mortality of patients with either hyponatremia or hypernatremia is approximately 30% to 40%, which is significantly greater than for normonatremic patients.

The most osmotically sensitive organ in the body is the brain. Therefore, it should not be surprising that symptoms of hyponatremia and hypernatremia predominantly involve the nervous system as water shifts into or out of neuronal cells. Hypotonicity results in water entry, leading to cell swelling within the fixed cranial vault (with risk of herniation), while hypernatremia results in cell shrinkage and tearing of the brain away from the meninges (with risk of hemorrhage). The severity of clinical symptoms often depends on the *acuity* of the disturbance and not just the *magnitude*, as neurons have the capability to adapt to gradual changes over 48 hours. Hyponatremia and hypernatremia can present with similar symptomatology and range from headache to confusion, stupor, or seizures and coma.

Hyponatremia

When evaluating a patient for hyponatremia (Algorithm 24.1), one should first confirm that the low [Na^+] truly reflects a hypotonic state by checking the serum osmolality.

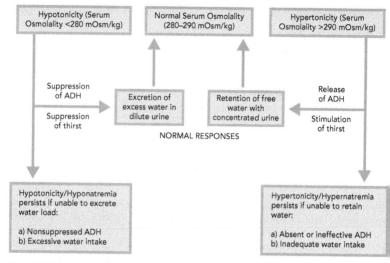

Figure 24.1. Regulation of osmolality. ADH, antidiuretic hormone.

When normal, "pseudohyponatremia," a measurement artifact, was likely present. However, if there is an elevated serum osmolality, a hypertonic disorder (e.g., hyperglycemia, mannitol) is responsible for water shifting out of cells, diluting the serum [Na+]. If there is indeed hypotonic hyponatremia, the patient's volume status can help determine if the cause of hypotonicity is from ADH secretion in response to a volume stimulus, such as from true hypovolemia or from a perceived decrease in effective circulating volume leading to an edematous state (e.g., heart failure, liver failure). If the patient is euvolemic, the cause is either from "inappropriate" ADH secretion (i.e., not mediated by an osmotic or volume stimulus) or from hypotonic fluid loading such as

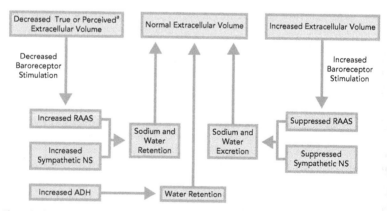

Figure 24.2. Regulation of extracellular volume. ADH, antidiuretic hormone; NS, nervous system; RAAS, renin–angiotensin–aldosterone system. aDecreased perceived extracellular volume occurs in decompensated congestive heart failure and cirrhosis, leading to a maladaptive sodium-avid state and edema.

ALGORITHM 24.1 Evaluation of Hyponatremia

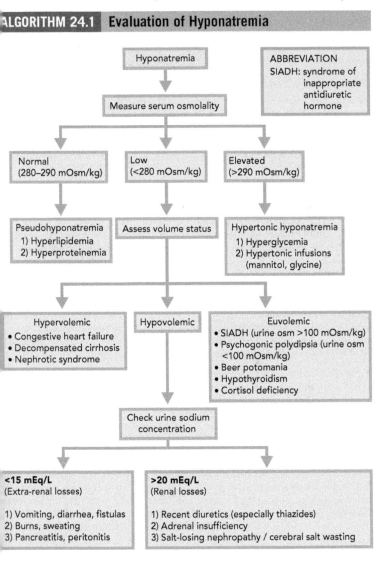

primary polydipsia; these can be distinguished by the urine osmolality, which should be maximally dilute (<50 to 100 mOsm/kg) if ADH is appropriately suppressed.

Etiologies of Special Importance in the Critically Ill Patient

Hyperglycemia (Hypertonic Hyponatremia)

Glucose acts as an osmotically active solute because it is restricted to the extracellular fluid (ECF) in states of insulin deficiency. In the marked hyperglycemia of diabetic ketoacidosis (DKA) and hyperosmolar hyperglycemic states, the ECF hyperosmolali (usually >290 mOsm/kg) causes water to shift from the intracellular fluid (ICF) cor partment to the ECF, and dilutional hyponatremia ensues. The plasma [Na^+] falls approximately 2 mEq/L for every 100 mg/dL rise in the plasma (glucose) above norm

Edematous States (Hypervolemic Hyponatremia)

Heart failure and cirrhosis result in a decreased "effective circulating volume." Giv the primacy of volume preservation, the body's response to this perceived threat is hold onto salt and water, with "nonosmotic" ADH release as part of the respons Thus, water excretion is submaximal. The degree of hyponatremia correlates wi the severity of the underlying condition, having been shown to be a poor prognost indicator in heart failure patients.

Syndrome of Inappropriate ADH (Euvolemic Hyponatremia)

Recall that ADH has overlapping roles in osmotic and volume balance. "Inappr priate" ADH secretion refers to release of ADH that is responding to neither these stimuli. Patients with the syndrome of inappropriate antidiuretic hormo (SIADH) are euvolemic, indicating that a true or perceived volume deficit is not t stimulus for ADH production. The urine osmolality is inappropriately concentrate (>100 mOsm/kg) for the prevailing hypotonic state, indicating the "inappropr ate" presence of ADH. Commonly associated conditions include neuropsychiatr disorders (e.g., meningitis, encephalitis, acute psychosis, cerebrovascular acciden head trauma), pulmonary diseases (e.g., pneumonia, tuberculosis, positive pressu ventilation, acute respiratory failure), malignant tumors (most commonly small ce lung cancer), and physical/emotional stress and pain. Before making the diagnosis SIADH, pharmacologic agents that enhance ADH action must be withdrawn.

- Nicotine, carbamazepine, antidepressants, narcotics, antipsychotic agents, and ce tain antineoplastic drugs may stimulate ADH release
- Chlorpropamide, methylxanthines, and nonsteroidal anti-inflammatory dru (NSAIDs) potentiate the action of ADH
- Oxytocin and desmopressin acetate are ADH analogs

Also, deficiencies of thyroid hormone or cortisol can present with euvolem hyponatremia and should be ruled out.

Many times, it is difficult to differentiate SIADH from true hypovolemia sinc both clinical scenarios are ADH driven and will have low serum osmolality and hig urine osmolality. Measuring the urine sodium (typically <20 mEq/L with volum depletion, >40 mEq/L with untreated SIADH) and serum uric acid (normal or ele vated with volume depletion, low with SIADH) may help in making this differentia tion, but if the diagnosis remains uncertain, one could challenge such a patient wit a normal saline fluid bolus. If the serum [Na^+] improves and the urine osmolalit decreases, one could attribute the hyponatremia to ADH release in setting of volum depletion, as opposed to SIADH where there may be a further drop in the serur [Na^+] and no change in the urine osmolality.

Cerebral Salt Wasting (Hypovolemic Hyponatremia)

Neurosurgery and central nervous system trauma, especially subarachnoid hemo rhage, may be associated with excessive renal Na^+ excretion. Although poorly unde stood, the mechanism may involve the release of a brain natriuretic peptide and/c the loss of renal sympathetic tone. The loss of Na^+ results in volume depletion, which leads to the "nonosmotic" release of ADH. This volume depletion is the main feature that distinguishes cerebral salt wasting from SIADH. The hyponatremia, however, does not always correct with volume resuscitation, perhaps, as a result of concomitant ADH release from the damaged brain. In some cases, the use of fludrocortisone can ameliorate the decline in $[Na^+]$.

Treatment

The hyponatremia in an *isotonic* state is usually of little clinical significance as fluid shifts and neuronal swelling do not occur or are readily corrected. With *hypertonic* hyponatremia, cellular dehydration may occur, and correction centers on metabolizing or removing the osmole responsible for the fluid shift. When true *hypotonic* hyponatremia occurs, treatment depends on eliminating the excess free water or suppressing the stimulus for ADH production. The rate of correction depends on the acuity with which it developed and the degree of symptomatology exhibited by the patient. Overly rapid correction can precipitate central pontine myelinolysis (CPM). In its most complete form, CPM is characterized by flaccid paralysis, dysarthria, dysphagia, and death.

Algorithm 24.2 outlines the standard treatment of hyponatremia. When the process is acute (duration of <2 days) or when severe neurologic dysfunction is present, correction of the serum $[Na^+]$ can be 1 to 2 mEq/L/hr until symptoms improve, then slowed to no more than 0.5 mEq/L/hr. When the hyponatremia has been present for at least 2 days, correction should begin at no more than 0.5 mEq/L/hr and no more than 10 to 12 mEq/L over a 24-hour period.

Most cases of hyponatremia can be corrected with free water restriction, except for those caused by true volume depletion. When more urgent correction is needed, 3% hypertonic saline can be used cautiously to raise the $[Na^+]$. The Adrogue–Madias equation (Box 24.1) can be used to estimate the expected change in $[Na^+]$ after 1 L of infusion; this anticipated change needs to be spread out over a number of hours to prevent overly rapid correction. However, this equation (and others) does not take into account the ongoing urinary losses and is notoriously inaccurate. It is therefore important to be aware that there is no substitute for measuring the serum $[Na^+]$ frequently (initially every 2 hours) to ensure a safe rate of correction.

A saline solution that is hypertonic to the *urine* can increase the $[Na^+]$ when oral water intake is restricted. Addition of intravenous (IV) loop diuretics can promote further water excretion by blocking the concentrating ability of the kidney. However, administering a fluid with an osmolality *less than urine osmolality* may actually worsen the hyponatremia, even if the fluid's $[Na^+]$ is greater than the serum $[Na^+]$. For example, if a patient with a serum $[Na^+]$ of 110 mEq/L and urine osmolality persistently >500 mOsm/kg from SIADH is given normal saline to attempt to correct the hyponatremia, the 308 mOsm (154 Na^+ + 154 Cl^-) contained in the liter of fluid will be extracted and concentrated down into a smaller volume of urine (fixed at 500 mOsm/kg in this example), resulting in the retention of further free water and worsening of the hyponatremia.

Hypernatremia

Hypernatremia is almost always the result of a relative water deficit (Algorithm 24.3). The three primary mechanisms are (a) decreased free water intake, (b) increased free water loss, or (c) excessive gain of hypertonic fluid.

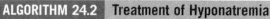

ALGORITHM 24.2 Treatment of Hyponatremia

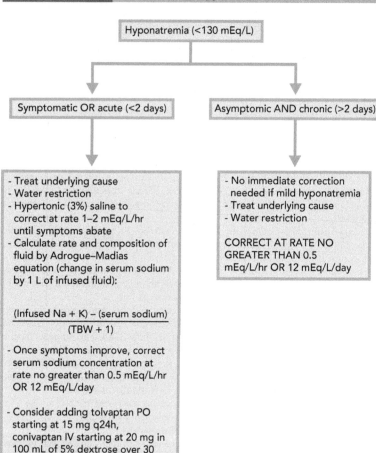

Hyponatremia (<130 mEq/L)

Symptomatic OR acute (<2 days)

- Treat underlying cause
- Water restriction
- Hypertonic (3%) saline to correct at rate 1–2 mEq/L/hr until symptoms abate
- Calculate rate and composition of fluid by Adrogue–Madias equation (change in serum sodium by 1 L of infused fluid):

$$\frac{(Infused\ Na + K) - (serum\ sodium)}{(TBW + 1)}$$

- Once symptoms improve, correct serum sodium concentration at rate no greater than 0.5 mEq/L/hr OR 12 mEq/L/day

- Consider adding tolvaptan PO starting at 15 mg q24h, conivaptan IV starting at 20 mg in 100 mL of 5% dextrose over 30 min, OR demeclocycline PO 300–600 mg bid if resistant to initial measures

Asymptomic AND chronic (>2 days)

- No immediate correction needed if mild hyponatremia
- Treat underlying cause
- Water restriction

CORRECT AT RATE NO GREATER THAN 0.5 mEq/L/hr OR 12 mEq/L/day

ABBREVIATION
TBW: total body water

Etiologies of Special Importance in the Critically Ill Patient

Decreased Water Intake

The most common etiology for hypernatremia in hospitalized patients is decreased free water intake. Although thirst is indeed a powerful stimulus, patients in certain circumstances may lack the ability to access or request water (i.e., a nursing home resident with dementia or sedated, intubated patient in the ICU). Thus, even at maximal

---

Box 24.1
Adrogue–Madias equation:

Change in [Na⁺] per liter = (infusate [Na⁺] + [K⁺] − serum [Na⁺])/(estimated total body water [kg] + 1)

Total body water = 60% of body weight
Infusate [Na⁺] for selected fluids:

3% Hypertonic saline: 513 mEq/L
Normal (0.9%) saline: 154 mEq/L
Ringer's lactate: 130 mEq/L (+4 mEq/L of potassium)
Half-normal (0.45%) saline: 77 mEq/L
5% dextrose (D5) water: 0 mEq/L

Example no. 1:
An obtunded 70-kg man presents with a serum [Na⁺] of 110 mEq/L. His clinician concludes that the [Na⁺] needs to be increased by 4 mEq/L in 2 hours using 3% hypertonic saline.

Expected change in [Na⁺] per liter of 3% saline = (513 − 110)/(42 + 1) = 9.37 mEq/L
Amount of fluid required to achieve desired change: 4/9.37 = 0.4 L (400 mL)
Rate of infusion: 400 mL/2 hrs = 200 mL/hr
To ensure safe rate of correction, check Na⁺ frequently.

ADH release and urinary concentration (urine osmolality >800 mOsm/kg), hypernatremia may ensue.

Insensible Free Water Loss

In ambulatory adults at room temperature, hypotonic fluid loss occurs from the skin and respiratory tract, each at a rate of approximately 400 to 500 mL/day. However, insensible water losses greatly depend on the respiratory rate, body temperature, ambient temperature, and humidity. These variables make losses much more difficult to predict in the ICU patient who may be mechanically ventilated. In general, water losses increase by 100 to 150 mL/day for each degree of body temperature more than 37°C. Fluid losses from the skin can vary enormously with sweating or in the setting of severe burns. If these insensible losses are not matched in addition to calculated free water loss, hypernatremia will develop.

Diabetes Insipidus

As noted above, the appropriate renal response to hypernatremia is excretion of maximally concentrated urine (>800 mOsm/kg) under the control of ADH. These responses are diminished in diabetes insipidus (DI), where there is either impaired ADH secretion (central DI) or resistance to its effect at the kidney (nephrogenic DI), resulting in an inappropriately dilute urine. Central DI is typically the result of damage to the neurohypophysis (posterior pituitary) from trauma, neurosurgery, granulomatous disease, neoplasms, vascular accidents, or infection. Nephrogenic DI can be classified into disorders associated with intrinsic renal diseases of the collecting duct where ADH acts (e.g., sickle cell nephropathy, polycystic kidney disease,

ALGORITHM 24.3 Evaluation of Hypernatremia

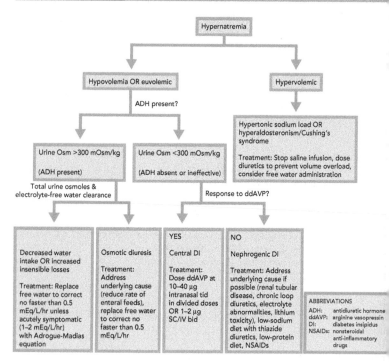

obstructive nephropathy, Sjögren's syndrome), drugs (e.g., lithium, demeclocycline, amphotericin, glyburide), electrolyte disorders (hypercalcemia and hypokalemia), and conditions that reduce renal medullary hypertonicity (e.g., excessive water intake and the chronic use of loop diuretics).

Osmotic Diuresis

Osmotic diuresis occurs when an osmolar load passes through the kidney, drawing out large amounts of electrolyte-free water into the urine. This commonly results from poorly controlled diabetes mellitus and its associated glycosuria. IV mannitol, retained uremic toxins in recovering renal failure, or large enteral solute loads with high osmolar tube feeds can also result in an osmotic diuresis. This cause of hypernatremia can resemble DI with its large urine volumes but is distinguished by the high total solute excretion, typically greater than 800 to 1000 mOsm per day. Urine osmolality is usually elevated (greater than 300 mOsm/kg) in an osmotic diuresis compared to DI, where it is quite low.

The workup for osmotic diuresis does deserve special attention as the mechanism for the development of hypernatremia is not readily intuitive. The urinary osmolality is elevated and typically higher than that of the serum osmolality. This would appear to be the proper physiologic response and might suggest that the hypernatremia will correct. However, the driving osmole in the urine is not sodium (nor its exchangeable ion, potassium), and instead, the offending osmole (e.g., glucose, urea) pulls out electrolyte-free water into the urine and leaves behind an even more hypertonic serum. The equation used to calculate this effect is the electrolyte-free water clearance, shown below. A positive value indicates the excessive water being lost.

$$\text{Electrolyte-free water clearance} = \text{Urine volume} - (U_{Na} + U_{K+})/P_{Na+}$$

Primary Na$^+$ Gain

Critically ill patients often require the administration of large amounts of saline solutions such as normal saline or sodium bicarbonate during cardiopulmonary resuscitation. Normally functioning kidneys have a large capacity to excrete this excess sodium load, and so iatrogenic hypernatremia is uncommon unless there is a concomitant urinary concentration defect.

Treatment

Hypernatremia treatment is outlined in Algorithm 24.3. The same principles as for hyponatremia apply here are well, since overly rapid correction (particularly if brain adaptation has occurred over 2 days) can result in dangerous fluid shifts. Excessive correction can result in water entering the cells, leading to cerebral edema and fatal brain herniation. Correction should not be faster than 0.5 mEq/L/hr unless acute symptoms are present or the disorder is of acute onset (<2 days), in which case correction can be 1 to 2 mEq/L/hr until symptoms abate.

The Adrogue–Madias equation (Box 24.2) used in correcting hyponatremia also applies to hypernatremia. The typical fluid used is 5% dextrose in water (D5W)containing no sodium, although in cases of concomitant volume depletion, normal saline or half-normal saline can be used initially to correct the volume deficit (note that even at an infusate [Na$^+$] of 154 mEq/L, the serum sodium concentration would improve if it starts above this level, albeit slowly). Alternatively, one can calculate the free water deficit by the equation below. However, one must also account for the ongoing water losses (sensible and insensible) to the total amount being replaced.

$$\text{Free water deficit} = \text{Total body water} \times [(\text{Serum } [Na^+]/140) - 1]$$

Once again, equations are not precise, and one must be sure to serially check the serum [Na$^+$] to ensure overly rapid correction is avoided. In an osmotic diuresis, calculating the electrolyte-free water clearance can also give an estimate for the amount of water required to offset the ongoing urinary losses, although treatment is generally centered on eliminating the offending osmole, such as metabolizing the glucose or reducing the protein content of the tube feeds.

DISORDERS OF VOLUME BALANCE

Control of the ECF volume depends on *total body sodium* (Fig. 24.2). Volume-depleted states result from total body sodium loss, while edematous states reflect total body sodium gain. As long as osmoregulatory mechanisms remain intact, the serum [Na$^+$] and serum osmolality remain normal.

Box 24.2

Adrogue–Madias equation:

Change in $[Na^+]$ per liter = (infusate $[Na^+]$ + $[K^+]$ − serum $[Na^+]$)/(estimated total body water [kg] + 1)

Total body water = 60% of body weight

Infusate $[Na^+]$ for selected fluids:

3% Hypertonic saline: 513 mEq/L
Normal (0.9%) saline: 154 mEq/L
Ringer's lactate: 130 mEq/L (+4 mEq/L of potassium)
Half-normal (0.45%) saline: 77 mEq/L
5% dextrose (D5) water: 0 mEq/L

Example no. 2:

A 70-kg woman presents with lassitude and a serum $[Na^+]$ of 160 mEq/L. She is having 2 L of diarrhea and 1 L of urine output each day. The replacement fluid chosen is 5% dextrose in water.

Expected change in $[Na^+]$ per liter of 5% dextrose = (0 − 160)/(42 + 1) = −3.72 mEq/L

1 L would need to be given over 7 to 8 hours to correct at a rate of 0.5 mEq/L (3.72/0.5 = 7.44)

Rate of infusion: 1000 mL over 8 hrs = 125 mL/hr

Then, to account for on-going water losses: (3000 mL/day)/24 = 125 mL/hr

Total fluid to be given: 125 + 125 = 250 mL/hr

Note some are more familiar with the calculation of the "free water deficit." This calculation can yield a similar answer, although it does not directly account for the rate of correction or fluid used.

Free water deficit: TBW [(serum $[Na^+]$/140) − 1] = 42[(160/140) − 1] = 6 L

If one was to correct this to 140 mEq/L with 5% dextrose, the change in 20 mEq/L would need to occur over roughly 40 to 48 hours to avoid overly rapid correction. Adding back the 3 L/day of on-going losses or 6 L over these 2 days, the total to be replaced is 12 L over 48 hours or 250 mL/hr.

True volume depletion, sensed by baroreceptors, results in the activation of the renin–angiotensin–aldosterone system, sympathetic nervous system, and to some degree, ADH to promote the retention of salt and water. Urinary sodium excretion is low (often <15 mEq/L). In congestive heart failure or decompensated cirrhosis, the "effective circulating volume" is diminished, and these same responses occur. However, instead of correcting the underlying state, this excess salt and water retention results in edema formation and ascites, while the salt-avid state persists to the point that it has become maladaptive.

Treatment of these edema-forming conditions is often centered on the underlying cause. Loop diuretics and potassium-sparing diuretics (spironolactone) in combination with salt and water restriction can alleviate the swelling. Renal function must be followed carefully, as overzealous diuresis can precipitate a drop in the glomerular filtration rate (GFR) and is particularly worrisome in the case of hepatorenal syndrome in decompensated cirrhosis. When advanced congestive heart failure compromises

al perfusion, diuresis may paradoxically improve renal function as cardiac perfor-
ance is enhanced.

DISORDERS OF POTASSIUM CONCENTRATION

he total body potassium in a normal adult is approximately 3000 to 4000 mEq, of
hich 98% is intracellular. Perturbations in the serum [K⁺] therefore are generally
e result of transcellular shifts and do not accurately reflect the total body K⁺ deficit
excess. Potassium excretion is primarily accomplished by the kidneys, at the level
the collecting duct under the influence of aldosterone. This process is coupled to
dium resorption and, therefore, volume repletion and blood pressure elevation.
dosterone activity in the collecting duct also stimulates H⁺ excretion.

Hypokalemia

Hypokalemia can result from (a) shifting of potassium into cells, (b) renal wasting,
(c) extrarenal losses (Algorithm 24.4). Calculating the transtubular K⁺ gradient
TKG) may help distinguish renal from extrarenal losses, although clues from the
story will often suffice. The TTKG is calculated as (urine [K⁺] × serum osmolality)/
erum [K⁺] × urine osmolality) and reflects potassium losses in the urine. The TTKG
ould be <3 *in the setting of hypokalemia*, reflecting renal conservation; a level greater
an this suggests inappropriate renal wasting of potassium. A recent analysis showed
at the central assumptions underlying the validity of the TTKG may not hold true,
articularly in hyperkalemia. One should be cautious in making a decision about
otassium balance entirely based on the TTKG.

Symptoms of hypokalemia seldom occur unless the potassium concentration is
3 mEq/L, with more acute changes having greater effect. Neuromuscular fatigue,
eakness, cramps, constipation, or ileus may occur and even progress to rhabdomy-
lysis or ascending paralysis when the potassium concentration falls to 2 mEq/L.
lthough the ECG does not correlate well with [K⁺], progressive changes may be
en in the individual patient. Moderate hypokalemia may have T-wave flattening,
T-segment depression, and the appearance of U waves. Severe hypokalemia shows
creased voltage, PR interval prolongation, and QRS widening.

Etiologies of Special Importance in the Critically Ill Patient
Transcellular Shifts

Movement of K⁺ into cells may transiently decrease the plasma [K⁺] without alter-
ng total body K⁺ content. The magnitude of the change is relatively small, often
1 mEq/L, but may exaggerate hypokalemia from other causes. Triggers of intracel-
lar shift include alkalemia, insulin activity, and catecholamine excess. The refeeding
ndrome, where nutritional support is initiated after a prolonged period of starva-
on, is a classic scenario where a transcellular shift exacerbates the hypokalemia in a
atient with deficient stores.

Renal Wasting

ncreased potassium loss by the kidney can be the result of increased urine flow
.g., loop or thiazide diuretic use, osmotic diuresis) or an elevated aldosterone state
usually with concomitant metabolic alkalosis). The presence of volume overload and
ypertension suggests that the aldosterone (or aldosterone-like) effect is driving the

ALGORITHM 24.4 Evaluation of Hypokalemia

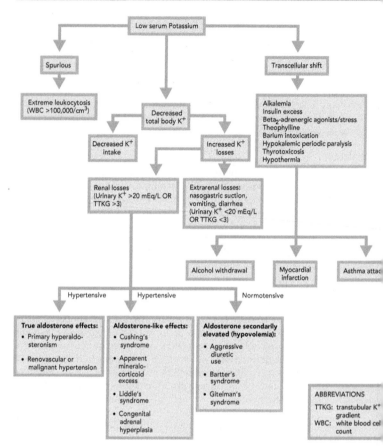

underlying process (e.g., primary hyperaldosteronism, apparent mineralocortico[...]
excess, Liddle's syndrome). When euvolemia and normal blood pressures are presen[...]
the aldosterone effect is secondary (or reactive) in response to a volume-depleted sta[...]
(e.g., Bartter's syndrome, Gitelman's syndrome, diuretic use).

Extrarenal K⁺ Loss

Gastrointestinal fluids (e.g., saliva, stomach secretions, diarrhea) have significant [...]
content and therefore excessive enteral losses may result in hypokalemia. Howeve[...]
if there is significant volume depletion, the renin–angiotensin–aldosterone system [...]
secondarily stimulated and may ultimately result in further potassium losses in th[...]
urine. When vomiting is the primary cause, there is often a concomitant metabol[...]
alkalosis from the acid loss. However, metabolic acidosis typically prevails when dia[...]
rhea is the prominent cause from the bicarbonate loss.

ALGORITHM 24.5 Treatment of Hypokalemia

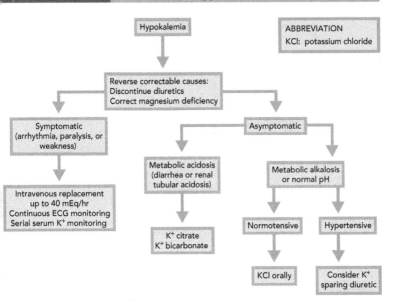

Treatment

Treatment of hypokalemia is outlined in Algorithm 24.5. Rapid correction of hypokalemia is required when symptoms or ECG changes are present. In these cases and when patients are unable to take oral medications, IV repletion is appropriate. Otherwise, it is generally safer to correct hypokalemia via the enteral route, and larger doses can be administered orally. Potassium chloride (KCl) is typically the preparation of choice regardless of the route of administration as it promotes more rapid correction of hypokalemia and concomitant metabolic alkalosis than the other preparations. Potassium bicarbonate or citrate may be useful in cases associated with metabolic acidosis (e.g., chronic diarrhea, renal tubular acidosis). Hypomagnesemia should be sought in all hypokalemic patients and corrected prior to or concurrently with K^+ repletion. A decrement of 1 mEq/L represents an estimated total body deficit of 200 to 400 mEq. However, the serum $[K^+]$ should be monitored frequently during therapy, as this total body deficit is difficult to estimate accurately.

Hyperkalemia

There are three main mechanisms of hyperkalemia (Algorithm 24.6): (a) transcellular shifts, (b) reduced glomerular filtration, (c) or effective aldosterone deficiency. Sustained hyperkalemia almost always requires decreased renal function, as normal kidneys have a tremendous capacity for K^+ excretion.

Symptoms of hyperkalemia are more pronounced when acute. Neuromuscular effects may manifest as weakness that can progress to flaccid paralysis and hypoventilation. As with hypokalemia, ECG changes do not correlate well with hyperkalemia,

ALGORITHM 24.6 Evaluation of Hyperkalemia

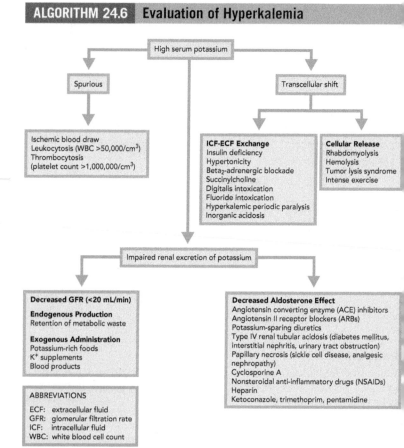

although progressive changes are seen within the individual. Moderate hyperkalemia shows peaked T waves with increased amplitude. More severe [K⁺] elevations cause prolonged PR intervals and QRS duration, atrioventricular delays, and loss of P waves. Profound hyperkalemia causes progressive widening of the QRS complex and merging with the T wave to produce sine waves; ventricular fibrillation and asystole may ultimately occur.

Etiologies of Special Importance in the Critically Ill Patient

Transcellular Shifts

The movement of K⁺ from the ICF to the ECF may transiently increase the plasma [K⁺] without altering total body K⁺ content, often amplifying the hyperkalemia resulting from other causes. Potential causes of extracellular shift include insulin deficiency, ECF hyperosmolality, inorganic acidemia, and cell breakdown (e.g., rhabdomyolysis, hemolysis, tumor lysis syndrome). DKA may promote hyperkalemia through relative

sulin deficiency, despite the presence of total body potassium depletion. Medica-
ons that cause extracellular shifts include nonselective beta blockers, digitalis, and
ccinylcholine. The hyperkalemia that occurs with succinylcholine is usually small
.5 mEq/L) and brief (resolving within 10 to 15 minutes), but it can be significantly
centuated in patients with massive trauma, burns, or neuromuscular disease.

educed Glomerular Filtration

reduced GFR in both acute and chronic kidney disease can predispose to the devel-
oment of hyperkalemia. Diseased kidneys respond to progressive insufficiency with
creased potassium excretion per functioning nephron. This compensation is typi-
lly adequate until the GFR falls to the point of oliguria. Thus, when hyperkalemia
evelops in a nonoliguric patient, there is usually a second contributing mechanism
r the renal injury is severe and acute. Diminished distal tubular sodium delivery, as
ccurs in volume depletion (prerenal azotemia), is a common contributing mech-
ism in the critically ill patient. Patients with underlying chronic kidney disease
ready have decreased functioning nephron mass, and any further decrease in GFR
n predispose to the development of hyperkalemia.

ffective Aldosterone Deficiency

ledications can account for the relative hypoaldosterone state that contributes to hyper-
alemia in the ICU patient. Heparin, ketoconazole, angiotensin-converting enzyme
ACE) inhibitors, and angiotensin II receptor blockers (ARBs) decrease aldosterone
roduction. Spironolactone and eplerenone are competitive aldosterone antagonists,
hile amiloride, triamterene, trimethoprim, and pentamidine block sodium resorption
nd thus potassium excretion) at the collecting duct where aldosterone would exert
s effect. NSAIDs inhibit renin secretion, a process that is several steps upstream of
ldosterone release; these medications can also decrease glomerular filtration in volume-
epleted states through the inhibition of local vasodilatory prostaglandins.

reatment

lyperkalemia treatment is outlined in Table 24.1. The presence of symptoms or
CG changes associated with hyperkalemia necessitates the prompt initiation of
leasures capable of rapidly lowering the serum [K^+]. Calcium serves to stabilize the
ardiac myocyte membrane but does not actually reduce the [K^+]; therefore, it is given
imultaneously with other therapies that shift potassium into the cell (insulin and
lbuterol) and promote its excretion (sodium polystyrene sulfonate, potassium-wasting
iuretics, and hemodialysis). The use of sodium bicarbonate to shift potassium intra-
ellularly is falling out of favor given its comparatively weak effect in the absence of
n inorganic metabolic acidosis. Dialytic therapies are generally reserved for cases of
evere hyperkalemia not responsive to medical management.

Another important component of therapy is to limit exogenous potassium
ntake. Each 8-oz can of high-protein tube feeds contains approximately 10 mEq of
K^+, and a single unit of packed red blood cells with a prolonged storage time may
ontribute approximately 5 mEq.

DISORDERS OF CALCIUM CONCENTRATION

The extracellular calcium concentration is tightly maintained and reflects the coordinated action of multiple hormones: parathyroid hormone (PTH), 1,25-(OH)$_2$

TABLE 24.1	Acute Therapies for the Management of Hyperkalemia			
Treatment	Dosing	Onset/Duration	Magnitude of [K^+] Decline	Comments
Ca^{2+}	1 g of 10% calcium gluconate or calcium chloride infused IV over 2–3 min; may repeat if no improvement in ECG by 5 min	Immediate onset, lasting 30–60 min	None	Calcium chloride should be administered via a central vein to decrease risk of extravasation and skin necrosis
Insulin	10 units of regular insulin IV (with one ampule of D50 IV if not significantly hyperglycemic)	Onset at 15 min, lasting 6–8 hrs	–1 mEq/L	Watch for hypo- or hyperglycemia (if dextrose given); the latter can offset insulin's K^+-lowering effect
Albuterol	10–20 mg given by nebulized inhalation over 15 min OR 0.5 mg in 100 mL of 5% dextrose infused IV over 15 min	Onset at 10–30 min, lasting 3–6 hrs	1–1.5 mEq/L	Tachycardia and variable effects on blood pressure may result; hyperglycemia may worsen and offset some K^+-lowering effect
$NaHCO_3$	2–4 mEq/min in drip (3 ampules $NaHCO_3$ in sterile water or 5% dextrose) until bicarbonate normalized	Onset at 4 hrs, lasting >6 hrs	0.5–0.75 mEq/L	Not effective unless concurrent inorganic metabolic acidosis; watch for volume overload and may lower serum ionized [Ca^{2+}] and make more susceptible to arrhythmias
Loop +/– thiazide diuretics	Widely variable dose depends on GFR	Onset at 30–60 min, lasting 4–6 hrs (duration prolonged in renal insufficiency)	Variable depending on diuretic response	Avoid in volume-depleted states until euvolemia restored
Sodium polystyrene sulfonate	25–50 g mixed in 100 mL 20% sorbitol PO OR 50 g in 200 mL 30% sorbitol per rectum	Onset at 1–2 hrs, lasting 4–6 hrs	0.5–1 mEq/L	Caution with use in the postoperative patient because of risk of intestinal necrosis; watch for worsening volume overload or hypernatremia from exchanged [Na^+]
Hemodialysis	Variable, based on starting [K^+]	Immediate onset, lasting until dialysis completion	Variable, based on dialysis dose and dialysate [K^+]	Watch for posttreatment K^+ rebound beginning immediately after dialysis completion

itamin D (calcitriol), and to a lesser extent, calcitonin. Approximately 99% of body alcium is in bone with most of the remaining 1% in the ECF. The total plasma alcium concentration consists of three fractions:

- Approximately 45% circulates as the physiologically active ionized (or free) calcium
- About 40% is bound to albumin, with greater binding in alkalemia
- The remaining 15% is bound to multiple organic and inorganic anions such as sulfate, phosphate, lactate, and citrate

The ionized Ca^{2+} concentration, which must lie within a narrow range (4.6 to 5.1 mg/dL) for optimal neuromuscular function, is under exquisitely tight minute-to-minute control by PTH. PTH increases serum $[Ca^{2+}]$ by stimulating bone resorption, calcium reclamation in the kidney, and renal conversion of 25-OH vitamin D to its more active form, 1,25-$(OH)_2$ vitamin D, which then promotes intestinal calcium absorption (Fig. 24.3). 1,25-$(OH)_2$ vitamin D in turn inhibits the production and secretion of PTH, closing the feedback loop.

Disorders of Ca^{2+} concentration are common among critically ill patients. Low ionized $[Ca^{2+}]$ has been observed in up to 88% of ICU patients. Furthermore, the presence of hypocalcemia serves as a marker of disease severity and patient mortality.

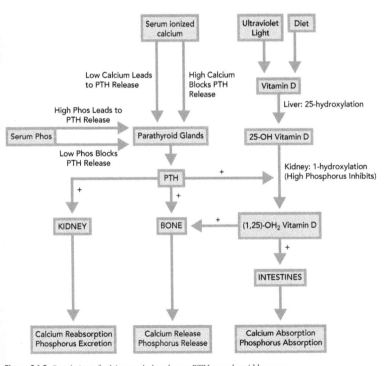

Figure 24.3. Regulation of calcium and phosphorus. PTH, parathyroid hormone.

ALGORITHM 24.7   Evaluation of Hypocalcemia

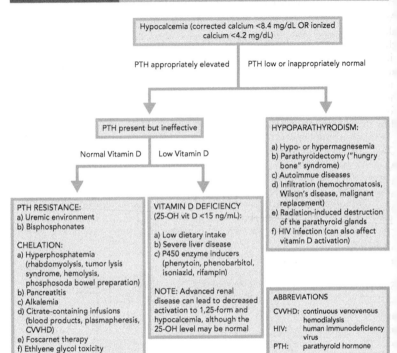

Hypocalcemia (corrected calcium <8.4 mg/dL OR ionized calcium <4.2 mg/dL)

PTH appropriately elevated   PTH low or inappropriately normal

PTH present but ineffective

Normal Vitamin D   Low Vitamin D

PTH RESISTANCE:
a) Uremic environment
b) Bisphosphonates

CHELATION:
a) Hyperphosphatemia (rhabdomyolysis, tumor lysis syndrome, hemolysis, phosphosoda bowel preparation)
b) Pancreatitis
c) Alkalemia
d) Citrate-containing infusions (blood products, plasmapheresis, CVVHD)
e) Foscarnet therapy
f) Ethlyene glycol toxicity

VITAMIN D DEFICIENCY (25-OH vit D <15 ng/mL):

a) Low dietary intake
b) Severe liver disease
c) P450 enzyme inducers (phenytoin, phenobarbitol, isoniazid, rifampin)

NOTE: Advanced renal disease can lead to decreased activation to 1,25-form and hypocalcemia, although the 25-OH level may be normal

HYPOPARATHYRODISM:

a) Hypo- or hypermagnesemia
b) Parathyroidectomy ("hungry bone" syndrome)
c) Autoimmue diseases
d) Infiltration (hemochromatosis, Wilson's disease, malignant replacement)
e) Radiation-induced destruction of the parathyroid glands
f) HIV infection (can also affect vitamin D activation)

ABBREVIATIONS

CVVHD: continuous venovenous hemodialysis
HIV: human immunodeficiency virus
PTH: parathyroid hormone

Hypocalcemia

Since the vast majority of calcium is stored in bone, hypocalcemia (corrected calcium <8.4 mg/dL or ionized calcium <4.2 mg/dL) reflects a defect in transferring this calcium into the ECF (Algorithm 24.7). Evaluation of such disorders always starts with measuring the PTH level, which should be elevated (even levels in the "normal" range are inappropriate in the setting of hypocalcemia). If the PTH level is appropriately elevated, then there is either resistance to its function at the level of bone, inadequate vitamin D activity, or chelation from the circulation.

Symptoms of hypocalcemia include circumoral or distal paresthesias and tetany. Latent tetany may be induced through several maneuvers. Trousseau's sign is positive when carpal spasm is induced after inflating a blood pressure cuff around the arm above systolic pressure for 3 minutes. Chvostek's sign is present when perioral muscle twitching is elicited with tapping the area of the facial nerve anterior to the ear. Acute, severe hypocalcemia may present with confusion, seizures, or bradycardia. ECG findings include QT interval prolongation, bradycardia, or complete heart block.

Etiologies of Special Importance in the Critically Ill Patient

Pseudohypocalcemia

Approximately 45% of serum Ca^{2+} exists in its free ionized form. Changes in serum albumin and serum anions alter total measured serum $[Ca^{2+}]$ without affecting the clinically relevant ionized $[Ca^{2+}]$. Hypoalbuminemia is very common in the ICU setting because albumin concentrations fall during the systemic inflammatory response and with large-volume fluid resuscitation. The total measured serum $[Ca^{2+}]$ is lowered in such situations, but ionized $[Ca^{2+}]$ remains within the normal range. It is recommended that the ionized $[Ca^{2+}]$ always be measured in this setting, since the equation for correction (adding back 0.8 mg/dL to the measured calcium for each 1 mg/dL drop in albumin from 4 mg/dL) may not correlate well.

Chelation

An increase in the availability of any anion that combines readily with Ca^{2+} may cause hypocalcemia, as ionized Ca^{2+} is chelated. The release of negatively charged fatty acids in severe pancreatitis or the spillage of large amount of phosphate in rhabdomyolysis or hemolysis can result in hypocalcemia. Tremendous deposition into bone after parathyroidectomy is termed the "hungry bone" syndrome and can persist for months. Chelation by citrate-containing fluids, such as blood products in massive transfusions or anticoagulants in some forms of continuous dialysis and plasmapheresis, can occur in the critically ill patient.

Sepsis

Hypocalcemia occurs commonly in sepsis, particularly when involving a gram-negative organism. Indeed, in one study, ionized calcium reduction was found in 30% of cases of gram-negative septicemia and in none of those cases caused by gram-positive bacteria. The pathogenesis is incompletely understood, but most patients have elevated PTH and low calcitriol levels. Elevated levels of procalcitonin have been found in many of these patients, suggesting that this hormone precursor may exert a hypocalcemic effect in the critically ill population.

Treatment

The management of symptomatic hypocalcemia or that associated with ECG abnormalities should be prompt and aggressive. IV Ca^{2+} replacement should be initiated in such situations. Treatment is outlined in Table 24.2.

Hypomagnesemia, if present, must be treated first for effective correction, as severe depletion of this electrolyte can impair PTH release. If the cause of low $[Ca^{2+}]$ is marked hyperphosphatemia, it is important to limit calcium replacement to those cases in which cardiac and neurologic symptoms are significant, since overaggressive correction may result in rebound hypercalcemia and metastatic calcification. In cases of profound hypocalcemia, clearance of the chelating species through the early initiation of hemodialysis with higher Ca^{2+} dialysate should be considered. For hypocalcemia occurring in the setting of profound sepsis or other shock states, therapy-guiding evidence is lacking. Although increases in cardiac contractility and blood pressure have been observed by Ca^{2+} administration, some animal data exist that suggest reperfusion injury and mortality may be worsened.

Asymptomatic hypocalcemia may be managed with oral calcium supplements along with vitamin D or its active metabolite, calcitriol, to increase intestinal

TABLE 24.2 Treatment of Hypocalcemia

General guidelines of therapy:
1. If ECG changes or symptoms present, begin IV replacement:
   a. Consider early initiation of hemodialysis when caused by hyperphosphatemia or hyperoxalemia
   b. Bolus 2 g $MgSO_4$ IV over 15 min if known hypomagnesemia or empirically if renal function is normal
   c. Bolus 2 g calcium gluconate (20 mL or 2 ampules of 10% calcium gluconate, 1 g = 93 mg elemental Ca^{2+}) in 50–100 mL of 5% dextrose or saline IV over 10–15 min
   d. Begin continuous Ca^{2+} infusion: dilute 6 g of calcium gluconate[a] in 500 mL of 5% dextrose or saline and infuse at 0.5–1.5 mg elemental Ca^{2+}/kg/hr
   e. Follow ionized $[Ca^{2+}]$ or corrected $[Ca^{2+}]$ q6h and continue infusion until $[Ca^{2+}]$ normalizes
   f. Overlap with PO replacement
2. Dose 1–2 g elemental Ca^{2+} PO tid to qid, separate from meals
3. Can add 0.25–4 µg/day calcitriol AND/OR ergocalciferol especially in vitamin D-deficient states
4. Can add salt restriction and hydrochlorothiazide if hypercalciuria occurs

[a]Alternatively, can use 2 g, 20 mL, or 2 ampules of 10% calcium chloride (1 g = 272 mg elemental Ca^{2+}) but should only be administered through a central vein.

absorption. Supplemental calcium should be administered between meals and away from other medications (particularly, thyroid hormone and iron) to maximize absorption.

Hypercalcemia

As with hypocalcemia, hypercalcemic disorders (corrected calcium >10.3 mg/dL or ionized calcium >5.2 mg/dL) are first evaluated by determining the PTH status (Algorithm 24.8). Levels should be maximally suppressed, and thus, even "normal" levels are inappropriately high, suggesting a hyperparathyroid state. the PTH level is indeed suppressed, hypercalcemia can still result from nutritional vitamin D overdose or excess formation of 1,25-$(OH)_2$ vitamin D (sarcoidosis granulomatous disease, or lymphoma). Malignancy can lead to hypercalcemia through production of a PTH-like substance (PTH-related peptide, PTHrP) or lytic destruction of bone with release of calcium into the circulation. Hypercalcemia itself, through its action in the kidneys, can induce significant volume depletion.

Symptoms of hypercalcemia can occur at levels >12 mg/dL and tend to be more severe with rapid elevations. Polyuria is common, leading to a volume depleted state. Gastrointestinal symptoms are also frequently seen, with anorexia, constipation, and abdominal pain, with pancreatitis a rare secondary complication. Neurologic symptoms include weakness, fatigue, confusion, stupor, or coma. The ECG may reveal a shortened QT interval or variable degrees of atrioventricular block.

ALGORITHM 24.8 Evaluation of Hypercalcemia

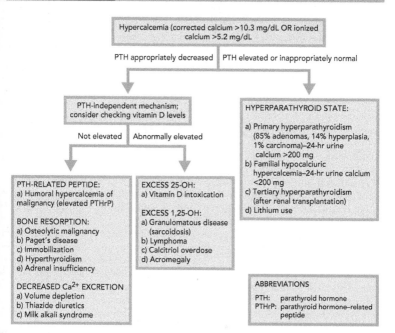

Etiologies of Special Importance in the Critically Ill Patient

Humoral Hypercalcemia of Malignancy

Certain malignancies, particularly squamous cell lung cancer; cancers of the head and neck, esophagus, genitourinary tract; and pheochromocytomas may produce a hormone that differs from PTH but retains its biologic activity. This PTHrP is not detected by standard PTH measurements and must be ordered separately when suspected. In most cases of humoral hypercalcemia of malignancy, patients have advanced disease.

Osteolytic Hypercalcemia of Malignancy

In this separate form of cancer-associated hypercalcemia, cytokines produced by tumor cells stimulate osteoclast bone resorption. Hypercalcemia and hyperphosphatemia occur with extensive bone involvement by tumor, and the serum alkaline phosphatase is often significantly elevated. The PTH is appropriately suppressed. The most frequently associated malignancies include breast carcinoma, nonsmall cell lung cancer, myeloma, and lymphoma.

Excess Calcitriol Production

Excess unregulated vitamin D activation can be produced by granulomatous disease such as sarcoidosis as well as the lymphocytes of some Hodgkin's and non-Hodgkin's lymphomas. These cells possess intrinsic 1-alpha hydroxylase activity, leading to excessive calcitriol production. The elevation in [Ca^{2+}] is usually less severe than in humoral hypercalcemia of malignancy.

Immobilization

Complete bed rest can result in hypercalcemia after several days. There is increased osteoclast activity as well as diminished bone formation, with resultant hypercalcemia.

It is usually more severe when renal function is impaired. Remobilization, when possible, leads to improvement and eventual resolution of the hypercalcemia.

Treatment

Hypercalcemia treatment is outlined in Table 24.3. Rapidly acting therapies for hypercalcemia are warranted if severe symptoms are present or with [Ca^{2+}] >12 mg/dL. First, the anticalciuric effect of hypovolemia should be corrected with IV isotonic fluid boluses. Continuing maintenance IV saline after achieving euvolemia further promotes calcium excretion. Loop diuretics add little to the calciuretic effect of saline administration and may prevent adequate volume restoration. However, they are useful if signs of hypervolemia develop. Calcitonin can also lower the serum [Ca^{2+}] within hours, and hemodialysis against a low calcium dialysate bath can be used if other medical maneuvers are unsuccessful.

While initiating the acute therapies, it is often necessary to simultaneously start long-term measures of Ca^{2+} control. Usually, this consists of administering an IV bisphosphonate, which decreases Ca^{2+} resorption from bone by osteoclasts. In situations of calcitriol excess and when hypercalcemia occurs as a result of hematologic malignancies, the administration of glucocorticoids is effective for lowering the serum [Ca^{2+}] and can be used alone or with bisphosphonates. Denosumab has been used to treat hypercalcemia related to malignancy; it is a monoclonal antibody to the receptor activator of nuclear factor kappa-B ligand (RANKL), inhibiting its interaction with RANK on the surface of osteocytes, resulting in decreased osteoclast differentiation. A potential side effect is symptomatic hypocalcemia which is more pronounced in patients with renal insufficiency and a creatinine clearance less than 30 mL/min.

DISORDERS OF PHOSPHORUS CONCENTRATION

Approximately 85% of total body phosphorus (as PO_4^{3-}) is in bone, and most of the remainder is within cells as the major intracellular anion. As only 1% of total body phosphorus is in the ECF, the serum PO_4^{3-} concentration may not reflect total body phosphorus stores. In addition to its importance in bone formation, phosphorus is an integral component of adenosine triphosphate (ATP) and thus critical for normal cellular metabolism. Furthermore, its presence in the red blood cell as 2,3-bisphosphoglycerate makes it important in the regulation of hemoglobin oxygen affinity and therefore tissue oxygen delivery.

Phosphorus balance is determined primarily by PTH, active vitamin D (calcitriol), fibroblast growth factor 23 (FGF23), and insulin. PTH lowers [PO_4^{3-}] through urinary excretion. Calcitriol increases [PO_4^{3-}] by enhancing intestinal phosphorus absorption. FGF23 is a hormone produced by osteocytes with a primary function of increasing phosphorus excretion by the kidney. It is stimulated by hyperphosphatemia, PTH, and calcitriol and in turn closes these feedback loops by inhibiting PTH production and by decreasing vitamin D activation. FGF23 has been shown to have off-target effects on cardiac remodeling and may in part be responsible for left ventricular hypertrophy seen

TABLE 24.3 | Treatment of Hypercalcemia

Treatment	Dosing	Onset/Duration	Comments
Isotonic saline	Bolus isotonic saline until euvolemic (may require up to 3–4 L), then adjust rate to achieve urine output of 100–150 mL/hr	Onset at 2–4 hrs	Watch for signs of volume overload; loop diuretics may help with calcium excretion, but should be held until volume deficits have first been corrected
Calcitonin	4–8 IU/kg IM or SC q6–12h	Onset at 4–6 hrs; tachyphylaxis develops after 2–3 days	Lowers serum Ca^{2+} 1–2 mg/dL; side effects include flushing, nausea, and, rarely, allergic reactions
Bisphosphonates	Zoledronate 4 mg IV over 15 min OR pamidronate 60–90 mg IV over 2–4 hrs	Onset at 2 days with peak effect at 4–6 days; lasts 2–4 wks	Decrease infusion rate of pamidronate or lower zoledronate dose in renal insufficiency
Denosumab	60–120 mg SC	Onset within 3 days, half-life of 25 days	Watch for hypocalcemia, risk for infection
Gallium nitrate	100–200 mg/m^2/day continuous infusion for up to 5 days	Onset after 2 days; lasts 1–2 wks	Significant risk of nephrotoxicity and is contraindicated if creatinine >2.5 mg/dL
Glucocorticoids	Prednisone 20–60 mg/day (or equivalent glucocorticoid dose)	Onset in 5–10 days	Effective only in cases of granulomatous disease and hematologic malignancies
Hemodialysis	Variable based on starting [Ca^{2+}]	Immediate onset, lasting until dialysis completion	Useful for cases of severe hypercalcemia (>16 mg/dL) and when diuretic-resistant volume overload prohibits saline administration

General guidelines of therapy:
1. Correct volume depletion FIRST, with isotonic normal saline
2. If ECG changes or severe symptoms are present, begin the most rapidly acting therapies in combination
3. If rapid improvement is not seen (or anticipated due to the underlying condition), consider adding the longer-acting treatments (bisphosphonates) early since their effects are delayed

TABLE 24.4		Interpretation of Calcium and Phosphorus Values	
Ca^{2+}	PO_4^{3-}	PTH	Diagnosis
↑	↓	↑	Primary hyperparathyroidism
↑	↓	↓	Humoral hypercalcemia
↑	↑	↓	Osteolytic malignancy (myeloma)
↑	↑	↓	Vitamin D excess, granulomas, lymphomas
↓	↑	↓	Hypoparathyroidism, Mg^{2+} disorders
↓	↑	↑	PTH resistance (pseudohypoparathyroidism)
↓	↑	↑	CKD (secondary hyperparathyroidism)
↓	↓	↑	Severe vitamin D deficiency

CKD, chronic kidney disease.

in chronic kidney disease and hyperphosphatemia, where levels are chronically elevated. Finally, insulin lowers serum levels by shifting PO_4^{3-} into cells. Hypophosphatemia is common in acutely ill patients, having been found to occur in 29% of surgical ICU patients. Hyperphosphatemia is frequently encountered in patients with renal failure.

Since many of the regulators of phosphorus are the same as those involved in calcium homeostasis, there is considerable overlap in the maintenance of an appropriate balance. In order to adequately assess phosphorus disorders, one must take into account the concurrent calcium concentration. This is summarized in Table 24.4 for the more common etiologies.

Hypophosphatemia

When evaluating a patient with hypophosphatemia, one should first rule out severe vitamin D deficiency and primary hyperparathyroidism (Algorithm 24.9). The remaining causes include gastrointestinal losses (e.g., phosphate binders, malnutrition, diarrhea), transcellular shifts (e.g., insulin, refeeding syndrome, respiratory alkalosis), or renal wasting. Losses by the kidney can be distinguished by the finding of a high fractional excretion of phosphorus (suggested by value greater than 5%), an inappropriate response to the prevailing hypophosphatemia. An elevated fractional excretion of phosphorus is associated with conditions of hyperparathyroidism, vitamin D deficiency, or tubular defects. Continuous renal replacement modalities used in the ICU setting can dramatically deplete serum phosphorus levels.

Symptoms typically occur only when there is total body PO_4^{3-} depletion and the serum $[PO_4^{3-}]$ is <1 mg/dL. Muscular weakness (including the diaphragm) can be seen, while paresthesias, seizures, stupor, or coma may develop when severe.

Etiologies of Special Importance in the Critically Ill Patient
Intracellular Shift

Respiratory alkalosis is a very common cause of redistributive hypophosphatemia as the intracellular rise in pH stimulates glycolysis and the subsequent phosphorylation of various intermediates in the pathway. The marked anabolism that occurs during the abrupt reversal of negative caloric states with dextrose-containing IV fluids or total parenteral nutrition (refeeding syndrome) similarly shifts PO_4^{3-} to the ICF and can occur after as little as 2 days of nutritional restriction. The accompanying surge in insulin further promotes the intracellular translocation.

ALGORITHM 24.9 Evaluation of Hypophosphatemia

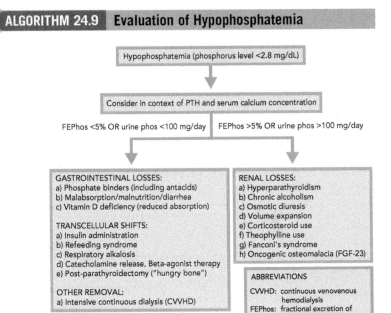

Hypophosphatemia (phosphorus level <2.8 mg/dL)

Consider in context of PTH and serum calcium concentration

FEPhos <5% OR urine phos <100 mg/day   FEPhos >5% OR urine phos >100 mg/day

GASTROINTESTINAL LOSSES:
a) Phosphate binders (including antacids)
b) Malabsorption/malnutrition/diarrhea
c) Vitamin D deficiency (reduced absorption)

TRANSCELLULAR SHIFTS:
a) Insulin administration
b) Refeeding syndrome
c) Respiratory alkalosis
d) Catecholamine release, Beta-agonist therapy
e) Post-parathyroidectomy ("hungry bone")

OTHER REMOVAL:
a) Intensive continuous dialysis (CVVHD)

RENAL LOSSES:
a) Hyperparathyroidism
b) Chronic alcoholism
c) Osmotic diuresis
d) Volume expansion
e) Corticosteroid use
f) Theophylline use
g) Fanconi's syndrome
h) Oncogenic osteomalacia (FGF-23)

ABBREVIATIONS

CVVHD: continuous venovenous hemodialysis
FEPhos: fractional excretion of phosphorus
FGF23: fibroblast growth factor-23
PTH: parathyroid hormone

Fractional excretion of phosphorus (FEPhos):
(urine phos × serum creatinine) / (serum phos × urine creatinine)

Renal Wasting

Hyperparathyroidism from any cause can increase renal PO_4^{3-} excretion. Chronic alcohol consumption also causes renal PO_4^{3-} wasting by an unknown mechanism. This, in combination with the usually poor nutritional status of these patients, contributes to a total body PO_4^{3-} deficit. Furthermore, the respiratory alkalosis of liver failure, the increased adrenergic tone of withdrawal, and the refeeding syndrome occurring with dextrose infusions can all lead to profound hypophosphatemia in the hospitalized alcoholic patient.

Increased renal tubular fluid flow from any cause can also lead to urinary PO_4^{3-} wasting. This can be seen with aggressive volume expansion or with osmotic diuresis, such as that which occurs with the glycosuria of DKA. Furthermore, insulin therapy in the management of DKA shifts PO_4^{3-} into cells and may worsen the hypophosphatemia.

Oncogenic osteomalacia involves tumor production of FGF23. An integral part of normal phosphorus homeostasis, FGF23 can lead to renal phosphorus wasting when overproduced through nonregulated ectopic production from tumors.

Continuous Hemodialysis

Standard intermittent hemodialysis is only able to inefficiently remove phosphorus from the intravascular space and thus rarely leads to hypophosphatemia on its own. However, with continuous hemodialysis modalities, there is a state of constant negative efflux that can result in significant hypophosphatemia. Patients on continuous venovenous hemodialysis (CVVHD) should have their phosphorus levels checked

TABLE 24.5	Treatment of Hypophosphatemia

1. If symptomatic, or intolerant to PO, begin IV replacement (reduce doses in setting of renal insufficiency):
   a. Severe (≤1 mg/dL): dose 0.6 mmol/kg ideal body weight (IBW) IV[a] over 6 hrs; if hypotension ensues, suspect hypocalcemia and discontinue infusion
   b. Moderate (1–1.8 mg/dL): dose 0.4 mmol/kg IBW IV[a] over 6 hrs
   c. Mild (1.9–2.5 mg/dL): dose 0.2 mmol/kg IBW IV[a] over 6 hrs
2. If asymptomatic, dose 0.5–1 g elemental phosphorus PO bid-tid; this should correct most deficits by 1 wk
   a. Neutra-phos: 250 mg (8 mmol) phosphorus and 7 mEq each of Na^+ and K^+
   b. Neutra-phos K: 250 mg phosphorus and 14 mEq K^+
   c. K-phos neutral: 250 mg phosphorus with 13 mEq Na^+ and 1.1 mEq K^+
   d. Treat vitamin D deficiency, if present

[a]Two IV preparations exist: use potassium phosphate if normal renal function and $[K^+]$ <4 mEq/L; use sodium phosphate if renal function is impaired or $[K^+]$ >4 mEq/L.

every 12 to 24 hours, and if hypophosphatemia develops, standard treatment measures should be employed.

Treatment

Hypophosphatemia treatment is outlined in Table 24.5. Mild hypophosphatemia (1.9 to 2.5 mg/dL) is common in the hospitalized patient and is often simply caused by transcellular shifts, requiring no specific treatment except correction of the underlying cause. Severe, symptomatic hypophosphatemia (<1.0 mg/dL), however, may require IV PO_4^{3-} therapy. Although the rapid administration of large doses of IV PO_4^{3-} (0.8 mmol/kg over 30 minutes) to critically ill patients has been shown to be safe and effective, care must be taken with parenteral therapy to avoid hyperphosphatemia, which may lead to hypocalcemia and metastatic calcification. In the presence of renal insufficiency, IV PO_4^{3-} should be given at lower doses (33% of usual doses in severe renal failure) and with even greater care. IV repletion can be transitioned over to oral therapy when the $[PO_4^{3-}]$ is >1.5 mg/dL. Enteral replacement may result in diarrhea and nausea. Because of the need to replenish intracellular stores, 24 to 36 hours of repletion may be required. There has been no demonstrated clear benefit to aggressive repletion of PO_4^{3-} in asymptomatic hypophosphatemia. Studies of PO_4^{3-} therapy in the treatment of DKA, for instance, have shown no improved outcomes and may even suggest increased morbidity, primarily through resultant hypocalcemia.

Hyperphosphatemia

When evaluating hyperphosphatemia (Algorithm 24.10), vitamin D levels and PTH activity should be assessed. The kidneys possess a remarkable ability to excrete phosphorus, but retention may result if there is acute or chronic renal damage. Chronic kidney disease often leads to secondary hyperparathyroidism, with increased phosphorus despite the elevated PTH, and with variable calcium concentrations. When increased intake or transcellular shifts are responsible for hyperphosphatemia, the urinary excretion is often quite high to attempt to correct the imbalance.

Symptoms of hyperphosphatemia primarily relate to the concomitant hypocalcemia that results. Metastatic calcification of soft tissue, vasculature, cornea, kidney,

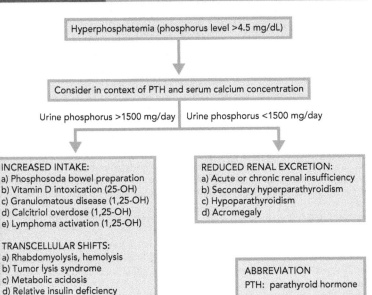

ALGORITHM 24.10 Evaluation of Hyperphosphatemia

Hyperphosphatemia (phosphorus level >4.5 mg/dL)

Consider in context of PTH and serum calcium concentration

Urine phosphorus >1500 mg/day | Urine phosphorus <1500 mg/day

INCREASED INTAKE:
a) Phosphosoda bowel preparation
b) Vitamin D intoxication (25-OH)
c) Granulomatous disease (1,25-OH)
d) Calcitriol overdose (1,25-OH)
e) Lymphoma activation (1,25-OH)

TRANSCELLULAR SHIFTS:
a) Rhabdomyolysis, hemolysis
b) Tumor lysis syndrome
c) Metabolic acidosis
d) Relative insulin deficiency

REDUCED RENAL EXCRETION:
a) Acute or chronic renal insufficiency
b) Secondary hyperparathyroidism
c) Hypoparathyroidism
d) Acromegaly

ABBREVIATION
PTH: parathyroid hormone

nd joints can occur. Calciphylaxis is skin ischemia and necrosis that can occur in atients with chronic kidney disease, resulting from calcium and phosphorus deposiion within small blood vessels and subsequent thrombosis.

Etiologies of Special Importance in the Critically Ill Patient

Transcellular Shifts

Since the majority of phosphorus is sequestered intracellularly, any process that leads to widespread cell destruction (e.g., rhabdomyolysis, hemolysis, tumor lysis syndrome) can lead to impressive hyperphosphatemia. The calcium concentration is often decreased as it complexes with the circulating phosphorus. Metabolic acidosis, especially lactic acidosis and DKA (with its concomitant relative insulin deficiency), can also result in phosphorus shifting out of cells.

Phosphate-rich Bowel Preparations

Hyperphosphatemia can occur from the use of bowel preparatory oral sodium phosphate formulations or phosphate-containing enemas. Cases of acute kidney injury via acute phosphate nephropathy have been reported following use of these laxatives. Volume depletion and underlying renal insufficiency are risk factors that may predispose toward acute kidney injury.

Treatment

Treatment of hyperphosphatemia is outlined in Table 24.6. Saline diuresis may help in excreting some of the excess phosphorus in the acute overload state. Acetazolamide is

TABLE 24.6	Treatment of Hyperphosphatemia

General guidelines of therapy:
1. Correct underlying cause (if normal renal function and phosphate handling are achieved, hyperphosphatemia will usually correct within 12 hrs)
2. Consider forced saline resuscitation with addition of acetazolamide (15 mg/kg q4h)
3. When severe, especially when renal insufficiency is not rapidly reversible, consider hemodialysis or continuous renal replacement therapy
4. When chronic, use phosphate binders (noncalcium based if concomitant hyper-calcemia) and dietary restriction

particularly effective at encouraging phosphorus elimination. If these conservative measures are unsuccessful and the underlying cause is not rapidly reversible, dialysis may become necessary for very severe hyperphosphatemia. For cases where chronic kidney disease is the cause, dietary restriction combined with oral phosphate binders is recommended.

DISORDERS OF MAGNESIUM CONCENTRATION

Approximately 60% of body magnesium is in bone, and most of the remainder within cells. Only 1% of the total magnesium is in the ECF. Mg^{2+} is not exchanged easily across the cell membrane, and therefore, there is little buffering of fluctuations in the serum Mg^{2+} concentration. Furthermore, the $[Mg^{2+}]$ is a poor predictor intracellular and total body stores. Unlike calcium and phosphorus, there are known hormones specifically delegated to the regulation of Mg^{2+} balance. The main determinant of Mg^{2+} balance is the serum $[Mg^{2+}]$ itself; hypomagnesemia stimulates renal tubular resorption of Mg^{2+}, whereas hypermagnesemia inhibits this process.

Hypomagnesemia

Hypomagnesemia occurs commonly in the ICU. As an important participant in most processes involving calcium flux and a cofactor in reactions consuming ATP, Mg^{2+} critical for many biologic processes. Algorithm 24.11 describes the primary etiologies of hypomagnesemia. Urinary losses in renal wasting have a fractional excretion magnesium >2%. This is calculated as (urine Mg^{2+} × serum creatinine)/(0.7 × serum Mg^{2+} × urine creatinine). Also, there may be gastrointestinal losses, reduced intake or chelation (similar process as in hypocalcemia).

Symptoms of hypomagnesemia generally do not occur until the $[Mg^{2+}]$ <1 mEq/L. Lethargy, confusion, ataxia, nystagmus, tremor, fasciculations, tetany, and seizures may occur. Atrial and ventricular arrhythmias may be seen, particularly patients on digoxin. The ECG may show prolonged PR and QT intervals with widened QRS complexes and U waves. Torsades de pointes is the classically associated arrhythmia with hypomagnesemia. There may be concurrent hypokalemia and hypocalcemia (particularly in alcoholic patients) and may contribute to the overall clinical picture.

Etiologies of Special Importance in the Critically Ill Patient
Gastrointestinal Loss
Intestinal secretions have significant Mg^{2+} content, with more magnesium present in lower intestinal fluids. Fistulas, prolonged gastrointestinal drainage, or diarrhea can therefore lead to negative Mg^{2+} balance.

ALGORITHM 24.11 Evaluation of Hypomagnesemia

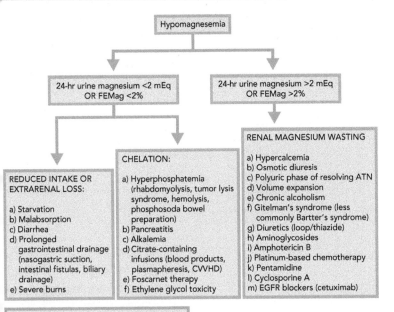

ABBREVIATIONS

ATN: acute tubular necrosis
CVVHD: continuous venovenous hemodialysis
EGFR: epithelial growth factor receptor
FEMag: fractional excretion of magnesium

Renal Wasting

Chronic alcoholism may lead to renal tubular dysfunction, resulting in inappropriate Mg^{2+} wasting, exacerbating the malnutrition that is often present. Numerous drugs have similarly been associated with urinary Mg^{2+} wasting. Prolonged dosing of aminoglycosides may cause renal tubular damage with characteristic Mg^{2+} wasting and polyuria. The development of hypomagnesemia may even be delayed until after completion of therapy, and the tubular transport defect can persist for months. Other common offenders are the platinum-based chemotherapies such as cisplatin and carboplatin. Cetuximab is an epithelial growth factor receptor (EGFR) antagonist used for colorectal and squamous cell head and neck can cause severe hypomagnesemia by its effect on the distal convoluted tubule.

Chelation

Because Mg^{2+} is an ion with similar charge and size as Ca^{2+}, similar causes of hypocalcemia from chelation can also result in hypomagnesemia, although usually to a lesser degree. This phenomenon has been described, for instance, in cases of severe acute pancreatitis. Hypomagnesemia worsens the hypocalcemia in this setting through its inhibition of PTH release.

TABLE 24.7 Treatment of Hypomagnesemia

General guidelines of therapy:

1. If ECG changes or symptoms present, begin IV replacement (reduce doses in renal insufficiency):
   a. 1–2 g MgSO$_4$ (1 g MgSO$_4$ = 96 mg elemental Mg^{2+} = 8 mEq Mg^{2+}) IV over 15 min, followed by an infusion of 6 g MgSO$_4$ in 1 L IV fluid over 24 hrs
   b. Continuous infusion may be required for 3–7 days to replenish total body stores; follow [Mg^{2+}] q24h (more frequently if renal insufficiency present) and adjust infusion to maintain [Mg^{2+}] <2.5 mEq/L
   c. Check deep tendon reflexes often to detect developing hypermagnesemia
2. If asymptomatic and no ECG changes:
   a. For mild hypomagnesemia: 240 mg PO elemental^a Mg^{2+} per day in divided doses
   b. For severe hypomagnesemia: up to 720 mg PO elemental^a Mg^{2+} per day in divided doses
   c. If PO not possible or diarrhea present: 2–6 g IV MgSO$_4$ infused at 1 g/hr or less
3. For chronic hypomagnesemia from renal wasting, consider high-dose amiloride

^{a}Magnesium oxide = 0.6 mg elemental Mg^{2+} per mg.

Treatment

Hypomagnesemia treatment is outlined in Table 24.7. The route of Mg^{2+} repletion depends on whether clinical manifestations from Mg^{2+} deficiency are present and not on the actual [Mg^{2+}]. Asymptomatic hypomagnesemia without ECG abnormalities can be treated orally, even if the deficiency is severe, unless malabsorption is present. Oral therapy avoids the abrupt increase in [Mg^{2+}] that occurs with IV repletion, which then increases renal excretion of part of the administered dose. The major side effect of enteral therapy is diarrhea. In scenarios with chronic urinary Mg^{2+} wasting, potassium-sparing diuretics like amiloride can be administered to reduce renal losses. Symptomatic hypomagnesemia should be treated parenterally initially to replenish intracellular stores. Deep tendon reflexes should be tested frequently during aggressive parenteral dosing, as hyporeflexia implies the development of hypermagnesemia. Reduced doses and more frequent monitoring must be used even in mild renal insufficiency.

Hypermagnesemia

The kidneys have a remarkable capacity to excrete excess magnesium, and therefore, it is uncommon to see hypermagnesemia unless concomitant renal insufficiency is present. Symptoms are typically seen only if the serum [Mg^{2+}] is >4 mEq/L, and patients present with neuromuscular manifestations including hyporeflexia (usually the first sign of magnesium toxicity), weakness, and lethargy that can progress to somnolence and paralysis. With diaphragmatic involvement, this can lead to respiratory failure. Cardiac manifestations include hypotension, bradycardia, and cardiac arrest. The ECG may show prolonged PR, QRS, and QT intervals when the magnesium is 5 to 10 mEq/L. With more severe hypermagnesemia (>15 mEq/L), complete heart block or asystole may ensue.

The diagnostic differential is summarized in Algorithm 24.12. Treatment is focused on the cardiac manifestations, with administration of calcium gluconate to stabilize the myocardium. Exogenous magnesium should be discontinued and

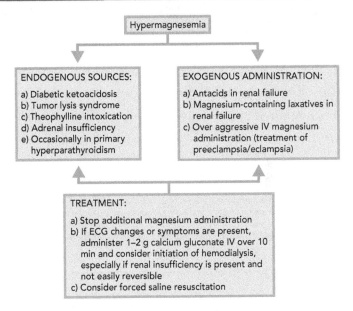

ALGORITHM 24.12 Evaluation and Treatment of Hypermagnesemia

Hypermagnesemia

ENDOGENOUS SOURCES:

a) Diabetic ketoacidosis
b) Tumor lysis syndrome
c) Theophylline intoxication
d) Adrenal insufficiency
e) Occasionally in primary hyperparathyroidism

EXOGENOUS ADMINISTRATION:

a) Antacids in renal failure
b) Magnesium-containing laxatives in renal failure
c) Over aggressive IV magnesium administration (treatment of preeclampsia/eclampsia)

TREATMENT:

a) Stop additional magnesium administration
b) If ECG changes or symptoms are present, administer 1–2 g calcium gluconate IV over 10 min and consider initiation of hemodialysis, especially if renal insufficiency is present and not easily reversible
c) Consider forced saline resuscitation

...alysis may be needed if renal insufficiency is present and not easily reversible ...lgorithm 24.12).

SUGGESTED READINGS

...drogue H, Madias N. Aiding fluid prescription for the dysnatremias. *Intensive Care Med.* 1997;23:309–316.

> *The original paper first presenting the use of the Adrogue–Madias equation for planning initial therapy in the dysnatremias. The concepts underlying the equation and its derivation are presented. Several examples with a comparison to the prior approach are also given.*

...lon M, Shanklin N. Effect of bicarbonate administration on plasma potassium in dialysis patients: interactions with insulin and albuterol. *Am J Kidney Dis.* 1996;28:508–514.

> *The time course of the acute therapies for hyperkalemia is studied and compared. This is one of several papers confirming the relative ineffectiveness of bicarbonate in the acute treatment of hyperkalemia.*

...manzadeh J, Reilly RF. Hypophosphatemia: an evidence-based approach to its clinical consequences and management. *Nat Clin Pract Nephrol.* 2006;2:136–148.

> *An excellent review of the effects of hypophosphatemia and its treatment based on the available clinical data.*

...raser CL, Arieff AI. Epidemiology, pathophysiology, and management of hyponatremic encephalopathy. *Am J Med.* 1997;102:67–77.

> *Review describing the pathophysiology of hyponatremia and factors linked with neurologic compromise based on case-control associations. Management guidelines differing from the traditional are offered. Includes a bibliography with most of the papers of significance on this topic.*

Kamel KS, Halperin ML. Intrarenal urea recycling leads to a higher rate of renal excretion potassium: an hypothesis with clinical implications. *Curr Opin Nephrol Hypertens.* 20 20:547–554.

Recent discoveries by developers of the transtubular potassium gradient equation affecting validity of this calculation.

Kraft MD, Btaiche IF, Sacks GS, et al. Treatment of electrolyte disorders in adult patients in t intensive care unit. *Am J Health Syst Pharm.* 2005;62:1663–1682.

An extensive topic review on the presentations and management of all of the electrolyte abn malities touched upon here. Whenever possible, clinical studies are cited by an extens bibliography.

Palevsky PM, Bhagrath R, Greenberg A. Hypernatremia in hospitalized patients. *Ann Inte Med.* 1996;124:197–203.

Describes the incidence of in-hospital hypernatremia and clinical characteristics, pathophys logic mechanisms, and outcomes for a cohort of hypernatremic patients.

Palmer BF. Hyponatremia in patients with central nervous system disease: SIADH versus CSV *Endocrinol Metab.* 2003;14:182–187.

A good review on the difficult topic of cerebral salt wasting.

Rose B, Post T. *Clinical Physiology of Acid–Base and Electrolyte Disorders.* 5th ed. New Yor McGraw-Hill; 2001.

A textbook which thoroughly describes the renal handling of sodium, potassium, and wat including normal physiology and pathophysiology. Many classic experiments in ren physiology are presented throughout the text to illustrate the described principles.

Zivin JR, Gooley T, Zager RA, et al. Hypocalemia: a pervasive metabolic abnormality in t critically ill. *Am J Kidney Dis.* 2001;37:689–698.

A study which defines the high incidence of hypocalcemia in a diverse population of the cri cally ill. Associations with increased illness severity are highlighted.

25

Metabolic Acid–Base Disorders

Usman Younus and Steven Cheng

Acid–base disorders are commonly encountered in the critical care setting. A stepwise approach to the evaluation of these disorders helps delineate underlying causes, compensatory mechanisms, and the correct approach to management. This section will review the diagnosis and management of metabolic acidosis and alkalosis. Respiratory acidosis and alkalosis are discussed separately (see Chapter 26).

The average individual generates a daily production of approximately 15,000 mmol of carbon dioxide (CO_2) and 50 to 100 mEq of hydrogen ions (H^+) from the catabolism of carbohydrates, fats, and proteins. An appropriate response to this acid load is essential because the range of extracellular H^+ concentration compatible with life (150 to 15 nmol/L and a respective pH of 6.8 to 7.8) is fairly narrow. Disorders of the acid–base system and the appropriate management are best understood by examining the equation for the bicarbonate–carbon dioxide buffer system:

$$H_2O + CO_2 \leftrightarrow H_2CO_3 \leftrightarrow H^+ + HCO_3^-$$

The enzyme carbonic anhydrase catalyzes the reaction of water (H_2O) and carbon dioxide (CO_2) to form carbonic acid (H_2CO_3). Carbonic acid dissociates into bicarbonate (HCO_3^-) and a hydrogen ion (H^+). The physiologic pH is thus balanced by respiratory processes, which adjust the partial pressure of CO_2 (PCO_2), and metabolic processes, which modulate the generation and excretion of bicarbonate and hydrogen ions in the kidney.

When acid–base homeostasis is disturbed by a metabolic acidosis or alkalosis, respiratory compensation is required to attenuate the degree of change in pH. In metabolic acidosis, this compensation begins immediately, although the full degree of compensation (a decrease in pCO_2 of 1.2 mm Hg for each 1 mEq/L decrease in the serum bicarbonate) may not be completely attained for 12 to 24 hours. In metabolic alkalosis the appropriate respiratory response is a 0.7 mm Hg increase in the pCO_2 for each 1 mEq/L increase in the serum bicarbonate (Table 25.1). However, the hypoventilation required for an increase in pCO_2 is often not possible for critically ill patients with underlying cardiac and pulmonary disorders.

The clinical identification of metabolic acid–base disorders, the evaluation of respiratory compensation, and the detection of mixed disorders requires a careful systematic approach. The following steps represent one such approach (Algorithm 25.1).

1. Determine the underlying abnormality—metabolic acidosis and/or metabolic alkalosis.

TABLE 25.1	Expected pCO_2 and Respiratory Compensation for Metabolic Acidosis and Alkalosis
Metabolic acidosis	pCO_2 is >10 mm Hg in a single disorder $pCO_2 = -1.2$ mm Hg for every 1 mEq/L fall in $[HCO_3^-]$ (below 24 mEq/L)
Metabolic alkalosis	pCO_2 is <60 mm Hg in a single disorder $pCO_2 = +0.7$ mm Hg for every 1 mEq/L rise in $[HCO_3^-]$ (above 24 mEq/L)

2. Determine the contributing factors and concomitant disorders (anion gap acidosis ± nonanion gap acidosis ± metabolic alkalosis).
3. Evaluate the appropriateness of respiratory compensation.
4. Determine the likely cause of the disorder and whether or not urgent intervention is necessary.

METABOLIC ACIDOSIS

Acidemia is the most common acute metabolic acid–base disturbance presenting in the critical care setting. The four main mechanisms used in an attempt to maintain homeostasis in this setting are:

1. Extracellular buffering primarily via HCO_3^-
2. Intracellular and bone buffering (buffers up to 55% to 60% of the acid load)
3. Renal excretion of H^+ and regeneration of bicarbonate
4. Respiratory excretion of CO_2 by alveolar ventilation

Metabolic acidosis may present as a single disturbance or as a more complex combined disorder due to various simultaneous processes with different effects on acid–base homeostasis. Double and triple metabolic disorders often reflect a metabolic alkalosis occurring with an anion gap acidosis (as can occur during diabetic ketoacidosis and vomiting) and/or a nonanion gap acidosis. Inappropriate respiratory compensation in any of these situations may add the additional component of respiratory acidosis or alkalosis.

Anion Gap Acidosis

The anion gap is a way of measuring "unmeasured" anions in the blood (as opposed to the "measured" chloride and bicarbonate anions typically identified in basic chemistry laboratory results). It can be calculated with the equation:

Anion Gap = [Serum Sodium (Na^+) – (Serum Chloride [Cl^-] + Serum HCO_3^-)]

Normal values are between 8 and 12 mEq/L.

An anion gap greater than this simply suggests that the patient has been exposed to an "unmeasured" anion, which increases the anion gap. For example, the accumulation of lactate, beta hydroxybutyrate, and acetoacetate—all of which are "unmeasured" anions—increases the anion gap. Thus common causes of an anion gap metabolic acidosis include lactic acidosis, toxic ingestions, ketoacidosis, rhabdomyolysis, and renal failure (Tables 25.2 and 25.3).

ALGORITHM 25.1 Approach to Metabolic Acidosis and Alkalosis

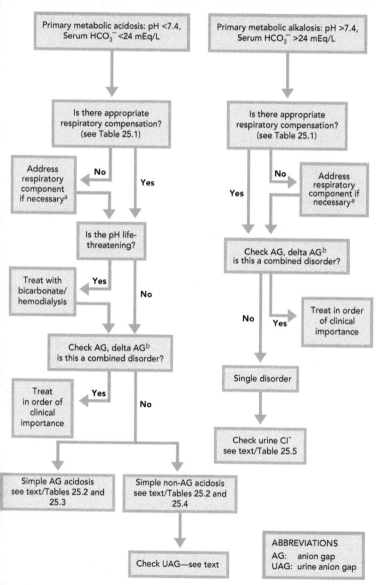

Primary metabolic acidosis: pH <7.4, Serum HCO₃⁻ <24 mEq/L

Primary metabolic alkalosis: pH >7.4, Serum HCO₃⁻ >24 mEq/L

Is there appropriate respiratory compensation? (see Table 25.1)

No → Address respiratory component if necessary[a]

Yes

Is the pH life-threatening?

Yes → Treat with bicarbonate/hemodialysis

No

Check AG, delta AG[b] is this a combined disorder?

Yes → Treat in order of clinical importance

No

Simple AG acidosis see text/Tables 25.2 and 25.3

Simple non-AG acidosis see text/Tables 25.2 and 25.4

Check UAG—see text

Is there appropriate respiratory compensation? (see Table 25.1)

No → Address respiratory component if necessary[a]

Yes

Check AG, delta AG[b] is this a combined disorder?

No

Yes → Treat in order of clinical importance

Single disorder

Check urine Cl⁻ see text/Table 25.5

ABBREVIATIONS
AG: anion gap
UAG: urine anion gap

[a] May require intubation and mechanical ventilation for patients with life-threatening acid–base disturbances unable to fully hyper- or hypoventilate appropriately.
[b] See text for details.

TABLE 25.2	Causes of Anion Gap and Nonanion Gap Metabolic Acidosis

Mechanism	Increased Anion Gap Acidosis[a]	Normal Anion Gap Acidosis

Increased acid production or administration	Lactic acidosis: lactate, D-lactate
	Ketoacidosis
	Massive rhabdomyolysis
	Intoxications:
	  Methanol/formaldehyde
	    → formate
	  Ethylene glycol → glycolate,
	    oxalate
	  Toluene → hippurate
	  Salicylates
	  Paraldehyde → organic anions
	  L-5 oxoprolinuria
		Ammonium chloride ingestion
		Hyperalimentation fluids/saline infusion

Increased bicarbonate loss or loss of bicarbonate precursors		GI losses (negative UAG)
		  Diarrhea
		  Pancreatic, biliary, intestinal
		    fistulas
		  Ostomy
		  Cholestyramine
		  Sevelamer
		Renal losses
		  Carbonic anhydrase inhibitors
		  Type 2 (proximal) RTA
		Treatment phase of
		  ketoacidosis

Decreased acid excretion (positive UAG)	Chronic renal failure	Acute renal failure Chronic renal failure Type 1 (distal) RTA Hypoaldosteronism (type 4 RTA)

[a]See Table 25.3 for further discussion.
GI, gastrointestinal; UAG, urine anion gap; RTA, renal tubular acidosis.

Of note, the normal range for the anion gap reflects the presence of physiologic unmeasured anions, such as albumin, in nonpathologic states. However, conditions that alter the concentrations of these unmeasured anions also alter the anion gap. For example, a 1 g/dL decrease in the serum albumin would be expected to decrease the anion gap by 2.5 to 3 mEq/L. It is important to adjust the anion gap for these changes in order to properly detect an anion gap acidosis that may be present despite a calculated anion gap that appears within the normal range of 8 to 12 mEq/L. The serum osmolal gap may also be of value when a toxic ingestion (ethanol, methanol, and ethylene glycol) is a suspected cause of an anion gap acidosis (Table 25.3). An increased osmolal gap is an otherwise nonspecific finding and may be seen in other forms of anion gap acidosis. The normal osmolal gap is approximately 10 mOsm/kg.

TABLE 25.3 Causes and Treatment of Anion Gap Metabolic Acidosis

Condition	Cause and Symptoms	Treatment	Comments
Lactic acidosis Pyruvate ↓ Lactate	*Increased lactate production* 1. Increased pyruvate production: enzymatic defects in glycogenolysis or gluconeogenesis 2. Decreased pyruvate utilization: enzymatic defects in pyruvate dehydrogenase or carboxylase 3. Increased conversion of pyruvate to lactate: Increased metabolic rate Grand mal seizure Severe exercise Hypothermic shivering Shock/cardiac arrest/acute pulmonary edema Severe hypoxemia CO poisoning Cyanide intoxication *Decreased lactate utilization* Hypoperfusion Alcoholism Liver disease	Correction of the underlying disorder and reversal of circulatory failure is the primary therapy Sodium bicarbonate is controversial; consider if pH <7.1 or loss of buffering capacity (bicarbonate <5 mEq/L). Hemodialysis may be indicated in resistant cases *Alternative therapies* (have not been demonstrated safe and effective in randomized controlled human studies) Tham (tromethamine)—inert amino alcohol that buffers acids without generating CO_2. Renally excreted and may produce hyperkalemia, hypoglycemia, and respiratory depression in anuric/oliguric patients Carbicarb—equimolar mixture of sodium carbonate and sodium bicarbonate. Diminished risk of hypercapnia and intracellular acidosis compared with sodium bicarbonate Dichloroacetate—activates pyruvate dehydrogenase, and increases oxidation of pyruvate thus decreasing its conversion to lactate	*Caution with bicarbonate therapy* Volume overload Postrecovery metabolic alkalosis Hypernatremia Increased CO_2 production and possible retention in setting of circulatory failure with worsening of mixed venous pCO_2 Intracellular acidosis Reduction in ionized calcium and worsening of cardiac contractility.

(continued)

TABLE 25.3 Causes and Treatment of Anion Gap Metabolic Acidosis (Continued)

Condition	Cause and Symptoms	Treatment	Comments
Propylene glycol toxicity	Converts to pyruvate and lactate Vehicle for lorazepam, etomidate, phenytoin and nitroglycerin, and other agents, and continuous infusion may result in lactate accumulation and increased osmolar gap	Discontinue infusion	
Ketoacidosis	In the setting of insulin deficiency Symptoms include vomiting, abdominal pain, severe volume depletion/dehydration	Insulin and fluids—acidosis will improve with insulin-induced metabolism of ketoacids and regeneration of serum HCO_3^-	
Salicylate toxicity	Toxicity when plasma level >40–50 mg/dL (therapeutic, 20–35 mg/dL). Mixed metabolic acidosis and respiratory alkalosis Increased ketoacid and lactate production Diagnosis—plasma salicylate level	Reduce salicylate levels to avoid neurotoxicity Alkalinization of plasma to a pH >7.45–7.5 converts salicylate to ionized form which lowers CNS levels Alkalinization of urine decreases renal tubular reabsorption of ionized salicylate Consider hemodialysis for plasma concentration >80 mg/dL	If respiratory alkalosis is the primary disturbance, then further alkalinization is not necessary
Methanol ↔ Formaldehyde ↔ Formic acid	Minimal lethal dose is 50–100 mL Symptoms include weakness, headache, blurred vision, and blindness Diagnosis—plasma methanol assay	The treatment for both methanol and ethylene glycol is identical Prompt treatment is necessary and includes: Oral charcoal Sodium bicarbonate	Simultaneous use of both ethanol and fomepizole is not recommended as fomepizole increases the half-life of ethanol

Ethylene glycol ↓ Glycolic and oxalic acid	Component of antifreeze and solvents Symptoms include neurologic and cardiopulmonary abnormalities, flank pain, and renal failure. Envelope- and needle-shaped oxalate crystals may be visible in the urine Diagnosis—plasma ethylene glycol assay	Administration of ethanol or fomepizole competes with or inactivates metabolism, respectively, of parent compound and prevents formation of toxic metabolites Administration of folic acid, thiamine, and pyridoxine. Hemodialysis for removal of toxic metabolites and parent compound
L-5 oxoproline toxicity	High anion gap acidosis in children secondary to congenital glutathione synthetase deficiency. Acquired oxoprolinuria associated with acetaminophen and other medications Renal dysfunction and sepsis predispose Diagnosis—negative toxicity screening and high plasma and urine levels of 5-oxoproline/urine organic acid screen	Treatment primarily includes cessation of the offending agent N-acetylcysteine may be beneficial; restoration of glutathione stores reduces L-5 oxoproline levels
D-Lactic acidosis (from bacterial overgrowth in the colon)	Associated with short gut syndrome and overproduction of D-lactate Symptoms: episodic anion gap acidosis (usually occurring after high-carbohydrate meals) and neurologic abnormalities including cerebellar ataxia, confusion, and slurred speech Diagnosis—enzymatic assay for D-lactate	Treatment includes sodium bicarbonate administration and antimicrobial agents

Osmolal gap = Measured serum osmolality − calculated serum osmolality

Calculated serum osmolality = 2[Na$^+$] + [BUN]/2.8 + [glucose]/18

Nonanion Gap Acidosis

Nonanion gap acidosis occurs in the setting of bicarbonate loss, but without the presence of an additional, pathologic anion. In a nonanion gap acidosis [Cl$^-$] increased to maintain electroneutrality and the calculated anion gap remains normal. The differential of nonanion gap acidosis includes gastrointestinal losses versus a renal etiology (Table 25.2).

The urine anion gap (UAG) is used to discern the source of bicarbonate loss in a nonanion gap acidosis when the cause is not clinically evident.

UAG = (Urine [Na$^+$] + Urine [K$^+$]) − (Urine [Cl$^-$])

The UAG is normally zero or slightly positive. In the setting of a nonanion gap acidosis, the appropriate renal response would be to increase ammonium excretion as NH$_4$Cl, which causes the UAG to become negative, usually ranging from −20 to −50 mEq/L. This is seen in nonrenal causes of nonanion gap acidosis, such as severe diarrhea. In conditions with impaired renal acid excretion, such as chronic kidney disease (CKD) and distal renal tubular acidosis (RTA), the UAG will remain positive or become only slightly negative. The UAG has no utility in the setting of hypovolemia, oliguria, low urine [Na$^+$], or in anion gap acidosis.

Renal Tubular Acidosis

These disorders are characterized by a hyperchloremic metabolic acidosis resulting from diminished capacity of the kidney to accommodate the acid load. A diagnosis of RTA cannot be made in the setting of acute renal failure or with moderate-to-severe CKD. Although RTA is generally a chronic condition and rarely causes acute critical illness, the identification of an RTA in the critical care setting is important as it may point clinicians toward underlying conditions which are associated with the various forms of RTA. Distal (type 1) RTA is associated with drugs such as amphotericin and autoimmune conditions such as lupus and Sjögren's syndrome. Proximal (type 2) RTA is associated with multiple myeloma and may manifest with profound wasting of solutes that are typically reabsorbed in the proximal tubule, such as glucose and phosphorus. Type 4 RTA, which is due to hyporeninemic hypoaldosteronism, is a commonly seen manifestation of diabetes and is closely linked to hyperkalemia. A detailed discussion of this topic is beyond the intent of this manual (Table 25.4).

Treatment

In patients with metabolic acidosis, the first goal of therapy is to identify and correct the underlying cause. The various causes and mechanisms of metabolic acidosis are listed in Table 25.2. Reversal of these underlying processes is of great importance and can often be sufficient to improve the acidemia. A common example of this can be illustrated in patients with diabetic ketoacidosis, who have prompt improvement with the administration of insulin and fluids.

However, not all causes can be rapidly reversed, and patients who are exposed to severe and/or prolonged acidemia are at risk for a variety of complications, including prolonged compensatory hyperventilation, deranged enzymatic activity, depressed cardiac contractility, reduced responsiveness to vasopressors, and arteriolar

	Distal (Type 1) RTA	Proximal (Type 2) RTA	Hyporeninemic Hypoaldosteronism (Type 4) RTA
Causes	Idiopathic, familial, Sjögren's syndrome, hypercalciuria, rheumatoid arthritis, sickle cell anemia, SLE, amphotericin	Idiopathic, multiple myeloma, carbonic anhydrase inhibitors, heavy metals (lead, mercury), amyloidosis, hypocalcemia, and vitamin D deficiency	Diabetes, ACE inhibitors, tubulointerstitial nephritis, NSAIDs, heparin, adrenal insufficiency, obstructive uropathy, K$^+$-sparing diuretics
Defect	Impaired distal tubular H$^+$ excretion (distal acidification)	Impaired proximal tubular bicarbonate absorption ± associated glycosuria, aminoaciduria, and phosphaturia	Aldosterone deficiency or resistance
Plasma HCO$_3^-$	Variable; usually more severe acidosis with level <10 mEq/L	Less severe acidosis than distal RTA; usually 12–20 mEq/L	Usually >15 mEq/L
Urine pH during acidemia[a]	>5.3	Variable; >5.3 if serum HCO$_3^-$ is above the reabsorptive threshold. The excessive bicarbonate "spills out" into the urine causing a high urine pH. <5.3 if serum HCO$_3^-$ is below threshold	Usually <5.3
Plasma K$^+$	Usually low; usually corrects with alkali therapy	Low; usually worsened by bicarbonaturia seen with alkali therapy	High
UAG	Positive	Variable; not helpful	Positive
Associated conditions	Renal stones/nephrocalcinosis	Rickets/osteomalacia/Fanconi's syndrome	None
Treatment	Alkali therapy: sodium citrate/potassium citrate/sodium bicarbonate	Alkali therapy: higher doses are needed because of bicarbonaturia. Thiazide diuretics may be tried in resistant cases	Treat the cause of hypoaldosteronism/low potassium diet/loop diuretics

[a]In metabolic acidosis with intact renal acid excretion, urine pH should be <5 to 5.3.

SLE, systemic lupus erythematosus; ACE, angiotensin-converting enzyme; NSAIDs, nonsteroidal anti-inflammatory drugs; UAG, urine anion gap.

Modified from Rose B, Post T. *Clinical Physiology of Acid-base and Electrolyte Disorders.* 5th ed. New York: McGraw-Hill; 2001.

vasodilation. Because these sequelae may result in severe respiratory, metabolic, an cardiovascular consequences, attenuation of the acidemia should be considered whe underlying causes cannot be immediately reversed.

The role of alkali therapy in attenuating acute metabolic acidosis depends o various factors including underlying etiology, chronicity, severity, and reversibilit Sodium bicarbonate therapy is controversial since bicarbonate therapy itself can resul in volume expansion, increased pCO_2 generation, hypernatremia, and hypocalce mia which all may contribute toward worsening cardiovascular depression. Howeve administration of bicarbonate is usually favored in life-threatening acidemia with pH less than 7.1. The total amount of bicarbonate required to correct a metaboli acidosis can be roughly approximated by calculating a patient's bicarbonate deficit.

$$\text{Bicarbonate deficit (mEq)} = \text{Apparent volume of distribution} \times \text{target change in } [HCO_3^-]$$

$$\text{Apparent volume of distribution} = \text{Total body weight (kg)} \times [0.4 + (2.4/[HCO_3^-])]$$

For example, to increase the serum bicarbonate to 12 mEq/L in a 60-kg patien with a serum bicarbonate level of 5 mEq/L:

$$\text{Apparent volume of distribution} = 60 \text{ kg} \times [0.4 + 2.4/5] = 53 \text{ L}$$

$$\text{Target change in } [HCO_3^-] = 12 \text{ mEq/L} - 5 \text{ mEq/L} = 7 \text{ mEq/L}$$
$$53 \text{ L} \times 7 \text{ mEq/L} = 371 \text{ mEq}$$

This amount of bicarbonate can be administered over a minimum of 4 to 8 hour with frequent monitoring of both $[HCO_3^-]$ and pH.

There are other agents which buffer H+ protons without increasing CO_2, includ ing tris-hydroxymethyl aminomethane (THAM) and dichloroacetate (via increasec oxidation of pyruvate). While THAM has been available for a number of years, there is little outcome data on mortality benefit, particularly in patients with lactic acidosis and its efficacy may be limited in patients with impaired renal function.

Continuous or intermittent hemodialysis may also be used to correct severe refractory acidosis particularly in patients with concomitant renal injury or in patients who cannot accommodate the volume associated with administration of intravenous bicarbonate-containing fluids. Most dialysate solutions have a bicarbonate concentration of 35 to 38 mEq/L.

Patients with chronic metabolic acidosis, often resulting from CKD or renal tubular dysfunction, are managed very differently from those with acute metabolic acidosis. While the degree of acidemia is generally less severe in patients with chronic acidosis, the persistently acidemic milieu is associated with bone demineralization, protein catabolism, and progression of CKD in untreated patients. Administration of oral alkali therapy, typically oral sodium bicarbonate, is usually sufficient to prevent these long-term complications. In small studies, correction of chronic metabolic acidosis has resulted in preservation of glomerular filtration rate (GFR), reduction in proteinuria, and a modest mortality benefit.

METABOLIC ALKALOSIS

Most cases of metabolic alkalosis encountered in the intensive care unit are induced by diuretics or the loss of gastric secretions due to vomiting or nasogastric suctioning. Other causes include bicarbonate administration, the posthypercapnic state,

ABLE 25.5	Chloride-Responsive and Chloride-Resistant Metabolic Alkalosis
Chloride Responsive (Urinary $Cl^- \leq 25$ **mEq/L)**	**Chloride Resistant (Urinary** $Cl^- > 25$ **mEq/L)**
Loss of gastric H^+—vomiting or gastric suction	Mineralocorticoid excess: primary hyperaldosteronism, Cushing's or Liddle's syndrome, exogenous steroid use, licorice ingestion
Prior loop/thiazide diuretic use	Active loop/thiazide diuretic use
Chloride-losing diarrhea: villous adenoma/some cases of factitious diarrhea due to laxative abuse	Bartter's or Gitelman's syndrome
Cystic fibrosis (high sweat Cl^-)	Alkali load: exogenous bicarbonate infusion, citrate-containing blood products, antacids (milk–alkali syndrome)
Posthypercapnia	Severe hypokalemia
Treatment includes administration of 0.9% or 0.45% NaCl and repletion of potassium stores.	**Treatment is disease specific and includes repletion of potassium stores.**

and citrate associated with centrifugal plasma exchange, massive transfusion, or fresh frozen plasma administration. The condition is often aggravated by renal insufficiency, which delays bicarbonate excretion. Because alkalemia promotes the release of protons bound to albumin, the negative charge of albumin can increase in metabolic alkalosis, resulting in a slight anion gap. Metabolic alkalosis can also be combined with other disorders, including gap and nongap acidosis, in mixed disorders. Metabolic alkalosis can be broadly categorized into a chloride-responsive or chloride-resistant process (Table 25.5).

Common Causes of Metabolic Alkalosis

Gastric Secretion Loss

Loss of gastric secretions occurs from removal of gastric contents by tube drainage or from vomiting. Normally, hydrogen ions released into the stomach reach the duodenum, where they stimulate pancreatic bicarbonate secretion into the gastrointestinal tract, maintaining acid–base balance. When gastric contents are lost, bicarbonate is not secreted, resulting in increased plasma bicarbonate and metabolic alkalosis. Self-induced vomiting is often denied by patients with eating or factitious disorders, and a low urine chloride supports the diagnosis.

Contraction Alkalosis

Contraction alkalosis occurs in the setting of excessive loss of chloride-rich, bicarbonate-free fluid. This is most commonly seen with the use of loop or thiazide diuretics, but can also occur with gastric losses or with cystic fibrosis (high sweat [Cl^-]). As a result of "contraction" of the extracellular volume, there is a relative increase in the bicarbonate concentration. Despite the relative intravascular volume depletion, there is an obligate urinary loss of sodium with bicarbonate in this setting. Therefore, urine chloride concentration is usually a better predictor of the volume status in this form of metabolic alkalosis than urine sodium.

Posthypercapnic Alkalosis

Chronic respiratory acidosis is associated with an appropriate compensatory incre
in the serum bicarbonate concentration. Sudden normalization of a chronic
elevated pCO_2 via mechanical ventilation can result in an acute, potentially let
increase in the pH. Therefore, the pCO_2 should not be decreased rapidly in
setting of a well-compensated chronic respiratory acidosis.

Refeeding Syndrome

Patients fed a high-carbohydrate diet after a prolonged fast can acutely develop me
bolic alkalosis. Intracellular hydrogen ion shift is the proposed mechanism. Refeed
may also be independently associated with hypophosphatemia.

Severe Hypokalemia

Severe hypokalemia via multiple renal mechanisms causes hydrogen ion secretion a
bicarbonate reabsorption. The ensuing metabolic alkalosis is refractory to treatme
until potassium stores are replaced.

Milk–Alkali Syndrome

Milk–alkali syndrome results from a chronic high calcium intake (usually in the fo
of calcium-containing antacids) and is usually associated with renal insufficiency.

Treatment

Intravenous sodium chloride fluid administration will reverse chloride-respons
metabolic alkalosis (Table 25.5). Response to treatment can be monitored via uri
pH and urine chloride concentration. Concomitant hypokalemia may also play
critical role in the maintenance of metabolic alkalosis, as it increases tubular secreti
of H^+ and reabsorption of bicarbonate. Patients with hypokalemia and alkalosis m
have a profound total body potassium deficit, and treatment of this will be necessa
in the correction of metabolic alkalosis. If the patient is able to take medication
mouth, oral supplementation is preferred with potassium chloride 40 mEq every
to 6 hours. Alternatively, if the patient is unable to take medication enterally, int
venous infusion of potassium chloride at a rate of 10 mEq/hr with close monitori
of serum potassium may be initiated.

Acetazolamide can be considered in cases of worsening metabolic alkalosis ass
ciated with volume overload complicated by the need for continued attempts
diuresis (nonchloride responsive). Acetazolamide inhibits carbonic anhydrase, t
enzyme that catalyzes the conversion of CO_2 and water into carbonic acid, causi
renal excretion of hydrogen ions and retention of bicarbonate. Decreased bicarbona
excretion from carbonic anhydrase inhibition causes a metabolic acidosis to count
the alkalosis. Acetazolamide has minimal diuretic effects as a single agent, but c
have additive effects when combined with loop and/or thiazide diuretics if the seru
bicarbonate concentration is elevated.

In cases of severe, refractory alkalosis (usually associated with bicarbonate admi
istration in the setting of renal failure), hydrochloric acid infusion through a centi
line is rarely needed, but can be used. Other alternatives include the use of intermitte
hemodialysis with the bicarbonate bath decreased to the lowest allowable value (lir
ited bicarbonate gradient available with most systems) or a continuous hemofiltratic
modality using primarily a nonbicarbonate, noncitrate replacement fluid.

MIXED ACID–BASE DISORDERS

The delta anion gap is useful in determining the presence of other metabolic disturbances superimposed on a known anion gap acidosis. It is calculated as follows:

$$\text{Delta Anion Gap } (\Delta/\Delta): \frac{\Delta * \text{AG (from normal, which is approximately 10)}}{\Delta * \text{HCO}_3 \text{ (from normal, which is approximately 25 mEq/L)}}$$

$$\Delta * \text{AG} = \text{Patient calculated AG} - \text{Normal AG}$$

$$\Delta * \text{HCO}_3 = \text{Serum HCO}_3 - \text{Normal HCO}_3$$

The delta gap is based on the principle that the change in AG should roughly approximate the change in serum bicarbonate in a simple anion gap acidosis. A ratio of <1 occurs if the change in serum bicarbonate is larger than the change in the anion gap, and indicates that a nonanion gap acidosis may be present, causing the disproportionate fall in serum bicarbonate. A ratio >1 suggests a combined anion gap acidosis and metabolic alkalosis (which both raises the anion gap and attenuates the expected drop in serum bicarbonate from the anion gap acidosis).

Elucidation of double or triple acid–base disturbances requires assessment of multiple metabolic parameters. Because complex acid–base disorders may at first manifest with several normal appearing lab values, a methodical evaluation of all data (including the calculation of anion gap and delta gap) should be done routinely. The following patterns are often suggestive of a combined acid–base disturbance despite a "normal" pH:

Normal pH + $\downarrow$ PCO$_2$ + $\downarrow$ HCO$_3$: respiratory alkalosis plus metabolic acidosis

Normal pH + $\uparrow$ PCO$_2$ + $\uparrow$ HCO$_3$: respiratory acidosis plus metabolic alkalosis

Normal pH + normal PCO$_2$ + normal HCO$_3$ + $\uparrow$ AG: metabolic acidosis and alkalosis

SUGGESTED READINGS

Arroliga AC, Shehab N, McCarthy K, et al. Relationship of continuous infusion lorazepam to serum propylene glycol concentration in critically ill adults. *Crit Care Med*. 2004;32(8): 1709–1714.
   Prospective observational study evaluating the dose relationship between lorazepam infusion and propylene glycol accumulation.

Gauthier PM, Szerlip HM. Metabolic acidosis in the intensive care unit. *Crit Care Clin*. 2002;18(2):289–308.
   An extensive review of diagnostic and therapeutic approach to metabolic acidosis with focus on critical care issues.

Gehlbach BK, Schmidt GA. Bench-to-bedside review: treating acid-base abnormalities in the intensive care unit—the role of buffers. *Crit Care*. 2004;8(4):259–265.
   This review article extensively discusses the role of bicarbonate therapy as well as alternative therapies in lactic acidosis.

Judge BS. Differentiating the causes of metabolic acidosis in the poisoned patient. *Clin Lab Med*. 2006;26(1):31–48.
   Describes toxicities due to methanol, ethylene glycol, and other ingestions, their effects on acid-base balance, diagnosis, and treatment.

Kimmoun A, Novy E, Auchet T, et al. Hemodynamic consequences of severe lactic acidosis in shock states: from bench to bedside. *Crit Care*. 2015;19:175.

Rose B, Post T. *Clinical Physiology of Acid Base and Electrolyte Disorders.* 5th ed. New York McGraw Hill; 2001.

An extremely comprehensive text book describing pathophysiologic mechanisms, diagnoses and treatment of metabolic acid–base disorders.

Tailor P, Raman T, Garganta CL, et al. Recurrent high anion gap metabolic acidosis secondary to 5-oxoproline (pyroglutamic acid). *Am J Kidney Dis.* 2005;46(1):e4–e10.

Case report and discussion of a common but underdiagnosed cause of high anion gap acidosis- oxoproline toxicity.

26 Respiratory Acid–Base Disorders

A. Cole Burks

INTRODUCTION

Respiratory acid–base disorders are commonly seen in the critical care setting, and can occur independently or coexist with metabolic acid–base disorders (metabolic disorders are discussed separately in Chapter 25). Evaluation of respiratory acid–base disorders can be relatively straightforward in patients with an isolated acute primary respiratory acidosis or alkalosis, or more complicated when superimposed metabolic acid–base disorders are present. Further complicating evaluation is the change that occurs in the serum bicarbonate in acute and chronic respiratory acidosis and alkalosis.

Respiratory acid–base disorders are defined by altered plasma carbon dioxide levels as measured on arterial blood gas (ABG) analysis by the partial pressure of carbon dioxide ($PaCO_2$). Respiratory acidosis is characterized by an elevated $PaCO_2$ and decreased pH; and respiratory alkalosis by a decreased $PaCO_2$ and elevated pH. The $PaCO_2$ in healthy adults is 35 to 45 mm Hg and the normal pH is 7.35 to 7.45. For calculation purposes, it is reasonable to use 40 mm Hg as the baseline normal $PaCO_2$ level and 7.4 as the baseline normal pH. In respiratory acid–base disorders, the kidneys compensate for changes in the $PaCO_2$ by adjusting excretion of bicarbonate (HCO_3^-) accordingly. In healthy adults, the serum HCO_3^- is generally 22 to 26 mEq/L. Thus, it is reasonable to use a level of 24 mEq/L for calculation purposes. Acute respiratory acid–base disorders result in small changes in the bicarbonate concentration, and cellular buffering predominates. Renal compensation occurs slowly, taking at least 24 to 72 hours to fully develop, and results in larger changes in serum HCO_3^-. Compensatory changes in serum HCO_3^- result in the pH shifting back toward, (but never reaching), normal. Mixed acid–base disorders do not include the renal bicarbonate compensation that occurs for acute and chronic respiratory acid–base disorders and are present any time the pH is normal with an abnormal $PaCO_2$. Algorithm 26.1 below can aid in analyzing a respiratory acid–base disorder.

Discussion

Carbon dioxide is excreted in the lung by simple diffusion and depends on the constant tidaling of alveolar air. Normal pH is maintained through the equilibrium between cellular CO_2 production and minute ventilation (respiratory rate × tidal volume). Chemoreceptors in the brain sense changes in cellular metabolism by increases in $PaCO_2$, and regulate respiratory drive by increases or decreases in tidal volume and respiratory rate. Disturbances in this equilibrium are the basis of the pathophysiology of respiratory acid–base disorders.

ALGORITHM 26.1 Approach to Respiratory Acid–Base Disorders

Step 1—Review ABG and basic metabolic panel and check for internal validity. Obtain an ABG and ensure the serum bicarbonate [HCO_3^-] is accurate using the Henderson–Hasselbach equation (Table 26.1).

$$[H^+] = 24\ [HCO_3^-]/PaCO_2$$

The [HCO_3^-] reported on the ABG and basic metabolic panel should also agree within 2 mmol/L.

Step 2—Determine the primary acid–base disturbance (metabolic acid–base disorders are discussed in Chapter 25). A primary respiratory acid–base disorder is present if the $PaCO_2$ is altered and the change in pH is in the opposite direction.

- Respiratory acidosis = $PaCO_2$ >45 mm Hg and pH <7.35
- Respiratory alkalosis = $PaCO_2$ <35 mm Hg and pH >7.45

Step 3—Determine if the respiratory acid–base disorder is uncompensated (acute) or compensated (chronic). *The pH will approach, but never reach normal* (see Table 26.2).

- A serum HCO_3^- or pH that deviates significantly from expected suggests a superimposed metabolic acid–base disorder.

Step 4—Determine if a mixed respiratory and metabolic acid–base disorder is present—if the change in pH is *more* than expected for the given $PaCO_2$ (see Table 26.2).

- A combined metabolic *and* respiratory acidosis is present if the *decrease* in pH is greater than expected based on the $PaCO_2$.

$$\Delta pH = \left(\frac{\Delta PaCO_2}{10}\right) \times 0.08$$

o Example—pH 7.1 with a $PaCO_2$ of 60 mm Hg. $\Delta pH = \left(\dfrac{20}{10}\right) \times 0.08 = 0.16$.

   7.4 – 0.16 = expected pH of 7.24. Thus a superimposed metabolic acidosis exists.

- A combined metabolic *and* respiratory alkalosis is present if the *increase* in pH is greater than expected.

o Example—pH 7.55 with a $PaCO_2$ of 30 mm Hg. $\Delta pH = \left(\dfrac{10}{10}\right) \times 0.08 = 0.08$.

   7.4 + 0.08 = expected pH of 7.48. Thus a superimposed metabolic alkalosis exists.

- A normal pH in the setting of an abnormal $PaCO_2$ indicates a mixed acid–base disorder.

o Example—pH 7.38 with a $PaCO_2$ of 60 mm Hg indicates a respiratory acidosis with a metabolic alkalosis.
o Example—pH 7.42 with a $PaCO_2$ of 30 mm Hg indicates a respiratory alkalosis with a metabolic acidosis.

Step 5—Correlate the above findings with clinical history and physical exam to arrive at the correct diagnosis (see Fig. 26.1 for select etiologies of respiratory acidosis and Table 26.3 for select causes of respiratory alkalosis).

Step 6—Treat appropriately (see discussion below).

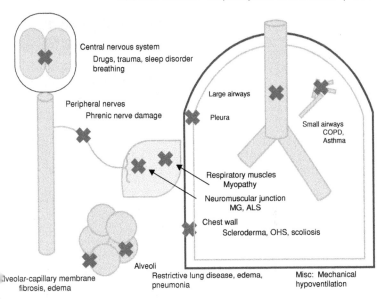

igure 26.1. Selected sites and causes of disease that can lead to hypoventilation. MG, myasthenia gravis; ALS, myotrophic lateral sclerosis; COPD, chronic obstructive lung disease; OHS, obesity hypoventilation syndrome.

Quite simply, the pathophysiology of respiratory acidosis is alveolar hypoventilation resulting in hypercapnia. The approach to and differential diagnosis of hypercapnia s outlined in chapter 7, Algorithm 7.1. Any component of the ventilatory mechanism may be involved, including both the central or peripheral nervous systems, neuromuscular junction, respiratory muscles, chest wall, pleura, large airways, small airways, or lung parenchyma (see Fig. 26.1).

Correcting alveolar hypoventilation is the main stay of treatment and requires treating the underlying cause of hypoventilation. This may include bronchodilators (for patients with asthma and chronic obstructive pulmonary disease), reversal of medication/drug effects, treatment of pulmonary edema, treatment of neuromuscular diseases, and mechanical ventilation (either via noninvasive positive pressure, or via endotracheal intubation). Special caution is required when mechanically ventilating patients with

TABLE 26.1	H⁺ Concentration and Corresponding pH
pH	[H⁺ mEq/L]
7.00	100
7.10	79
7.20	63
7.30	50
7.40	40
7.50	32
7.60	25

TABLE 26.2	Expected [HCO₃⁻] Change in Acute and Chronic Respiratory Acid–Base Disorders (Assume a Baseline [HCO₃⁻] of 24 mEq/L)
Acute respiratory acidosis	Increase in $[HCO_3^-] = \Delta PaCO_2/10$ +/− 3 Decrease in pH = $0.08*[\Delta PaCO_2/10]$
Chronic respiratory acidosis (3–5 days)	Increase in $[HCO_3^-] = 3*[\Delta PaCO_2/10]^a$ Decrease in pH = $0.03*[\Delta PaCO_2/10]$ to $0.08*[\Delta PaCO_2/10]$
Acute respiratory alkalosis	Decrease in $[HCO_3^-] = 2*[\Delta PaCO_2/10]$ Increase in pH = $0.08*[\Delta PaCO_2/10]$
Chronic respiratory alkalosis	Decrease in $[HCO_3^-] = 5*[\Delta PaCO_2/10]$ to $7*[\Delta PaCO_2/10]$ Increase in pH = $0.03*[\Delta PaCO_2/10]$ to $0.08*[\Delta PaCO_2/10]$

[a]Some authors use 3.5 mEq/L for chronic respiratory acidosis.

compensated, chronic respiratory acidosis—with an elevated serum HCO_3^-, as rapid correction can cause life-threatening metabolic alkalosis. Sodium bicarbonate is not recommended in respiratory acidosis as it may worsen hypercapnia and pulmonary edema, or cause a metabolic alkalosis. Small doses of sodium bicarbonate can be considered in cases of intractable hypercapnia with severe acidosis (pH <7.1).

Causes of respiratory alkalosis are listed in Table 26.3. The underlying pathophysiologic mechanism for each is alveolar hyperventilation. Respiratory alkalosis

TABLE 26.3	Select Causes of Respiratory Alkalosis	
Normal P(A-a) O₂ Gradient		Drugs
Mechanical hyperventilation		Salicylates
		Progesterone
		Catecholamines
Central nervous system		Tissue hypoxia
Psychogenic hyperventilation		High altitude
Fever		Severe anemia
Pain		
Encephalitis/meningitis		
Tumors		
Pregnancy		Endotoxinemia
Hyperthyroidism		Cirrhosis
Elevated P(A-a) O₂ Gradient[a]		
V/Q mismatch and stimulation of chest receptors		Pulmonary embolism
Right to left shunt		Pneumonia
Pneumothorax		Edema
Congestive heart failure		

[a]The differential diagnosis of respiratory alkalosis with an elevated alveolar–arterial oxygen gradient (P[A-a]O₂) is the same as hypoxia with an elevated P(A-a)O₂ listed in Chapter 7, Algorithm 7.2.
P[A-a]O₂, alveolar–arterial oxygen gradient; V/Q, ventilation/perfusion.

be associated with either normal or increased alveolar–arterial oxygen gradient [A-a]O$_2$ gradient, abbreviated A-a gradient, and is discussed in more detail in apter 7). In patients with an elevated A-a gradient, the differential diagnosis is the ne as for patients with hypoxia with an elevated A-a gradient (see Algorithm 7.2). patients with a normal A-a gradient, causes include hyperventilation due to central rvous system disorders, fever, severe anemia, hypoxia from altitude, endocrine disders, drugs, and iatrogenic hyperventilation in patients on mechanical ventilatory pport.

Similar to respiratory acidosis, the treatment of respiratory alkalosis is directed the underlying etiology. Causes of hypoxia should be identified and treated. In echanically ventilated patients, minute ventilation should be decreased by decreasg the respiratory rate and/or tidal volume. For psychogenic hyperventilation, reasrance and anxiolytics can be used.

Acetazolamide can be used to induce a metabolic acidosis to compensate for the spiratory alkalosis caused by high altitudes.

UGGESTED READINGS

stein SK, Singh N. Respiratory acidosis. *Respir Care.* 2001;46(4):366–383.
   Review of the pathophysiology, evaluation, and causes of respiratory acidosis.
ster GT, Vaziri ND, Sassoon CS. Respiratory alkalosis. *Respir Care.* 2001;46(4):384–391.
   Review of the pathophysiology, evaluation, and causes of respiratory alkalosis.
ufman D, Kitching AJ, Kellum JA. Acid–base balance. In: Hall JB, Schmidt GA, Wood LD,
   eds. *Principles of Critical Care.* 3rd ed. New York: McGraw Hill; 2002:1202–1208.
   Comprehensive textbook review of acid–base disorders.

Thyroid Disorders

William E. Clutter

HYPERTHYROIDISM

Major clinical findings in hyperthyroidism are listed in Table 27.1. Cardiac findings may be prominent including tachycardia, atrial fibrillation, heart failure, and exacerbation of coronary artery disease. Rarely, severe hyperthyroidism may be associated with fever and delirium, sometimes called "thyroid storm."

Major causes of hyperthyroidism are listed in Table 27.2. Graves' disease (which may also cause proptosis) is the most common.

When hyperthyroidism is suspected in a critically ill patient, plasma thyroid stimulating hormone (TSH) and free thyroxine (T_4) should be measured. Clinical hyperthyroidism suppresses TSH to <0.1 µU/mL, so a normal plasma TSH excludes the diagnosis of hyperthyroidism. Plasma TSH may also be suppressed to below normal by severe nonthyroidal illness (about 10% of patients in intensive care units have plasma TSH <0.1 µU/mL) and by therapy with dopamine or high-dose glucocorticoid. Thus, a suppressed plasma TSH alone does not establish the diagnosis.

If plasma TSH is suppressed and plasma-free T_4 is elevated, the diagnosis of hyperthyroidism is established. If plasma-free T_4 is not elevated, one of the other causes of suppressed plasma TSH listed earlier is more likely.

Treatment

The etiology of hyperthyroidism determines the best long-term therapy, but differential diagnosis can be deferred in the critically ill patient. Emergency therapy

TABLE 27.1	Major Clinical Findings in Hyperthyroidism
Common	Seen Primarily in Severe Hyperthyroidism
• Heat intolerance • Weight loss • Palpitations • Sinus tachycardia • Atrial fibrillation • Brisk tendon reflexes • Fine tremor • Lid lag • Proximal muscle weakness	• Heart failure • Exacerbation of coronary artery disease • Fever and delirium ("thyroid storm")

TABLE 27.2	Major Causes of Hyperthyroidism

Associated with Increased Radioactive Iodine Uptake
- Graves' disease
- Toxic multinodular goiter
- Thyroid adenoma

Associated with Decreased Radioactive Iodine Uptake
- Iodine-induced hyperthyroidism (due to amiodarone or iodine-containing contrast media[a])
- Painless thyroiditis
- Subacute thyroiditis
- Factitious hyperthyroidism (ingestion of thyroid hormone)

Iodine excess can cause both hyper- and hypothyroidism depending on the patients' underlying thyroid function and basal iodine consumption.

Table 27.3) is indicated when hyperthyroidism exacerbates heart failure or an acute coronary syndrome, or when thyroid storm is present. It includes rapid inhibition of thyroid hormone synthesis (and conversion of T_4 to triiodothyronine [T_3]) by the thioamide propylthiouracil (PTU), inhibition of thyroid hormone secretion by iodine, and inhibition of the cardiovascular effects of hyperthyroidism by beta-adrenergic antagonists. Hydrocortisone is usually recommended because it also inhibits T_4 conversion to T_3. Fever and concomitant illness must be vigorously treated.

Some authors have advocated treatment of amiodarone-induced hyperthyroidism with glucocorticoids alone, but the regimen described above has a high success rate in this disorder.

Plasma-free T_4 should be measured every 3 to 7 days. When free T_4 approaches the normal range, the doses of PTU and iodine should be gradually decreased. Iodine can usually be stopped at the time of hospital discharge, and radioactive iodine (RAI) therapy for Graves' disease or toxic multinodular goiter can be scheduled 2 to 3 weeks later. If long-term thioamide therapy is chosen instead of RAI, PTU should be stopped and methimazole used instead.

HYPOTHYROIDISM

Major clinical findings in hypothyroidism are listed in Table 27.4. Severe hypothyroidism may contribute to hypothermia, hypoventilation, bradycardia, hypotension, and hyponatremia in the setting of concomitant critical illnesses.

TABLE 27.3	Emergency Therapy of Hyperthyroidism

Propylthiouracil (PTU) 300 mg PO q6h
Iodine (supersaturated potassium iodide, SSKI) 2 drops PO q12h
(start 1 hr after first dose of PTU)
Beta antagonist, with the dose adjusted to control tachycardia; initially:
    Propranolol 40 mg PO q6h, or
    Esmolol 500 µg/kg IV followed by 50 µg/kg/min IV
Hydrocortisone 100 mg IV q8h

TABLE 27.4	Major Clinical Findings in Hypothyroidism
Common	Seen Primarily in Severe Hypothyroidism
• Cold intolerance • Fatigue • Somnolence • Constipation • Weight gain • Slow tendon reflexes • Nonpitting edema (myxedema) • Dry skin	• Hypothermia • Bradycardia • Hypoventilation • Hypotension • Hyponatremia • Pericardial or pleural effusion

Major causes of hypothyroidism are listed in Table 27.5. More than 90% of case are primary hypothyroidism, most often iatrogenic or due to chronic autoimmune thyroiditis. Any pituitary or hypothalamic disorder can cause secondary hypothyroidism, but these disorders are usually clinically apparent because of other manifestations

When the diagnosis of hypothyroidism is suspected in a critically ill patient plasma TSH and free T_4 should be measured. Even mild primary hypothyroidism causes elevation of plasma TSH, so a normal plasma TSH excludes this diagnosis Plasma TSH values >20 μU/mL establish the diagnosis of primary hypothyroidism Milder elevations of plasma TSH are usually due to primary hypothyroidism, but may also occur transiently during recovery from severe nonthyroidal illness.

If plasma-free T_4 is low and plasma TSH is not elevated, the patient may have secondary hypothyroidism, but in a critically ill patient, this pattern of test result is more likely to be due to functional suppression of TSH and T_4 secretion by the nonthyroidal illness (the "euthyroid sick syndrome"). If the patient has clinical findings that may be due to hypothyroidism, empiric treatment with T_4 should be started and the diagnosis should be reassessed after recovery. Otherwise, the patient can be observed with periodic measurement of plasma TSH and free T_4 to determine whether the abnormalities resolve with recovery.

Treatment

Emergency therapy of hypothyroidism (Table 27.6) is indicated if the patient has clinical signs that could be contributed to by hypothyroidism, such as bradycardia

TABLE 27.5	Major Causes of Primary Hypothyroidism

- Chronic lymphocytic thyroiditis (Hashimoto's disease)
- Iatrogenic (after radioactive iodine therapy or thyroidectomy)
- Drugs
  - Iodine excess (e.g., amiodarone, iodine-containing contrast media[a])
  - Lithium
  - Interferon alpha
  - Interleukin-2; other immunomodulatory drugs

[a]Iodine excess can cause both hyper- and hypothyroidism depending on the patients' underlying thyroid function and basal iodine consumption.

TABLE 27.6	Emergency Therapy of Hypothyroidism

Thyroxine 50–100 µg IV q6–8h for 24 hrs, then
Thyroxine 75–100 µg IV q24h until oral intake is possible
Hydrocortisone 100 mg IV q8h

hypoventilation, hypothermia, or hypotension. Each of these abnormalities should also be treated in the standard fashion, since they are rarely due to hypothyroidism alone. Vital signs and cardiac rhythm should be monitored since the treatment can exacerbate underlying heart disease. Hydrocortisone should be given because adrenal failure may be associated with chronic autoimmune thyroiditis.

No clinical trials have determined the optimum method of emergency treatment of hypothyroidism, but this method rapidly alleviates T_4 deficiency while minimizing the risk of adverse events. There is no evidence to support treatment of the functional suppression of TSH and T_4 by nonthyroidal illness.

SUGGESTED READINGS

Adler SM, Wartofsky L. The nonthyroidal illness syndrome. *Endocrinol Metab Clin North Am.* 2007;36(3):657–672.
    Review of the pathophysiology, diagnosis, and management of the changes in thyroid function in nonthyroidal illness.
Bahn Chair RS, Burch HB, Cooper DS, et al; American Thyroid Association; American Association of Clinical Endocrinologists. Hyperthyroidism and other causes of thyrotoxicosis: management guidelines of the American Thyroid Association and American Association of Clinical Endocrinologists. *Thyroid.* 2011;21(6):593–646.
    Comprehensive guide to management of hyperthyroidism.
Kaptein EM, Beale E, Chan LS. Thyroid hormone therapy for obesity and nonthyroidal illnesses: a systematic review. *J Clin Endocrinol Metab.* 2009;94(10):3663–3675.
    The data do not support treatment of thyroid test abnormalities due to nonthyroidal illness.
Osman F, Franklyn JA, Sheppard MC, et al. Successful treatment of amiodarone-induced thyrotoxicosis. *Circulation.* 2002;105:1275–1277.
    Case series showing a high success rate with thioamide treatment alone.

28 Adrenal Insufficiency in Critical Illness

Marin H. Kollef

An increase in circulating and tissue corticosteroid levels during critical illness is a important adaptive response. Normally, severe illness and stress stimulate the hypothalamic–pituitary–adrenal (HPA) axis, causing release of corticotropin-releasing hormone (CRH) from the hypothalamus. CRH stimulates the anterior pituitary to release adrenocorticotropic hormone (ACTH or corticotropin), with ACTH causing increased cortisol production by the adrenal cortex's zona fasciculata. With acute illness such as severe infection, trauma, and burns, there is an increase in cortisol production by as much as a factor of 6. Normally, circulating cortisol is bound to corticosteroid-binding globulin (CBG) and albumin, with <10% in the free, bioavailable form. During acute illness, however, CBG and albumin levels decrease by as much as 50%, with unbound cortisol levels increasing. Although it is the unbound cortisol that is physiologically active, current laboratory assays only measure total cortisol. In a healthy, unstressed person, the HPA axis undergoes diurnal variation, but this is lost in critical illness. The major physiologic actions of circulating cortisol include increasing blood sugar levels; facilitating the delivery of glucose to cells during stress; facilitating normal cardiovascular reactivity to angiotensin II, epinephrine, and norepinephrine; contributing to the maintenance of cardiac contractility, vascular tone, and blood pressure; and anti-inflammatory and immunosuppressive effects.

Chronic adrenal insufficiency (Addison's disease) is a rare cause of intensive care unit admission and is distinct from the HPA axis dysfunction that occurs during critical illness, which has been termed *critical illness-related corticosteroid insufficiency* (CIRCI). CIRCI is characterized by an inappropriately low increase in cortisol during acute illness, also referred to as *relative adrenal insufficiency*. It is mediated in part by inflammatory cytokine inhibition of (a) CRH and ACTH release, (b) adrenal cortisol synthesis, and (c) glucocorticoid receptor translocation and transcription. In addition to CIRCI, adrenal insufficiency in critical illness may also be separated into two categories: *primary* if it is due to adrenal gland dysfunction, or *secondary* if it caused by central disruption of CRH or ACTH release. Causes of primary adrenal insufficiency in acute illness include direct injury to the adrenal glands from trauma, infarction, infection, malignancy, and hemorrhage; drug-induced suppression of cortisol synthesis; and autoimmune adrenalitis. Secondary causes include discontinuation of exogenous corticosteroids in patients on chronic immunotherapy, central nervous system malignancies, and head trauma. Causes of adrenal insufficiency are listed in Table 28.1.

Signs and symptoms of corticosteroid insufficiency resulting from HPA dysfunction are listed in Table 28.2. In pre-existing hypoadrenalism, these findings may

TABLE 28.1	Causes of Adrenal Insufficiency
Cause	Example
Infection	Sepsis/septic shock HIV Cytomegalovirus *Staphylococcus aureus,* toxin-producing strain Fungal disorders (histoplasmosis, blastomycosis, cryptococcus) Tuberculosis

Medications	Suppressing release of corticotropin-releasing hormone from the hypothalamus and pituitary:
	  Corticosteroids
	  Megestrol acetate
	Inhibition of enzymes involved in cortisol synthesis:
	  Etomidate
	  Ketoconazole
	  Metyrapone
	Increased metabolism of cortisol:
	  Rifampin
	  Phenytoin

Malignancy	Adrenal metastases

Adrenal hemorrhage	Secondary to shock
	  Anticoagulation
	  Meningococcemia (Waterhouse–Friderichsen syndrome)
	  Disseminated intravascular coagulation
	  Antiphospholipid syndrome

Autoimmune	Addison's disease

Hypothalamic and pituitary disorders	Resulting in secondary adrenal insufficiency:
	  Infection
	  Pituitary tumor or metastases
	  Infiltrative disorders (sarcoidosis, histiocytosis)
	  Postpartum pituitary necrosis
	  Trauma (blunt, radiation, surgical)

HIV, human immunodeficiency virus.

be present before the onset of acute illness. However, in critically ill patients, adrenal insufficiency should be suspected in all patients with hypotension that is unresponsive to intravenous (IV) fluid administration and vasopressor support.

Although it is well documented that acute illness increases cortisol through stimulation of the HPA axis, it is less clear what defines an adequate stress response to acute illness. In addition, although CIRCI should be considered in all critically ill patients, most of the studies have focused on patients with sepsis and septic shock. Previous studies have suggested that a random serum cortisol >25 to 34 mcg/dL in critically ill patients makes relative adrenal insufficiency unlikely. However, recent

TABLE 28.2	Signs and Symptoms of Adrenal Insufficiency
Sign	Symptoms
Cardiovascular	Hypotension that is usually not responsive to fluid administration requiring use of vasopressors; hyperdynamic hemodynamic profile is common; tachycardia unless severe hypothyroidism is also present
Metabolic/electrolyte	Hypoglycemia, hyponatremia, hyperkalemia, fever
Hematologic	Eosinophilia and anemia
Neuromuscular	Weakness, fatigue, myalgia, arthralgia, headache, memory impairment, depression
Gastrointestinal	Anorexia, diarrhea, nausea, salt craving, weight loss
Cutaneous	Vitiligo, alopecia

studies have suggested that random cortisol measurements may have limited utility in the diagnosis of adrenal insufficiency, except in patients with a baseline cortisol <10 to 15 mcg/dL, and have highlighted the diagnostic value of a cortisol increase of ≤9 mcg/dL 60 minutes after stimulation with 250 mcg of IV cosyntropin (synthetic ACTH) as making adrenal insufficiency likely in critical illness.

In a prospective inception cohort study performed by Annane et al. in 2000 of 189 patients with septic shock, it was noted that an intermediate or poor prognosis occurred in patients with a cortisol increase in response to cosyntropin of ≤9 mcg/dL, with the highest mortality found in those patients who, in addition to a cosyntropin response of ≤9 mcg/dL, had an initial cortisol >34 mcg/dL. Another study by Annane et al. in 2006 of 101 patients with sepsis, 41 patients without sepsis, and 32 healthy controls, employed the overnight metyrapone stimulation test to investigate the diagnostic value of various markers of adrenal function, and found that adrenal insufficiency was likely if the baseline cortisol level was <10 mcg/dL or change in cortisol after cosyntropin was ≤9 mcg/dL, and unlikely when cosyntropin-stimulated cortisol levels were ≥44 mcg/dL and the change in cortisol after cosyntropin was ≥16.8 mcg/dL. These diagnostic values were explored further in 2007 by Lipiner-Friedman et al. in the retrospective arm of the CORTICUS study group. This retrospective multicenter cohort study included 477 patients with sepsis and septic shock who had undergone an ACTH stimulation test on the first day of sepsis, and found that random cortisol levels ≥15 mcg/dL, regardless of the cutoff, were not independent predictors of shock reversal, hospital mortality, or survival duration. However, patients with a baseline cortisol level <15 mcg/dL or change in cortisol ≤9 mcg/dL after cosyntropin, had a longer duration of shock and a shorter survival time. Corticosteroids were used to treat 44% of patients and were associated with a strong reduction in the risk of dying (OR, 0.21; 98% CI, 0.08 to 0.52). Measuring serum cortisol 30 and 60 minutes after cosyntropin added no significant diagnostic value to checking cortisol at 60 minutes alone.

Randomized studies have been performed to determine if corticosteroid replacement therapy is beneficial in patients with varying diagnostic definitions of adrenal

ufficiency. In a placebo-controlled, randomized, double-blind study by Annane
al. in 2002, 300 patients with septic shock were randomized to receive hydro-
tisone 50 mg every 6 hours and fludrocortisone 50 mcg once daily for 7 days,
placebo, after undergoing a 250-mcg cosyntropin test. Of the 229 patients with
ative adrenal insufficiency (115 placebo and 114 corticosteroid), defined as an
crease after cosyntropin of ≤9 mcg/dL, there was significantly reduced mortality
3 patients vs. 60 patients, $p = 0.02$) and withdrawal of vasopressor therapy within
days (46 patients vs. 65 patients, $p = 0.001$) in the corticosteroid-treated patients,
thout increasing adverse events. In the 70 patients who had a cosyntropin response
mcg/dL, corticosteroid replacement therapy had no significant effect on the same
tcomes and no trend toward efficacy.

However, the CORTICUS study found no benefit to treating patients with
tic shock, including the subgroup with a cosyntropin response ≤9 mcg/dL. This
dy differed from the initial randomized study by Annane in 2002 in that patients
the CORTICUS study were randomized up to 72 hours after the onset of septic
ock rather than within 8 hours, patients in the CORTICUS study included those
th sepsis and septic shock rather than septic shock alone (i.e., could be included
the study without hypotension requiring vasopressors), received 11 days of cor-
osteroid replacement rather than 7 days, and were not given fludrocortisone.
lditionally, the CORTICUS study lacked clinical equipoise resulting in a selection
as whereby patients least likely to benefit from corticosteroids were enrolled in
e study.

Glucocorticoids, however, may not be appropriate for all critically ill patients
highlighted in a case-control study by Britt et al. in 2006 in 100 patients (six
th septic shock) in a burn trauma ICU who received steroids, compared with
0 matched control patients, showing that corticosteroid use was associated with
creased infection rates, increased ICU and ventilator duration, and a trend toward
creased mortality.

Thus, although our understanding of relative adrenal insufficiency in the crit-
ally ill continues to evolve, nearly all evidence agrees that adrenal insufficiency
likely when the baseline cortisol is <10 to 15 mcg/dL in critically ill patients,
d that cosyntropin stimulation testing may have additional diagnostic value in
entifying which patients are likely to respond to corticosteroid replacement, at
ast in the setting of volume unresponsive hypotension in patients with septic shock.
owever, given the often unreliable nature of cortisol concentrations in blood and
eir response to cosyntropin stimulation, we recommend that critically ill patients
th septic shock unresponsive to IV fluids and vasopressor support be managed as
ustrated in Algorithm 28.1. Patients should be started on hydrocortisone (200 to
0 mg/day) for 5 to 7 days. Once treatment is initiated, the cause of adrenal insuf-
ciency can be explored further. Many patients with adrenal insufficiency related
critical illness can be expected to regain normal function of the HPA axis with
covery from their illness. Some experts, however, still use the random cortisol alone,
eling that adrenal insufficiency is unlikely when the random cortisol is ≥25 mcg/dL
d that corticosteroids can be withheld in that setting. However, most meta-anal-
es of corticosteriod therapy in critical illness suggest a decrease in mortality with
eatment, especially in severely ill septic shock patients. These same meta-analyses
ggest that shock reversal is improved with corticosteroids. Therefore, corticosteroid
placement should be provided to all patients with septic shock that is not responsive
IV fluids and vasopressors.

ALGORITHM 28.1 | Therapeutic Approach to Relative Adrenal Insufficiency in the Critically Ill Patient

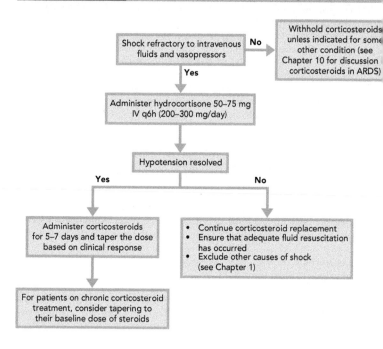

SUGGESTED READINGS

Annane A, Bellissant E, Bollaert PE, et al. Corticosteroids for severe sepsis and septic shock systematic review and meta-analysis. *BMJ.* 2004;329(7464):480–489.

> *Meta-analysis of 16 randomized and quasirandomized trials involving 2063 patients w severe sepsis and septic shock showing that long courses (≥5 days) with low-dose corti steroids (≤300 mg hydrocortisone or equivalent) reduced 28-day and hospital mortal*

Annane D, Bellissant E, Bollaert PE, et al. Corticosteroids in the treatment of severe sepsis a septic shock in adults: a systematic review. *JAMA.* 2009;301(22):2362–2375.

> *A systematic review of 17 trials with 12 trials investigating prolonged low-dose corticoster therapy, with the latter subgroup suggesting a beneficial effect in terms of short-te mortality.*

Annane D, Bellissant E, Bollaert PE, et al. Corticosteroids for treating sepsis. *Cochrane Datab. Syst Rev.* 2015;12:CD002243.

> *In an updated meta-analysis, low-quality evidence indicates that corticosteroids can red mortality among patients with sepsis. Moderate-quality evidence suggests that a lo course of low-dose corticosteroid can reduce 28-day mortality without inducing ma complications.*

Annane D, Maxime V, Ibrahim F, et al. Diagnosis of adrenal insufficiency in severe sepsis a septic shock. *Am J Respir Crit Care Med.* 2006;174(12):1319–1326.

> *An update on the diagnosis of adrenal insufficiency using cosyntropin stimulation.*

Annane D, Sebille V, Charpentier C, et al. Effect of treatment with low doses of hydrocortisone and fludrocortisone on mortality in patients with septic shock. *JAMA.* 2002;288(7):862–871.

> *A placebo-controlled, randomized, double-blind study showing a 7-day treatment with low doses of hydrocortisone and fludrocortisone in patients with septic shock and relative adrenal insufficiency, significantly reduced the risk of death without an increase in adverse events.*

Annane D, Sebille V, Troche G, et al. A 3-level prognostic classification in septic shock based on cortisol levels and cortisol response to corticotropin. *JAMA.* 2000;283(8):1038–1045.

> *A prospective inception cohort study evaluating the prognostic value of cortisol and the cosyntropin stimulation test in patients with septic shock.*

Cooper MS, Stewart PM. Corticosteroid insufficiency in acutely ill patients. *N Engl J Med.* 2003;348(8):727–734.

> *A focused review on the pathogenesis and treatment of adrenal insufficiency in the critically ill.*

Lipiner-Friedman D, Sprung CL, Laterre PF. Adrenal function in sepsis: the retrospective Corticus cohort study. *Crit Care Med.* 2007;35(4):1012–1018.

> *Retrospective cohort study from 20 European intensive care units examining the relationship between baseline and cosyntropin-stimulated cortisol levels and mortality in patients with severe sepsis and septic shock showing that delta cortisol and not basal cortisol levels were associated with clinical outcomes.*

Marik PE. Critical illness-related corticosteroid insufficiency. *Chest.* 2009;135(1):181–193.

> *Concise review of the causes, pathophysiology, diagnosis and treatment of adrenal insufficiency in critically ill patients.*

Marik PE, Pastores SM, Annane D, et al. Recommendations for the diagnosis and management of corticosteroid insufficiency in critically ill adult patients: consensus statements from an international task force by the American College of Critical Care Medicine. *Crit Care Med.* 2008;36(6):1937–1949.

> *Evidence-based guidelines for the diagnosis and medical management of adrenal insufficiency in critically ill patients. This guideline recommends that adrenal insufficiency in critical illness is best diagnosed by a delta cortisol (after 250 mcg cosyntropin) of <9 mcg/dL or a random total cortisol of <10 mcg/dL. Treatment with hydrocortisone (200 to 300 mg/day) is recommended for patients with septic shock who have responded poorly to fluid resuscitation and vasopressor agents.*

Minneci PC, Deans KJ, Eichacker PQ, et al. The effects of steroids during sepsis depend on dose and severity of illness: an updated meta-analysis. *Clin Microbiol Infect.* 2009;15(4):308–318.

> *An updated analysis of 21 trials. There was no effect of response to adrenocorticotropic hormone (ACTH) stimulation testing concerning the effects of steroids. Low-dose steroids appeared to be associated with improved mortality rates in patients with septic shock.*

Sligl WI, Milner DA Jr, Sundar S, et al. Safety and efficacy of corticosteroids for the treatment of septic shock: a systematic review and meta-analysis. *Clin Infect Dis.* 2009;49(1):93–101.

> *This meta-analysis observed that in patients with septic shock, corticosteroid therapy proved to be safe and significantly reduced the incidence of vasopressor-dependent shock. However, no effect on 28-day all-cause mortality was found.*

Sprung CL, Annane D, Keh D, et al. Hydrocortisone therapy for patients with septic shock. *N Engl J Med.* 2008;358(2):111–124.

> *The prospective CORTICUS study which demonstrated that hydrocortisone did not improve survival or reversal of shock in patients with septic shock, either overall or in patients who did not have a response to corticotropin, although hydrocortisone hastened reversal of shock in patients in whom shock was reversed.*

29 Diabetic Ketoacidosis and Hyperosmolar Hyperglycemic State

Tracy Trupka, Marin H. Kollef, and Garry S. Tobin

Diabetic ketoacidosis (DKA) and hyperosmolar hyperglycemic state (HHS) are life-threatening hyperglycemic complications of diabetes mellitus (DM) and common reasons for admission to the intensive care unit. The annual incidence of DKA is approximately 7.1 episodes per 1000 patients with DM (22.0 episodes per 1000 patients when age adjusted), resulting in a total of more than 140,000 hospitalizations per year with an ongoing upward trend. The annual incidence of HHS is lower than DKA and accounts for less than 1% of primary diabetic admissions. The mortality rate is 2% to 5% in DKA (in children <1%) and 15% in HHS, notably most often mortality in HHS is due to the underlying condition which precipitated the decompensation rather than the metabolic derangements related to the hyperglycemic state. Worse outcomes are seen at extremes of age and with the presence of coma, hypotension, and severe comorbidities. Precipitating factor is most commonly an infection (most commonly pneumonia and urinary tract infections, accounting for 30% to 50% of cases). Other common causes include inadequate insulin treatment or noncompliance, new-onset DM, cardiovascular events, cerebral vascular accident (CVA), pancreatitis, drugs/alcohol abuse, pulmonary embolism, trauma, and pregnancy. DKA typically occurs in patients with type 1 DM but does occur in patients with type 2 DM (as high as 1/3 of DKA cases). HHS is typically confined to patients with type 2 DM. Severity of the condition at time of presentation is often exacerbated by limited intake of water in the elderly or chronically ill. DKA and HHS are the result of insulin deficiency in patients with DM. In both disorders, insulin deficiency causes increased hepatic glycolysis, gluconeogenesis, and impaired glucose utilization by peripheral tissues, leading to hyperglycemia. The hyperglycemia in turn causes an osmotic diuresis. Table 29.1 highlights the differences between DKA and HHS.

DIABETIC KETOACIDOSIS

DKA is characterized by hyperglycemia (blood glucose [BG] typically 250 to 800 mg/dL), anion gap metabolic acidosis (arterial pH ≤7.3), and ketosis (positive urine and plasma ketones), along with dehydration and electrolyte abnormalities in varying degrees. Common ketone assays use nitroprusside, measuring acetoacetate and acetone, but not beta hydroxybutyrate which requires a separate assay. Prominent presenting symptoms include nausea/vomiting, abdominal pain, labored breathing (Kussmaul's respirations), and polyuria. A mixed acid–base disorder may also be present, such as a concomitant severe contraction metabolic alkalosis elevating the serum bicarbonate level, masking the underlying metabolic acidosis.

TABLE 29.1	Initial Laboratory Values in Diabetic Ketoacidosis and Hyperosmolar Hyperglycemic State			
	DKA			
Value	Mild	Moderate	Severe	HHS
Plasma glucose (mg/dL)	>250	>250	>250	>600
Arterial pH	7.25–7.30	7–7.24	<7	>7.30
Serum bicarbonate (mEq/L)	15–18	10–14	<10	>15
Urine and serum ketones	Positive	Positive	Positive	Trace/small
Serum osmolarity (mOsm/L)	Variable	Variable	Variable	>320
Anion gap	>10	>12	>12	<12
Mental status	Alert	Alert/drowsy	Stupor/coma	Stupor/coma
Sodium (mmol/L)	125–135	125–135	125–135	135–145
Potassium (mmol/L)	Normal to ↑	Normal to ↑	Normal to ↑	Normal
Creatinine (mg/dL)	Slight ↑	Slight ↑	Slight ↑	Moderate ↑

DKA, diabetic ketoacidosis; HHS, hyperosmolar hyperglycemic state.

In patients with DKA, the absolute lack of insulin causes an increase in counter regulatory hormones (cortisol, growth hormone, catecholamines, and glucagon), which promote lipolysis in adipose tissue and the release of free fatty acids. In the liver, the free fatty acids are converted to ketones. These patients suffer from a metabolic acidosis as a result of these circulating ketoacids. Ketone bodies and hyperglycemia contribute to the osmotic diuresis, resulting in a loss of sodium and potassium. Although initial laboratory values are variable (often with a state of seemingly hyperkalemia due to potassium efflux into the extracellular space in the acidotic environment), total body sodium and potassium are depleted.

While prompt management of DKA as described below is essential, finding and treating the precipitating cause should not be forgotten or delayed. Blood, urine, and sputum cultures; chest x-ray; EKG; and empiric treatment based on clinical suspicion should be part of the initial management of DKA. One should further evaluate the cause of abdominal pain if this symptom does not resolve with correction of the dehydration and metabolic acidosis.

Treatment of DKA requires reversal of the hyperglycemia by administering insulin and replacing the circulating and total body volume and electrolyte deficits (Algorithm 29.1). Fluid deficits in DKA can be more than 6 L. Mainstay of therapy consists of normal saline boluses for acute volume resuscitation, followed by ½ NS replacement of the remaining fluid deficit, and later 5% dextrose-containing fluids are continued from the time the glucose falls below 250 mg/dL, until the anion gap normalizes and the patient is able to tolerate oral intake. Insulin should be given as an IV bolus, followed by continuous infusion. Hyperglycemia resolves faster than

ALGORITHM 29.1 **Management of Diabetic Ketoacidosis and Hyperosmolar Hyperglycemic State**

INSULIN TREATMENT

1) Bolus 0.1–0.15 U/kg regular insulin intravenously (IV) (subcutaneous [SC]/intramuscular [IM] can be given if no IV access).
2) Start continuous IV insulin infusion via an infusion pump.
   Standard infusion is 100 U **regular human insulin** (IV t $^{1}/_{2}$ 5–9 minutes) in 100 mL 0.9% NaCl.
   For **DKA** start at 0.1 U/kg/hr.
   For **HHS** start at 0.05 U/kg/hr; delay insulin in **HHS** until at least 1 L NS infused.

BLOOD GLUCOSE MONITORING

1) Check initial blood glucose (BG) q1h. **Goal decrease in BG is 50–75 mg/dL/hr.**
2) Once stable (three consecutive values decreased in target range), change BG monitoring to q2h. Resume q1h BG monitoring for each change in the insulin infusion rate (see below)
3) Add dextrose 5% to IV fluids when BG <250 mg/dL
   For **DKA goal BG 150–200 mg/dL until anion gap closed.**
   For **HHS goal BG is 250–300 mg/dL until mental status improves.**

CHANGING THE INSULIN INFUSION RATE

1) ↓ IV insulin by 50%/hr if BG decreases by >100 mg/dL/hr in any 1-hour period.*
2) ↑ insulin drip by 50%/hr if change in BG is <50 mg/dL/hr.
3) For **DKA and HSS**, when BG decreases to 250 mg/dL, insulin infusion may need to be decreased 50% to maintain glucose at target levels (see Blood Glucose Monitoring above).

Start SC insulin when:
1) Anion gap closed (DKA)
2) Serum bicarbonate increases to >15 mEq/L (DKA)
3) Patient able to eat
4) Mental status improves (HHS)

Stop the insulin drip after all of the following are done**
1) Give short-acting insulin (aspart or lispro) SC at twice the hourly IV rate (e.g., if IV rate is 5 U/hr, give 10 U short-acting insulin SC).
2) Give long-acting insulin (NPH or glargine) SC at 0.2–0.3 U/kg (divided q8 for NPH), or home insulin dose.
3) Ensure patient has a meal and is eating.

*Lowering glucose >100 mg/dL/hr may cause osmotic encephalopathy.
**Failure to give SC insulin may result in rebound hyperglycemia and ketosis due to the short t $^{1}/_{2}$ of IV regular insulin (5–9 min).

ALGORITHM 29.1 **Management of Diabetic Ketoacidosis and Hyperosmolar Hyperglycemic State (Continued)**

FLUID MANAGEMENT*

Fluid replacement varies based on age, weight, hemodynamics, and comorbidities. A reasonable approach follows:

1) **Replace intravascular volume**
   Give 1 L 0.9% NaCl over 30–60 min. Give an additional 1–2 L q30–60min until hemodynamically stable and urine output increased.
2) **Replace total body water deficit**
   Change to 0.45% NaCl and infuse at 150–500 mL/hr.
   When BG <250 mg/dL, add dextrose 5% and decrease to 100–200 mL/hr.

*Fluid is replaced over 12–24 hrs and patients are generally depleted 3–6 L in DKA and 8–12 L in HHS.
*Monitor urine output, heart rate, blood pressure, and respiratory status. Care must be taken in patients with congestive heart failure and kidney disease.

ELECTROLYTE MANAGEMENT

1) Check basic metabolic panel (BMP), arterial blood gas, magnesium (Mg^{2+}), and phosphorus (PO_4^{3-}).
2) Repeat BMP, Mg, PO_4^{3-} q2–4h depending on degree of electrolyte imbalance.

Potassium (K^+)
K^+ ≥5.5 mEq/L: leave potassium supplement out of IVF
K^+ 4–5.4 mEq/L: add 20 mEq KCl/L to IVF
K^+ 3–3.9 mEq/L: add 40 mEq KCl/L to IVF
K^+ <3 mEq/L: add 60 mEq KCl/L to IVF
In DKA, if initial K^+ is <3.3 mEq/L, **DO NOT** give IV insulin until the serum K^+ is supplemented to >3.3 mmol/L due to the risk of severe hypokalemia.

Sodium (Na^+)
Hypoglycemia causes an artifactually low serum sodium, and the correct value must be calculated. Corrected Na^+ = Measured Na^+ [mmol/L] + (1.6 [Measured BG (mg/dL) – 100]/100)
Na^+ replaced with IV fluids initially as 0.9% NaCl for first 1–3 L and then as 0.45% NaCl (see Fluid Management).

Bicarbonate (HCO_3^-)
Usually in DKA only.
Replacement generally not necessary as insulin will reverse the HCO_3^- deficit with its inhibition of lipolysis.
Consider HCO_3^- in the following situations (see Chapter 25; metabolic acidosis):
1) Severe acidosis with pH <7 (the HCO_3^- should be stopped once the pH is >7.1)
2) Severe loss of buffering capacity when serum HCO_3^- <5–10 mEq/L
3) Acidosis-induced cardiac or respiratory distress
4) Severe hyperkalemia

Magnesium and Phosphorus
Severe hypomagnesemia and hypophosphatemia are not common complications of DKA and HHS (see Chapter 29 if they occur) and supplementation is usually not necessary.

PRECIPITATING FACTOR TREATMENT

The cause of the DKA or HHS should be sought and treated. Common precipitants include missed insulin therapy, infections such as pneumonia, sepsis, and urinary and upper respiratory tract infections, trauma, myocardial infarction, pregnancy, or as the initial presentation of DM.

acidosis, and supraphysiologic insulin doses are needed to overcome hyperglycemia-induced insulin resistance to achieve euglycemia. After this is achieved, insulin is still required to drive peripheral ketone use, resolving the remaining acidosis. Therefore, the BG should be kept between 150 and 200 mg/dL with 5% dextrose, until the anion gap is closed. Intermediate- or long-acting subcutaneous insulin must be given before insulin drip discontinuation. Failure to do this properly can lead to rebound hyperglycemia and recurrence of DKA. The patient should be able to tolerate PO fluids, and dextrose-containing IV fluids should be stopped at that time.

Initially, insulin should be given IV. If IV administration cannot be achieved, an intramuscular or subcutaneous (SC) route is an option. However, this is a less reliable method to achieve the insulin levels needed in seriously ill patients. In adults, the BG should be decreased by 50 to 100 mg/dL/hr. Decreasing the BG more than 75 to 100 mg/dL/hr can cause an osmotic encephalopathy (0.3% to 1% of DKA in children, extremely rare in adults). Glucose lowering in the first 2 hours may be more rapid as a result of initial volume expansion.

Insulin and intravenous (IV) fluids will correct the acidosis in patients with DKA but can rapidly produce hypokalemia, as potassium shifts intracellularly. The patient is total body potassium deficient at presentation, even if serum potassium is elevated (caution in concomitant chronic kidney disease). Successful treatment requires frequent monitoring and decision-making based on the patient's clinical condition and laboratory data as it becomes available.

HYPEROSMOLAR HYPERGLYCEMIC STATE

HHS is characterized by hyperglycemia (BG typically 600 to greater than 1200 mg/dL), hyperosmolarity (serum osmolarity 320 to 380 mOsm/L), pronounced dehydration (hemodynamic instability, prerenal azotemia, decreased urine output), and neurologic sequelae ranging from mild lethargy to coma. HHS has an insidious onset, typically over weeks, with patients experiencing polyuria, polydipsia, weight loss, and neurologic changes, including fatigue, confusion, or coma. Even in the absence of exogenous insulin, there is typically enough intrinsic insulin production by beta cells to suppress hepatic lipoprotein lipase and ketoacid production. As a result, HHS lacks the metabolic acidosis prominent in DKA; however, small amounts of ketoacids may still be present from concomitant alcoholic or starvation ketosis. In HHS, the hyperglycemia is more pronounced than in DKA, resulting in greater diuresis (average fluid deficit of 9 L vs. 6 L in DKA). The resulting dehydration impairs renal function, decreasing glucose excretion, and worsening hyperglycemia. IV insulin should not be given until fluid resuscitation with 1 to 2 L of normal saline has been completed to prevent rapid hyperglycemia correction and hemodynamic collapse from intracellular fluid shifts. Patients with HHS are often more responsive to insulin than patients with DKA and a lower dose is often used. The blood glucose should be kept slightly higher, generally between 250 and 300 mg/dL, to allow gradual correction of intracranial fluid shifts. These levels should be maintained until the patient's mental status improves. When this happens, IV insulin can be converted to SC insulin as listed in Algorithm 29.1. Failure to give SC insulin when the IV insulin is stopped can result in rebound hyperglycemia with worsening mental status in HHS. Of note, mental status has been shown to correlate with elevated serum osmolality at presentation but not with acidosis. Stupor or coma while serum osmolality is less than 320 mOsm/L warrants immediate consideration of other causes of altered mental status.

ABLE 29.2	Treatment of Cerebral Edema Complicating DKA or HHS

itiate treatment as soon as cerebral edema is clinically suspected.

ve mannitol 0.5–1 g/kg IV over 20 min and repeat if there is no initial response in 30 min to 1 hr.

mediately reduce the rate of fluid administrated by one-third.

ypertonic saline (3%), 5–10 mL/kg over 30 min, may be an alternative to mannitol, especially if there is no initial response to mannitol.

evate the head of the bed.

tubation for airway protection and impending respiratory failure. Hyperventilation to a PCO_2 <22 mm Hg has been associated with poor outcomes and is not recommended.

fter treatment for cerebral edema is initiated, a brain CT should be obtained to rule out other possible causes of intracerebral deterioration, especially thrombosis or hemorrhage.

EREBRAL EDEMA

hile hypoglycemia is the most common complication of treatment for DKA/HS, cerebral edema, occurring in less than 1% of cases, remains a far more serious mplication. This devastating consequence is observed more frequently in children an in adults and accounts for 60% to 90% of all DKA-related deaths. Symptoms clude headache, altered mental status, or a sudden deterioration in mental status er an initial improvement. Bradycardia, hypertension, and papilledema can be en. Cerebral edema usually develops 4 to 12 hours after treatment has started but n occur before treatment has begun or, uncommonly, may develop as late as 24 to hours after start of treatment. The risk factors for cerebral edema are excessive correction with free H_2O and a rapid decline in the BG. Effective osmolality and water ficit can be calculated to replete at an appropriate rate (Algorithm 29.1). Failure the serum sodium to rise during treatment is a clue to excess hydration with free O. Prompt recognition and treatment with IV mannitol, hypertonic saline, and rticosteroids is essential to prevent neurologic sequelae. Computed tomography aging can show the presence of cerebral edema. Morbidity and mortality are high ce cerebral edema is recognized (Table 29.2).

UGGESTED READINGS

ich GA, Fishbein HA, Ellis SE. The epidemiology of diabetic acidosis: a population based study. *Am J Epidemiol.* 1983;177:551–558.

    A 12-month epidemiologic study conducted from 1979 to 1980 of all acute care centers in Rhode Island, which examined the incidence, mortality rates, precipitating factors, and cost for patients admitted with DKA.

aser N. Cerebral injury and cerebral edema in children with diabetic ketoacidosis: could cerebral ischemia and reperfusion injury be involved? *Pediatr Diabetes.* 2009;10:534–541.

    A concise review of the pathogenesis of cerebral edema in DKA and how this is related to treatment.

itabchi AE, Guillermo EU, Miles JM, et al. Hyperglycemic crises in adult patients with diabetes. *Diabetes Care.* 2009;32:1335–1343.

    An extensive review of the definitions, causes, manifestations, pathophysiology, and treatment of DKA and HHS.

Kitabchi AE, Umpierrez GE, Fisher JN, Murphy MB, Stentz FB. Thirty years of personal experience in hyperglycemic crises: diabetic ketoacidosis and hyperglycemic hyperosmolar state. *J Clin Endocrinol Metab.* 2008;93(5):1541–1552.
  Diabetic ketoacidosis and hyperglycemic hyperosmolar syndrome.
Magee MF, Bhatt BA. Management of decompensated diabetes. Diabetic ketoacidosis hyperglycemic hyperosmolar syndrome. *Crit Care Clin.* 2001;17(1):75–106.
  Review of DKA and HHS.
Wolfsdorf JI, Allgrove J, Craig ME, et al. Diabetic ketoacidosis and hyperglycemic hyperosm state. *Pediatric Diabetes.* 2014;15:154–179.
  ISPAD Clinical Practice Consensus Guidelines 2014 Compendium.
Wolfsdorf JI, Craig ME, Daneman D, et al. Diabetic ketoacidosis. *Pediatr Diabetes.* 200 28–43.
  Consensus guidelines from the International Society for Adolescent and Adolescent Diabetes the management of DKA.

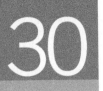

30 Glucose Control in the ICU

Marin H. Kollef, Paulina Cruz Bravo, and Garry S. Tobin

Hyperglycemia is a common finding in up to 90% of patients in the intensive care unit (ICU), occurring in both diabetic and nondiabetic patients. Factors contributing to hyperglycemia in critically ill patients include increased counterregulatory hormones (cortisol and glucagon), hepatic insulin resistance, decreased physical activity with resultant decrease in insulin-stimulated glucose uptake in the heart and skeletal muscle, glucocorticoid therapy, dextrose-containing intravenous (IV) fluids, and dense caloric enteral and parenteral nutrition. Numerous observational studies have shown that hyperglycemia is an independent risk factor for morbidity and mortality in patients in the medical, surgical, neurology, and cardiac ICUs, including postoperative cardiac and general surgery patients, patients with acute myocardial infarction and stroke, and general medicine patients.

A few earlier single-center randomized trials have suggested that treating hyperglycemia in critically ill patients could reduce morbidity and mortality. However, which patients benefit the most from treatment and the optimal glucose targets were unclear from those studies. More recently, multicenter trials, have demonstrated that hypoglycemia and intensive glycemic control were associated with adverse outcomes including increased hospital mortality. The following discussion addresses the current evidence, recommendations, and areas of uncertainty in regard to glucose control in the ICU.

TRIALS

The seminal randomized study treating hyperglycemia in critically ill patients was published by Van den Berghe et al. in 2001 and included 1548 intubated patients (13% with known diabetes) in a surgical ICU who were randomly assigned to intensive glycemic control with a target glucose between 80 and 110 mg/dL ($n = 765$), versus a standard care group that was treated with insulin when the blood glucose was >215 mg/dL, with a target glucose between 180 and 200 mg/dL ($n = 783$). The study found that the intensive care mortality rate was 42% lower (8% vs. 4.6%, $p <0.04$) in the intensive treatment group, with the benefit reaching statistical significance in patients who remained in the ICU for more than 5 days. The major difference in mortality was attributed to a decrease in the development of multiorgan failure with sepsis.

Van den Berghe et al. addressed nonsurgical patients in 2006 with a follow-up trial limited to patients in a medical ICU, which randomized 1200 patients (16.9% with known diabetes) to intensive glucose control versus standard care utilizing the same protocol as in their 2001 trial. The study did not replicate the mortality benefit seen in the surgical ICU study. Overall, there was no significant difference in the in-hospital mortality rate (37.3% vs. 40%, $p = 0.33$). While the study did show decreased in-hospital mortality for the 767 patients who stayed in the ICU ≥3 days (43% vs. 52.5%, $p = 0.009$), there was increased mortality in the patients who stayed in the ICU <3 days (12.9% vs. 9.6%, $p = 0.41$ after correcting for baseline risk factors). This difference did not reach statistical significance. Despite no overall mortality benefit, there was reduced morbidity in the intensive treatment group, including less newly acquired kidney injury, reduced duration of mechanical ventilation, shorter ICU stay, and shorter hospital stays. There were no significant differences in bacteremia rates or duration of antibiotics.

In the two trials by Van ben Berghe et al., hypoglycemic episodes were increased in the intensive treatment group (5.2% vs. 0.7% in the surgical ICU, 18.7% vs. 3.1% in the medical ICU). Despite the high incidence of hypoglycemia, serious immediate side effects such as hemodynamic compromise and seizures were not reported. While hypoglycemia is more common in patients with renal and hepatic failure, which may partially explain the increased incidence of hypoglycemia in the medical ICU, hypoglycemia was identified as an independent risk factor for death in the medical ICU population. However, the effect was not seen until at least 24 hours after the hypoglycemic episode. The reason for this is unclear. The first Van den Berghe trial utilized arterial blood and arterial blood gas analyzers, not capillary glucose or point of care (POC) glucometers. The second trial utilized capillary blood glucose normalized to whole blood and a Hemo Cue meter which has less variance than other POC techniques. Patients in these trials also consistently received early caloric intervention, often with total parenteral nutrition (TPN).

Brunkhorst et al. randomized patients to an intensive insulin treatment arm (mean morning blood glucose level 112 mg/dL) and a conventional insulin treatment arm (mean morning blood glucose level 151 mg/dL) in a multicenter randomized trial. No significant difference in 28-day mortality or mean organ failure score was observed between treatment groups. However, the intensive insulin treatment arm was associated with a statistically greater incidence of severe hypoglycemia, defined as ≤40 mg/dL, (17.0% vs. 4.1%; $p < 0.001$) and serious adverse events (10.9% vs. 5.2%; $p = 0.01$) compared to the conventional insulin treatment arm.

The NICE-SUGAR study randomized critically ill patients expected to remain in the ICU >3 days to intensive glucose control (81 to 108 mg/dL) versus conventional glucose control (180 mg/dL or less) in a multinational randomized trial. They found that severe hypoglycemia was more common in the intensive glucose control group (6.8% vs. 0.5%; $p < 0.001$) and that 90-day all-cause mortality was increased (27.5% vs. 24.9%; $p = 0.02$). The treatment effect did not differ significantly between surgical patients and medical patients. Trauma patients and those on corticosteroids showed a trend for mortality benefit with intensive control. These authors concluded that a blood glucose target of 180 mg/dL or less resulted in lower morbidity and mortality compared to a more aggressive glucose control target.

The Glucontrol Study was another recent randomized control trial of intense versus intermediate glucose control in medicosurgical ICUs. The trial was stopped early due to a high rate of unintended protocol violations. They only studied one-third of their intended number of patients, and the study was therefore underpowered. The intense group did have significantly more hypoglycemia, and no difference in ICU mortality was seen. Twenty out of 111 hypoglycemic events were attributed inappropriate continuation of insulin infusion, seen more in the intense therapy group. Other trials over the years have tried to determine benefits of intense glucose control in specific patient populations with conflicting results. What is consistent, however, is the increase in hypoglycemic events with more intense therapy, making hypoglycemia the limiting factor in lower target glucose protocols.

Several meta-analyses of intensive insulin therapy in critically ill patients have come up with similar conclusions. These analyses found that medical and surgical patients receiving intensive insulin therapy had similar mortality and greater occurrence of hypoglycemia compared to those who received less stringent glucose control.

MANAGEMENT

The conclusions and current recommendations based on these studies are still somewhat controversial. Table 30.1 lists the most recent recommendations for glucose control in the ICU by the American Diabetes Association (Position Statement 2016), Society of Critical Care Medicine, and the American College of Endocrinology, which includes patients in all ICUs and hospital wards. The authors of the Surviving Sepsis Campaign advocate blood sugar goals of less than 180 mg/dL in critically ill patients in large part to limit hypoglycemia and to simplify management. Overall, some studies support intensive glucose control in patients who are expected to stay in the ICU more than 3 to 5 days, and those on corticosteroids or suffering from recent trauma. The postulated reason for this is that preventing hyperglycemia prevents complications from hyperglycemia, and complications take time to develop. It seems reasonable to exclude medical ICU patients who are eating and who are expected to be in the ICU <3 days. However, it is not always possible to predict the length of ICU stays, and physician discretion is needed.

The benefits seen in the surgical ICU study by Van den Berghe were not replicated in later studies. Potential reasons for this include the strict use of blood gas analyzers on arterial blood (which would increase the accuracy of the readings compared to POC bedside analyzers on capillary blood), and the use of early parenteral

TABLE 30.1	Recommended Target Blood Glucose for Patients in the Intensive Care Unit

American Diabetes Association
- Initiate insulin starting at ≤180 mg/dL.
- Once insulin has started, a target glucose range of 140–180 mg/dL is recommended for most patients.
- More stringent targets may be appropriate for certain populations (110–140 mg/dL) providing a lower target does not confer increased hypoglycemic risk.

American College of Endocrinology
<180 mg/dL

Surviving Sepsis Campaign
<180 mg/dL

Society of Critical Care Medicine
100–150 mg/dL

nutrition, which may increase morbidity/mortality from blood stream infections the conventional group.

Another difference noted is the premorbid diabetes status. In nondiabeti maintaining euglycemia and decreasing glucose variability have been independen associated with a reduced mortality risk. This benefit has not been seen in patie with diabetes, and furthermore, they appear to have an increased risk of mortal with a mean glucose of 80 to 110 mg/dL compared to less than 180 mg/dL (Krins et al. [PMID: 23452622. doi: 10.1186/cc12547]).

In critically ill patients admitted to the ICU, all oral antihyperglycemic age and subcutaneous insulin should be stopped. Insulin in critically ill patients shou be given intravenously. The half-life of IV insulin is 5 to 9 minutes, which allows rapid reversal of hypoglycemia when it occurs. Most ICUs now have standardiz glucose algorithms, generally managed by nurses, which have been shown to be val ways to manage glucose. The most effective glucose algorithms are dynamic ar incorporate the rate of glucose change into the insulin dose adjustments. Table 3C contains a validated insulin-infusion protocol outlining how to initiate an insul infusion, monitor blood glucose, and manage hypoglycemia. Algorithm 30.1 ar Table 30.3 show how to manage the insulin-infusion rate. It is important that o does not draw the wrong conclusions from trials examining intensive glucose contr in the ICU. The standard of care in all of these studies is IV insulin to prevent hype glycemia in critically ill, intubated patients. What is in dispute is the target bloc glucose range to achieve. NICE-SUGAR and other trials mentioned here should n be used to support the decision to use subcutaneous insulin over IV insulin, or allow persistent hyperglycemia >180 mg/dL, in a critically ill patient.

In managing glucose, one must make insulin-infusion adjustments based c changes in carbohydrate intake. For example, a change in the dextrose 5% rate fro 150 mL/hr (180 g carbohydrates normalized during a 24-hour period) to 75 mL/ (90 g carbohydrates normalized during a 24-hour period) will require a decrease in th insulin-infusion rate in order to prevent hypoglycemia. In critically ill patients, mul ple sources of carbohydrate need to be taken into consideration when calculating th insulin dose such as parenteral nutrition, enteral tube feeds, and glucose-containi IV fluid. Nutrition, whether enteral or parenteral, should be given as a continuo infusion rather than intermittent boluses to prevent significant fluctuations in bloc glucose. It is often critical to reassess caloric intake every 12 to 24 hours. The patien mostly at risk for hypoglycemia are those with renal failure and hepatic failure. Clo attention to details and a less aggressive upward titration schedule in patients wi liver and renal failure should allow insulin drips to be safely used. Meticulous atter tion must also be paid to patients with impaired mental status who are unable perceive and respond to low glucose levels.

The implementation of any protocol, whether taken from the literature c developed locally, especially one as complex as an IV insulin drip protocol, requires significant amount of education and training. Even under controlled conditions, th protocol can be violated frequently, as seen in the Gluncontrol Study. The violation could be as simple as missed blood glucose or as serious as a failure to adjust the insuli infusion rate. Human error has to be taken into consideration when evaluating bloc glucose control.

Computerized calculation of the drip rate has been shown to minimize mistak and may improve outcomes. Multiple computerized programs are available. Our inst tution has studied EndoTool in patients undergoing elective cardiac surgery, requirir

TABLE 30.2	Insulin-Infusion Protocol

Initiating Insulin Infusion

Standard insulin infusion 100 U *regular human insulin* in 100 mL 0.9% normal saline.
Preferred administration IV (t½ 5–9 min) via an infusion pump.
Give initial bolus if blood glucose (BG) >180 mg/dL;
   Divide initial BG by 70 and round to nearest 0.5 U (e.g., BG 250: 250/70 = 3.57,
     rounded to 4, so IV bolus 4 U).
After bolus, start infusion at same hourly rate as bolus (4 U/hr IV in above example).
If *BG less than 180 mg/dL*, divide by 70 for initial hourly rate with *NO bolus* (e.g.,
  BG 150 would be 150/70 = 2.15, rounded to 2, so start at 2 U/hr IV).
Go to Algorithm 30.1 for instructions on changing the insulin-infusion rate.

Blood Glucose Monitoring

Check BG q1h until stable (three consecutive values in target range).
Once stable can change BG monitoring to q2h.
If stable q2h for 12–24 hrs can change to q3–4h if
  no significant change in nutrition or clinical status
Resume q1h BG monitoring for BG >70 mg/dL with any of the following;
  Change in insulin-infusion rate.
  Initiation or cessation of corticosteroid or vasopressor therapy.
  Significant change in clinical status.
  Change in nutritional support (initiation, cessation, or rate change).
  Initiation or cessation of hemodialysis or CVVHD.

Hypoglycemia (BG <70 mg/dL)

If *BG <50 mg/dL*, stop infusion and give 25 g dextrose 50% (1 amp D50) IV.
  Recheck BG q10–15min.
When BG >90 mg/dL, recheck in 1 hr. If still >90 mg/dL after 1 hr, resume insulin
  infusion at *50% most recent rate.*
If *BG 50–69 mg/dL*, stop infusion.
  If symptomatic or unable to assess, give 25 g dextrose 50% (1 amp D50) IV.
    Recheck BG q15min.[a]
  If asymptomatic, consider 12.5 g dextrose 50% (1/2 amp D50) or 8 oz. fruit juice
    PO.
    Recheck q15–30min.[a]

---

[a]When, BG >90 mg/dL, recheck in 1 hr. If still >90 mg/dL after 1 hr, resume insulin infusion at
75% most recent rate.
BG, blood glucose; CVVHD, continuous venovenous hemodialysis; IV, intravenous; PO, by mouth.
Modified from Goldberg PA, Siegel MD, Sherwin RS, et al. Implementation of a safe and effective
insulin-infusion protocol in a medical intensive care unit. *Diabetes Care.* 2004;27(2):461–467,
with permission.

cardiopulmonary bypass and compared glycemic control to a paper-based protocol using a target of 100 to 150 mg/dL. The computerized protocol resulted in a higher proportion of patients achieving the desired target for longer time and quicker than the paper-based protocol with no significant difference in hypoglycemia. (Other computerized based protocols include eMPC [*BMC Anesthesiol.* 2016;16:8. doi: 10.1186/s12871–016–0175–4], Glucocare IGC system [*Diabetes Technol Ther.* 2013;15(3):246–252. doi: 10.1089/dia.2012.0277. Epub 2013 Jan 4] and Glucommander.)

ALGORITHM 30.1 Changing the Insulin Infusion Rate

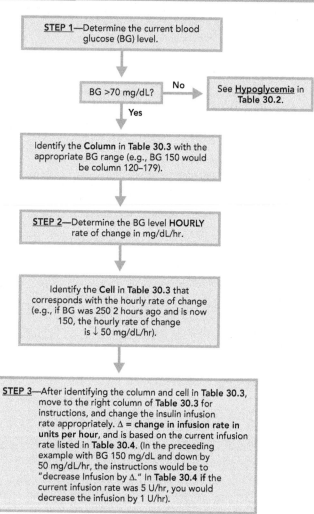

STEP 1—Determine the current blood glucose (BG) level.

BG >70 mg/dL? → **No** → See <u>Hypoglycemia</u> in Table 30.2.

Yes

Identify the **Column** in **Table 30.3** with the appropriate BG range (e.g., BG 150 would be column 120–179).

STEP 2—Determine the BG level **HOURLY** rate of change in mg/dL/hr.

Identify the **Cell** in **Table 30.3** that corresponds with the hourly rate of change (e.g., if BG was 250 2 hours ago and is now 150, the hourly rate of change is ↓ 50 mg/dL/hr).

STEP 3—After identifying the column and cell in **Table 30.3**, move to the right column of **Table 30.3** for instructions, and change the insulin infusion rate appropriately. Δ = **change in infusion rate in units per hour**, and is based on the current infusion rate listed in **Table 30.4**. (In the preceeding example with BG 150 mg/dL and down by 50 mg/dL/hr, the instructions would be to "decrease Infusion by Δ." In **Table 30.4** if the current infusion rate was 5 U/hr, you would decrease the infusion by 1 U/hr).

Once patients improve and are ready to be discharged from the ICU, IV insulin needs to be switched to subcutaneous insulin. Using an insulin sliding scale alone results in rebound hyperglycemia. The development of diabetic ketoacidosis and hyperglycemic hyperosmolar state in the hospital is considered "never events" by Centers for Medicare and Medicaid Services (CMS). Using basal long-acting insulin (NPH, glargine, or detemir) combined with prandial and sliding scale short-acting insulin (aspart, lispro, glulisine) will lead to better glycemic control. When calculating dosage, one needs to take into account the prior history of diabetes, type of betes, stress level, prior insulin dosage, steroid use, and general clinical status. ng-acting insulin needs to overlap with discontinuation of the drip to prevent ound hyperglycemia. We give short-acting insulin at two times the drip rate plus g-acting insulin (generally starting with 0.3 U/kg of body weight/day) and turn e drip off immediately. If short-acting insulin is not given, then the drip should erlap 2 to 4 hours to allow the long-acting insulin to be effective.

Attention should be paid to what glucose analyzer is used (blood gas, core labo-ory, POC glucose oxidase, or POC glucose dehydrogenase), the source of patient nple (arterial, capillary, central venous), and what conditions the patient has (ane-ia, hypoxia, poor peripheral perfusion) or medications they are receiving (acetamin-hen, oxygen, vasopressors, mannitol, ascorbic acid, IVIG, peritoneal dialysis) that use changes in glucose results.

Anemia (Hct <34%) has been shown to cause significant error, overestimating cose with some POC glucometers. Dosing insulin based on falsely elevated glucose ues could contribute to hypoglycemia in intensively treated patients in ICU set-gs. The use of formulas correcting for the level of anemia has been shown to reduce poglycemic events in ICU patients and has been incorporated into most meters mmonly in use in the hospital setting. Meters using glucose dehydrogenase strips e affected by maltose in IVIG, and icodextrin from peritoneal dialysis, and therefore ould not be used in health care facilities until these problems are corrected.

The FDA has issued an off-label designation for POC glucose meters not proved for their use in critically ill patients. However, the FDA did not define itical illness, which has allowed institutional discretion of choice of meter. To date, o POC glucose meters that automatically correct for hematocrit, hypoxia, and terfering reducing substances have been approved by the FDA to be used in these lnerable population (Nova StatStrip and Nova StatStrip Xpress Systems). By the d of 2015, approximately 50% of the hospitals in the United States reported using em. Off-label use of other meters can result in regulatory burden with mandatory aining and certification of the staff.

Even without an identified clinical interference, glucose meters can have an error argin of up to 20%, where as laboratory analyzers must be below 10% to meet DA standards. Arterial blood measured by POC glucometers is more accurate than pillary glucose, and should be used when available in ICU patients on IV insulin. "stat" blood sample should be sent to the laboratory when in doubt of the glucose ading.

As the use of continuous glucose monitors (CGM) expands, two randomized inical trials have evaluated its impact on glycemic control and risk of hypoglycemia critically ill patients. Holziger et al. randomized 124 patients on mechanical ven-lation to real-time (RT) CGM with glucose values given every 5 minutes ($n = 63$) rsus a control group ($n = 61$), selective arterial glucose measurements were obtained ased on an algorithm. Both groups were treated to normoglycemia, target 80 to 00 mg/dL. A modified version of the Leuven protocol was used in both groups. the intervention group, nurses utilized RT-CGM values to guide insulin therapy. lean glucose level was not improved using CGM, but the risk of severe hypoglycemia as reduced (1.6 vs. 11.7%, $p = 0.031$) with an absolute risk reduction of 9.9% and a umber to treat of 10.1.

De Block et al. studied 35 patients in the medical ICU that were randomized to T-CGM ($n = 16$) or blinded CGM with a normoglycemic target of 80 to 100 mg/dL

TABLE 30.3 Current Blood Glucose Level and Rate of Change[a]

BG 70–89 mg/dL	BG 90–119 mg/dL	BG 120–179 mg/dL	BG >180 mg/dL	Instructions (See Table 30.4 for Δ)
		BG ↑ by >40 mg/dL/hr	BG ↑	INCREASE INFUSION by 2Δ
	BG ↑ by >20 mg/dL/hr	BG ↑ by 1–40 mg/dL/hr OR BG UNCHANGED	BG UNCHANGED OR BG ↓ by 1–40 mg/dL/hr	INCREASE INFUSION by Δ
BG ↑	BG ↑ by 1–20 mg/dL/hr, BG UNCHANGED, OR BG ↓ by 1–20 mg/dL/hr	BG ↓ by 1–40 mg/dL/hr	BG ↓ by 41–80 mg/dL/hr	NO INFUSION CHANGE
BG UNCHANGED OR BG ↓ by 1–20 mg/dL/hr	BG ↓ by 21–40 mg/dL/hr	BG ↓ by 41–80 mg/dL/hr	BG ↓ by 81–120 mg/dL/hr	DECREASE INFUSION by Δ
BG ↓ by >20 mg/dL/hr See below[b]	BG ↓ by >40 mg/dL/hr	BG ↓ by >80 mg/dL/hr	BG ↓ by >120 mg/dL/hr	HOLD INFUSION × 30 min then DECREASE by 2Δ

[a]See Algorithm 30.1 for instructions.

[b]Hold insulin infusion; check BG q15–30min; when >90 mg/dL, restart infusion at 75% most recent rate.

TABLE 30.4	Changes in Insulin Infusion Rate (Δ) in Units per Hour	
Current Infusion Rate (U/hr)	Δ = Rate Change (U/hr)	2Δ = 2 × Rate Change (U/hr)
<3	0.5	1
3–6	1	2
6.5–9.5	1.5	3
10–14.5	2	4
15–19.5	3[a]	6[a]
20–24.5[a]	4[a]	8[a]
>25[a]	5[a]	10[a]

Infusions typically range 2 to 10 U/hr. Doses in excess of 20 U/hr are unusual and a physician should be notified to explore potential contributing factors such as errors in insulin dilution and administration.

using a modified version of the Yale infusion protocol for a median time of 96 hours. CGM data were only used to obtain additional arterial blood samples if the rate of change in glucose exceeded 25 mg/dL per 30 minutes. Mean glucose averaged 119 +/− 17 mg/dL in the intervention group versus 122 +/− 11 mg/dL in the control group. Glucose variability and time spent at target glycemia and hypoglycemia were similar between groups. The insulin-infusion protocol provided very good control that further improvement was difficult. Therefore, CGM use did not improve glucose control, neither did it reduce hypoglycemia.

Recently, the FDA has approved the first hybrid closed loop system for insulin delivery, as these technologies become available in the outpatient setting, we anticipate increased patient's expectations in the inpatient and ICU settings.

In summary, although the current recommendations for glucose targets are widespread, evidence supporting the goal of <180 mg/dL is still lacking. Treating hyperglycemia in critically ill patients can lead to decreased morbidity and mortality. Available data suggest medical and postsurgical patients who are in the ICU more than 3 to 5 days are most likely to benefit from a lower target range, but mortality benefit is lessened or eliminated when hypoglycemic events increase. Insulin in critically ill patients should be given intravenously to allow rapid reversal of hypoglycemia if it occurs, with early data suggesting that critically ill medical and cardiac patients may be most sensitive to the effects of hypoglycemia. Insulin-infusion protocols implemented by well-trained staff can be effective ways to manage blood glucose. Paying careful attention to changes in patients' clinical condition and nutritional status, as well as vigorous glycemic monitoring by hospital staff, will minimize hypoglycemic events. Standardizing the glucose monitoring methods and using more accurate technologies may reduce hypoglycemic events and allow for safer intense glucose management, resulting in better outcomes in future trials.

SUGGESTED READINGS

American Diabetes Association. Standards of medical care in diabetes-2016. *Diabetes Care.* 2016;39:S1–S106.
  ADA summary and recommendations for diagnosing and treating diabetes and hyperglycemia.

Brunkhorst FM, Engel C, Bloos F, et al. Intensive insulin therapy and pentastarch resuscitation in severe sepsis. *N Engl J Med*. 2008;358(2):125–139.

Randomized trial demonstrating increased incidence of hypoglycemia and adverse events among patients receiving intensive glucose control.

Dellinger RP, Levy MM, Rhodes A, et al. Surviving Sepsis Campaign: international guidelines for management of severe sepsis and septic shock: 2012. *Crit Care Med*. 2013;41(2):580–637.

Recommendations from the authors of the Surviving Sepsis Campaign for glucose control in critically ill septic patients.

Fahy BG, Sheehy AM, Coursin DB. Glucose control in the intensive care unit. *Crit Care Med*. 2009;37(5):1769–1776.

A recent comprehensive review summarizing the recommendations for glucose control in critically ill patients and the evidence in support of these recommendations.

Goldberg PA, Siegel MD, Sherwin RS, et al. Implementation of a safe and effective insulin infusion protocol in a medical intensive care unit. *Diabetes Care*. 2004;27(2):461–467.

Results of a nurse-implemented insulin-infusion protocol which incorporated the velocity of glycemic change, showing it to be a safe and effective protocol for managing blood glucose in critically ill patients.

Griesdale DE, de Souza RJ, van Dam RM, et al. Intensive insulin therapy and mortality among critically ill patients: a meta-analysis including NICE-SUGAR study data. *CMAJ*. 2009;180(8):821–827.

Intensive insulin therapy significantly increased the risk of hypoglycemia and confirmed no overall mortality benefit among critically ill patients.

Handelsman Y, Bloomgarden ZT, Grunberger G, et al. American Association of Clinical Endocrinologists and American College of Endocrinology- clinical practice guidelines for developing a diabetes mellitus comprehensive care plan- 2015. *Endocr Pract*. 2015;21 (suppl 1):1–87.

Summary of current evidence and recommendations for glycemic targets in diabetic and non-diabetic critically ill patients.

Inzucchi SV. Management of hyperglycemia in the hospital setting. *N Eng J Med*. 2006;355: 1903–1911.

A review of glycemic control in hospitalized and critically ill patients, including evidence for treatment, strategies for glucose control, and current recommendations.

Kansagara D, Fu R, Freeman M, et al. Intensive insulin therapy in hospitalized patients: a systematic review. *Ann Intern Med*. 2011;154(4):268–282.

Meta-analysis demonstrating no consistent evidence to favor the use of strict glycemic control over less strict glycemic control.

Krinsley JS. Association between hyperglycemia and increased hospital mortality in a heterogeneous population of critically ill patients. *Mayo Clin Proc*. 2003;78(12):1471–1478.

Retrospective analysis of blood glucose levels in intensive care unit patients showing the lowest hospital mortality (9.6%) among patients with mean glucose values between 80 and 99 mg/dL, with mortality increasing progressively as glucose values increased (42.5% in patients with mean glucose values above 300 mg/dL).

Krinsley JS, Egi M, Kiss A, et al. Diabetic Status and the relation of the three domains of glycemic control to mortality in critically ill patients: an international multicenter cohort study. *Crit Care*. 2013;17(2):R37. doi: 10.1186/cc12547.

Retrospective analysis of prospectively collected data involving 44,964 patients admitted to 23 intensive care units (ICUs) from nine countries showed that among patients without diabetes, mean BG bands between 80 and 140 mg/dL were independently associated with decreased risk of mortality. Among patients with diabetes, mean BG from 80 to 110 mg/dL was associated with increased risk of mortality and mean BG from 110 to 180 mg/dL with decreased risk of mortality.

Malmberg K, Ryden L, Efendic S, et al. Randomized trial of insulin–glucose infusion followed by subcutaneous insulin treatment in diabetic patients with acute myocardial infarction (DIGAMI study): effects on mortality at 1 year. *J Am Coll Cardiol*. 1995;26(1):57–65.

Randomized trial of patients with acute MI showing a 29% reduction in 1-year mortality in patients assigned to intensive glucose control starting in-hospital and continuing for 3 months when compared with standard glucose control.

Imberg K, Ryden L, Wedel H, et al. Intensive metabolic control by means of insulin in patients with diabetes mellitus and acute myocardial infarction (DIGAMI 2): effects on mortality and morbidity. *Eur Heart J.* 2005;26(7):650–651.

Randomized trial of patients with acute MI comparing intensive inpatient glucose control to intensive outpatient glucose control compared to standard care which showed no difference in 1-year mortality. However, the study was underpowered and the difference in mean glucose values was small.

CE-SUGAR Study Investigators, Finfer S, Chittock DR, et al. Intensive versus conventional glucose control in critically ill patients. *N Engl J Med.* 2009;360(13):1283–1297.

A multinational study of intensive versus conventional glucose control in critically ill patients. Demonstrated increased incidences of hypoglycemia and mortality in the intensive glucose control group.

Icoke HF, Wade CE, Mann EA, et al. Anemia causes hypoglycemia in intensive care unit patients due to error in single-channel glucometers: methods of reducing patient risk. *Crit Care Med.* 2010;38(2):471–476.

to DS, Skolnick AH, Kirtane AJ, et al. U-Shaped relationship of blood glucose with adverse outcomes among patients with ST-segment elevation myocardial infarction. *J Am Coll Cardiol.* 2005;46(1):178–180.

Report on pooled data from the TIMI 10-A/B, LIMIT-AMT, and OPUS studies showing significantly higher 30-day mortality in patients with acute STEMI who had hypoglycemia (BG <81 mg/dL), with only 8.7% of the hypoglycemic patients diagnosed with diabetes.

eiser JC, Devos P, Ruiz-Santana S, et al. A prospective randomised multi-centre controlled trial on tight glucose control by intensive insulin therapy in adult intensive care units: the Glucontrol study. *Intensive Care Med.* 2009;35(10):1738–1748.

Randomized trial in a medicosurgical ICUs showed increased hypoglycemia but no change in mortality with intense (target BG 4.4 to 6.1 mmol/L) compared to intermediate (target BG 7.8 to 10.0 mmol/L) glucose control. Stopped early for protocol errors.

ott MG, Bruns DE, Boyd JC, et al. Tight glucose control in the intensive care unit: are glucose meters up to the task? *Clin Chem.* 2009;55(1):18–20.

n Den Berghe G, Wilmer A, Hermans G, et al. Intensive insulin therapy in the medical ICU. *N Eng J Med.* 2006;354(5):449–461.

Randomized trial in a medical ICU which showed significantly reduced morbidity but not in-hospital mortality in patients assigned to intensive glucose treatment (goal 80 to 110 mg/dL) compared with standard care (goal 180 to 200 mg/dL).

n Den Berghe G, Wouters P, Weekers F, et al. Intensive insulin therapy in critically ill patients. *N Engl J Med.* 2001;345(19):1359–1367.

Randomized trial in a surgical ICU which showed decreased ICU mortality in hyperglycemic patients assigned to intensive glucose treatment (goal 80 to 110 mg/dL) compared with standard care (goal 180 to 200 mg/dL).

iener RS, Wiener DC, Larson RJ. Benefits and risks of tight glucose control in critically ill adults: a meta-analysis. *JAMA.* 2008;300(8):933–944.

Tight glycemic control was not associated with reduced hospital mortality, but was associated with an increased risk of hypoglycemia.

31 Oncologic Emergencies

Eric Knoche

Cancers can cause metabolic, space occupying, and hematologic complications whi
require immediate recognition and treatment to prevent death or significant mo
bidity. This chapter will review the acute management of spinal cord compressio
tumor lysis syndrome (TLS), superior vena cava (SVC) syndrome, and leukostas
which can occur in patients with known malignancy or at initial presentation. Acu
management of other serious complications of malignancy such as airway and ga
trointestinal obstruction, cardiac tamponade, hypercalcemia, adrenal insufficien
hematologic abnormalities, increased intracranial pressure, and febrile neutropenia
discussed in other chapters.

SPINAL CORD COMPRESSION

Back pain is the most frequent presenting symptom associated with spinal co
compression. This symptom commonly precedes neurologic impairment. The pa
may be localized to the back or radiate unilaterally or bilaterally in the distributio
of spinal roots. Movement or cough can often exacerbate the pain secondary
radiculopathy. Patients may also report paresthesias such as burning, skin sensitivit
and numbness. Compression of the long sensory tracts in the cervical cord may cau
paresthesias to appear in various lower dermatomes. Motor symptoms more ofte
precede sensory symptoms. Common motor symptoms include weakness or heav
ness of the affected limbs, flaccid paralysis, and loss of bladder and bowel control.

The most important aspect of the patient's evaluation is suspicion for the pre
ence of cord compression by the examining health care provider. New-onset bac
pain in a patient at risk mandates a careful history and neurologic examination. Co
compression symptoms may present abruptly or progress gradually. In cases of grad
ual cord compression, patients may be unaware of sensory deficits but they may b
noted on neurologic exam. Regions distal to the cord compression may be weak an
hyperreflexic with up-going (extensor plantar) reflexes in the toes, while reflexes
the level of a lesion are decreased. Patients with voiding symptoms may have urinar
retention and should be evaluated by obtaining a postvoid bladder residual volume
by ultrasound examination. Anal sphincter function is usually preserved until late i
cord compression but should be evaluated by digital rectal examination. Acute, sever
cord compression can cause spinal shock, with hyporeflexia and flaccid paralysis i
all regions below the lesion.

All patients with suspected cord compression should undergo urgent spin
imaging. Magnetic resonance imaging (MRI) with contrast is the modality of choic

hen available. Contrast computed tomography (CT) or CT myelography is recom-
ended if MRI is not available or cannot be performed. It is important to image the
ntire spine, as some patients may have compression or metastases at multiple levels.
lain films and bone scans have a limited role, since they may miss the soft tissue
omponents of tumors. If the nature of the compressing mass is uncertain, surgical
r image-guided biopsy for tissue diagnosis is essential. When cord compression is
e initial presentation of cancer, further examination or imaging studies may reveal
lesion such as a lymph node, which may be more accessible for biopsy.

reatment

he general approach to the evaluation and management of the patient with spinal
ord compression is outlined in Algorithm 31.1. The importance of early recognition
nd intervention is to preserve or improve the patient's neurologic function. This is
uly a medical urgency and should receive urgent evaluation and treatment.

Corticosteroids should be started if spinal cord compression is suspected
nd may be started in the absence of a tissue diagnosis. Steroids decrease edema
ssociated with spinal cord compression and transiently improve symptoms. One
ommon approach is dexamethasone given as a loading dose of 10 mg IV or PO
llowed by 4 mg IV or PO every 6 hours. Prophylactic gastric acid suppression
with an H2 blocker or proton pump inhibitor) should be considered to prevent
e development of stress ulcers. Dexamethasone should be continued during the
itial evaluation and treatment period and then tapered over the subsequent 2 to
weeks regardless of symptom improvement. Longer duration of steroids may be
eneficial in patients with cord compression due to multiple myeloma or lymph-
proliferative disorders.

Because early studies of surgical decompression through posterior laminectomy
llowed by radiation therapy (XRT) seemed equivalent to XRT alone, external beam
RT became the treatment of choice. Commonly recommended radiation doses
ange from 2500 to 4000 cGy delivered in 10 to 20 fractions. Traditional indications
or surgical intervention have included the need for a tissue diagnosis, resection of
elatively "radioresistant" tumors, tumors primarily treated by surgery (such as sarco-
nas), spinal instability, and cord compression in a previously irradiated spine. A later
andomized study comparing surgical decompression followed by XRT to XRT alone
as led to a major change in the approach to patients with spinal cord compression.
he study was stopped after an interim analysis revealed significantly better outcomes
or patients treated surgically, with more patients remaining ambulatory (84% vs.
7%) and nonambulatory patients regaining the ability to walk (62% vs. 19%). For
hese reasons, surgery should be considered initially in all patients presenting with
ord compression. Our approach at Washington University is to have all patients pre-
enting with spinal cord compression evaluated by spine surgery, radiation oncology,
nd medical oncology to determine optimal therapy.

Hyperacute onset of neurologic symptoms and back pain suggest the possibility
f vertebral burst fracture causing bony impingement on the cord. This requires
rgent surgical intervention to remove bone fragments from the spinal canal. Patients
vith extensive bony destruction by tumor and vertebral instability may be at risk
or further compression fractures and symptom recurrence after completing XRT.
hese patients should be considered for vertebral stabilization. Surgical patients usu-
lly require 7 to 10 days for wound healing before beginning postoperative XRT.
ystemic therapy using hormonal therapy or chemotherapeutic agents should be

ALGORITHM 31.1 Approach to the Evaluation and Management of Patients with Suspected or Documented Spinal Cord Compression from Cancer

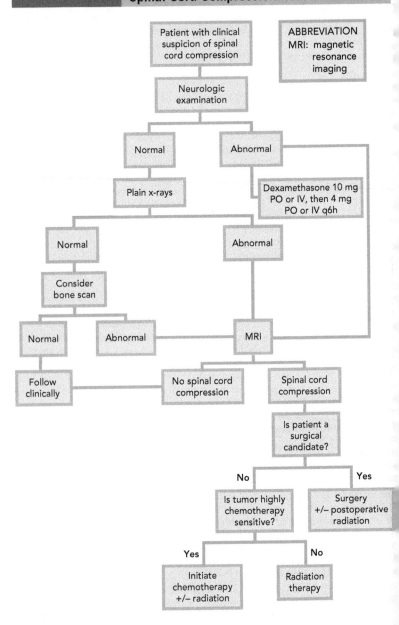

ciated when appropriate, especially in highly sensitive tumors such as prostate cancer, germ cell tumors, small cell lung cancer, multiple myeloma, and lymphoma.

TUMOR LYSIS SYNDROME

The TLS refers to the metabolic consequences resulting from the sudden release of potassium, phosphates, and purine metabolites from tumor cells undergoing cell death. TLS is classically associated with malignancies such as acute lymphoblastic leukemia (ALL) or Burkitt's lymphoma, which are characterized by a high growth fraction, present with substantial systemic tumor burden, and which respond rapidly to cytotoxic chemotherapy. Patients with other "treatment-sensitive" malignancies such as chronic lymphocytic leukemia (CLL) and small cell lung cancer and high tumor burden should also be considered at risk. TLS can, however, occur in any situation in which considerable tissue bulk is rapidly destroyed within the body and may occur after cytotoxic chemotherapy, biologic treatments, corticosteroids, radiation, and chemoembolization. Clinical manifestations are variable and should not be used to monitor the course of TLS but may include arrhythmias, mental status changes, tetany, stupor, renal failure, and even cardiac arrest from hyperkalemia. Treating physician should anticipate TLS and intervene before the patient develops symptoms or serious metabolic complications.

TLS is diagnosed by analysis of venous blood and is characterized by acute renal failure and electrolyte derangements including hyperkalemia, hyperuricemia, hyperphosphatemia, and hypocalcemia. Renal failure occurs from the precipitation of phosphate and urate salts in the renal tubules. The resulting renal impairment leads to further accumulation of phosphorus and uric acid, creating an escalating destructive cycle. In addition to patients with high-grade or bulky lymphoid malignancies (ALL, Burkitt's), patients with some degree of renal insufficiency prior to chemotherapy are at increased risk of developing TLS.

Treatment

The general approach to the prevention and management of TLS is summarized in algorithm 31.2. The best approach is prevention. Patients at high risk of TLS should volume repleted before initiating chemotherapy, and isotonic fluids should be infused at 200 to 300 mL/hr to achieve a brisk diuresis during the first 2 to 3 days of treatment. The goal of hydration is to preserve renal function and to eliminate cellular breakdown products as they are released. Patients should have blood chemistries (especially potassium, phosphorous, calcium, creatinine, uric acid, and lactate dehydrogenase [LDH]) monitored every 8 to 12 hours during the first 2 to 3 days of treatment. Furosemide may be given to maintain urine output and may also increase excretion of potassium. The utility of urine alkalization is not established, as evidence supporting its clinical benefit is lacking. In addition, urine alkalization has a theoretical risk of promoting soft tissue deposition of calcium phosphate. For this reason, we do not recommend the routine use of urine alkalization over hydration alone. In situations when urine alkalization is considered, we recommend administration of IV fluids containing 1 amp $NaHCO_3$ in 0.45% NaCl or 2 to 3 amps $NaHCO_3$ in 5% dextrose in water solution (D5W). Bicarbonate should be cautiously used in severe hyperphosphatemia, as this may exacerbate renal failure by causing calcium phosphate crystallization in the renal microvasculature and renal tubules.

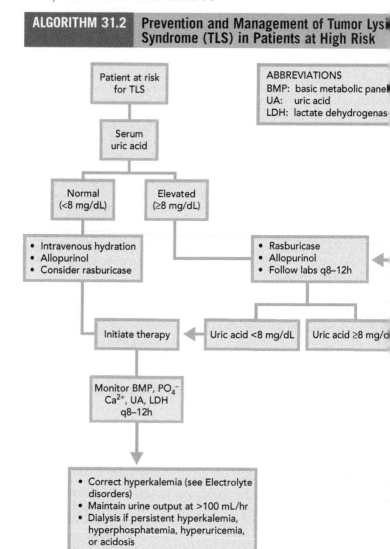

ALGORITHM 31.2 Prevention and Management of Tumor Lysis Syndrome (TLS) in Patients at High Risk

Patient at risk for TLS

↓

Serum uric acid

ABBREVIATIONS
BMP: basic metabolic panel
UA: uric acid
LDH: lactate dehydrogenase

Normal (<8 mg/dL) / Elevated (≥8 mg/dL)

Normal (<8 mg/dL):
- Intravenous hydration
- Allopurinol
- Consider rasburicase

Elevated (≥8 mg/dL):
- Rasburicase
- Allopurinol
- Follow labs q8–12h

Uric acid <8 mg/dL / Uric acid ≥8 mg/dL

Initiate therapy

↓

Monitor BMP, PO_4^- Ca^{2+}, UA, LDH q8–12h

↓

- Correct hyperkalemia (see Electrolyte disorders)
- Maintain urine output at >100 mL/hr
- Dialysis if persistent hyperkalemia, hyperphosphatemia, hyperuricemia, or acidosis

If the serum uric acid is <8 mg/dL, allopurinol should be given PO at 300 600 mg/day starting 24 to 48 hours before chemotherapy, as it requires 2 to 3 da to decrease uric acid levels. Allopurinol blocks xanthine oxidase and thus prevents t conversion of xanthine to uric acid. Xanthine is more soluble and easily excreted. T allopurinol dose should be decreased in patients with pre-existing renal insufficien and as tumor bulk decreases.

Urate oxidase (uricase) is a proteolytic enzyme absent in humans, which converts uric acid into allantoin. Allantoin is highly soluble and is readily excreted by the kidney. Recombinant urate oxidase, rasburicase, should be given to all patients with a serum uric acid level ≥8 mg/dL as well as to patients at high risk for TLS. Dosing is 0.15 to 0.2 mg/kg IV and can be repeated daily for a maximum of 7 days for uric acid levels above 8 mg/dL. Please note: repeated dosing is rarely required. Rasburicase induces a rapid decline in serum uric acid levels often with normalization of uric acid levels within 4 hours and improvement in renal function. Rasburicase also causes phosphate reabsorption, and calcium phosphate deposition can be a persistent problem requiring aggressive hydration and diuresis even after uric acid levels are undetectable.

Hyperkalemia may develop rapidly and patients at risk should have serum electrolytes checked at least every 8 to 12 hours and more frequently if TLS develops. Mild hyperkalemia (>5.5 to 6 mmol/L) may be managed with Kayexalate (sodium polystyrene sulfonate) resin and hydration. Kayexalate cation exchange resin should be avoided in the setting of hypotension and shock, as it may increase the risk of bowel ischemia. More serious hyperkalemia (>6 mmol/L or with ECG changes) may be treated acutely with 2 amps of calcium gluconate IV rapidly to stabilize the cardiac membrane potentials, followed by 50 mL of 50% glucose solution IV with 10 units regular insulin IV, to transport extracellular potassium intracellularly. This should be followed by Kayexalate to decrease total body potassium, as insulin and calcium gluconate transiently improve hyperkalemia as potassium shifts intracellularly. Other interventions for hyperkalemia including loop diuretics, bicarbonate, inhaled beta agonists, and hemodialysis should be considered based on the individually assessed risks and benefits (see "Hyperkalemia" section of Chapter 24, Electrolyte Abnormalities, for more detailed treatment).

Hyperphosphatemia may be treated with noncalcium-based phosphate binders, and patients should be placed on a renal diet with restricted phosphorous and potassium intake.

Indications for hemodialysis include volume overload, serum uric acid >10 mg/dL despite multiple doses of rasburicase, or rapidly rising phosphorus and uncontrolled hyperkalemia. Renal failure caused by TLS is usually reversible, and even patients requiring hemodialysis often regain normal kidney function as the TLS resolves.

SUPERIOR VENA CAVA SYNDROME

Patients with SVC syndrome commonly present with dyspnea, cough, headaches, chest pain, and swelling of the face, neck, and upper extremities. These symptoms may develop acutely or gradually. Bending forward or lying flat may worsen symptoms. Even in the presence of severe symptoms, patients are rarely critically ill as a result of SVC syndrome alone. While SVC occlusion is usually not a life-threatening emergency, it can cause significant discomfort and morbidity and mandates immediate attention. Potentially life-threatening complications of SVC syndrome that warrant urgent intervention are cerebral edema causing coma and laryngeal edema causing central airway obstruction.

On physical examination, dilated neck veins are usually present, as is edema of the face, arms, neck, and supraclavicular region. Gradual occlusion of the SVC allows the development of collateral veins that may be easily visible over the upper chest. The chest radiograph can reveal a right suprahilar mass or mediastinal widening but can be normal in some patients.

Contrast CT or MRI of the chest can provide information regarding the patency of the SVC. Imaging may reveal the presence of thrombus or compressive mass lesions and is useful in planning subsequent diagnostic or therapeutic interventions. A surgical or percutaneous biopsy of an accessible site should be performed in patients who present with SVC syndrome as the initial manifestation of malignancy. A tissue diagnosis is essential in the management of SVC syndrome, as the tumor type will influence the specific treatment. Only in very rare circumstance should therapy be initiated without histologic diagnosis.

Treatment

The general approach to the management of SVC syndrome is outlined in Algorithm 31.3. Radiotherapy is one of the mainstays of treatment for SVC syndrome. While success depends on the tumor type, 87% of patients respond when treated with regimens delivering 2000 cGy or more. Patients with "chemo responsive" tumors, such as germ cell carcinoma, small cell lung cancer, and lymphoma, can be treated with chemotherapy, followed by radiation if clinically indicated. Expandable vena caval stents can provide immediate relief to patients who are not expected to have a rapid response to radiation or chemotherapy and to patients who have symptom recurrence after therapy.

A subset of patients develop SVC syndrome from benign causes, and stenting should be considered in these patients. Occlusive SVC thrombosis may occur as a complication of central venous catheters. At Washington University, we generally recommend leaving the central catheter in place to prevent dislodging of the clot and initiate therapeutic anticoagulation as with any DVT. Anticoagulation should be continued as long as the patient has active cancer and for 6 months after the removal of the catheter in patients who are cancer free. Central venous catheters may also lead to stenosis of the SVC, which can be treated with fluoroscopy-guided balloon dilatation with or without stenting.

LEUKOSTASIS

Leukostasis is a syndrome usually associated with high numbers of immature leukocytes (blasts) in the peripheral circulation. Symptoms may include shortness of breath, headache, confusion, stupor, or focal neurologic deficits. Leukostasis is a clinical diagnosis, as the symptoms are nonspecific and may be attributed to infection, heart failure, or vascular disease. However, without prompt recognition and treatment, mortality rates may be as high as 40% and can occur within hours of presentation.

Leukostasis is associated with high and rapidly rising blast counts, usually over 100,000/mL, but may occur with blast counts as low as 50,000/mL. Although patients with leukostasis are frequently hypoxemic, spuriously low PaO_2 levels, commonly in the setting of normal pulse oximetry hemoglobin oxygen saturation, can result from the high metabolic rate of blasts in the arterial blood sample if the specimen is not processed in a timely fashion (leukocyte larceny). On chest radiograph, a nonspecific diffuse infiltrate is often present. There may be impairment of other end organs, including the eye, kidney, and liver. Lactic acidosis can occur as a late event. The classic pathologic finding in leukostasis is occlusive intravascular aggregates of blasts blocking the microcirculation in multiple organs, especially the lungs and the brain.

LGORITHM 31.3 **Evaluation and Management of Patients with Suspected or Confirmed Superior Vena Cava (SVC) Syndrome**

ABBREVIATION
XRT: radiation therapy

```
                              SVC
                            syndrome
                               |
                        CT or MRI evidence
                        of intrathoracic
                              mass?
              No                              Yes
               |                               |
        Central venous                   Known cancer
          catheter?                        diagnosis?
      Yes          No                  Yes          No
       |            |                   |            |
   Evidence of      |             Sensitivity to   Obtain tissue
   thrombosis?      |             chemotherapy       biopsy
  Yes      No       |
   |        |       |
 Begin    SVC fibrosis
nticoagulation present?
        Yes      No
         |        |
    Consider    Evaluate for other
    dilation    causes of upper
    +/- stent   body swelling

                        Highly          Not highly
                       sensitive         sensitive
                          |                  |
                     Chemotherapy          XRT
                       +/- XRT           +/- stent
                       +/- stent
```

Although leukostasis is most commonly seen in patients with acute leukemia sub-
pes such as myelomonocytic (M4) and monocytic (M5), it has also been described
other forms of myeloid leukemias and chronic myelogenous leukemia. It is not very
mmon in ALL or CLL even in the presence of very high lymphocyte counts.

eatment

he general approach to the patient with hyperleukocytosis is outlined in
gorithm 31.4. Initiation of leukapheresis should not be delayed while a pathologic

ALGORITHM 31.4 Evaluation and Management of Patients Presenting with Hyperleukocytosis

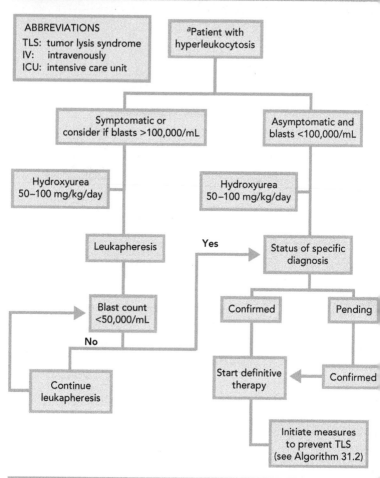

ABBREVIATIONS
TLS: tumor lysis syndrome
IV: intravenously
ICU: intensive care unit

[a]Patient with hyperleukocytosis

Symptomatic or consider if blasts >100,000/mL

Asymptomatic and blasts <100,000/mL

Hydroxyurea 50–100 mg/kg/day

Hydroxyurea 50–100 mg/kg/day

Leukapheresis

Yes

Status of specific diagnosis

Blast count <50,000/mL

Confirmed

Pending

No

Continue leukapheresis

Start definitive therapy

Confirmed

Initiate measures to prevent TLS (see Algorithm 31.2)

[a]For all patients:
- If cerebral edema is present, start dexamethasone 10 mg IV, then 4 mg every 6 hours
- If significant hypoxia, monitor in ICU and consider mechanical ventilatory support
- Correct coagulopathy if present
- Hydroxyurea should be initiated if chemotherapy not immediately planned but should not take place of definitive therapy

iagnosis is being determined. Initial management includes IV hydration, allopuri-
ol and/or rasburicase, and hydroxyurea at a dose of 50 to 100 mg/kg/day in three
ivided doses as long as the blast count remains above 50,000/mL. Red blood cell
ansfusion should be resisted if possible, even in patients with significant anemia,
s this increases whole blood viscosity and may exacerbate symptoms of leukostasis.
eukapheresis should be initiated, with a goal of rapidly reducing the blast count to
50,000/mL. Leukapheresis can attenuate or reverse the symptoms of leukostasis,
nd patients who undergo leukapheresis have a decreased incidence of central nervous
ystem complications. Since blast counts may rebound rapidly after leukapheresis, a
efinitive treatment plan must be initiated as soon as possible.

Coexisting disorders should be sought and reversed. If present, disseminated
ntravascular coagulation or thrombocytopenia should be corrected to minimize the
sk of central nervous system bleeding. Platelet counts should be monitored closely
fter leukapheresis, as the procedure often removes a significant number of platelets.
'atients suspected of having coexisting infection should have blood drawn for culture
nd be treated with broad-spectrum antibiotics, as local inflammatory processes may
ncrease the expression of cellular adhesion molecules and contribute to leukostasis,
ven in the setting of moderate blast counts.

SUGGESTED READINGS

hmann FR. A reassessment of the clinical implications of the superior vena cava syndrome.
J Clin Oncol. 1984;2(8):961–969.
> *Review of 1986 cases of SVC syndrome, where therapy was initiated without a cancer diagnosis,
> which determined that treatment without a histologic diagnosis was not advised.*

atchell RA, Tibbs PA, Regine WF, et al. Direct decompressive surgical resection in the treatment of spinal cord compression caused by metastatic cancer: a randomized trial. *Lancet.*
2005;366:643–648.
> *Randomized, multi-institutional, nonblinded trial, which randomly assigned patients with
> spinal cord compression from metastatic cancer to surgery followed by radiotherapy
> (n = 50) or radiotherapy alone (n = 51), prematurely stopped after it was found that
> decompressive surgery with postoperative radiotherapy was superior to treatment with
> radiotherapy alone (as discussed in text).*

ampello E, Fricia T, Malaguarnera M. The management of tumor lysis syndrome. *Nat Clin
Pract Oncol.* 2006;3(8):438–447.
> *Review of tumor lysis syndrome management.*

ilverman P, Distelhorst CW. Metabolic emergencies in clinical oncology. *Semin Oncol.* 1989;
16(6):504–515.
> *Review of metabolic complications of malignancy, including tumor lysis syndrome.*

anigawa N, Sawada S, Mishima K, et al. Clinical outcome of stenting in superior vena cava
syndrome associated with malignant tumors. *Acta Radiol.* 1998;39:669–674.
> *Small study of 33 patients with SVC syndrome, with 23 receiving an expandable metallic stent
> and 10 receiving radiation therapy alone. The study showed no difference in survival and
> similar improvements in clinical symptoms.*

Wilson E, Lyn E, Lynn A, et al. Radiological stenting provides effective palliation in malignant
central venous obstruction. *Clin Oncol (R Coll Radiol).* 2002;14(3):228–232.
> *Review of 18 patients presenting with SVC obstruction from tumor or thrombus, all undergo-
> ing stenting or thrombolysis, showing a mean duration of palliation of 87 days with no
> procedure-related complications.*

Zarkovic M, Kwaan HC. Correction of hyperviscosity by apheresis. *Semin Thromb Hemost.*
2003;29(5):535–542.
> *Review of apheresis principles, methods, indications for, and complications.*

32 Temperature Alterations

A. Cole Burks and Derek E. Byers

TEMPERATURE REGULATION

Temperature regulation involves a balance between heat production and dissipation. Basic metabolic processes generate heat, and various adaptive processes ranging from vasodilation and sweating to vasoconstriction and shivering help to maintain the normal core body temperature at 37°C (98.6°F). Maintenance of euthermia is controlled by the hypothalamus, the brainstem's serotonergic system, and cellular mitochondrial oxidative phosphorylation. Interruption or alterations in any of these processes can lead to temperature dysregulation.

FEVER AND HYPERTHERMIA

Fever is a preserved evolutionary response to infection. It involves an increase in the hypothalamic temperature set point resulting in an increase in body temperature. Studies have shown that immune activity is augmented at elevated temperatures, while bacterial growth is suppressed, and that blocking the body's normal increase in body temperature in response to infection (by forced cooling or antipyretic therapy) may prolong the duration of infectious symptoms. However, abnormally high fever (prolonged above 103°F/39.4°C, or any fever above 105°F/40.5°C) can have undesired consequences including seizures, disseminated intravascular coagulation, renal failure, and death.

A task force including societies in critical care medicine and infectious disease defines *fever* as a temperature ≥38.3°C (≥101°F) measured from a reliable site (oral, rectal, auditory, intravenous, or bladder thermistor). Temperatures above 38.3°C warrant a thorough physical examination to determine if infection is the cause. The initial workup should include at a minimum, two sets of blood cultures drawn from two different sterile sites, chest radiograph (especially for intubated patients), and urinalysis with microscopy. Additional cultures and testing should be ordered as indicated. See Algorithm 32.1 for more information. The decision to begin antibiotic therapy is based on the patient's clinical stability, likelihood of infection, and immune status. Immunocompromised patients should be quickly administered empiric broad-spectrum antibiotic coverage while awaiting further workup (see Chapter 40). Stable patients without an obvious infectious source may be monitored closely for fever recurrence and culture results prior to initiating therapy.

Table 32.1 lists infectious and noninfectious causes of fever and hyperthermia in the ICU. Most fevers are the result of infection, and appropriate antibiotic therapy

ALGORITHM 32.1 Workup for Fever/Hyperthermia

Temp ≥38.3°C (101°F)

↓

Review possible causes (Table 32.1)
and
Draw two sets sterile blood cultures

No obvious cause
and clinically stable

↓

Monitor closely

↓

If fever recurs →

Possible infectious source:
  Intubated
  Intravenous/arterial catheter
  Foley catheter
  Nasogastric tube
  Surgical drain
  Diarrhea

↓

Immunosuppressed
or clinically unstable

↓

Chest x-ray
Culture possible source

↓

Broad empiric antibiotic coverage based
on likely pathogens

Improvement ←   → No improvement after
48 hours or worsening

↓   ↓

Monitor closely

ABBREVIATION
CT: computed tomography

Change lines/catheters
Consider;
  Antifungal treatment
  CT imaging
  Venous dopplers
  Noninfectious cause (Table 32.1)

TABLE 32.1	Causes of Fever and Hyperthermia

Infectious Causes
- Ventilator-associated pneumonia
- *Clostridium difficile* colitis
- Intravenous catheter infection
- Urinary tract infection
- Nosocomial pathogen (gram-negative bacteria, *Candida* species)
- Sinusitis
- Abscess formation (intra-abdominal and elsewhere)
- Wound infection (decubitus ulcer)

Noninfectious Causes
- Posttransfusion
- ARDS
- Deep vein thrombus
- Chemical thrombophlebitis
- Fat embolism
- Pancreatitis
- Acalculous cholecystitis
- Subarachnoid hemorrhage
- Alcohol/drug withdrawal
- Hyperthyroidism/thyroid storm
- Acute adrenal insufficiency
- Pheochromocytoma
- Transplant rejection
- Rhabdomyolysis/tetanus
- Connective tissue diseases
- Thrombotic thrombocytopenic purpura
- Malignancy ("B symptoms")
- Central/hypothalamic fever
- Drugs (antibiotics, chemotherapeutic agents, cytokines)
- Baclofen withdrawal
- Hyperthermic syndromes:
  - Malignant hyperthermia (halothane, isoflurane, succinylcholine)
  - Serotonin syndrome (SSRIs, mixed reuptake inhibitors)
  - Neuroleptic malignant syndrome (antipsychotic phenothiazines: haloperidol, metoclopramide, and prochlorperazine)
  - Anticholinergic toxicity (atropine, TCAs, antihistamines)
  - Sympathomimetic poisoning (MAOIs, cocaine, amphetamines, methamphetamines)

ARDS, acute respiratory distress syndrome; SSRI, selective serotonin reuptake inhibitors; TCAs, tricyclic antidepressants; MAOIs, monoamine oxidase inhibitors.

should lead to improvement within a few days. However, a temperature ≥38.3° (≥101°F) can be associated with several noninfectious sources and these should considered in the initial workup to avoid unnecessary antibiotics, diagnostic testin and loss of time. Temperatures >38.9°C (>102°F) are uncommon for noninfectio auses, with the exception of drugs (including hyperthermic syndromes), transfusion eactions, and hematologic malignancies.

Damage to the hypothalamus from trauma, tumor, hemorrhage, or ischemia can aise the hypothalamic temperature set point, causing what is termed a *hypothalamic* r *central fever.* This is a true fever as opposed to a hyperthermic process. Clues to sug-est a central fever include a plateau fever curve, poor response to antipyretics, lack f sweat, and suspected or confirmed hypothalamic injury. However, hypothalamic esions are most commonly associated with hypothermia.

In contrast to fevers, hyperthermia refers to an increase in body temperature lespite normal thermoregulatory center (hypothalamic) activity, and can be due o increased heat production or decreased heat loss. Hyperthermia is not a normal physiologic response, and when left untreated, can result in serious morbidity and nortality.

Although numerous drugs can cause hyperthermia, certain drugs cause specific syperthermic syndromes. Diagnosis of drug-induced hyperthermic syndromes can e made based on medication history and clinical signs (Table 32.2). See Chapter 33 or more information regarding toxidromes including drug-induced hyperthermic yndromes.

Treatment

The priority in treating a patient with fever is to treat the underlying cause. The deci-ion to pharmacologically (i.e., antipyretics) or physically lower the body temperature s based on the cause, clinical situation, and severity of temperature elevation. Treat-nent options are listed in Table 32.3. There is no clear benefit to treating low-grade evers, and treatment can mask characteristic disease-specific fever patterns, like the ertian and quartan fevers of plasmodium infections, or the Pel–Ebstein fevers of ymphoma. Lowering the body temperature is warranted in cases of high fevers asso-iated with mental status changes, seizures, and in critically ill patients with severe underlying pulmonary or cardiovascular disease. Hyperthermic syndromes typically lo not respond well to antipyretic therapy, and as such, require removal of the incit-ng agent and targeted pharmacologic therapy as outlined in Table 32.3. In addition, external (or noninvasive) cooling methods should be started immediately, and severe cases may require internal (invasive) cooling methods.

HYPOTHERMIA

Hypothermia is defined as core body temperature <35°C (<95°F). Table 32.4 lists possible causes. Excessive cold exposure is the most common etiology in emer-gency department settings, but severe sepsis, intoxications, and endocrinopathies are frequent causes seen in the ICU. The majority of cases occur in patients with chronic underlying illness, the elderly, and in debilitated, homeless, or intoxicated patients.

Hypothermia can be divided into three grades of severity when based on a reliable core body temperature measurement: mild (32°C to 35°C [90°F to 95°F]), moderate (28°C to 32°C [82°F to 90°F]), and severe (<28°C [<82°F]). The charac-teristics of patients with mild hypothermia are shivering, cool extremities, and pallor. Shivering decreases as hypothermia worsens and moderate to severe hypothermia is characterized by depressed mental status, ataxia, cardiac arrhythmias (i.e., bradycardia or supraventricular arrhythmias), hyporeflexia, hypoventilation, dilated pupils, and

TABLE 32.2	Selected Drug-Induced Hyperthermic Syndromes				
Clinical Syndrome	Associated Precipitants	Time Course	Signs/Symptoms	Complications	Notes
Malignant hyperthermia	Volatile anesthetic gases and depolarizing paralytics (halothane, isoflurane, succinylcholine)	Minutes to hours after exposure	Dramatically high fever, muscle rigidity, tachycardia, hypercarbia	Rhabdomyolysis, hemodynamic collapse, and death	Inherited defect in skeletal muscle calcium metabolism
Serotonin syndrome	Serotonergic pathway medications (SSRI, MAOI, SNRI, TCA), linezolid, fentanyl, meperidine, dextromethorphan	Hours after exposure	Triad: 1. cognitive problems (confusion, agitation) 2. autonomic instability 3. neuromuscular abnormalities (clonus, hyperreflexia, and tremor)	Rhabdomyolysis, renal failure	Hyperthermia is present in ~50% and is due to increased muscle activity (agitation and tremor)
Neuroleptic malignant syndrome (NMS)	Neuroleptic medications (phenothiazines, haloperidol, metoclopramide, and prochlorperazine), or acute withdrawal of dopamine agonists (L-dopa)	Several hours to days after exposure	Hyperthermia, "lead-pipe" muscle rigidity, autonomic instability, and altered mental status (stupor, depression)	*Neuro:* seizures *Cardiac:* cardiac arrhythmias including torsades de pointes, cardiac arrest, MI, cardiomyopathy *Pulm:* respiratory failure, aspiration pneumonia, pulmonary embolism	Hyperthermia results from muscle activity and central hypothalamic dysregulation

				...nal dehydration, electrolyte imbalance, ARF due to rhabdomyolysis; *Heme:* DVT and phlebitis, thrombocytopenia, DIC, sepsis	
Anticholinergic toxicity	Central and peripheral muscarinic receptor blockers (antihistamines, atropine, and tricyclic antidepressants)	Hours after exposure	confusion, tremor, hallucinations, mydriasis, xerostomia, constipation, urinary retention, and coma	Similar to NMS	Hyperthermia results from decreased sweating
Sympathomimetic toxicity poisoning	MAOI and drugs of abuse (cocaine, amphetamine, methamphetamine and derivatives, i.e., ecstasy)	Hours after exposure	hyperthermia, diaphoresis, tachycardia, ataxia, insomnia, rhabdomyolysis, and seizures	Cerebral edema, seizures, cardiac arrest, ARF	Serotonergic and dopaminergic pathways involved. Central and peripheral dysregulation leads to hyperthermia

SSRI, selective serotonin reuptake inhibitors; MAOI, monoamine oxidase inhibitors; SNRI, serotonin–norepinephrine reuptake inhibitors; TCA, tricyclic antidepressants; MI, myocardial infarction; ARF, acute renal failure; DVT, deep vein thrombosis.

TABLE 32.3	Therapeutic Options for Fever and Hyperthermia

Antipyretics
 Acetaminophen (preferred if no contraindications)
 Nonsteroidal anti-inflammatory drugs

External cooling
 Cooling blankets
 Sponging
 Fans
 Ice baths

Internal cooling
 Gastric or peritoneal lavage
 Intravenous fluid replacement
 Hemodialysis
 Endovascular cooling catheter
 Sedation with paralysis if necessary

Drug-induced hyperthermia
 Remove inciting agent

Pharmacologic therapies (and specific indications)[a]
 Dantrolene (MH and NMS)
 Bromocriptine (NMS)
 Cyproheptadine (SS)
 Physostigmine (AS)
 Procainamide (VF prophylaxis in NMS)

[a]See common drug dosages and side effects in Appendix.
MH, malignant hyperthermia; NMS, neuroleptic malignant syndrome; SS, serotonin syndrome; AS, anticholinergic syndrome; VF, ventricular fibrillation.

TABLE 32.4	Causes of Hypothermia

Cold exposure
Fulminant sepsis
Drugs (alcohol intoxication, sedatives, general anesthetics, antihypertensives)
Hypothyroidism/myxedema coma
Diabetic ketoacidosis
Multisystem trauma
Prolonged cardiac arrest
Kidney failure
Liver failure
Aggressive intravenous fluid replacement
Continuous or intermittent hemodialysis
Hypothalamic lesions (multiple sclerosis)

peripheral vasoconstriction resulting in impalpable pulses. Severe cases can lead to coma, pulmonary edema, cardiac arrest, and death.

Laboratory studies may include renal failure, liver dysfunction, acidosis, and coagulopathy. Typically, electrolyte changes are unpredictable. End-organ dysfunction results from decreased cardiac output and diminished clearance of toxins and drugs. Electrocardiographic abnormalities include J (a.k.a. Osborn) waves and prolonged PR, QRS, and QT intervals. J waves are positive deflections at the QRS-ST junction in the left ventricular leads, can be found in up to 80% of hypothermic patients, and may be mistaken for new right bundle branch block. Unlike other EKG changes in hypothermia (which resolve with resolution of hypothermia), J waves can persist for 12 to 24 hours after restoration of euthermia.

Treatment

Initial treatment follows the ABCs (airway, breathing, circulation) of advanced cardiac life support and begins with removal of wet clothing, protection from heat loss, and avoiding excessive movement to prevent cardiac dysrhythmias. Patients should be connected to a cardiac monitor to identify the cardiac rhythm, as hypothermia-induced bradycardia and peripheral vasoconstriction can make palpation of peripheral pulses difficult.

Passive rewarming is usually sufficient for mild hypothermia, but aggressive active external and internal rewarming is the mainstay of therapy for more severe cases, as outlined in Table 32.5. The goal temperature increase is 1°C to 2°C (2°F to

TABLE 32.5	Therapies for Hypothermia and Expected Change in Core Body Temperature
Warming Method	Temperature (°C/hr)
Passive external	0.5–4
Blankets	
Warmed ambient environment	
Humidified inspired air	
Active external	1–4
Blankets (prewarmed or heated with forced air or fluid)	
Warm water immersion	
Warm water packs	
Active internal	Variable
Warmed (42°C) humidified air	
Warmed (42°C) intravenous fluids	
Body cavity lavage with warm saline (GI, bladder, peritoneal, pleural)	
Extracorporeal	
Hemodialysis/hemofiltration	2–3
Continuous arteriovenous rewarming	3–4
Cardiopulmonary bypass	7–10

GI, gastrointestinal.

Modified from Aslam AF, Aslam AK, Vasavada BC, et al. Hypothermia: evaluation, electrocardiographic manifestations, and management. *Am J Med.* 2006;119(4):297–301, with permission.

4°F) per hour, and should be monitored with a continuous core body temperature probe. More rapid rewarming may be necessary for patients in the event of cardiac arrest associated with severe hypothermia.

Active external rewarming alone can cause temperature "afterdrop" as cold peripheral blood is circulated back to the core. This can be avoided by the concomitant use of internal rewarming. Hypotension may occur during rewarming due to reactive peripheral vasodilation. Patients should therefore be treated with warm intravenous fluids and blood pressure should be monitored frequently. Continuous cardiac monitoring and frequent serum electrolyte tests with prompt correction can help with early detection of and minimize the risk for arrhythmias.

As hypothermia progresses the risk of cardiac arrest due to arrhythmias increases, and these arrhythmias become more refractory to cardioversion. In addition, cardiovascular drug efficacy is reduced and metabolism is decreased in hypothermic patients. As such, advanced cardiac life support management is modified in these circumstances. When the core temperature is <30°C and ventricular tachycardia or fibrillation occurs, a single initial defibrillation attempt is appropriate, but further attempts should be withheld until the core temperature is increased to >30°C. Similarly, cardioactive medications are often held until body temperatures rise above 30°C and when given, the interval between drug administrations should be increased to avoid toxic buildup.

The prognosis depends on cause, comorbidities, and complications. Mortality rates up to 100% are reported in the most severe cases but death should not be proclaimed until the patient has been successfully rewarmed.

In the patients also affected by frostbite, affected body parts should be manipulated as little as possible. Affected areas should be thawed by warm water immersion, no warmer than 40°C to 42°C. Water above this temperature can cause additional damage. Blisters may form during the rewarming process. Clear blisters can be debrided to avoid continued tissue damage, but hemorrhagic blisters should be left intact to avoid infection. Thawed body parts should be kept on sterile sheets and evaluated by a surgeon to assess tissue viability. Urgent amputation is rarely indicated, but patients should be monitored frequently for the development of compartment syndrome.

INDUCED HYPOTHERMIA AS THERAPY

Iatrogenic hypothermia can help minimize the neurologic sequelae due to ischemia–reperfusion injury to the brain following cardiac arrest, traumatic cerebral edema, or cerebral edema related to acute liver failure. The American Heart Association recommends active temperature management (<36°C) or induced hypothermia (32°C to 34°C) for comatose patients following cardiac arrest, and some medical centers have made induced hypothermia a standard of care for cerebral edema associated with traumatic brain injury, acute liver failure, and neonatal asphyxiation.

In cardiac arrest, therapeutic hypothermia should be considered for all patients who are nonresponsive and have a return of spontaneous circulation (ROSC), and fevers should be strictly avoided. Failure to actively control core body temperature to avoid hyperthermia can result in fevers and subsequent irreversible neurologic damage. Contraindications to therapeutic hypothermia include more than 8 hours since ROSC, imminent cardiovascular collapse, life-threatening bleeding or infection, an underlying terminal condition, or advanced directive precluding aggressive therapeutic measures.

Treatment protocols vary, but generally include initiation of hypothermia as ⁙n as possible by active external and/or intravascular cooling, sedation, paralysis, ⅃ mechanical ventilation with a goal core temperature of 32°C to 34°C, and at ⁙t less than 36°C. Maintenance of hypothermia is continued with close ICU mon⁙ring for up to 24 hours, and controlled rewarming (decooling) at a rate of 0.2°C ⁙0.33°C per hour may minimize hemodynamic complications. Fluid boluses, ino⁙pes, and vasopressors may be required to maintain adequate cerebral perfusion, ⅃ combinations of sedatives, analgesics, and neuromuscular blockade can help to ⁙ntrol shivering (which is counterproductive to the attainment of hypothermic tem⁙ratures). For these reasons, therapeutic hypothermia should be reserved for centers ⁙uipped to closely monitor hemodynamic and neurologic side effects that can occur.

UGGESTED READINGS

⁙5 American Heart Association Guidelines for cardiopulmonary resuscitation and emergency cardiovascular care, part 10.4: hypothermia. *Circulation.* 2005;112(suppl 24):IV136–IV138.
Current AHA guidelines for modifications of ACLS in hypothermic patients.

⁙am AF, Aslam AK, Vasavada BC, et al. Hypothermia: evaluation, electrocardiographic manifestations, and management. *Am J Med.* 2006;119(4):297–301.
A review of the causes, diagnostic signs, and management of patients with hypothermia.

⁙nnino MW, Andersen LW, Berg KM, et al; ILCOR ALS Task Force. Temperature management after cardiac arrest: an advisory statement by the Advanced Life Support Task Force of the International Liaison Committee on Resuscitation and the American Heart Association Emergency Cardiovascular Care Committee and the Council on Cardiopulmonary, Critical Care, Perioperative and Resuscitation. *Circulation.* 2015;132(25):2448–2456.

⁙dad E, Weinbroum AA, Ben-Abraham R. Drug-induced hyperthermia and muscle rigidity: a practical approach. *Eur J Emerg Med.* 2003;10(2):149–154.
A review of the drug-induced hyperthermic syndromes, help in differential diagnosis, and therapeutic options.

⁙arik PE. Fever in the ICU. *Chest.* 2000;117(3):855–869.
A review of the causes of fever in the ICU and rational approach to management.

⁙Grady NP, Barie PS, Bartlett J, et al. Practice parameters for evaluating new fever in critically ill adult patients. Task Force of the American College of Critical Care Medicine of the Society of Critical Care Medicine in collaboration with the Infectious Disease Society of America. *Crit Care Med.* 1998;26(2):392–408.
Consensus statement from a panel of 13 experts from the Society of Critical Care Medicine and Infectious Disease Society of America that provides a rational and cost-effective approach to diagnosis and management of patients with fevers in the ICU.

⁙der DB, Van der Kloot TE. Methods of cooling: practical aspects of therapeutic temperature management. *Crit Care Med.* 2009;37(suppl 7):S211–S222.
From a supplemental publication that focuses on the clinical and biologic aspects of therapeutic hypothermia and temperature management.

33 Toxicology

Jesse L. Mecham and Steven L. Brody

More than 2.1 million cases of accidental or intentional poisoning were record by U.S. poison control centers in 2015. Among fatalities, 92% were 20 years of or older. Deaths were most common following ingestion of sedatives/hypnoti antipsychotics (13.7%), cardiovascular drugs (13.3%), acetaminophen alone or combination (9.9%), opioids (7.9%), stimulants and street drugs (7.39%), alcoh (5.6%), and antidepressants (4.7%). More recently, ICU admissions and deaths fr opioids have been rapidly increasing. Although much of the initial managemen provided in the emergency department (ED), critical care physicians often sub quently manage the poisoned patient. Additionally, the intensivist may encoun iatrogenic intoxications due to drugs used in an intensive care unit.

KEY STEPS IN THE MANAGEMENT OF THE POISONED PATIENT

Algorithm 33.1 presents an outline for managing the poisoned patient.

1. Before all else, address the "ABCs" (airway, breathing, and circulation):
   - Provide oxygen, intubate and mechanically ventilate for airway protection respiratory failure
   - Obtain intravenous access and give crystalloid for hypotension. Obtain elect cardiogram (EKG) and routine labs. Obtain extra tubes of blood for serum dr and toxin levels
   - Perform a secondary trauma survey
2. Treat potentially reversible causes of altered mental status or coma with:
   - Rapid glucose assessment and treatment, if indicated
   - Thiamine 100 mg IV
   - Naloxone 0.4 to 2 mg IV/IM or 2 to 4 mg intranasal if possible opioid toxic
3. Assess for and treat toxidrome and give specific antidotes or therapy when in cated (Tables 33.1 to 33.4). Call the regional Poison Control Center at 1-80 222-1222 for management advice.
4. Block absorption of toxins when appropriate (see "Gastric Decontamination").
5. Enhance elimination of toxins when appropriate (see "Enhancing Drug Elimination

INITIAL EVALUATION

The initial assessment of the poisoned patient should begin with the ABCs: airw breathing, and circulation. Respiratory depression, loss of airway protective reflex

ALGORITHM 33.1 Key Steps in the Initial Management of the Poisoned Patient

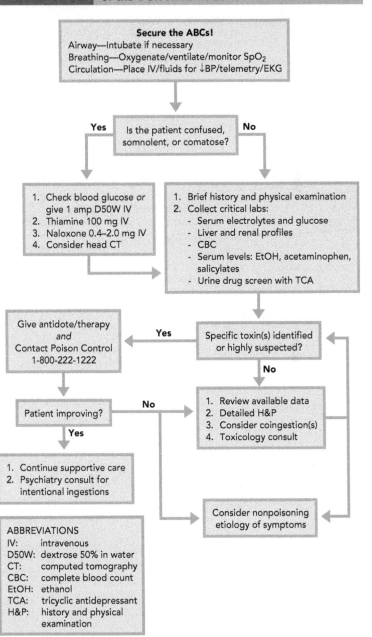

Secure the ABCs!
Airway—Intubate if necessary
Breathing—Oxygenate/ventilate/monitor SpO₂
Circulation—Place IV/fluids for ↓BP/telemetry/EKG

Is the patient confused, somnolent, or comatose?

Yes

1. Check blood glucose *or* give 1 amp D50W IV
2. Thiamine 100 mg IV
3. Naloxone 0.4–2.0 mg IV
4. Consider head CT

No

1. Brief history and physical examination
2. Collect critical labs:
   - Serum electrolytes and glucose
   - Liver and renal profiles
   - CBC
   - Serum levels: EtOH, acetaminophen, salicylates
   - Urine drug screen with TCA

Specific toxin(s) identified or highly suspected?

Yes

Give antidote/therapy *and* Contact Poison Control 1-800-222-1222

No

1. Review available data
2. Detailed H&P
3. Consider coingestion(s)
4. Toxicology consult

Patient improving?

No

Yes

1. Continue supportive care
2. Psychiatry consult for intentional ingestions

Consider nonpoisoning etiology of symptoms

ABBREVIATIONS
IV: intravenous
D50W: dextrose 50% in water
CT: computed tomography
CBC: complete blood count
EtOH: ethanol
TCA: tricyclic antidepressant
H&P: history and physical examination

TABLE 33.1	Clinical Toxidromes	
Toxidrome	Features	Offending Agents
Sympathomimetic	Hypertension, tachycardia, tachypnea, hyperthermia, mydriasis, agitation, hallucinations, diaphoresis	Cocaine Amphetamines 3,4-Methylenedi-oxymeth-amphetamine (MDMA) Bath salts Ephedrine Pseudoephedrine Theophylline Caffeine Cannabinoids Energy drinks
Anticholinergic "hot as a hare, dry as a bone, red as a beet, mad as a hatter"	Hypertension, tachycardia, tachypnea, hyperthermia, mydriasis, agitation, delirium, hallucinations, dry skin, dry mouth, ileus, urinary retention	Tricyclic antidepressants Antihistamines Atropine Phenothiazines Scopolamine Belladonna alkaloids
Cholinergic "SLUDGE"	Salivation, lacrimation, urination, diarrhea, gastrointestinal distress, emesis; also bradycardia, miosis, confusion, coma, bronchoconstriction	Organophosphates Physostigmine Pyridostigmine Edrophonium
Opioid	Hypotension, bradycardia, hypopnea, bradypnea, hypothermia, miosis, CNS depression/coma, decreased bowel sounds, pulmonary edema	Heroin Oxycodone Morphine Meperidine Fentanyl Codeine Methadone Loperamide
Sedative-hypnotic	Hypotension, bradycardia, hypopnea, bradypnea, CNS depression, coma	Benzodiazepines Barbiturates Alcohols
Extrapyramidal	Rigidity, torticollis, opisthotonos, trismus, oculogyric crisis, dysphoria	Prochlorperazine Haloperidol Chlorpromazine Other antipsychotics

TABLE 33.1	Clinical Toxidromes (*Continued*)	
Toxidrome	Features	Offending Agents
Serotonin syndrome	Triad of cognitive (agitation, confusion), autonomic (hyperthermia, diarrhea, nausea, vasoconstriction), and somatic (myoclonus, hyperreflexia) symptoms	Monoamine oxidase inhibitor Selective serotonin reuptake inhibitor (SSRI) Serotonin–norepineph-rine reuptake inhibitor (SNRI) Trazodone Opioids Amphetamines Cocaine Linezolid

TABLE 33.2	Selected Causes of an Elevated Anion Gap
Toxic Ingestions	Other Causes
Salicylate	Lactic acidosis
Ethylene glycol	Ketoacidosis
Methanol	Diabetic
Paraldehyde	Starvation
Isoniazid	Alcoholic
Iron	Uremic acidosis
	Oxoproline
	D-Lactate
Selected causes of a low anion gap	
Lithium	Hypoalbuminemia
	Elevated immunoglobulin G (IgG, e.g., myeloma)

TABLE 33.3	Selected Causes of an Elevated Osmolal Gap
With Normal Anion Gap	With Elevated Anion Gap
Isopropanol	Methanol
Acetone	Ethylene glycol
Mannitol	Formaldehyde
Diethyl ether	Paraldehyde

TABLE 33.4	Specific Antidotes for Selected Toxins
Toxin	Antidotes
Acetaminophen	N-acetylcysteine—Table 33.10
Beta blocker	Atropine 0.5 mg q3–5min, max 3 mg;
Calcium channel blockers	Glucagon 5–10 mg IV bolus followed by 1–10 mg/hr infusion; High-dose insulin IV 0.5–1.0 units/kg/hr (with dextrose); Intralipid 20% 1.5 mL/kg bolus followed by 0.25–0.5 mL/kg/min until recovery of vital signs; Consider transcutaneous pacing, cardiopulmonary bypass
Carbon monoxide	100% O_2, hyperbaric O_2 in some cases
Cholinesterase inhibitors (e.g., organophosphates)	Atropine 1–5 mg IV, repeat q5–10min for ongoing wheezing or bronchorrhea Pralidoxime 1–2 g IV over 30 min, repeat after 1 hr if ongoing weakness or fasciculations
Cyanide	Sodium nitrite 300 mg IV over 2–5 min
Digoxin	Digoxin-specific antibody fragments (Fab) Acute: 10–20 vials; chronic: 3–6 vials
Ethylene glycol Methanol	Fomepizole 15 mg/kg IV over 30 min (first dose), then 10 mg/kg every 12 hrs × 4 doses, then 15 mg/kg every 12 hrs as needed
Iron	Deferoxamine start at 5 mg/kg/hr, titrate as tolerated to 15 mg/kg/hr, max daily dose 6–8 g/day
Methemoglobinemia	Methylene blue 1–2 mg/kg IV over 5 min followed by 30-mL saline flush
Opioids	Naloxone 0.04–2 mg IV (IM, SC, or endotracheally)
Sulfonylureas	Octreotide 50 mcg SC q6h, dextrose 10% IV
Snake bite	CroFab 4–6 vials in 250 mL NS, infused over 1 hr. Double the dose if shock or serious active bleeding. Reevaluate every hour for progression of symptoms and repeat dosing until control is achieved. Call physician expert.
Tricyclic antidepressants	Sodium bicarbonate 1–2 mEq/kg bolus, followed by 1–2 mEq/kg/hr Intralipid 20% 1.5 mL/kg bolus followed by 0.25–0.5 mL/kg/min until recovery of vital signs

IV, intravenously; IM, intramuscularly; SC, subcutaneously.

d aspiration are common consequences of ingestion. Awake patients may need
ose monitoring for delayed drug effects. Lethargic patients or those with recurrent
izures may require endotracheal intubation. When in doubt, the airway should be
cured by intubation.

Ventilatory failure in the poisoned patient may be a consequence of aspiration,
spiratory depression (e.g., from sedatives), muscle paralysis/weakness (e.g., from
otulism), or pulmonary edema. Arterial blood gas (ABG) measurement may reveal
1 elevated $PaCO_2$ as a marker of early respiratory failure. Somnolence in the setting
f a rising $PaCO_2$ (detected by monitoring end-tidal CO_2) is an indication for intu-
ation. Bronchospasm may be observed in inhalational injury and other toxins, and
ronchodilators may be useful.

Arrhythmias, hypotension, and circulatory failure/shock can occur with poison-
gs. Venous access should be obtained and IV fluids given for hypotension. Con-
nuous EKG monitoring should be initiated and an EKG obtained. Pulseless or
emodynamically unstable patients should receive standard advanced cardiac life
pport therapies. However, toxin-induced cardiac arrest may at times require specific
erapies. For example, suspected calcium channel blockers may be preferentially
eated with adrenergic agonists and high-dose insulin. Also, some common ther-
pies should be avoided with certain intoxications (e.g., beta blockers in cocaine
toxication).

All patients with altered mental status should be screened for hypoglyce-
ia or treated empirically with IV dextrose (25 g or 1 amp of D50W). Thiamine
100 mg IV) and naloxone (0.4 to 2 mg IV) should also be given to these patients
or possible Wernicke's encephalopathy and opiate intoxication, respectively. Patients
eceiving thiamine should also receive IV dextrose. A head CT should be considered.

DIAGNOSTIC STRATEGIES

Important Principles

All overdoses are considered to be polysubstance overdoses until proven otherwise.
Ethanol and opiates are common components of polysubstance overdose.
The following lethal ingestions with specific therapies should always be ruled out:
- Acetaminophen (serum level)
- Tricyclic antidepressants (EKG)
- Salicylates (serum level)

Pre-existing illnesses and coingestions can confound a "classic" poisoning presentation.
Toxins screened on "drug screens" vary among institutions and are often insensitive
and nonspecific. Avoid reliance on drug screens in the face of a clinical toxidrome.

Toxidromes

A *toxidrome* is a constellation of signs and symptoms that may be seen after exposure
o a specific class of intoxicant (Table 33.1). The physical examination should be
erformed with particular attention to vital signs, mental status, pupillary size, and
sychomotor state that may suggest a specific toxidrome.

Ingestion History

An accurate accounting of the ingestion should be obtained. Specific details including
he specific drug name, the formulation (e.g., sustained release), time of ingestion

(and if acute or chronic), and quantity of ingestion should be sought. An outpatient medication profile should be established. Relevant details may come from first responders (e.g., emergency medical services) or patient contacts. Be aware that the history obtained may be unreliable or incomplete.

The Optimal Use of Laboratory Tests

Basic tests should include a comprehensive metabolic panel, complete blood cell count, coagulation studies, ethanol, acetaminophen, and salicylates. Arterial blood should be analyzed by co-oximetry in the presence of respiratory distress, altered mental status, somnolence, coma, or cyanosis. A urine toxin screen may be used to support a history of cocaine, opiate, or benzodiazepine use. Serum levels of digoxin, lithium, theophylline, phenytoin, and iron should be obtained if the patient is known to take or have immediate access to these medicines. Do not delay treatment awaiting test results if a toxic ingestion is suspected.

Be cautious with the use and interpretation of toxicology screening tests. Many substances are not included on screens for drugs of abuse, and other substances may be present but not causative. Further, depending on the timing of the ingestion, coingestions, and the sensitivity of the test used, results may be falsely negative even in the presence of intoxication. Some tests evaluate for metabolites of a drug, and others may test for only some drugs in a particular drug class (e.g., some opiate screens are negative in the presence of methadone or fentanyl). Thus, toxicology screening tests may support clinical suspicion, but management should be guided by a careful history, identification of a toxidrome, and therapy driven by clinical findings.

Evaluation of Laboratory Abnormalities

Clues to specific poisonings may be found by attention to the "three gaps": the anion gap, the osmolal gap, and the oxygen saturation gap.

Anion gap elevations may indicate the ingestion of toxins such as ethylene glycol, methanol, or salicylates. The formula for calculating the serum anion gap follows, and causes of an elevated or low anion gap are included in Table 33.2.

$$\text{Anion gap} = [Na^+] - ([Cl_2^-] + [HCO_3^-])$$

The normal range is 8 to 13 mEq/L and varies with albumin levels.

Osmolal gap elevations may be present following toxic ingestions of alcohols. The serum osmolal gap is the difference between the measured and calculated serum osmolality. Thus, an elevated osmolal gap reflects the presence of an osmotically active substance in the blood that is not accounted for by routine calculation of osmolality. Formulas necessary for calculating the osmolal gap follow, and a list of causes of an elevated osmolal gap is included in Table 33.4.

$$\text{Osm}_{\text{calculated}} = 2[Na^+] + [\text{urea}]/2.8 + [\text{glucose}]/18 + [\text{ethanol}]/4.6$$

where $[Na^+]$ is in mmol/L and [urea], [glucose], and [ethanol] are in mg/dL.

$$\text{Osmolal gap} = \text{Osm}_{\text{measured}} - \text{Osm}_{\text{calculated}} \ (\text{normal} < 10)$$

Oxygen saturation gap describes differences between oxyhemoglobin percentages as measured by pulse oximetry (SpO_2) or as estimated from arterial oxygen tension (PaO_2) when compared with the oxyhemoglobin percentage (SaO_2) as measured by co-oximetry. An oxygen saturation gap may indicate poisoning from

bon monoxide (CO), cyanide, or hydrogen sulfide, or the presence of an acquired
moglobinopathy, as occurs with methemoglobinemia. If these toxins are suspected,
erial blood must be analyzed by a co-oximeter, which is capable of measuring the
acentrations of oxyhemoglobin, deoxyhemoglobin, methemoglobin, and carboxy-
moglobin in the specimen.

REATMENT STRATEGIES

atidotes

ecific antidotes are available for relatively few toxins. Although potentially lifesav-
, many of these antidotes have adverse effects and can be harmful if used inappro-
ately. Consultation with a poison control center or a medical toxicologist is advised
en prescribing an antidote with which one is unfamiliar. A select list of antidotes
included in Table 33.4.

astric Decontamination

mong methods for blocking the absorption of drugs in the gastrointestinal (GI)
ict, activated charcoal and whole-bowel irrigation (WBI) are recommended for
e in limited circumstances. Induced emesis and cathartics are not recommended
cause of the lack of proven efficacy and interference with enterally administered
ecific antidotes. Gastric lavage is rarely indicated, such as for massive ingestion of
stained-release medications.

Single-dose activated charcoal, given orally or through a nasogastric tube,
adily binds many toxins to prevent systemic toxicity. The efficacy of activated
arcoal is greatest when given within 1 hour of ingestion and is generally ineffec-
e by 4 hours postingestion. Substances that are not well adsorbed by activated
arcoal are alcohols, iron, and lithium. Recommended single dose of activated
arcoal is 1 g/kg for adolescents and adults. Contraindications include an unpro-
cted airway and the ingestion of a hydrocarbon. Caution should be taken in the
tting of significant GI pathology or recent GI surgery.

Multiple-dose activated charcoal (MDAC) refers to the repeated enteral
lministration of activated charcoal, which may enhance the elimination of certain
xins (Table 33.5); however, evidence of efficacy is limited. Dosing regimens vary,
it a typical regimen would include a 1 g/kg loading dose, followed by 0.5 g/kg

TABLE 33.5	Potential Indications for Activated Charcoal (Severe Poisoning)
Carbamazepine	
Dapsone	
Phenobarbital	
Quinine	
Theophylline	
Contraindications	
Unprotected airway	
Coadministration of cathartic with activated charcoal	

TABLE 33.6	Potential Indications for Whole-Bowel Irrigation

Indications
Iron poisoning
Lithium poisoning
Sustained-release or enteric-coated medication toxicity
Retained illicit drug packets (i.e., from "body packing")

Contraindications
Unprotected airway (relative)
Bowel obstruction
Ileus
Bowel perforation
Uncontrolled vomiting
Hemodynamic instability
Toxic colitis

every 2 to 4 hours, for at least three doses. Cathartics should not be coadministe with MDAC.

WBI is the enteral administration of large volumes of an osmotically balan polyethylene glycol electrolyte solution to induce diarrhea with rapid expulsion unabsorbed toxins from the GI tract. No controlled studies have been publish but WBI may be considered in the management of certain ingestions (Table 33. WBI is best performed using a nasogastric tube, and a recommended regimer 1500 to 2000 mL/hr of enterally administered fluid, continued until the rectal effent is clear. Contraindications include an unprotected airway, bowel perforation obstruction, ileus, significant GI hemorrhage, toxic colitis, uncontrolled vomiti and hemodynamic instability.

Enhancing Drug Elimination

Urine alkalinization is a method of enhancing the renal elimination of certain poiso by increasing urine pH to levels ≥7.5 (e.g., pH 8.0) through the administration IV sodium bicarbonate (e.g., 1 to 2 mEq/kg IV during 3 to 4 hours). The strong indication is moderately severe salicylate toxicity not meeting criteria for hemodia sis. Other possible indications are included in Table 33.7. Potassium supplementati may be required in the setting of hypokalemia to ensure effective urine alkalinizatio Urine pH should be monitored frequently (every 1 hour initially) to ensure that t target pH ≥7.5 is reached. Serum electrolytes should be monitored every 2 to 4 hou as well. Complications of therapy include alkalemia and hypokalemia. Renal fail is a contraindication.

Hemodialysis and hemoperfusion are extracorporeal methods of toxin remo that may be required to treat life-threatening toxicity (Table 33.8). General in cations for use include clinical deterioration despite intensive alternative thera impairment of normal toxin elimination capacity (e.g., liver or renal failure), a severe toxicity from drugs that can be removed faster by extracorporeal methods th by other means. Prompt nephrology and medical toxicology consultation should obtained when hemodialysis or hemoperfusion is being considered.

TABLE 33.7 | **Potential Indications for Urine Alkalinization (With Selected Comments)**

Goal urine pH ≥8 and urine output 2–3 mL/kg/hr

Salicylates: severe cases not meeting criteria for hemodialysis

Methotrexate: consider hemoperfusion instead

2,4-Dichlorophenoxyacetic acid (2,4-D herbicide): urine pH >8, urine output >500 mL/hr

Chlorpropamide: dextrose infusion alone usually adequate

Phenobarbital: multiple-dose activated charcoal may be more effective

Diflunisal

Fluoride

Contraindications

Renal failure

TABLE 33.8 | **Selected Toxins Removable by Hemodialysis or Hemoperfusion With Potential Indications**

Hemodialysis	Indications
Salicylates	Serum salicylate level >100 mg/dL for acute ingestions; hemodynamic deterioration; persistent CNS derangement; severe acid–base or electrolyte disturbances despite appropriate therapy; renal failure; acute lung injury
Lithium	Renal failure, coma, seizures, cardiovascular instability, myoclonus
Methanol	New visual deficit, severe acidosis, level >50 mg/dL
Ethylene glycol	Severe acidosis, renal failure, level >50 mg/dL
Isopropanol	Hypotension, clinical worsening, level >400 mg/dL; rarely needed
Calcium channel blockers	Nicardipine, nifedipine, and nimodipine with severe cardiotoxicity, heart block requiring pacing, refractory hypotension
Beta blockers	Limited to acebutolol, atenolol, and especially sotalol with cardiovascular instability, renal failure
Hemoperfusion	
Barbiturates	Clinical deterioration or renal failure
Carbamazepine	Life-threatening ingestion or clinical deterioration; consider activated charcoal
Theophylline	Seizures, arrhythmias, persistent hypotension
Valproic acid	Rapid deterioration, hepatic dysfunction, level >1000 mg/L

Emerging evidence suggests a therapeutic role for intravenous lipid emulsion (e.g., lipid parenteral nutrition, 20% lipid) in overdoses with lipophilic drugs (e.g., bupivacaine, verapamil, chlorpromazine, clomipramine). It is theorized that the intravenous lipid sequesters toxins from physiologic binding sites. The American Society of Anesthesiology currently recommends 1.5 mL/kg bolus of 20% lipid followed by a 0.25 mL/kg/min infusion until hemodynamic stability is achieved. This group and the American Heart Association now recommend lipid infusion as a therapy in local anesthetic toxicity. Lipid infusion may have benefit in multiple other toxicities although data are limited.

SPECIFIC INTOXICATIONS AND MANAGEMENT STRATEGIES

The following toxins are commonly managed in the intensive care unit. In addition, drugs used in the hospital, and specifically in the intensive care unit, may result in toxicity with specific features and therapies resulting from drug combinations (e.g., linezolid contributing to serotonin syndrome), sedatives (e.g., opiates, gabapentin), propofol infusion syndrome, and others (Table 33.9).

TABLE 33.9	Hospital-Acquired Intoxications	
Drug	Clinical Setting and Symptoms	Management
Propofol infusion syndrome	History of propofol infusion with hyperlipidemia (triglycerides), lactic acidosis, hyperkalemia, renal failure, and heart failure. Associated with high mortality (30–50%).	Discontinue propofol Supportive care
Gabapentin	Confusion or lethargy, recent change in renal function.	Discontinuation of medication Hemodialysis
Propylene glycol intoxication	Prolonged infusion with medication containing propylene glycol as a preservative (e.g., lorazepam). Anion gap (lactic) metabolic acidosis, renal failure, hypotension.	Hemodialysis Supportive care
Methemoglobinemia	Multiple causes including local anesthetic toxicity (e.g., bedside Cetacaine spray left with patient), antibiotics (trimethoprim, dapsone, sulfonamide), metoclopramide, rasburicase, nitrates.	Diagnosis with co-oximetry Methylene blue

Acetaminophen

- Sx: Asymptomatic early nausea and vomiting, liver failure
- Dx: Serum acetaminophen level
- Tx: *N*-acetylcysteine (NAC), liver transplantation

The majority of acetaminophen ingestions cause no significant clinical toxicity, but life-threatening liver injury and death can occur with overdose. Acute ingestions of 150 mg/kg (or 10 g) or the chronic ingestion in excess of 4 g/day may result in clinical toxicity. The generation of a toxic metabolite, *N*-acetyl-p-benzoquinone imine (NAPQI), by the cytochrome P-450 mixed function oxidase system (specifically the CYP2E1 enzyme) in the setting of overwhelmed hepatic glutathione results in hepatic and renal injury. Induction of CYP2E1 (e.g., by ethanol, rifampin, isoniazid, or carbamazepine) or decreased glutathione stores, as occurs with chronic malnutrition from alcoholism, increases the risk for acetaminophen toxicity.

The clinical presentation of acetaminophen overdose depends on the time of presentation and amount of acetaminophen taken. Patients may be entirely asymptomatic, but early symptoms include anorexia, nausea, and vomiting. Liver injury usually occurs within 24 to 36 hours of ingestion as evidenced by elevations in blood levels of aspartate aminotransferase (AST) and alanine aminotransferase (ALT) and abnormal coagulation tests. Maximal hepatotoxicity is usually seen 72 to 96 hours after ingestion and may result in encephalopathy, coagulopathy, renal failure, hypoglycemia, and shock. Elevations in pancreatic enzymes and acute myocardial injury have also been described.

In all cases of known or potential acetaminophen overdose, the serum level of acetaminophen should be measured 4 hours after ingestion or as soon as possible thereafter and plotted against time using the Rumack–Matthew nomogram (Fig. 33.1). Plasma concentrations above the lower line ("possible risk") are an indication for treatment with NAC. Administration of NAC should not be delayed while awaiting the serum level in cases of witnessed ingestions, delayed presentation, hepatotoxicity, or pregnancy. Repeating the serum acetaminophen level should be considered in cases of ingestion of extended-release products if the initial value is below the treatment line. Although the nomogram assesses risk of toxicity with levels obtained from 4 to 24 hours post-ingestion, patients who present after 24 hours with detectable acetaminophen levels or elevated liver enzymes should receive NAC therapy while awaiting further data or input from poison control.

NAC enhances both the synthesis of glutathione (which acts as an antioxidant) as well as the conversion of acetaminophen to (nontoxic) acetaminophen sulfate, rather than NAPQI. Several different NAC protocols have been used and are of similar efficacy (Table 33.10).

A specific pitfall of acetaminophen overdose management arises in patients with chronic ingestions or an unknown time of ingestion because they cannot be plotted on the Rumack–Matthew nomogram. Considering the relatively safe profile of NAC therapy and the disastrous consequences of failing to treat acetaminophen toxicity, early NAC treatment is recommended. Any patient with a clinically suspected toxic acetaminophen ingestion with unknown time of ingestion should be treated if either: (a) the presenting acetaminophen level is detectable (even if below the Rumack–Matthew treatment line), or (b) the serum hepatic transaminases (e.g., AST) are elevated above baseline. In general, discontinuation of NAC

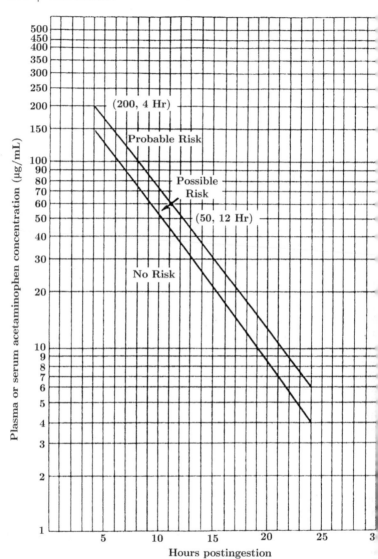

Figure 33.1. Rumack–Matthew acetaminophen toxicity nomogram. (From Green GB, Harris IS, Lin G, et al. The Washington Manual of Medical Therapeutics, 31st Edition, Philadelphia: Lippincott Williams Wilkins, 2014. Adapted from Rumack BH, Peterson RC, Koch GG, et al. Acetaminophen overdose: 662 cas with evaluation of oral acetylcysteine treatment. *Arch Intern Med.* 1981;141:380.)

TABLE 33.10	N-Acetylcysteine Protocols for the Treatment of Acetaminophen Toxicity
20-hr intravenous (IV) regimen as a continuous infusion (preferred protocol)	150 mg/kg IV given over 15 min, then 50 mg/kg IV given over 4 hrs, then 100 mg/kg IV given over 20 hrs
72-hr oral (PO) regimen	140 mg/kg PO once, then 70 mg/kg PO every 4 hrs × 17 doses
52-hr IV regimen	140 mg/kg given over 60 min, then 70 mg/kg IV every 4 hrs × 12 doses

therapy is appropriate in communication with a medical toxicologist either after a complete treatment course, normalization of serum transaminases, or clarification of the patient's ingestion history.

NAC therapy is available in both IV and oral formulations. Although neither has superior efficacy, most centers use the IV formulation for simplicity of administration. In general, NAC therapy is continued for the duration of therapy (20 hours for IV, 72 hours for oral), except in cases of hepatic failure when longer treatment is usually recommended. Severe acetaminophen toxicity resulting in fulminant hepatic failure should be managed with early hepatology consultation or transfer to a tertiary center capable of liver transplantation. A suspected suicide attempt and drug or ethanol abuse alone may not preclude transplantation, but formal psychiatric assessment may be required. The most often used predictor of the need for liver transplantation after acetaminophen overdose is the King's College Hospital criteria: (a) pH <7.25 in spite of adequate fluid resuscitation or (b) the combination of grade III to IV hepatic encephalopathy, serum creatinine >3.4 mg/dL, and prothrombin time >100 seconds. Acute renal failure is common in the setting of acetaminophen-induced fulminant hepatic failure and is likely multifactorial in nature. Intravascular volume status should be assessed.

Opioids

- Sx: Lethargy, hypercarbic respiratory failure, miosis
- Dx: Clinical diagnosis
- Tx: Naloxone, mechanical ventilation

Opioid-intoxicated patients typically present with lethargy, miosis, decreased GI motility, and respiratory depression ranging from hypoventilation to apnea. ABG analysis may reveal an elevated $PaCO_2$, and hypoxemia in severe intoxication. Hypotension (resulting from histamine release) is more common with certain agents (e.g., meperidine). Noncardiogenic pulmonary edema may occur. Seizures may occur as a result of the accumulation of the neurotoxic metabolites of certain opioids (specifically meperidine, propoxyphene, and tramadol). Acetaminophen or aspirin toxicity may complicate the patient presentation and management when combination analgesics have been ingested. Drug screens may not detect some opiate medications (e.g., fentanyl, methadone). As such, patients with a toxidrome consistent with opioid toxicity should be treated regardless of toxicology screening tests.

Management of opioid intoxication is primarily directed at ensuring adequate airway control and ventilation and the early use of the opioid antagonist naloxone.

TABLE 33.11	Half-Life of Selected Opioids
Opioid	Half-life
Codeine	3 hrs
Fentanyl	2–4 hrs (intravenous); 3–14 hrs (transdermal); 3–14 hrs (transmucosal); 15–25 hrs (nasal spray)
Heroin	2–6 min, metabolized to monoacetylmorphine in 2–6 min, then to morphine
Hydrocodone	3–4.5 hrs
Hydromorphone	2–3 hrs (immediate release); 11 hrs (extended release)
Methadone	8–59 hrs
Meperidine	2–4 hrs active metabolite 15–30 or longer with renal failure
Morphine	2–4 hrs (immediate release); 11–24 hrs (extended release)
Opium tincture	36 hrs
Oxycodone	2–4 hrs
Oxymorphone	7–9 hrs (immediate release); 9–11 hrs (extended release)
Tramadol	4–6 hrs

Naloxone is given initially at doses of 0.04 to 2 mg IV every 2 minutes until effect to a maximum of 10 mg. Naloxone should be viewed as an agent to prevent intubation, not for use after mechanical ventilation is initiated. The duration of naloxone action is 1 to 2 hours, which may be shorter than the activity of the opioid intoxicant, mandating a several hour monitoring period after response (Table 33.11). Intoxication with long-acting opioids may require repeated doses of naloxone. Continuous naloxone infusions can be used at a dose of two-thirds the original response dose per hour (dosing assistance from a pharmacist or toxicologist is recommended). Opioid-dependent patients may suffer opioid withdrawal with naloxone treatment. Pregnant patients may develop uterine contractions and induction of labor with naloxone administration. Body packers should be treated with activated charcoal, WBI, and naloxone infusion if symptomatic.

Beta Blockers

- Sx: Bradycardia, hypotension, AV blockade, confusion, hypoglycemia, hyperkalemia
- Dx: Clinical diagnosis
- Tx: Atropine, high-dose insulin, intravenous glucagon, cardiac pacing, cardiopulmonary bypass, lipid infusion

a-adrenergic receptor antagonists can result in life-threatening toxicity when taken doses even two to three times the therapeutic range. Beta blockers include agents h different degrees of beta-1, 2, and 3 receptor antagonism, additional alpha-ptor antagonism (e.g., carvedilol, labetalol), and intrinsic sympathomimetic activity. sentation and management of intoxication is generally similar for all drugs. Potential diovascular manifestations of toxicity include bradycardia and hypotension, heart ck of any degree, and cardiogenic shock. Central nervous system (CNS) toxicity luding confusion, seizures, and coma may occur, particularly with lipid-soluble medi-ions (e.g., propranolol, metoprolol, timolol). Bronchospasm can be life-threatening patients with underlying chronic obstructive pulmonary disease or asthma. Metabolic angements such as hypoglycemia and hyperkalemia may occur. Many beta blockers ve long half-lives, potentially resulting in prolonged effects. Toxicity may even be seen h ocular preparations.

Treatment is directed at the specific clinical manifestation and may include opine, isoproterenol, high-dose insulin (1 unit/kg continuous infusion), cardiac cing, and nebulized bronchodilators for bronchospasm. Refractory bradycardia or potension may be treated with glucagon, starting with a 5- to 10-mg IV bolus, lowed by continuous infusion at 1 to 10 mg/hr. Adrenergic agents such as dobuta-ne, dopamine, epinephrine, and norepinephrine may be ineffective at usual thera-utic doses. External or transvenous pacing should instead be considered early in the anagement of significant toxicity or large ingestions. Refractory cases may require modynamic support by cardiopulmonary bypass.

Activated charcoal may be useful to block absorption in early presentations. ost beta blockers have very large volumes of distribution, making them less sus-ptible to clearance by extracorporeal techniques. Acebutolol, atenolol, and sotalol e exceptions that are amenable to extracorporeal removal in cases of severe toxicity, rticularly in the patient with renal failure.

lcium Channel Blockers

Sx: Hypotension, bradycardia, AV nodal blockade, hypoglycemia, seizures
Dx: Clinical diagnosis
Tx: IV calcium, glucagon, high-dose insulin, lipid infusion, extracorporeal mem-brane oxygenation (ECMO)

lcium channel antagonists can result in significant toxicity, particularly in patients th underlying cardiovascular disease or when coingested with other cardiovascular edicines (e.g., beta blockers). Clinical manifestations of calcium channel blocker toxic-are primarily cardiovascular. Hypotension is common. Bradycardia and cardiac con-iction disturbances may occur, typically with nondihydropyridines (e.g., verapamil). contrast, dihydropyridines (e.g., amlodipine) may result in hypotension with reflex chycardia due to a lack of activity on the sinoatrial and atrioventricular nodes. oncardiovascular effects include nausea and vomiting, depressed mental status, oncardiogenic pulmonary edema, hyperglycemia, and seizures. Sustained-release eparations may result in prolonged or delayed toxicity.

Diagnosis is made based on a typical presentation with a history of ingestion. omprehensive urine toxicology screening may detect diltiazem and verapamil.

Treatment is directed at the particular manifestation of toxicity. IV fluid should e given initially for hypotension. IV calcium is given for hypotension or cardiac nduction disturbances. A typical dose is 10 mL of 10% $CaCl_2$ given over 2 to

3 minutes, with additional doses every 5 to 10 minutes for ongoing instabi
followed by continuous infusion of 10% $CaCl_2$ at 10 mL/hr. IV dopamine, nor
nephrine, or epinephrine may be needed for refractory hypotension. Glucagon
phosphodiesterase inhibitors should also be considered in these cases. Insulin-gluc
infusions (to a target serum glucose between 100 and 200 mg/dL) may be usefu
cases refractory to these measures. Invasive hemodynamic monitoring is encoura
in patients not responding to initial resuscitative measures. Severely poisoned patic
may require support using ventricular pacing, ventricular assist devices, and e
cardiopulmonary bypass, depending on the scenario.

Activated charcoal may be given to block absorption in early presentations
with sustained-release preparations. Most calcium channel blockers have large
umes of distribution and are highly protein bound, making them poor candid
for removal by hemodialysis, although lipid emulsion therapy has been describ
Nicardipine, nifedipine, and nimodipine have lower volumes of distributions a
are potentially removable by hemoperfusion in cases of severe toxicity (Table 33.8

Cocaine and Amphetamine-Related Toxins

* Sx: Sympathomimetic toxidrome
* Dx: Clinical history, urine drug screen
* Tx: Benzodiazepines and antihypertensives (except beta blockers)

Cocaine intoxication can result in life-threatening cardiovascular, pulmonary, a
CNS complications. Mechanisms of toxicity include inhibited monoamine reupt
and enhanced catecholamine release (together resulting in increased levels of catech
amines) as well as blockade of Na^+ channel activity. In addition, cocaine prome
thrombogenesis and vasoconstriction. Many features of cocaine intoxication a
management strategies are shared with amphetamine toxicity, and methamphetami
3,4-methylenedioxymethamphetamine (MDMA), and synthetic cannabinoids ("b
salts"). The clinical presentations of cocaine intoxication and sympathomime
may be quite varied. Hyperthermia, hypertension, and tachycardia are comm
Neuropsychiatric presentations may include agitation and confusion ("agitated de
ium"), dystonic reactions, acute cerebrovascular thrombosis or bleeding, and seizu
Cardiovascular complications include acute myocardial infarction and arrhythm
Pulmonary complications of cocaine include pulmonary edema (cardiogenic
noncardiogenic), alveolar hemorrhage, inhalational heat or burn injury to the aero
gestive tract mucosa, and barotrauma (e.g., pneumothorax, pneumomediastinu
from coughing or intranasally inhaling cocaine. Vasoconstriction can cause inte:
nal, hepatic, or renal ischemia. Rhabdomyolysis is common in those with agita
delirium. Cocaine or amphetamine use during pregnancy may result in fetal toxic
abruptio placentae, spontaneous abortion, and premature labor.

Urine drug-of-abuse screens may be positive for cocaine for 2 to 3 days af
use and false-negative test results can occur. Markers for cardiac injury and creatini
phosphokinase levels as well as urinalysis should be obtained in patients with sigr
icant intoxication.

Management of cocaine toxicity depends on the presentation. Benzodiazepi
(e.g., diazepam 5 to 10 mg every 5 minutes as needed) function as first-line thera
for agitation and most manifestations of toxicity. If seizures are present, IV lorazep
is recommended. Treatment of hyperthermia includes adequate sedation and, if ne
essary, external cooling. Hypertension is best treated with sedation, and if necessa

TABLE 33.12	Medications Contraindicated in the Setting of Cocaine Use
Drug or Class	Complication of Use
Pure beta blockers (absolute contraindication)	Unopposed alpha-adrenergic activity may cause hypertension or coronary vasospasm
Phenothiazines and butyrophenone anti-psychotics (absolute contraindication)	Increase seizure risk, prolong QT interval, promote dystonic reactions
Succinylcholine	Exacerbation of rhabdomyolysis-induced hyperkalemia
Class Ia antiarrhythmics (e.g., procainamide)	Increased QRS and QT prolongation and potentiate cocaine effects

calcium channel blockers (e.g., titrated clevidipine or nicardipine infusion), sodium nitroprusside, or phentolamine. Pure beta blockers are contraindicated. Other contraindicated medications are listed in Table 33.12.

Chest pain should be thoroughly evaluated. Possible causes include acute coronary events, aortic dissection, and pneumothorax. Cocaine may impair the coronary artery perfusion by vasoconstriction via alpha-adrenergic stimulation, prothrombotic effects via thromboxane, and promotion of atherosclerosis in chronic use. Cardiac ischemia occurs in at least 5% of those with cocaine use presenting to the ED, so a high index of suspicion should prompt the use of oxygen, aspirin, nitroglycerin, and benzodiazepines. An EKG and serial troponin measurements should be obtained. Further diagnostic evaluation for cardiac ischemia, (e.g., stress testing, cardiac catheterization), is pursued when there is active infarction (ST elevations) or significant clinical suspicion of fixed coronary lesions that may benefit from intervention.

Supraventricular arrhythmias are treated with calcium channel blockers (e.g., diltiazem) and pure beta blockers are contraindicated. Ventricular arrhythmias should be treated with benzodiazepines, oxygen, control of ischemia, correction of electrolytes, and if necessary, lidocaine. Class Ia antiarrhythmics (e.g., procainamide) should be avoided. Management of body packing by drug smugglers may include activated charcoal and WBI if asymptomatic, but immediate surgical removal is required in patients with any signs of cocaine intoxication, suggesting packet rupture. Attempts to retrieve drug packets by endoscopy risk drug spillage and are not recommended, particularly in the asymptomatic patient.

Alcohols

- Sx: All alcohols present similarly–ataxia, dysarthria, somnolence, respiratory depression, odor on breath
- Dx: Elevated osmolal gap, elevated anion gap (methanol, ethylene glycol), serum levels
- Tx: Fomepizole

Ethanol is widely abused and is a common component of mixed ingestions, particularly in suicide attempts. Toxicity may present with ataxia, dysarthria, CNS depression, and respiratory depression. The diagnosis should be suspected based on presence of symptoms with characteristic ethanol odor and can be confirmed b measuring the blood ethanol level. Treatment is largely supportive and is directed ensuring a patent airway and ventilation. Three nonethanol toxic alcohol ingestion are important to diagnose quickly in critically ill patients: isopropanol, methanol, an ethylene glycol. The key to diagnosis for these ingestions is maintaining a high inde of suspicion and measuring the anion and osmolal gaps.

Isopropanol is a component of rubbing alcohol and other household con pounds that may be intentionally ingested as an alternative to ethanol. Clinical mar ifestations include GI irritation, upper GI bleeding, CNS depression, respirator depression, and ketosis. Diagnosis should be considered in patients with these symp toms, particularly when presenting with fruity breath (due to acetone production unexplained ketosis (with an anion gap), or an elevated serum osmolal gap. The diag nosis can be confirmed by measuring the serum level. As with ethanol intoxicatior treatment is largely supportive. Confused or comatose patients should be screene for hypoglycemia and treated with thiamine 100 mg followed by 25 g dextrose, I\ Isopropanol may be removed by hemodialysis, but this is rarely necessary. Uppe GI bleeding should be managed with adequate volume resuscitation, correction c coagulopathies, and usual therapies for GI mucosal injury (proton pump inhibitor: endoscopic interventions as needed).

Methanol is found in many household solvents and may be ingested as a subst tute for ethanol. Patients may present initially with inebriation. After a characterist latent period of 12 or more hours, severe manifestations of toxicity including anio gap acidosis, visual disturbance, blindness, respiratory failure, seizures, and coma ma occur. Physical examination should include assessment of the pupillary light refle and funduscopic exam to assess optic nerve injury and vision. Methanol ingestio should be considered in all cases of elevated anion gap. The screening test of choic is the osmolal gap. Definitive diagnosis may be made by measuring the serum meth anol level, although later presentations may reveal undetectable methanol levels (bu elevated formate levels). Toxicity results when methanol is converted to formaldehyd and then to formate by alcohol dehydrogenase. Fomepizole (or ethanol) should b given as a competitive inhibitor of alcohol dehydrogenase in cases of methanol leve >20 mg/dL, acidemia, or an elevated osmolal gap. Fomepizole is dosed at 15 mg/kg I\ over 30 minutes, followed by 10 mg/kg IV every 12 hours for four doses, followed b 15 mg/kg IV every 12 hours as needed until the serum methanol level is <20 mg/dL Folic acid (e.g., 50 mg IV every 6 hours) should be given to promote conversion o formate to CO_2 and water. Hemodialysis should be implemented in cases of visua disturbances, serum methanol levels >50 mg/dL, or severe acidosis. Treatment shoul be initiated rapidly without waiting for definitive measurement of a methanol level.

Ethylene glycol is found in antifreeze and may be ingested during suicid attempts or as a substitute for ethanol. Early toxicity manifests with CNS depression As with methanol, delayed toxic manifestations (after 4 to 12 hours) are often mor severe and may include metabolic acidosis, renal failure, seizures, coma, and death Toxicity arises from the formation of toxic metabolites (glycolaldehyde and oxalate generated by alcohol dehydrogenase activity. Ethylene glycol should be considere in all cases of elevated anion gap and elevated osmolal gap. The patient's urine may fluoresce under a Wood's lamp (ultraviolet-A light) or reveal oxalate crystals unde microscopy. Diagnosis can be confirmed by measuring the serum level, but treatmen should not be delayed if clinical suspicion of ingestion is high. Therapy with fome pizole should be used as described for methanol poisoning. Indication for therapy includes a serum ethylene glycol levels >20 mg/dL, the presence of acidosis, or an elevated osmolal gap. Hemodialysis should be instituted in the setting of renal failure, serum level >50 mg/dL, or severe acidosis. Seizures should be treated with benzodiazepines and correction of hypocalcemia, if present.

Carbon Monoxide

Sx: Nausea and vomiting, headache, lethargy, confusion.
Dx: Exposure history, oxygen saturation gap, elevated carboxyhemoglobin.
Tx: 100% oxygen, hyperbaric oxygen (HBO_2) when indicated.

CO competes with O_2 for hemoglobin-binding sites (forming carboxyhemoglobin, COHb) and has an affinity for hemoglobin that is greater than 200 times that of O_2. Subsequently, COHb dissociates extremely slowly, resulting in inadequate oxygen delivery to peripheral tissues.

Neurologic symptoms of toxicity include headache, confusion, vision changes, and coma. Nausea and vomiting are common. Cardiac manifestations include arrhythmias and myocardial ischemia or infarction. Less commonly, rhabdomyolysis, pancreatitis, and hepatic injury may be seen. Pulmonary edema may occur as a consequence of primary cardiac disturbance or from associated smoke inhalation. Delayed neurologic manifestations (e.g., impaired concentration, amnesia, and depression) are common months later.

CO poisoning should be suspected after certain exposures (e.g., smoke or poorly ventilated car exhaust, gas stoves, and space heaters). The diagnosis can be confirmed by analyzing arterial blood by co-oximetry, which will allow measurement of COHb. Symptoms and signs of CO toxicity may correlate poorly with the measured COHb levels. Oxyhemoglobin assessments by pulse oximetry (SpO_2) or by estimates made from the partial pressure of oxygen (as reported by some ABG analyzers) can be misleading in CO poisoning. A device for measuring carboxyhemoglobin noninvasively using light transmitted through a capillary bed (similar to pulse oximetry) is available for screening but lacks accuracy, and laboratory co-oximetry confirmation is required.

The treatment of CO toxicity is 100% oxygen. The half-life of COHb varies inversely with the inspired partial pressure of O_2. For this reason, HBO_2 therapy has been used to treat CO toxicity since the 1960s. The threshold indications to institute HBO_2 therapy are not well defined, but most experts recommend this therapy for patients who have had loss of consciousness, neurologic abnormalities, cardiac ischemia, or pregnancy. There is a lower threshold for treatment of pregnant patients due to increased affinity of CO by fetal hemoglobin. The benefits of HBO_2 therapy are thought to be greatest when administered promptly (within 6 hours of exposure) to mitigate late neurologic sequelae.

Salicylates

Sx: Abdominal pain, nausea and vomiting, respiratory alkalosis, anion gap acidosis
Dx: Salicylate level
Tx: Alkalinization of the urine, hemodialysis

Salicylate toxicity results from both direct corrosive injury to the GI tract and multiple metabolic effects (e.g., respiratory stimulation, uncoupling of mitochondrial oxidative phosphorylation, inhibition of the tricarboxylic acid cycle, enhanced lipolysis with ketone generation). Patients may present with GI symptoms (e.g., abdominal

TABLE 33.13	Indications for Hemodialysis in Acute Salicylate Poisoning

Progressive hemodynamic deterioration
Persistent CNS derangement
Severe acid–base or electrolyte disturbances despite appropriate therapy
Renal failure
Acute lung injury
Serum salicylate level >100 mg/dL for acute ingestions

pain, nausea and vomiting, and GI bleeding), diaphoresis, respiratory alkalosis wi[th] anion gap metabolic acidosis, deranged glucose regulation, tachycardia, ventricul[ar] arrhythmias, pulmonary edema/acute lung injury, prolonged prothrombin tim[e,] CNS effects (e.g., agitation, confusion, seizures, and coma), tinnitus, rhabdomyolys[is] and renal failure. The clinical course may be dynamic. The finding of coincide[nt] CNS changes with tachycardia and diaphoresis suggests severe toxicity and warrar[ts] immediate and aggressive action. Many salicylate overdoses are accidental, so labo[ra]tory screening should be performed on any patient with an uncertain diagnosis wh[o] has nonspecific symptoms and a significant anion gap metabolic acidemia.

The diagnosis of salicylate exposure can be confirmed by obtaining a seru[m] salicylate level. Activated charcoal may be administered within an hour of suspected [or] confirmed salicylate poisoning unless a contraindication exists. Serum glucose shou[ld] be measured or dextrose given empirically if confusion or seizures occur. Benzodiaz[e]pines should be administered for recurrent seizures. Fluid deficits may be substant[ial] because of vomiting and insensible losses and should be treated with IV fluid. [In] addition, sodium bicarbonate should be given intravenously to a target serum p[H] of approximately 7.50 (to limit tissue redistribution of salicylate) and urine pH [of] approximately 8 (to enhance renal elimination of salicylate). Effective alkaluria w[ill] require correction of hypokalemia and potassium supplementation in the setting [of] normokalemia should be considered. ABG analysis, urine pH, and serum chemi[s]tries should be followed serially (every 1 to 4 hours) to guide therapy in the most [ill] patients. Hemodialysis is indicated in severe intoxication (see Table 33.13). Dela[y] in initiating hemodialysis when indicated may result in unnecessary morbidity ar[d] mortality.

Digoxin

- Sx: Nausea, vomiting, altered mental status, arrhythmias
- Dx: Serum digoxin level
- Tx: Digoxin-specific antibody (Fab) fragments

Digoxin toxicity may occur from acute or chronic ingestion owing to a narrow the[r]apeutic window. Digoxin and related cardiac glycosides reversibly inhibit sodium[–]potassium–ATPase, causing an increase in intracellular sodium and a decrease i[n] intracellular potassium. Changes in volume of distribution, diminished prote[in] binding from hypoalbuminemia, and renal impairment can result in decreased elim[i]ination and increased risk for toxicity. Clinical features of toxicity include anorexi[a,] nausea, vomiting, and abdominal pain; and if severe, lethargy and delirium. Chron[ic] toxicity tends to be more insidious and includes the classic visual changes of blurre[d]

sion and alterations in color vision. Cardiac toxicity, predisposing to arrhythmias, is
e most concerning effect. Digoxin toxicity may induce almost any cardiac arrhyth-
ia (except for atrial fibrillation, atrial flutter, or Mobitz II heart block). Hypokale-
ia is more common with chronic ingestion, while hyperkalemia often occurs with
ute toxicity and is correlated with increased mortality.

When digoxin toxicity is suspected, initial management includes acute stabiliza-
on, obtaining an EKG with continuous monitoring, measuring serum electrolytes
d a digoxin level. The normal therapeutic range for digoxin is 0.8 to 2.0 ng/mL;
owever, "toxic" levels have been described in asymptomatic patients, while toxicity
s also been described in the setting of "normal" levels. Symptoms of severe intoxica-
on (life-threatening arrhythmia, acute renal failure, altered mental status, or hyperka-
mia >5.5 mEq/L) are indications for treatment with digoxin-specific antibody (Fab).
vidence to support the administration of Fab in patients without these symptoms
lacking, although some advocate use when digoxin levels are >10 ng/L in acute
gestions and >4 ng/mL in chronic ingestions based on the potential to develop
mptoms. Hyperkalemia should be treated conservatively since hypokalemia can
ropagate lethal arrhythmias in the setting of high digoxin levels. Thus primary treat-
ent with bicarbonate, insulin and glucose, or ion exchange resins is seldom war-
nted. Maintenance of normal serum levels of magnesium is also important. There
no proven beneficial role for oral activated charcoal and/or hemodialysis.

on

Sx: Vomiting, diarrhea, GI bleeding
Dx: Serum iron level
Tx: Deferoxamine

on toxicity results from both direct corrosive effects to the GI mucosa and from
npairment of cellular respiration with resultant lactic acidosis. Doses of >60 mg/kg
f elemental iron are potentially lethal. Patients may initially be asymptomatic or
resent with GI symptoms or hypovolemia. After 6 to 72 hours, anion gap metabolic
cidosis, shock, hepatotoxicity, and multiorgan failure may occur. Diagnosis of iron
oisoning can be made based on an ingestion history with an appropriate clinical
resentation.

Abdominal radiographs should be obtained to evaluate for radiopaque tablets.
he serum iron level should be measured on presentation (and followed serially up to
2 hours after ingestion), with toxicity likely if the iron level is ≥450 μg/dL. WBI is
ndicated (in the absence of bowel perforation or obstruction) as the first-line method
f gastric decontamination, as activated charcoal will not adsorb iron. Patients pre-
enting with altered mental status, shock, metabolic acidosis, or serum iron levels
500 μg/dL at 4 to 6 hours after ingestion should be treated with the iron chelator
eferoxamine. Deferoxamine is given at 10 to 15 mg/kg/hr by continuous infusion
vith a recommended maximum daily dose of 6 to 8 g, and therapy should not be
elayed while awaiting iron levels in the setting of clinical toxicity. Deferoxamine may
ause infusion rate-related hypotension, and adequate IV fluid replacement is needed
s prophylaxis against acute renal failure. Deferoxamine therapy may be stopped
vhen the serum iron level normalizes (as measured by atomic absorption spectros-
opy, as deferoxamine interferes with most routine assays), when systemic toxicity
nd acidosis resolve, or when the urine is no longer reddish brown (an indication of
he presence of chelated deferoxamine–iron complex). GI or surgical consultation

is warranted in cases of tablet concretion/bezoar, continued GI bleeding, or bowel perforation.

Tricyclic Antidepressants

- Sx: Anticholinergic toxidrome (especially, tachycardia, confusion)
- Dx: Prolonged QT interval, tricyclic antidepressant (TCA) use history
- Tx: IV sodium bicarbonate

Although the use of TCAs for the treatment of psychiatric disease has declined in recent years, drugs in this class are increasingly used as a treatment for chronic pain or insomnia. TCA overdose can result in life-threatening cardiovascular and CNS effects due to the narrow therapeutic window for these agents. Toxicity may vary with the class of TCA, but amitriptyline is particularly toxic. Symptoms from TCA toxicity are a result of anticholinergic effects, alpha-adrenergic blockade, inhibition of norepinephrine and serotonin reuptake, and blockade of the fast sodium channel in myocardium, resulting in a quinidine-like effect. Cardiotoxicity may manifest with tachycardia; prolongation of the PR, QRS, or QT intervals; atrioventricular block; arrhythmias; depressed myocardial contractility; or hypotension. Seizures are a common consequence of TCA overdose and when coupled with impaired sweating, can lead to life-threatening hyperthermia.

TCA overdose should be considered in any patient with an anticholinergic toxidrome or with confusion or coma, especially if accompanied by tachycardia, QRS prolongation, rightward axis deviation of the terminal 40 ms of the QRS complex or QT interval prolongation. Specific drug levels are neither valuable nor required to make the diagnosis of acute intoxication. Qualitative urine and serum screens can retrospectively support the diagnosis of intoxication.

Initial management of TCA overdose is directed at emergent management of airway, hemodynamic instability, and treatment of ongoing seizures. Sodium bicarbonate infusion should be given as an antidote for cardiotoxicity in the setting of ventricular arrhythmias or QRS prolongation >100 ms or in the presence of hypotension with acidosis (pH <7.20). A typical regimen would be an initial bolus of 1 to 2 mEq/kg, followed by an infusion of 150 mEq of sodium bicarbonate in 1 L of D5W given at 2 to 3 mL/kg/hr IV, adjusted to a target arterial pH of 7.45 to 7.50. The benefits of sodium bicarbonate therapy are multifactorial, related in part to the effect of sodium on myocardial channels. Hypertonic saline has been used in refractory cases. Combination therapy with bicarbonate infusion and hyperventilation should be avoided because of the risk of induction of a life-threatening alkalosis and hypokalemia. Type 1a and 1c antiarrhythmics (e.g., procainamide and flecainide) should be avoided in the management of arrhythmias and lidocaine has not been shown to have efficacy. Although the evidence is limited, magnesium sulfate has been shown to be effective for TCA-induced wide complex tachycardia unresponsive to other agents. Benzodiazepines should be used to treat TCA-induced seizures, with phenytoin, barbiturates, and propofol used for refractory cases. Activated charcoal should be given if no contraindication exists. Infusion of lipid emulsion (20%) may be used (1.5 mL/kg over 1 minute, followed by an infusion of 0.25 to 5 mL/kg/hr) in unstable patients, refractory to sodium bicarbonate. Hemodialysis and hemoperfusion are not shown to be beneficial in TCA overdose. Physostigmine should not be given in the management of TCA overdose because of significant toxicity associated with use.

Synthetic Cannabis (Cannabinoids)

Sx: Variable, sympathomimetic toxidrome
Dx: Clinical history and symptoms
Tx: Supportive, benzodiazepines

Cannabinoids (i.e., K2, "Spice," synthetic marijuana) are increasingly popular in the United States. They are often purchased online (not regulated) and used by inhalation. These agents bind to the cannabinoid receptor in the brain and spinal cord. Synthetic cannabinoids are not detected with a urine drug screen, so the diagnosis is based on clinical features. Patients typically will present with tachycardia, agitation, and vomiting. Those with severe symptoms may present with hyperthermia, seizures, psychosis, cardiac ischemia, renal failure (with rhabdomyolysis), resulting in metabolic derangements. Management is supportive, as determined by the clinical features. Acute agitation should be treated with repeated dosing with benzodiazepines. Antipyretic agents are not effective, but fluids should be aggressively repleted and electrolytes monitored closely.

Dextromethorphan

Sx: Agitation, mydriasis, dizziness, and hallucinations
Dx: Clinical history and symptoms
Tx: Naloxone for respiratory depression

Dextromethorphan is a nonnarcotic derivative of morphine used as an antitussive in some over-the-counter cough and cold preparations (e.g., Robitussin DM, NyQuil Cold/Flu). It is an N-methyl d-aspartate (NMDA) receptor antagonist and sigma-1 receptor agonist, which are sites for the binding of many psychoactive drugs. As such, dextromethorphan-containing products are often intentionally abused for their psychoactive properties. Intoxicated patients may present with restlessness, mydriasis, ataxia, dizziness, and hallucinations. Psychomotor agitation, coma, and seizure can occur in more severe cases. Mixed ingestions must be ruled out as over-the-counter cold remedies often contain other ingredients (e.g., acetaminophen, aspirin). Dysphoria associated with dextromethorphan intoxication may be treated with benzodiazepines, and naloxone is partially effective for reversal of respiratory depression. A serotonin syndrome of hyperthermia, hypertension, and muscle rigidity may occur in dextromethorphan-intoxicated patients also taking monoamine oxidase inhibitors.

Snake Envenomation

Sx: Pain and swelling, coagulopathy, renal failure, paralysis
Dx: History
Tx: Antivenin, supportive

Snakebites account for approximately 1.8 to 2.5 million cases of envenomation and many as 100,000 deaths per year worldwide, but only 4000 to 6000 bites and <5 fatalities per year in the United States. The majority of bites occur in males. Most snakes are nonvenomous, and often even venomous snakes cause no clinical symptoms ("dry bites"). Venomous snakes are grouped into two families: Elapidae (eastern coral snake) and Viperidae (pit vipers: rattlesnake, water moccasin or cottonmouth, copperhead). As a general rule, venomous rattlesnakes have a triangular shaped head, elliptical pupils, and hollow, retractable fangs. Coral snakes are identified by the adage "red on yellow, kill a fellow; red on black, venom lack."

Clinical manifestations of Viperidae envenomation include rapidly increas tissue swelling, ecchymosis, nonspecific systemic symptoms (nausea, vomiting, phoresis, diarrhea, weakness), coagulopathy, rhabdomyolysis, hypotension. C snakes envenomation consists of moderate local effects with rapid onset neurot icity (ptosis, ophthalmoplegia, dysarthria, dysphagia, unusual taste, fasciculatic paralysis, seizures).

Treatments that are no longer recommended include tourniquets, prophyla antibiotics, prophylactic fasciotomy, pressure immobilization, cutting or suction the wound. Approximately 70% of all reported snake bites in the United Sta receive antivenom therapy. Be aware that exotic collectors may have snakes that not respond to CroFab antivenom.

Recommended treatment of North American snake envenomation includes access; laboratory testing including CBC, PT/PTT, fibrinogen, analgesia; and clin reevaluation every 15 minutes. The leading edge of edema should be marked, extremity elevated, and poison control or an expert in management should be c tacted to guide crotaline Fab administration. In general, if angioedema, hypotensi refractory vomiting, neurotoxicity, respiratory distress are absent, then antiven need not be given. If any of these are present, options include observation for to 24 hours with serial labs every 4 to 6 hours or administration of crotaline I antivenom (CroFab). CroFab (4 to 6 vials) is infused in saline over 1 hour. Do should be doubled if shock or serious active bleeding is present. If symptoms pre ress, initial CroFab dosing should be repeated until control is achieved, after wh maintenance antivenom dosing (2 vials every 6 hours) with accompanying labo tory testing for coagulopathy may be considered. Upon discharge, patient should advised of increased bleeding risk for at least 2 weeks.

SUGGESTED READINGS

Brent J, Burkhart K, Dargan P, et al., eds. *Critical Care Toxicology: Diagnosis and Managemen the Critically Poisoned Patient.* New York, NY: Springer; 2017.
   A comprehensive and well-referenced toxicology textbook with a critical care focus.
Brooks DE, Levine M, O'Connor AD, et al. Toxicology in the ICU: part 2: specific toxins. *Ch* 2011;140(4):1072–1085.
   Part 2 of review of toxicology in the ICU.
Fertel BS, Nelson LS, Goldfarb DS, et al. Extracorporeal removal techniques for the poiso patient: a review for the intensivist. *J Intensive Care Med.* 2010;25:139–148.
   A review of indications for extracorporeal removal of toxins.
Flomenbaum NE, Goldfrank LR, Hoffman RS, et al., eds. *Goldfrank's Toxicologic Emergenc* 9th ed. New York: McGraw-Hill; 2010.
   A classic toxicology reference.
Heard KJ. Acetylcysteine for acetaminophen poisoning. *New Engl J Med.* 2008;359:285–292
   Clearly written perspectives regarding the management of acetaminophen overdose.
Levine M, Brooks DE, Truitt CA, et al. Toxicology in the ICU: part 1: general overview a approach to treatment. *Chest.* 2011;140(3):795–806.
   Part 1 of a review of toxicology in the ICU.
Levine M, Ruha AM, Graeme K, et al. Toxicology in the ICU: part 3: natural toxins. *Ch* 2011;140(5):1357–1370.
   Part 3 of a review of toxicology in the ICU.
Olson KR, ed. *Poisoning and Drug Overdose.* 6th ed. New York: McGraw-Hill; 2012.
   A condensed and handy paperback toxicology reference.

34

Central Nervous System Infections

Caline S. Mattar and Keith F. Woeltje

Meningitis and encephalitis cause significant morbidity and mortality, often requiring intensive care unit–level care. Approximately 50% of patients with bacterial meningitis require endotracheal intubation, usually because of altered mental status. Physiologically, *meningitis* is characterized by the inflammation of the meninges surrounding the brain and spinal cord, while *encephalitis* refers to the inflammation within the brain parenchyma. Clinically, patients with encephalitis are more likely to have altered level of consciousness or confusion, although the clinical presentations of encephalitis and meningitis overlap considerably. The distinction between meningitis and encephalitis has important implications in the etiology, treatment, and prognosis of the illness. Table 34.1 identifies the most common etiologies of meningitis and encephalitis.

The initial evaluation of patients with any type of suspected central nervous system (CNS) infection usually takes place outside the intensive care unit, but a thorough understanding of the workup is essential. An approach to the initial evaluation of CNS infections is presented in Algorithm 34.1. The sensitivity of the classic triad of fever,

TABLE 34.1	Common Etiologies of Meningitis and Encephalitis
Type	Etiology
Bacterial meningitis	*Streptococcus pneumoniae*
	Neisseria meningitidis
	Haemophilus influenzae
	Listeria monocytogenes[a]
Viral meningitis	Enteroviruses[b]
	HSV
	Lymphocytic choriomeningitis virus
Encephalitis	Enteroviruses[b]
	HSV
	Arboviruses[b]
	West Nile virus
	St. Louis encephalitis virus
	Eastern equine virus
	Western equine virus

[a]More common in patients >50 years of age and immunocompromised individuals.
[b]Seasonal predominance in summer and fall.
HSV, herpes simplex virus.

ALGORITHM 34.1 Initial Evaluation for Possible Central Nervous System (CNS) Infection

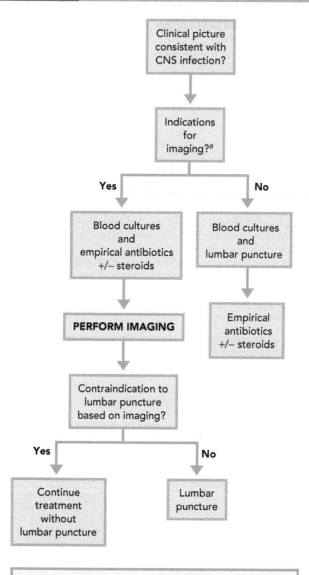

^aHistory of CNS disease, history of recent seizure, altered level of consciousness, new focal neurologic deficits, or neurologic deficits in the setting of immunosuppression.

neck, and altered mental status in predicting bacterial meningitis is <50%, but absence of all three symptoms makes CNS infection unlikely. In one large series 493 episodes of meningitis, fever was found to be present in 95% of patients at sentation, neck stiffness in 88% of cases, and altered mental status in 78% (mostly argy and confusion). Retrospective studies have shown that almost all patients with terial meningitis have at least two of four critical symptoms, including fever, neck fness, headache, and altered mental status. Until the diagnosis of CNS infection is firmed or rejected, antimicrobials should be administered empirically.

There is little evidence to suggest that imaging prior to lumbar puncture impacts nagement or outcomes in patients with CNS infection. Clinical and historical fea- es suggestive of possible abnormalities on computed tomography include history CNS disease, history of recent seizure, altered level of consciousness, new focal urologic deficits on examination, or neurologic findings in the setting of immuno- pression. Many physicians will perform imaging in the presence of these findings. e presence of an abnormality on imaging is not predictive of brain herniation, a -threatening complication of lumbar puncture, and the decision to obtain imaging uld never delay the initiation of empirical antimicrobial treatment.

Because clinical history and physical examination can be unreliable in diagnos- CNS infection, analysis of cerebrospinal fluid (CSF) is crucial. CSF findings are ential in distinguishing bacterial from viral causes of infection. When performed an experienced technician, Gram stain of the CSF is positive in approximately % to 75% of cases of bacterial meningitis. Sensitivity of the test varies by organism; is positive in 90% of untreated cases of *Streptococcus pneumoniae* versus 30% to % of cases of *Listeria* meningitis. Although receipt of antibiotics prior to lumbar ncture will decrease the sensitivity of the cultures, antibiotic treatment should not delayed to increase culture yield.

In addition to routine Gram stain and culture, CSF should be examined for cose and protein quantitation, and cell count should be examined from the last be of fluid obtained. Although rarely seen, cryptococcal meningitis may present acute meningitis even in immunocompetent individuals. A cryptococcal antigen ay should be ordered on all patients. Fungal, viral, and acid-fast bacilli cultures are ry low yield in the setting of acute meningitis or encephalitis and should not be utinely ordered. The laboratory can hold a quantity of CSF for additional testing if dicated from the initial CSF findings. Typical CSF findings for viral and bacterial eningitis as well as encephalitis are presented in Table 34.2.

Encephalitis caused by herpes simplex virus is most often seen in young children d individuals older than 50 years. Patients may present with altered level of con- ousness, focal cranial nerve findings, or focal seizures and may have abnormal tem- ral lobe findings on imaging. Because herpes simplex virus encephalitis is associated th high morbidity and mortality when treatment is delayed, patients aged 50 years d older with symptoms of encephalitis should be given acyclovir empirically until e results of CSF polymerase chain reaction for herpes virus are obtained. Table 34.3 tlines specific recommendations for empirical and specific treatment regimens of NS infection.

The use of adjuvant steroids in the treatment of bacterial meningitis remains con- oversial. A Cochrane meta-analysis published in 2015 did not show any difference in ortality between patients who received steroids and those who did not. A subgroup alysis however, did show that mortality was decreased in patients with *S. pneumoniae* eningitis but not with *Haemophilus influenzae* or *Neisseria meningitidis*. In that same

TABLE 34.2	CSF Findings in Meningitis and Encephalitis		
CSF Finding	Bacterial Meningitis	Viral Meningitis	Encephalitis
WBC/mm³	≥1000	100–10,000	<250
Differential	PMN predominance (≥80%)	Lymphocyte predominance[a] (≥50%)	Lymphocyte predominance
Protein	>250	50–250	<150
CSF to serum glucose ratio	≤0.4	Normal to decreased	>0.5
Opening pressure (mm Hg)	>200	Usually normal	Normal to slight increased

[a]May have neutrophilic predominance initially.
CSF, cerebrospinal fluid; WBC, white blood cell; PMN, polymorphonuclear cells.

TABLE 34.3	Treatment Recommendations for CNS Infection
Etiology	Suggested Therapy
Empirical	Vancomycin 10–15 mg/kg IV q8h[a] PLUS Ceftriaxone 2 g IV q12h Addition of steroids if indicated[b] If ≥50 years, addition of ampicillin 2 g IV q4h[a] If suspicion for HSV, addition of acyclovir 10 mg/kg q8h[a]
Streptococcus pneumoniae	If PCN MIC ≤1 µg/mL, ceftriaxone 2 g IV q12h If PCN MIC ≥2 µg/mL OR ceftriaxone MIC ≥1 µg/mL, vancomycin 10–15 mg/kg IV q8h[a] AND Ceftriaxone 2 g IV q12h
Neisseria meningitidis	If PCN MIC <0.1 µg/mL, ampicillin 2 g IV q4h[a] If PCN MIC ≥0.1 µg/mL, ceftriaxone 2 g IV q12h
Listeria monocytogenes	Ampicillin 2 g IV q4h[a] If PCN allergy, use trimethoprim/sulfamethoxazole 5 mg/kg q8h[c]
Viral meningitis	Supportive measures
Herpes encephalitis	Acyclovir 10 mg/kg IV q8h[a]
Other viral encephalitis	Supportive measures

[a]Dose adjustment required for impaired renal function.
[b]Dexamethasone 0.15 mg/kg every 6 hours × 4 days.
[c]Dosing based on trimethoprim component.
IV, intravenous; HSV, herpes simplex virus; PCN, penicillin; MIC, mean inhibitory concentration.
Adapted from Infectious Diseases Society of America Guidelines.

dy, steroids were shown to reduce severe hearing loss in high-income countries only. urrently, the recommendation based on the Infectious Diseases Society of America idelines is to administer steroids to all patients with suspected or proven pneumo- ccal meningitis. However, since improvement in clinical outcomes using steroids in cterial meningitis due to other pathogens (e.g., *N. meningitidis*, *H. influenzae*) is not ident, it is not recommended as the preferred therapy. Although in patients with spected or proven *S. pneumoniae* meningitis, steroids prior to, or concurrent with, e initial dose of antibiotics should be given, timely diagnosis of definite bacterial eningitis and prompt pathogen identification is a challenge. The benefit of steroids arted after antibiotics is less certain, although one study suggests that it may be ben- icial in patients with microbiologically proven diseases.

Nosocomial meningitis accounts for only 0.4% of all hospital infections and almost ways occurs in the setting of neurosurgical intervention. In contrast to community- quired bacterial meningitis, nosocomial meningitis is typically caused by gram-negative ganisms, coagulase-negative staphylococcal species, or *Staphylococcus aureus*. Empirical eatment should include vancomycin for gram-positive organisms plus cefepime, ceftazi- me, or meropenem to cover the possibility of aerobic gram-negative bacilli including eudomonas aeruginosa. Recommendations regarding length of treatment are often ised on historical practices rather than specific evidence from clinical trials. Given the ariable absorption of certain oral antimicrobials, treatment should be given intrave- ously for the duration of therapy. The choice of intravenous antimicrobial therapy for icterial meningitis is also influenced by its penetration to CSF. Suggested lengths of eatment for various CNS infections are shown in Table 34.4.

There is often confusion about the need for isolation in patients diagnosed ith meningitis. Two common causes of bacterial meningitis, *H. influenzae* and *. meningitidis*, are spread via large particle droplets >5 μm in size. Infection with ther of these organisms warrants droplet precautions for the first 24 hours of treat- ient. Health care workers, who examine (i.e., funduscopic exam) or perform proce- ures (intubation, bronchoscopy, and suctioning endotracheal secretes) on patients ith suspected bacterial meningitis, should wear surgical mask to prevent potential xposure to droplet particles. Individuals entering the room should wear standard iasks when working within 3 ft of the patient as well. Patient movement should be imited if possible; however, if transport is required, the patient should wear a mask to

TABLE 34.4	Suggested Length of Therapy for CNS Infection by Etiology
Etiology	Length of Treatment (days)
Listeria monocytogenes	≥21
Gram-negative bacilli	21
Group B *Streptococcus*	14–21
HSV encephalitis	14[a]
Streptococcus pneumoniae	14
Haemophilus influenzae	7
Neisseria meningitidis	7

Extend therapy to 21 days if there is immunosuppression.
HSV, herpes simplex virus.
Adapted from Infectious Diseases Society of America Guidelines.

minimize potential spread of infection. Because the etiology of bacterial meningitis typically unknown at the time of presentation, all patients with suspected mening should initially be placed on droplet precautions in addition to standard precaution

SUGGESTED READINGS

Brouwer MC, McIntyre P, Prasad K, et al. Corticosteroids for acute bacterial meningitis. *Coch Database Syst Rev.* 2015; CD004405. doi: 10.1002/14651858.CD004405.pub5.

> *A systematic review of 25 studies looking at benefits of steroids in bacterial meningitis. Fin ings showed that steroids did not affect mortality but decreased neurologic sequelae high-income countries only.*

de Gans J, van de Beek D; European Dexamethasone in Adulthood Bacterial Mening Study Investigators. Dexamethasone in adults with bacterial meningitis. *N Engl J Me* 2002;347(20):1549–1556.

> *A recent, randomized, placebo-controlled trial of adjuvant steroid therapy in bacterial meni gitis concluding that early steroid therapy decreases mortality and morbidity in patier with bacterial meningitis.*

Durand ML, Calderwood SB, Weber DJ, et al. Acute bacterial meningitis in adults. A review 493 episodes. *N Engl J Med.* 1993;328(1):21–28.

> *A review of 493 episodes of meningitis, suggesting a high proportion of nosocomial infectio and reporting clinical findings on presentation.*

Flores-Cordero JM, Amaya-Villar R, Rincón-Ferrari MD, et al. Acute community-acquire bacterial meningitis in adults admitted to the intensive care unit: clinical manifestation management and prognostic factors. *Intensive Care Med.* 2003;29(11):1967–1973.

> *A focused look at patients with bacterial meningitis requiring admission to the intensive ca unit suggesting that clinical course of disease over the first 24 hours of hospitalization a major predictor of morbidity and mortality.*

Hasbun R, Abrahams J, Jekel J, et al. Computed tomography of the head before lumbar pun ture in adults with suspected meningitis. *N Engl J Med.* 2001;345(24):1727–1733.

> *Large prospective study of CT scan prior to lumbar puncture in patients with clinical suspici of meningitis that shows certain clinical features are predictive of normal head CT patients with suspected meningitis.*

Korinek AM, Baugnon T, Golmard JL, et al. Risk factors for adult nosocomial meningitis aft craniotomy: role of antibiotic prophylaxis. *Neurosurgery.* 2006;59(1):126–133.

> *Brief review of nosocomial meningitis with evaluation of perioperative antibiotic prophylax Findings demonstrate that antibiotic prophylaxis at the time of neurosurgery improv surgical site infection rates but does not have significant impact on rates of postoperativ meningitis.*

Nguyen TH, Tran TH, Thwaites G, et al. Dexamethasone in Vietnamese adolescents and adul with bacterial meningitis. *N Engl J Med.* 2007;357(24):2431–2440.

> *A recent, randomized controlled trial for dexamethasone use in patients with bacterial men ingitis concluded that the dexamethasone does not improve outcome for patients wit suspected bacterial meningitis although the benefit of dexamethasone use was observe for patients with microbiologically proven bacterial meningitis even those who receive the prior antibiotic treatment.*

Palabiyikoglu I, Tekeli E, Cokca F, et al. Nosocomial meningitis in a university hospital betwee 1993 and 2002. *J Hosp Infect.* 2006;62(1):94–97.

> *Retrospective evaluation of 51 cases of nosocomial meningitis which showed the major ris factor for hospital-acquired meningitis was neurosurgical procedure. The most commo causative organisms were gram-negative bacilli and Staphylococcus species.*

Rotbart HA. Viral meningitis. *Semin Neurol.* 2000;20(3):277–292.

> *Complete review of all aspects of viral meningitis including epidemiology, pathogenesis, clinica presentations, diagnosis, and treatment options.*

ar JJ. The evolving epidemiology of viral encephalitis. *Curr Opin Neurol.* 2006;19(4):350–357.

    A current look at emerging causes of viral encephalitis which shows ongoing transmission of West Nile Virus in the United States and explores transfusions and transplants as potential sources of transmission for viral encephalitis.

kel AR, Hartman BJ, Kaplan SL, et al. Practice guidelines for the management of bacterial meningitis. *Clin Infect Dis.* 2004;39(9):1267–1284.

    A thorough review of evidence-based treatments for bacterial meningitis with evaluation and treatment guidelines endorsed by the Infectious Diseases Society of America.

de Beek D, de Gans J, Tunkel AR, et al. Community-acquired bacterial meningitis in adults. *N Engl J Med.* 2006;354(1):44–53.

    An up-to-date review of recent studies and advances in bacterial meningitis including management of complications.

de Beek D, Drake JM, Tunkel AR. Nosocomial bacterial meningitis. *N Engl J Med.* 2010; 362(2):146–154.

    A thorough review of current evidence of nosocomial meningitis.

35 Community-Acquired Pneumonia

Lemuel R. Non and Rupa R. Patel

Community-acquired pneumonia (CAP) has an annual incidence of about 5 to 11 cases per 1000 persons. Although mortality is relatively low (<1%) for nonhospitalized patients, the 30-day mortality among hospitalized patients can be as high as 23%, with the majority of deaths occurring in patients admitted to the intensive care unit (ICU). It is essential to determine if the patient truly has CAP as opposed to health care–associated pneumonia (HCAP). CAP refers to pneumonia that occurs in the community or within 48 hours of hospital admission, and lacks risk factors for HCAP. Please see Chapter 36 for the HCAP criteria.

An essential step in managing patients with CAP is the initial assessment of severity, which could guide diagnostic and treatment decisions. The physician assessment supplemented by severity-of-illness scores, such as the CURB-65 criteria (1 point each for: confusion, BUN >7 mmol/L [>20 mg/dL], respiratory rate ≥30, systolic blood pressure <90 mm Hg or diastolic blood pressure ≤60 mm Hg, age ≥65 years) or prognostic models, such as Pneumonia Severity Index (PSI) can be used to identify CAP patients who may need hospitalization (Table 35.1). Hospitalization is recommended for patients with CURB-65 scores ≥2. Direct admission to the ICU is recommended for patients with severe CAP. The American Thoracic Society and the Infectious Diseases Society of America (ATS/IDSA) CAP guidelines define severe CAP as patients presenting with any of the major criteria or at least three minor criteria (see Table 35.2). The decision to admit a patient to the ICU can have significant implications since studies have shown that patients who are admitted to a hospital ward but later require admission to the ICU have a higher morbidity and mortality than patients directly admitted to the ICU.

Streptococcus pneumoniae remains the most commonly identified cause of CAP, although its frequency is declining, in part due to the widespread use of pneumococcal vaccines and decreased rates of cigarette smoking. Other pathogens implicated in CAP include *Haemophilus influenzae, Staphylococcus aureus, Moraxella catarrhalis, Pseudomonas aeruginosa,* other gram-negative bacilli, and atypical bacteria (*Mycoplasma pneumonia, Legionella pneumophila,* and *Chlamydophila pneumoniae*). Viruses, such as influenza, respiratory syncytial virus, parainfluenza, human metapneumovirus, adenovirus, coronavirus, and rhinovirus, have also been implicated in CAP.

While not recommended for all patients with CAP, routine testing to determine the etiology of CAP is recommended for hospitalized patients or in those suspected to have pathogens that would alter decisions regarding empirical treatment. These tests should at least include Gram staining and culture of sputum or endotracheal aspirate

TABLE 35.1	Criteria for Severe Community-Acquired Pneumonia[a]

Major criteria
  Invasive mechanical ventilation
  Septic shock with the need for vasopressors

Minor criteria
  Respiratory rate ≥30 breaths/min[b]
  PaO_2/FIO_2 ratio ≤250[b]
  Multilobar infiltrates
  Confusion/disorientation
  Uremia (BUN level ≥20 mg/dL)
  Leukopenia from infection (WBC count <4000 cells/mm³)
  Thrombocytopenia (platelet count <100,000 cells/mm³)
  Hypothermia (core temperature <36°C)
  Hypotension requiring aggressive fluid resuscitation

[a]Patients who meet one major criterion or at least three minor criteria are recommended to be admitted to the ICU.
[b]Noninvasive ventilation can be substituted for respiratory rate ≥30 breaths/min or PaO_2/FIO_2 ratio ≤250.
Adapted from Mandell LA, Wunderink RG, Anzueto A, et al. Infectious Diseases Society of America/American Thoracic Society consensus guidelines on the management of community-acquired pneumonia in adults. *Clin Infect Dis.* 2007;44:S27–72.

for intubated patients, blood cultures, *Legionella* and pneumococcal urinary antigens, and multiplex PCR assays for *Mycoplasma pneumonia, Chlamydophila pneumonia,* and respiratory viruses. For patients who undergo bronchoscopy, bronchial washings, and bronchoalveolar lavage can be sent and tested for Gram stain, cultures, and multiplex polymerase chain reaction (PCR) assays as above. Antibiotic therapy should not be delayed in favor of collecting samples for laboratory testing. Sputum culture results are particularly helpful when an organism that is not part of the normal flora is recovered. Blood cultures should preferably be obtained prior to the administration of antibiotics. Obtaining blood cultures within 24 hours of admission has been shown to reduce mortality simply because resistant pathogens are identified earlier with the availability of culture results. A *Legionella* urine antigen test is recommended for all immunocompromised patients with CAP or any patient with severe CAP admitted to the ICU. This diagnostic test only detects *Legionella pneumophila* serogroup 1, so a negative result does not rule out *Legionella* pneumonia. A pneumococcal urinary antigen assay may also help in the diagnosis of pneumococcal pneumonia. However, this test is not as reliable as the *Legionella* urine antigen assay because it only has a sensitivity of 50% to 80%. Finally, during influenza season, rapid antigen or PCR assay testing for presence of influenza A or B virus is recommended for both treatment and epidemiologic purposes.

For patients deemed adequate for outpatient treatment (i.e., those with nonsevere pneumonia, CURB-65 score <2, and those who can reliably take oral medications) and no comorbidities, macrolides or doxycycline is recommended. Patients with other comorbidities, such as diabetes mellitus, chronic renal and liver disease, heart failure, and other immunocompromising conditions, respiratory fluoroquinolone

TABLE 35.2	Antibiotic Recommendations for the Intensive Care Unit Patient With Bacterial Community-Acquired Pneumonia
No risk factors for *Pseudomonas* or CA-MRSA	Recommended antibiotics β-Lactam[a] + azithromycin OR β-Lactam[a] + respiratory fluoroquinolone[b] OR Respiratory fluoroquinolone[b] + aztreonam (if penicillin allergic)
Risk factors for *Pseudomonas* infection present[c]	Recommended antibiotics Antipseudomonal β-lactam[d] + ciprofloxacin OR levofloxacin (750-mg dose) OR Antipseudomonal β-lactam[d] + an aminoglycoside + azithromycin OR Antipseudomonal β-lactam[d] + an aminoglycoside + respiratory fluoroquinolone[b] OR Aztreonam + an aminoglycoside + respiratory fluoroquinolone[b] (if penicillin allergic)
Risk factors for CA-MRSA infection present[e]	Vancomycin or linezolid (daptomycin cannot be used)

[a]Cefotaxime, ceftriaxone, ampicillin-sulbactam.
[b]Levofloxacin (750 mg) or moxifloxacin.
[c]Severe structural lung disease (e.g., bronchiectasis, severe COPD), recent antibiotic therapy, recent stay in the hospital, malnutrition, chronic corticosteroid therapy (e.g., prednisone >10 mg/day).
[d]Cefepime, piperacillin-tazobactam, imipenem, or meropenem.
[e]End-stage renal disease, prior known colonization with CA-MRSA, injection drug use, or prior recent viral influenza infection.
DRSP, drug-resistant *Streptococcus pneumoniae*.
CA-MRSA, community-acquired methicillin-resistant *Staphylococcus aureus*.
Adapted from Mandell LA, Wunderink RG, Anzueto A, et al. Infectious Diseases Society of America/American Thoracic Society consensus guidelines on the management of community-acquired pneumonia in adults. *Clin Infect Dis*. 2007;44:S27–72.

(e.g., moxifloxacin, levofloxacin) or a β-lactam plus macrolide is preferred. For patients who are hospitalized in a non-ICU setting, respiratory fluoroquinolone or β-lactam plus macrolide can be given. Patients admitted to the ICU should receive at least the combination of a β-lactam plus macrolide, which should cover the overwhelming majority of pathogens associated with CAP. In the rare instance that community-acquired methicillin-resistant *S. aureus* (CA-MRSA) or *P. aeriginosa* is suspected based on epidemiologic patterns and clinical presentation, anti-MRSA (vancomycin or linezolid) or antipseudomonal antibiotics, respectively, should be given and diagnostic tests should be pursued. In patients with complicated influenza infection, oseltamivir or zanamavir is recommended, ideally within 48 hours of symptoms set. In patients with influenza for whom bacterial superinfection is considered, ibiotic coverage for *S. aureus,* such as with ceftriaxone or an anti-MRSA antibiotic ncomycin or linezolid), should be considered as there are high rates of coinfection th this organism. Daptomycin does not achieve therapeutic concentrations in lung and should not be considered for *S. aureus* pneumonia treatment. Serum ocalcitonin level, which has been found to have a high negative predictive value excluding concomitant bacterial infection in patients with viral pneumonia, can o be used to guide discontinuation or withholding of antibiotics.

In patients admitted to the hospital, the first dose of the antibiotic should be ministered at the first point of contact; in hospitalized patients, the first dose ould be given in the emergency department. In terms of duration of therapy, a cent prospective trial has shown that 5 days of antibiotic therapy was as effective as 0-day course. A meta-analysis has also shown that patients treated with antibiotics r 7 days or less and patients treated with 8 days or more showed no differences in tcomes. The recommendation for treatment is usually for 5 to 7 days in patients to are receiving treatment in the outpatient setting or in hospitalized patients th prompt response. CAP from *S. aureus* or gram-negative bacilli tend to cause ore severe disease than the usual pathogens, so clinicians generally choose a more olonged course. *S. aureus* pneumonia is generally treated for 2 to 4 weeks; *S. aureus* AP with bacteremia, without evidence of endocarditis, is usually treated for weeks. Patients should be assessed daily and treatment should be switched from ' to oral when they are clinically improving, hemodynamically stable, and are able ingest medications.

If there is clinical deterioration after 24 hours of therapy, several possibilities ould be considered. Infection with a pathogen not covered by the empiric antibi- ic regimen or with resistant pathogen is a major cause of apparent antibiotic fail- e, which could be addressed by a reassessment of microbiologic results. Antibiotic erapy should be tailored based on culture and sensitivity results. Further testing for her pathogens can be performed as indicated by specific risk factors or exposures. he patient's history should be reviewed again for certain exposures: cattle, sheep, or at for *Coxiella burnetii,* birds for *Chlamydophila psittaci,* and rabbits for tularemia. espiratory tract viruses are common causes of pneumonia. Viral pneumonia may severe in the elderly, immunocompromised, or patients with chronic obstructive ng disease and other comorbid illnesses. Although the results are varied, previous idies have shown that 4% to 39% of patients hospitalized for CAP have evidence a viral infection. There should also be a low threshold in screening for human munodeficiency virus (HIV) infection, especially those with epidemiologic risk ctors, as HIV predisposes to a whole gamut of opportunistic pathogens that can use pneumonia, such as *Pneumocystis jirovecii, Nocardia,* tuberculosis, cryptococcus, id endemic mycosis.

Complications of CAP should also be suspected in patients who fail to respond initial therapy. About 10% of patients with pneumococcal pneumonia have met- tatic diseases such as meningitis, arthritis, endocarditis, and peritonitis. A parap- eumonic effusion or empyema may require drainage with a chest tube. A repeat est x-ray or a computed tomography scan may be warranted in patients who fail respond to therapy. Finally, noninfectious causes such as pulmonary embolus and/ infarction, lung malignancy, hypersensitivity pneumonitis, granulomatosis with olyangiitis (Wegener's granulomatosis), acute respiratory distress syndrome (ARDS), ilmonary edema, or eosinophilic pneumonia can be misdiagnosed as CAP.

SUGGESTED READINGS

Gadsby NJ, Russell CD, McHugh MP, et al. Comprehensive molecular testing for respiratory pathogens in community-acquired pneumonia. *Clin Infect Dis.* 2016;62(7):817–823.
  Comprehensive molecular testing improves pathogen detection in those with CAP, potentially leading to early deescalation from empiric therapy to pathogen-directed therapy.

Isturiz R, Webber C. Prevention of adult pneumococcal pneumonia with the 13-valent pneumococcal conjugate vaccine: CAPiTA, the community-acquired pneumonia immunization trial in adults. *Hum Vaccin Immunother.* 2015;11(7):1825–1827.
  Large, randomized, and placebo-controlled trial demonstrating efficacy of the pneumococcal conjugate vaccine (PCV13) in adults 65 years and older.

Jain S, Self WH, Wunderink RG, et al. Community-acquired pneumonia requiring hospitalization among U.S. adults. *N Engl J Med.* 2015;373:415–427.
  Population-based surveillance study showing the incidence of CAP requiring hospitalization in the adult population.

Longo DL, Musher DM, Thorner AR, et al. Community-acquired pneumonia. *N Engl J Med.* 2014;371(17):1619–1628.
  Review article on current understanding, clinical presentation, diagnosis, and treatment of CAP.

Mandell LA, Wunderink RG, Anzueto A, et al. Infectious Diseases Society of America/American Thoracic Society consensus guidelines on the management of community-acquired pneumonia in adults. *Clin Infect Dis.* 2007;44 Suppl 2:S27–S72.
  Guideline from the Infectious Diseases Society of American and the American Thoracic Society on CAP in adults.

Rodríguez AH, Avilés-Jurado FX, Díaz E, et al. Procalcitonin (PCT) levels for ruling-out bacterial coinfection in ICU patients with influenza: A CHAID decision-tree analysis. *J Infect.* 2015;72(2):143–151.
  Secondary analysis from a prospective, multicenter study showing the potential utility of procalcitonin in the ICU setting in excluding coinfection in influenza-infected patients.

36

Nosocomial Pneumonia

Kristen Fisher and Marin H. Kollef

ospital-acquired pneumonia (HAP) is defined as a nosocomial pneumonia (NP) that
:curs 48 hours or more after hospital admission, which was not incubating at the time
° hospital admission and is not associated with mechanical ventilation (Table 36.1).
entilator-associated pneumonia (VAP) refers to NP that develops more than 48
⸱ 72 hours after endotracheal intubation. Prevention strategies for HAP and VAP
iould be routinely employed to minimize the occurrence of this nosocomial infection
[able 36.2). It is important to thoroughly evaluate patients with suspected NP in order
⸱ exclude other conditions that can mimic the presentation of NP (Table 36.3). NP is
ne second most common nosocomial infection in the United States after urinary tract

TABLE 36.1	Definitions of Pneumonia[a] (With Focus on Bacterial Pathogens)
Pneumonia Category	Definition
Community-acquired pneumonia (CAP)	Patients with a first positive bacterial culture obtained within 48 hrs of hospital admission lacking risk factors for health care–associated pneumonia
Health care–associated pneumonia (HCAP)	Patients with a first positive bacterial culture within 48 hrs of admission and any of the following: admission source indicates a transfer from another health care facility (e.g., hospital, nursing home); receiving hemodialysis, wound, or infusion therapy as an outpatient; prior hospitalization for at least 3 days within 90 days; immunocompromised state due to underlying disease or therapy (human immunodeficiency virus, chemotherapy)
Hospital-acquired pneumonia (HAP)	Patients with a first positive bacterial culture >48 hrs after hospital admission
Ventilator-associated pneumonia (VAP)	Mechanically ventilated patients with a first positive bacterial culture >48 hrs after hospital admission or tracheal intubation, whichever occurred first

Criteria for pneumonia include new or progressive lung infiltrate and at least two of the following
inical criteria: hyperthermia or hypothermia, elevated white blood cell count, purulent tracheal
ecretions or sputum, and worsening oxygenation.

TABLE 36.2 Strategies for the Prevention of Nosocomial Pneumonia

Strategy	Recommendation	Evidence Level
Orodigestive decontamination[a] (Topical/topical plus intravenous antibiotics)	No	1
Oral chlorhexidine[b]	—	—
Aerosolized antibiotics[a]	No	1
Intravenous antibiotics[a]	No	1
Specific stress ulcer prophylaxis regimen	No	1
Short-course antibiotic therapy (when clinically applicable)	Yes	1
Routine antibiotic cycling/rotation/heterogeneity[c]	No	2
Use of noninvasive positive pressure ventilation in select populations	Yes	1
Avoid reintubation	Yes	2
Minimize sedation	Yes	2
Spontaneous awakening trials daily	Yes	1
Assess readiness to extubate daily	Yes	1
Early mobility	Yes	2
Avoid patient transports	Yes	2
Orotracheal intubation preferred for airways	Yes	1
Orogastric intubation preferred for feeding tubes	Yes	2
Routine ventilator circuit changes	No	1
Use of heat–moisture exchanger	Yes	1
Closed endotracheal suctioning	Yes	1
Subglottic secretion drainage	Yes	1
Shortening the duration of mechanical ventilation	Yes	1
Adequate intensive care unit staffing	Yes	2
Silver-coated endotracheal tube	Yes	1
Polyurethane endotracheal tube cuff	Yes	1
Semierect positioning	Yes	1
Rotational beds	Yes	1
Chest physiotherapy	No	1
Early tracheostomy	No	1
Use of protocols/bundles incorporating multiple prevention elements	Yes	2

[a]Routine antibiotic prophylaxis not recommended due to potential emergence of antibiotic-resistant bacteria.
[b]Because of concerns related to excess mortality a firm recommendation cannot be provided to recommend routine use.
[c]May be useful in specific clinical circumstances (as an adjunct to controlling an outbreak of a multidrug-resistant bacterial infection).
Evidence levels: 1, supported by randomized trials; 2, supported by prospective or retrospective cohort studies.

TABLE 36.3	Noninfectious Causes of Fever and Pulmonary Infiltrates Mimicking Nosocomial Pneumonia

Chemical aspiration without infection
Atelectasis
Pulmonary embolism
Acute respiratory distress syndrome
Pulmonary hemorrhage
Lung contusion
Infiltrative tumor
Radiation pneumonitis
Drug reaction
Cryptogenic organizing pneumonia

infection, but is the leading cause of mortality attributed to nosocomial infections. The incidence of NP is between 5 and 10 cases per 1000 hospital admissions and, although the incidence of VAP is difficult to determine because of differences in the case definition, it is estimated that 9% to 27% of patients undergoing mechanical ventilation for 48 hours are affected. "Attributable mortality" from NP is estimated to be between 5% and 15%, with the higher mortality occurring in patients with bacteremia or infections with *Pseudomonas aeruginosa* or *Acinetobacter* species (Table 36.4).

The American Thoracic Society and the Infectious Diseases Society of America published guidelines for the management of adults with HAP and VAP pneumonia

TABLE 36.4	Most Common Pathogens Associated With Various Pneumonia Categories
Infection Site	**Pathogens**
Pneumonia (immunocompetent) 1. Community-acquired pneumonia (nonimmunocompromised host)	*Streptococcus pneumoniae* *Haemophilus influenzae* *Moraxella catarrhalis* *Mycoplasma pneumoniae* *Legionella pneumophila* *Chlamydia pneumoniae* Methicillin-resistant *Staphylococcus aureus* (MRSA) Influenza virus/other respiratory viruses[a]
2. Health care–associated pneumonia	Methicillin-resistant *S. aureus* *Pseudomonas aeruginosa* *Klebsiella pneumoniae* *Acinetobacter* species *Stenotrophomonas* species *L. pneumophila*

(continued)

TABLE 36.4	Most Common Pathogens Associated With Various Pneumonia Categories (Continued)
Infection Site	Pathogens

Infection Site	Pathogens	
3. Pneumonia (immunocompromised host)		
a. Neutropenia	Any pathogen listed above *Aspergillus* species *Candida* species	
b. Human immunodeficiency virus	Any pathogen listed above *Pneumocystis carinii* *Mycobacterium tuberculosis* *Histoplasma capsulatum* Other fungi Cytomegalovirus	
c. Solid-organ transplant or bone marrow transplant	Any pathogen listed above (Can vary depending on timing of infection to transplant)	
d. Cystic fibrosis	*H. influenzae* (early) *S. aureus* *Pseudomonas aeruginosa* *Burkholderia cepacia*	
4. Lung abscess	*Bacteroides* species *Peptostreptococci* *Fusobacterium* species *Nocardia* (in immunocompromised patients) Amebic (when suggestive by exposure)	
5. Empyema	*S. aureus* *S. pneumoniae* Group A Streptococci *H. influenzae*	Usually acute
	Anaerobic bacteria *Enterobacteriaceae* *M. tuberculosis*	Usually subacute or chronic

[a]Respiratory syncytial virus (RSV), parainfluenza virus, adenovirus, human metapneumovirus, corona virus, rhinovirus/enterovirus.

in 2016. The definition of health care–associated pneumonia was removed from the most recent guidelines with a recommendation to base antibiotic decisions based upon the institution's individual resistance patterns. However, this is controversial as it remains important to recognize individuals who are at risk for multidrug-resistant infections. Recommendations for the antibiotic management of NP as summarized in Table 36.5 and Algorithm 36.1. It is imperative for clinicians treating patients with suspected NP to prescribe initial antimicrobial regimens that are likely to be active against the offending pathogen in order to optimize the outcome. Clinicians

Category of Pneumonia	Organisms	Empiric Therapy	Additional Information
HCAP/HAP/VAP Not at Risk for MDR pathogens and hospitalized <5 days	Nonmultidrug-resistant (MDR) potential pathogens: *Streptococcus pneumonia* *Haemophilus influenza* Methicillin-sensitive *Staphylococcus aureus* *Escherichia coli* *Klebsiella pneumoniae* *Enterobacter* species *Proteus* species *Serratia marcescens*	Third-generation cephalosporin (ceftriaxone) Or Ampicillin–sulbactam Or Respiratory fluoroquinolone (levofloxacin or moxifloxacin) Or Nonantipseudomonal carbapenem (ertapenem)	Azithromycin should be considered for atypical coverage in very ill patients or ones with a high suspicion for atypical organisms or *Legionella* who are not on a respiratory fluoroquinolone.
HCAP/HAP/VAP At Risk for MDR pathogens or hospitalized for =>5 days	Potential MDR pathogens: *Pseudomonas aeruginosa* *Klebsiella pneumonia* (extended-spectrum β-lactamase+) *Acinetobacter* species *Legionella pneumophila* Methicillin-resistant *S. aureus*	Antipseudomonal cephalosporin (cefepime, ceftazadime) Or Antipseudomonal carbapenem (imipenem or meropenem) Or Antipseudomonal penicillin with β-lactamase inhibitor (pipercillin–tazobactam, ceftazidime-avibactam, or ceftolozane-tazobactam) Plus Aminoglycoside (gentamycin, tobramycin, or amikacin)[b] Plus Anti-MRSA agent (linezolid, vancomycin, or ceftaroline)	Carbapenems are often effective against ESBL organisms (*E. coli, Klebsiella*) or Acinetobacter. Antipseudomonal cephalopsporin with β-lactamase inhibitor (Ceftazidime-avibactam or ceftolozane-tazobactam) can be used for multidrug-resistant infections but should be reserved only for culture-proven infections. For patients with penicillin allergy consider substituting β-*lactam* with: • Aztreonam • Meropenem (<1% cross reactivity to penicillin allergy) Inhaled antibiotics (colistin and aminoglycosides) have been used in select populations and should be used only after consultation with a subspecialist.

[a]Clinicians should be aware of the prevailing bacterial pathogens associated with nosocomial pneumonia and the antibiotic susceptibility patterns of these pathogens locally in order to optimize clinical outcomes.

[b]Aminoglycoside is recommended as the choice of additional coverage for patients at risk of multidrug-resistant pathogens over fluoroquinolones as most institutions have high resistance rates for fluoroquinolones.

ALGORITHM 36.1 A Step-by-Step Approach to the Management of Nosocomial Pneumonia

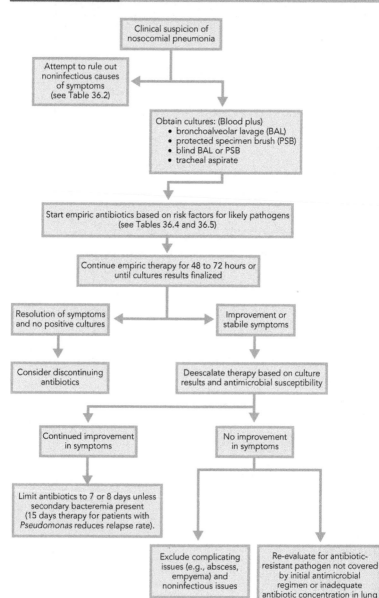

uld be aware of the prevailing bacterial pathogens associated with NP, and their imicrobial susceptibility, in order to optimize antimicrobial treatment. Once the hogens and antimicrobial susceptibilities are known, narrowing or deescalation of antimicrobial regimen can occur.

UGGESTED READINGS

erican Thoracic Society; Infectious Diseases Society of America. Guidelines for the management of adults with hospital-acquired, ventilator-associated, and healthcare-associated pneumonia. *Am J Respir Crit Care Med.* 2005;171(4):388–416.
Management guidelines for nosocomial pneumonia.

astre J, Fagon JY. Ventilator-associated pneumonia. *Am J Respir Crit Care Med.* 2002;165(7): 867–903.
State-of-the-art review of nosocomial pneumonia.

il AC, Metersky ML, Klompas M, et al. Management of adults with hospital-acquired and ventilator-associated pneumonia: 2016 clinical practice guidelines by the Infectious Diseases Society of America and the American Thoracic Society. *Clin Infect Dis.* 2016;63(5):e61–e111.

mpas M, Branson R, Eichenwald EC, et al. Strategies to prevent ventilator-associated pneumonia in acute care hospitals: 2014 update. *Infect Control Hosp Epidemiol.* 2014;35(8): 915–936.

rrow LE, Kollef MH. Recognition and prevention of nosocomial pneumonia in the ICU and infection control in mechanical ventilation. *Crit Care Med.* 2010;38(8 Suppl):S352–S362.

res A, Niederman MS, Chastre J, et al. International guidelines for the management of hospital-acquired pneumonia (HAP) and ventilator-associated pneumonia (VAP). Guidelines for the management of HAP/VAP of the European Respiratory Society (ERS), European Society of Intensive Care Medicine (ESCIM), European Society of Clinical Microbiology and Infectious Diseases (ESCMID) and Asociación Latino-americana del Tórax (ALAT). *Eur Respir J.* (In Press).

37 Cellulitis/Fasciitis/ Myositis

Jason P. Burnham

Severity of illness due to skin and soft tissue infections (SSTIs) loosely correlate with depth of skin structure involvement. Terminology based on anatomic dep continues to be widely used (Fig. 37.1). Patients with superficial infections involvi only the epidermis and dermis, such as impetigo, ecthyma, erysipelas, folliculi furuncles, and carbuncles rarely need admission to the intensive care unit. In co trast, deeper soft tissue infections, including cellulitis, fasciitis, and myositis, a associated with significant morbidity and mortality, particularly in immunoco promised hosts.

CELLULITIS

Cellulitis is an acute bacterial infection involving the skin and subcutaneo tissue that is characterized by diffuse-spreading erythema and can be associat with lymphangitis. The disease most commonly involves the lower extremiti other areas that may be affected include the periorbital regions, areas near bo piercings, incisions, puncture wounds ("skin-popping"/illicit drug injection site

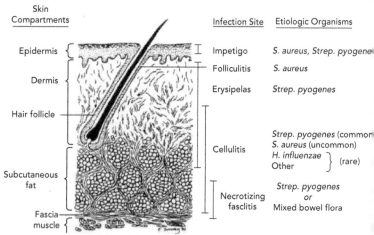

Figure 37.1. Anatomic classification of soft tissue infections.

TABLE 37.1	Less Common Sources of Soft Tissue Infections
History	Source
Fresh or brackish water with laceration or abrasion	*Aeromonas hydrophila*
Salt water or seafood contamination of wound, seafood consumption	*Vibrio* species (especially *Vibrio vulnificus*)
Cat/dog bite	*Pasteurella multocida, Capnocytophaga canimorsus* (dogs), polymicrobial anaerobes
Human bite	Streptococci, *Eikenella* spp., polymicrobial anaerobes

bites, and areas with any preexisting skin condition such as venous stasis, ischemia, or decubitus ulcers. Critically ill patients may have increased susceptibility to these infections because of their impaired immune status and altered skin flora. The most common causative organisms are beta-hemolytic streptococci (BHS) and *Staphylococcus aureus*. In patients with cellulitis and no culture evidence of BHS infection, the vast majority respond to therapy directed against BHS. Less common causes of cellulitis may be suspected based on the patient's history or comorbidities (Table 37.1).

NECROTIZING FASCIITIS

Necrotizing fasciitis is a rare SSTI that involves the deep fascia and always requires surgical intervention and broad-spectrum intravenous antimicrobials. Rates of necrotizing fasciitis vary widely based on region (0.18 to 15.5 per 100,000) and seem to be increasing over time. Type I necrotizing fasciitis is polymicrobial, including aerobic and anaerobic organisms. Type II necrotizing fasciitis is classically caused by *Streptococcus pyogenes*, though *S. aureus* also falls into this category. There are a variety of case reports and case series of less frequently encountered agents causing necrotizing fasciitis, making it important for practitioners to realize the importance of surgical debridement with attendant bacterial cultures in combination with broad-spectrum antimicrobials as the first lines of therapy.

Though the classic teaching for necrotizing fasciitis is pain out proportion to physical examination findings, it is important to remember that superficial nerves can undergo necrosis, resulting in anesthesia of affected areas (see Table 37.2). Eliciting a history may be problematic due to the severity of illness and alterations in sensorium, requiring maintenance of a high degree of suspicion for necrotizing SSTIs. Imaging findings cannot rule out necrotizing fasciitis (due to unacceptably low sensitivity) and may delay surgical intervention, which is associated with poor outcomes. Necrotizing fasciitis predominantly occurs in the lower extremities and the predisposing conditions (diabetes, abnormalities of venous return or arterial insufficiency, and intravenous drug use) explain the predilection for this anatomical localization. Due to the relative rarity, heterogeneity of microbiologic causes, and severity of disease, no clinical trials are available to guide duration of therapy, though guidelines based on expert opinion suggest continuation of therapy directed against cultured organisms

TABLE 37.2	Characteristics Associated With Increased Likelihood of Necrotizing Infection
Pain out of proportion to examination	
Bullae	
Systemic toxicity	
Serum sodium <135 mmol/L	
WBC >15,400 cell/mm^3	
Tenderness beyond the area of erythema	
Crepitus	
Cutaneous anesthesia	
Cellulitis refractory to antibiotic therapy	

WBC, white blood count.

for at least 48 to 72 hours after patients are clinically stable and require no further operative interventions.

MYOSITIS/PYOMYOSITIS/GAS GANGRENE

Myositis involves infection down to muscle and is generally differentiated into myonecrosis or pyomyositis. Myonecrosis is associated with gas gangrene and clostridial infections, and pyomyositis is almost universally due to *S. aureus*. The distinction is vital, as myonecrosis necessitates immediate operative debridement, whereas pyomyositis may be amenable to antibiotics and percutaneous drainage. Pyomyositis is characterized by localized pain in a single muscle group associated with fever. Magnetic resonance imaging (MRI) is the imaging study of choice for diagnosis of pyomyositis, though bedside ultrasound may be a useful rapid diagnostic alternative.

Gas gangrene or myonecrosis is caused by *Clostridium* species. *Clostridium perfringens* is classically associated with traumatic injuries; *C. septicum* with neutropenic patients or those with gastrointestinal malignancies or abnormalities; *C. sordellii* with childbirth and "home" abortions; and *C. perfringens, C. novyi,* and *C. sordellii* with drug users who "skin pop." Though rare, *C. sordellii* infections are notable as they can be associated with a toxic-shock–like syndrome, particularly in patients with recent parturition or abortion.

ECTHYMA GANGRENOSUM

Ecthyma gangrenosum is an uncommon necrotizing, hemorrhagic cutaneous vasculitis that is classically associated with *Pseudomonas aeruginosa* septicemia, though many other pathogens have been implicated, including other gram-negative bacilli, *S. aureus, S. pyogenes,* fungi, molds, atypical mycobacteria, and viruses. The lesions typically begin as painless erythematous nodules that evolve into painful necrotic ulcers with eschar, predominantly seen between the umbilicus and knees. Necrosis results from invasion of the medial and adventitial blood vessel walls by the implicated microbe. Patients suspected of having ecthyma gangrenosum should be given broad-spectrum antimicrobials, including an agent with antipseudomonal activity.

AGNOSIS AND TREATMENT OF
CROTIZING INFECTIONS

termining whether or not a necrotizing infection is present can be challenging, ause physical examination is often unreliable (Table 37.2). Patients with these ections frequently have normal overlying skin. Overt signs of necrotic tissue, h as crepitus, occur in only 30% of patients. Laboratory abnormalities, including reactive protein, hemoglobin, sodium, creatinine, glucose levels, and white blood l counts, have been used to construct risk scores, but these are not in widespread e.

Radiographic imaging may assist in the diagnosis of necrotizing soft tissue infec-ns. However, plain radiography shows soft tissue gas in only 15% to 30% of crotizing infections. Computed tomography and ultrasound are sometimes helpful cillary studies to identify soft tissue gas or necrotic tissue. MRI may delineate the ent of the infection and has a high sensitivity for detection of necrotizing soft sue infections; however, specificity is somewhat low, and logistic difficulties in dy availability limit its utility in critically ill patients. In equivocal cases, biopsy h frozen section has been recommended for definitive diagnosis, but is associated h significant logistical difficulties when needed urgently. An alternative means of ablishing the severity of the infection is to make a bedside incision under local esthesia and digitally examine the tissue planes; facile separation of the subcutane-s tissue from the fascia is pathognomonic sign for necrotizing soft tissue infection. the suspicion for a necrotizing infection is high, imaging studies should not delay gical exploration. A potential management algorithm for distinguishing necrotiz-g from nonnecrotizing infections is presented in Algorithm 37.1.

Antibiotic therapy directed against streptococci and staphylococci has gen-lly been used for initial therapy of nonnecrotizing soft tissue infections. How-er, one-third of isolates from patients with soft tissue infections are gram-negative ganisms, so additional antibiotic therapy directed against common gram-negative ganisms may be needed, particularly with infections involving the axillae or rineum. Gram-negative antimicrobials are also recommended in patients with vere infections and those that are immunocompromised. Antimicrobial manage-ent of nonnecrotizing infections is complicated by the increased prevalence of sistant organisms such as methicillin-resistant *S. aureus* (MRSA), including those sitive for the Panton–Valentine leukocidin. MRSA was responsible for 59% of e skin/soft tissue infections of patients presenting to emergency departments at 11 cilities across the country. Therefore, it is generally appropriate to include an anti-icrobial agent that has activity against this organism. Vancomycin has traditionally en used for this, but linezolid, daptomycin, and ceftaroline may be alternatives in tically ill patients.

Necrotizing soft tissue infections are lethal disorders, associated with a 20% 70% mortality. Patients with necrotizing infections require immediate surgical bridement and broad-spectrum antibiotics directed against gram-positive cocci, am-negative bacilli, and anaerobes. For patients with monomicrobial infections due *S. pyogenes* or clostridia, penicillin PLUS clindamycin are the definitive treatment. gents that can decrease toxin production, such as clindamycin or linezolid, may also useful in selected patients with necrotizing soft tissue infections.

SSTIs have a variety of presentations and can be severe enough to require inten-ve care. Practitioners should be familiar with the spectrum of clinical presentations

ALGORITHM 37.1 Algorithm for Managing Soft Tissue Infection

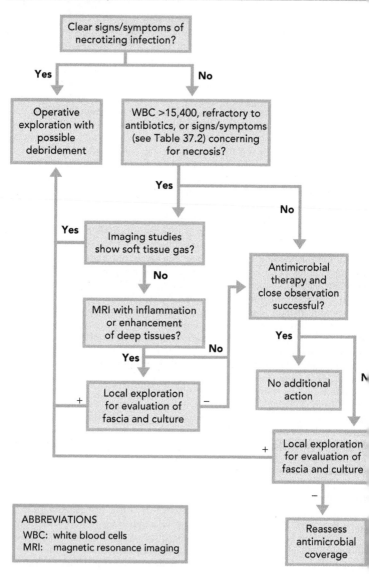

ABBREVIATIONS
WBC: white blood cells
MRI: magnetic resonance imaging

or SSTIs that require urgent surgical debridement to avoid delays in surgery as is can lead to worsened outcomes. Aggressive source control and broad-spectrum ntimicrobials are essential for all severe SSTIs, with empiric therapy guided by nowledge of patient risk factors and the local antibiogram.

SUGGESTED READINGS

ldape MJ, Bryant AE, Stevens DL. Clostridium sordellii infection: epidemiology, clinical findings, and current perspectives on diagnosis and treatment. *Clin Infect Dis.* 2006;43(11):1436–1446.

angsberg DR, Rosen JI, Aragon T, et al. Clostridial myonecrosis cluster among injection drug users: a molecular epidemiology investigation. *Arch Intern Med.* 2002;162(5):517–522.

olognia JL, Jorizzo J, Schaffer JV. *Dermatology.* Philadelphia, PA: Elsevier Saunders; 2012.

> *These references review the salient features of diagnosis and treatment of ecthyma gangrenosum.*

urnham JP, Kirby JP, Kollef MH. Diagnosis and management of skin and soft tissue infections in the intensive care unit: a review. *Intensive Care Med.* 2016;42(12):1899–1911.

> *This article reviews the clinical presentation, diagnosis, and treatment of skin and soft tissue infections commonly encountered in the intensive care unit.*

Centers for Disease Control and Prevention (CDC). Update: Clostridium novyi and unexplained illness among injecting-drug users–Scotland, Ireland, and England, April-June 2000. *MMWR Morb Mortal Wkly Rep.* 2000;49(24):543–545.

> *These articles describe multiple cases of clostridial myonecrosis and gas gangrene.*

Cheng NC, Yu YC, Tai HC, et al. Recent trend of necrotizing fasciitis in Taiwan: focus on monomicrobial Klebsiella pneumoniae necrotizing fasciitis. *Clin Infect Dis.* 2012;55(7):930–939.

Cohen AL, Bhatnagar J, Reagan S, et al. Toxic shock associated with Clostridium sordellii and Clostridium perfringens after medical and spontaneous abortion. *Obstet Gynecol.* 2007;110(5):1027–1033.

Das DK, Baker MG, Venugopal K. Increasing incidence of necrotizing fasciitis in New Zealand: a nationwide study over the period 1990 to 2006. *J Infect.* 2011;63(6):429–433.

Ellis Simonsen SM, van Orman ER, Hatch BE, et al. Cellulitis incidence in a defined population. *Epidemiol Infect.* 2006;134(2):293–299.

Fischer M, Bhatnagar J, Guarner J, et al. Fatal toxic shock syndrome associated with Clostridium sordellii after medical abortion. *N Engl J Med.* 2005;353(22):2352–2360.

eng A, Beheshti M, Li J, et al. The role of beta-hemolytic streptococci in causing diffuse, nonculturable cellulitis: a prospective investigation. *Medicine.* 2010;89(4):217–226.

> *This article describes the role of beta-hemolytic streptococci in cellulitis and treatment outcomes.*

Khamnuan P, Chongruksut W, Jearwattanakanok K, et al. Necrotizing fasciitis: epidemiology and clinical predictors for amputation. *Int J Gen Med.* 2015;8:195–202.

Kimura AC, Higa JI, Levin RM, et al. Outbreak of necrotizing fasciitis due to Clostridium sordellii among black-tar heroin users. *Clin Infect Dis.* 2004;38(9):e87–e91.

Kumar MP, Seif D, Perera P, et al. Point-of-care ultrasound in diagnosing pyomyositis: a report of three cases. *J Emerg Med.* 2014;47(4):420–426.

Lopez FA, Lartchenko S. Skin and soft tissue infections. *Infect Dis Clin North Am.* 2006;20(4):759–772.

> *A review article which emphasizes microbiology and emergence of MRSA in soft tissue infections.*

Moran GJ, Krishnadasan A, Gorwitz RJ, et al. Methicillin-resistant S. aureus infections among patients in the emergency department. *N Engl J Med.* 2006;355(7):666–674.

> *Multicenter trial showing the emergence of MRSA in soft tissue infections.*

Oud L, Watkins P. Contemporary trends of the epidemiology, clinical characteristics, and resource utilization of necrotizing fasciitis in Texas: a population-based cohort study. *Crit Care Res and Pract.* 2015;2015:618067.

> *These articles demonstrate the increasing incidence of necrotizing fasciitis over time.*

Reich HL, Williams Fadeyi D, Naik NS, et al. Nonpseudomonal ecthyma gangrenosum. *J Am Acad Dermatol.* 2004;50(suppl 5):S114–S117.

Sauler A, Saul T, Lewiss RE. Point-of-care ultrasound differentiates pyomyositis from cellulit. *Am J Emerg Med.* 2015;33(3):482.e3–482.e5.

Shaked H, Samra Z, Paul M, et al. Unusual "flesh-eating" strains of Escherichia coli. *J Cl Microbiol.* 2012;50(12):4008–4011.

These articles describe some rare causes of necrotizing fasciitis.

Sinave C, Le Templier G, Blouin D, et al. Toxic shock syndrome due to Clostridium sordellii: dramatic postpartum and postabortion disease. *Clin Infect Dis.* 2002;35(11):1441–144?

Stevens DL, Bisno AL, Chambers HF, et al. Practice guidelines for the diagnosis and manag ment of skin and soft tissue infections: 2014 update by the Infectious Diseases Society America. *Clin Infect Dis.* 2014;59(2):147–159.

This article is a review of all SSTIs, including presentation, diagnosis, and treatment.

Theodorou SJ, Theodorou DJ, Resnick D. MR imaging findings of pyogenic bacterial mye sitis (pyomyositis) in patients with local muscle trauma: illustrative cases. *Emerg Radi* 2007;14(2):89–96.

These articles illustrate the imaging studies helpful in diagnosis of pyomyositis.

Vaiman M, Lazarovitch T, Heller L, et al. Ecthyma gangrenosum and ecthyma-like lesion review article. *Eur J Clin Microbiol Infect Dis.* 2015;34(4):633–639.

Wall DB, Klein SR, Black S, et al. A simple model to help distinguish necrotizing fasciitis fro nonnecrotizing soft tissue infection. *J Am Coll Surg.* 2000;191(3):227–231.

This article describes the use of serum sodium and white blood cell count to identify patien with necrotizing infections.

Weigelt J, Itani K, Stevens D, et al. Linezolid versus vancomycin in treatment of complicate skin and soft tissue infections. *Antimicrob Agents Chemother.* 2005;49(6):2260–2266.

This article describes the role of linezolid and vancomycin in complicated SSTIs.

Wong CH, Chang HC, Pasupathy S, et al. Necrotizing fasciitis: clinical presentation, micr biology, and determinants of mortality. *J Bone Joint Surg Am.* 2003;85-A(8):1454–1460.

The salient feature of this article is the description of poor outcomes when debridement delayed.

Wong CH, Khin LW, Heng KS, et al. The LRINEC (Laboratory Risk Indicator for Necrotizin Fasciitis) score: a tool for distinguishing necrotizing fasciitis from other soft tissue infec tions. *Crit Care Med.* 2004;32(7):1535–1541.

This article describes the use of common laboratory values in predicting the presence of a ne rotizing infection.

38 Bacteremia and Catheter-Related Bloodstream Infections

David K. Warren

cteremia is a common complication in the critically ill. Bloodstream infections can secondary to a recognized infection site, primary infections without an obvious urce, or from the intravascular devices commonly used in critical care. Central 10us catheters (CVCs) are the most common source of primary bloodstream infec- n in critically ill patients, and provide a unique opportunity for pathogens to enter ε bloodstream. CVCs become infected through multiple mechanisms. Bacteria can lonize the intra- and extraluminal portions of the catheter or the catheter hub(s) at then enter the bloodstream. Contaminated intravenous solutions can create e outbreaks of bacteremia with uncommon pathogens. Hematogenous seeding the catheter from bacteremia originating at another source can occur. Successful atment of catheter-associated bloodstream infection is more difficult than simple cteremia, as organisms on intravascular catheters exist within a slimelike biofilm, lucing their susceptibility to antimicrobial therapy and host defenses, which often cessitates removal of the CVC for definitive treatment.

A high degree of clinical suspicion is necessary to diagnose CVC-related bactere- ia because local catheter insertion site inflammation and/or purulent drainage from ε site are typically absent in catheter-associated bacteremia. Embolic phenomena stal to the catheter (e.g., septic pulmonary emboli) are highly suggestive of a catheter- sociated infection, although not commonly seen. More commonly, the clinician is :ed with a critically ill patient who is febrile without an obvious source and has a VC in place.

Determining if a CVC is the source of a new fever presents a diagnostic and anagement challenge. A conservative strategy of removing all catheters and replac- g them at new sites at the first sign of fever would benefit some patients, but also ids to the removal of many uninfected CVCs, unnecessarily exposing patients to e risks of line replacement. A reasonable approach would be to draw blood cultures :fore any antibiotics are given, and then immediately remove the catheter if there are ovious signs of infection at the insertion site (especially in the case of nontunneled theters) or the patient is in septic shock. If a thorough evaluation does not reveal source of infection and the patient is stable, it is reasonable to leave the catheter place, follow the blood cultures, and start empirical antibiotics at the clinician's scretion. If the cultures become positive, the catheter can be removed and a new theter placed at a different site, if still indicated.

The sensitivity and specificity of blood cultures are imperfect. For example, the nsitivity of blood cultures in detecting bacteremia is increased by the number of ood cultures drawn. Multiple strategies have been studied in an attempt to improve

ALGORITHM 38.1 Evaluation of Suspected Catheter-Associated Bacteremia

New fever in patient with central venous catheter (CVC)

↓

- Evaluate for other potential sources of infection
- Draw two sets of blood cultures, at least one peripherally

↓

Inflammation at CVC insertion site or patient with clinical sepsis?

Yes →
- Remove CVC
- Send catheter tip culture
- Start appropriate antibiotics

No

↓

- Consider empirical antibiotics if fever persists or patient clinically worsens
- Follow blood cultures

↓

Blood culture results

Likely pathogen:
- *Staphylococcus aureus*,
- Gram negative bacilli
- Coagulase-negative Staphylococci from ≥2 blood cultures
- *Candida* spp.

Possible contaminant:
- i.e., Coagulase-negative *Staphylococci*, *Bacillus spp*, *Corynebacterim spp*. from a single blood culture
- Repeat blood cultures

No growth

Repeat blood cultures positive for same organism?

Yes → Remove CVC (box above)

No → Evaluate for another source of infection

the diagnosis of catheter-associated bloodstream infection. Currently, two metho
are practical for widespread application. The first takes advantage of the continuo
monitoring system for blood cultures used in most modern microbiology laborat
ries. Blot et al. found that, in cases of catheter-associated bloodstream infection,

TABLE 38.1	Management of Bloodstream Infections by Common Pathogens

Staphylococcus aureus
  Use parenteral β-lactams (oxacillin or nafcillin) for susceptible strains
  Use vancomycin for MRSA only
  Linezolid and daptomycin are acceptable alternatives for MRSA if unable to tolerate vancomycin
  Transesophageal echocardiogram (TEE) recommended, if possible, evaluating for endocarditis
  Remove catheters
  If endocarditis ruled out by TEE, blood cultures are negative within 72 hrs of treatment, no prosthetic material in place and catheter removed, treat for 14 days; otherwise treat for ≥4 wks
  Treat complicated infections (endocarditis, septic thrombophlebitis, prolonged bacteremia) for 4–6 wks (6–8 wks for osteomyelitis)

Coagulase-negative Staphylococci
  If catheter removed, treat with vancomycin for 5–7 days after removal
  If catheter must be retained, treat for 10–14 days with vancomycin, consider antibiotic lock, and repeat blood cultures if signs/symptoms recur

Enterococci
  Ampicillin for susceptible isolates
  Vancomycin for ampicillin-resistant, vancomycin-sensitive isolates
  Linezolid or daptomycin for vancomycin-resistant, ampicillin-resistant isolates
  Consider addition of synergy-dosed gentamicin (1 mg/kg IV q8h)
  Remove catheters if possible
  Treat for 7–14 days of systemic antibiotic therapy for uncomplicated infection

Gram-negative bacilli
  Empiric therapy should include agents active against *Pseudomonas aeruginosa*
  Tailor antibiotics to sensitivity results
  Remove catheter, especially with *Pseudomonas, Acinetobacter, Stenotrophomonas* spp.
  If catheter removed, treat for 10–14 days of systemic antibiotic therapy; if catheter must be retained consider antibiotic lock therapy

Candida species
  An echinocandin is preferred for empirical therapy in critically ill patients; liposomal amphotericin B is an alternative therapy
  Antifungal susceptibility can be inferred from the species identification
  Repeat blood cultures on therapy until negative
  Remove catheters
  Dilated ophthalmologic examination on treatment to exclude endophthalmitis
  Treat for 14 days after first negative culture in uncomplicated infections

MRSA, methicillin-resistant staphylococcus aureus; IV, intravenous.

blood culture drawn from a catheter became positive for growth faster than a paired sample from a peripheral venipuncture. If a catheter-drawn blood culture becomes positive for growth at least 2 hours earlier than a peripherally drawn culture obtained at the same time, this strongly suggests the catheter as the source of the bacteremia. The other common method is culturing segments of catheters after their removal. A variety of techniques have been studied, but the semiquantitative roll plate technique described by Maki et al. remains the most common. Documenting significant colonization of a catheter with the same organism isolated from blood cultures provides strong evidence that the catheter is the source of infection. An approach to suspected catheter-associated bloodstream infection in the intensive care unit is presented in Algorithm 38.1.

Management strategies for specific pathogens can be found in Table 38.1. Special care should be taken in the case of *Candida* species (discussed in Chapter 39) and *Staphylococcus aureus,* given their ability to establish metastatic foci of infection. *S. aureus* bacteremia should prompt a thorough examination for metastatic sites of infection. High rates of endocarditis have been reported in catheter-associated *S. aureus* bacteremia, and transesophageal echocardiography should be considered if no contraindications exist.

The decision to remove a tunneled catheter or implanted port in the face of bacteremia is more difficult, given the expense and risk involved and often these patients may have limited options for vascular access. In general, these devices should be removed when there is a soft tissue infection of the tunnel or the port reservoir, when there are systemic complications (i.e., septic shock, septic thromboembolic disease, endocarditis, osteomyelitis, or other metastatic foci of infection), when infection is due to *S. aureus* or *Candida* spp., and prolonged bacteremia not responding to appropriate antibiotic therapy. If salvage of the catheter is deemed necessary, there is evidence that use of high-concentration antibiotic lock therapy may improve success rates. Consultation with an infectious disease specialist is recommended for complicated cases.

SUGGESTED READINGS

Beutz M, Sherman G, Mayfield J, et al. Clinical utility of blood cultures drawn from central vein catheters and peripheral venipuncture in critically ill medical patients. *Chest.* 2003; 123(3):854–861.
  Blood cultures drawn from central venous catheters or from peripheral venipuncture had similar positive and negative predictive values for detected bloodstream infection.
Blot F, Schmidt E, Nitenberg G, et al. Earlier positivity of central-venous-versus peripheral-blood cultures is highly predictive of catheter-related sepsis. *J Clin Microbiol.* 1998;36(1):105–109.
  Paired sets of blood cultures from a catheter and peripheral venipuncture can be used to diagnose catheter-related bacteremia.
Fowler VG Jr, Li J, Corey GR, et al. Role of echocardiography in evaluation of patients with Staphylococcus aureus bacteremia: experience in 103 patients. *J Am Coll Cardiol.* 1997;30(4):1072–1078.
  Transesophageal echocardiography found a surprisingly high rate of endocarditis in patients with S. aureus bacteremia who had negative transthoracic echocardiograms.
Lee A, Mirrett S, Reller LB, et al. Detection of bloodstream infections in adults: how many blood cultures are needed? *J Clin Microbiol.* 2007;45(11):3546–3548.
  Three 20 mL blood cultures obtained in a 24-hour period detected over 96% of all episodes of bacteremia in a multicenter study.

i DG, Weise CE, Sarafin HW. A semiquantitative culture method for identifying intrave-
nous-catheter-related infection. *N Engl J Med.* 1977;296(23):1305–1309.

The original paper describing the commonly used roll plate culture technique.

mel LA, Allon M, Bouza E, et al. Clinical practice guidelines for the diagnosis and management of intravascular catheter-related infection: 2009 update by the Infectious Diseases
Society of America. *Clin Infect Dis.* 2009;49(1):1–45.

The most recent evidence-based guidelines for managing catheter-associated bacteremia.

vart PS, William Costerton J. Antibiotic resistance of bacteria in biofilms. *Lancet.* 2001;
358(9276):135–138.

A review of possible mechanisms of bacterial resistance within biofilms.

nstein MP, Towns ML, Quartey SM, et al. The clinical significance of positive blood cultures
in the 1990s: a prospective comprehensive evaluation of the microbiology, epidemiology,
and outcome of bacteremia and fungemia in adults. *Clin Infect Dis.* 1997;24(4):584–602.

*A prospective study of bacteremia from three large medical centers; appropriate antibiotic ther-
apy was associated with lower mortality.*

39 Invasive Fungal Infection

Krunal Raval and Andrej Spec

INTRODUCTION

Invasive fungal infections are a significant cause of morbidity and mortality wo wide and the incidence is steadily increasing. Fungi are major pathogens in critic ill patients, and even though the incidence is lower than bacterial infections, the case mortality is higher and resistance appears to be on the rise.

There are several reasons for the increase in invasive fungal infectic including an increase in the use of antineoplastic and immunosuppressive age broad-spectrum antibiotics, prosthetic devices, and grafts, as well as more aggres surgical interventions. Patients with burns, neutropenia, HIV infection, and pan atitis are also predisposed to fungal infection.

The fungi of clinical significance are divided into three clinically relevant gro based on morphology: yeasts, dimorphic fungi, and molds. This classification d not represent a true phylogeny, as for example, *Cryptococcus* and *Candida* are b classified as yeasts, but *Cryptococcus* is more closely related to edible mushrooms th it is to *Candida. Candida spp.* and *Cryptococcus spp.* represent the vast majority yeasts found in clinical practice. Pneumocystis is an important cause of a multifo pneumonia in immunocompromised hosts.

Most common dimorphic fungi are *Blastomyces, Histoplasma, Coccidioides,* a *Penicillium.* Their distribution is geographically restricted but due to increased tr and weather change, they are increasingly diagnosed outside of their traditional ran

The most frequently isolated molds are *Aspergillus* and the *Zygomycetes,* but th are over 200 clinically important species, with complex and varied presentatio treatment considerations, and clinical outcomes.

YEAST

Candida Spp.

Candida is a commensal organism of the skin, gastrointestinal and genitourin tract. There are many species of *Candida* but only a few species are commo encountered in clinical care.

Overall, *Candida albicans* remains the most common species isolated fr patients, accounting for 44% to 79.4% of disease. This is fortunate as *C. albican* not commonly resistant to commonly used antifungals.

However, an epidemiologic shift toward nonalbicans species may be occurri with the most important nonalbicans isolates being *C. glabrata* and *C. krusei.* T

TABLE 39.1	Risk Factors for Invasive Candidiasis

Prolonged ICU stay
Candida colonization
Central venous catheterization
Broad-spectrum antimicrobials
Renal failure
Hemodialysis
Diabetes
Parenteral nutrition
Malignancy
Chemotherapy/immunosuppressive medications
Surgery (particularly abdominal)
Transplantation
APACHE II score ≥20
Acute pancreatitis

ICU, intensive care unit; APACHE, acute physiology and chronic health evaluation.

shift has particularly important implications for therapy because of various intrinsic resistance patterns associated with nonalbicans *Candida*.

C. krusei is intrinsically fluconazole resistant while *C. glabrata* has higher minimum inhibitory concentration (MICs) and the ability to develop resistance to all azoles as well as echinocandins, especially after exposure. Azole and echinocandin resistant *C. glabrata* isolates are rare, but are exceedingly difficult to treat, requiring administration of Amphoterin B. *C. lusitaniae* is resistant to Amphotericin B, but is very rare and still retains sensitivity to the azoles and echinocandins. *C. parapsilosis* have been noted to have increased MICs to echinocandins.

When visceral or normally sterile body fluids are infected via hematogenous spread or direct invasion the resultant syndrome is referred to as invasive candidiasis. However, it is important to note that *Candida* is commonly isolated from the lungs and urine, where it is most commonly a colonizer, and does not represent true disease. However, these are associated with increased risk for invasive candidiasis. Invasive candidiasis is associated with overall mortality in excess of 40%. Most common and clinically significant invasive candidiasis in ICU includes candidemia, endocarditis, abdominal infections, and endophthalmitis (Table 39.1).

The presence of *Candida* in a blood culture should never be treated as a contaminant and should prompt further investigation and treatment. However, blood cultures are positive in only 50% to 70% of patients with invasive candidiasis. Because of these limitations, a reliable, nonculture-based method has been vigorously sought. 1,3-β-D-glucan, which is a major component of fungal cell wall, can be detected and is recently approved by the Food and Drug Administration (FDA). This test has sensitivity of 75% to 100% and a specificity of 88% to 100%. However, it is a broad-spectrum assay that detects *Aspergillus, Fusarium, Acremonium,* and *Saccharomyces* species in addition to *Candida,* necessitating careful interpretation. None of the currently available tests have adequate sensitivity and specificity for reliable diagnosis.

Candida endocarditis is one of the most serious manifestations of candidiasis and is the most common cause of fungal endocarditis. It should be suspected with persistently positive blood cultures and echocardiography frequently shows veget tions that are larger than those caused by bacteria, and much more likely to emboli

Around 2% to 26% of cases of candidemia are complicated by endophthalmit which can affect the choice of antifungals and the duration of therapy. The minimu treatment is extended to 4 weeks in presence of endophthalmitis, and echinocandi should be avoided due to low penetration into vitreal fluid. Thus, due to a significa risk of endophthalmitis, early-dilated retinal examination by an ophthalmologi should be performed in all candidemic patients. Biopsy of a specific lesion (from normally sterile site) demonstrating characteristic histopathology can be consider definitive, but this is often not feasible in critically ill patients.

Cryptococcus Spp.

Cryptococcus neoformans is the most common cause of cryptococcosis, with the va majority of the remaining cases by *C. gattii*. Respiratory tract is the most likely port of entry. The organism disseminates hematogenously and has a propensity to locali to the central nervous system (CNS) and skin. Recovery from any site other than tl lungs should lead to treatment of disseminated disease, as local inoculation or anoth mode of entry is much less likely than dissemination.

C. neoformans is mostly contracted by inhalation of spores. Subsequently, it is di seminated to melanin-rich regions like skin and CNS. Cryptococcal infection shoul be suspected in any immunocompromised patient with fever, headache, and CN symptoms. Conversely any patient with cryptococcal infection should be evaluated f underlying immunocompromised condition including undiagnosed HIV and for ev dence of dissemination, including CNS disease, as this will significantly affect therap

Meningoencephalitis is the most frequently encountered manifestation of cryp tococcosis in ICU patients, especially in patients with T-cell dysfunction such HIV-seropositive patients and solid-organ transplant recipients. Clinically it presen as a subacute to chronic meningitis, and the patients are often septic.

Lumbar puncture is necessary to definitively diagnose cryptococcal meningo encephalitis. Lymphocytic pleocytosis accompanied by elevated protein and elevate opening pressure are the classic presentation. Subsequent evaluation of CSF wit measurement of cryptococcal antigen is sufficient evidence to initiate treatmen Symptomatic patients should be treated with amphotericin B and flucytosine whil evaluation for dissemination is underway. If further workup is negative, patient ca be deescalated to fluconazole.

Cryptococcal antigen is very sensitive and specific in the CSF with sensitivitie ranging from 93% to 100% and specificities from 93% to 98%. But false-positiv tests can result from infection due to the fungus *Trichosporon asahii* (formerl *T. beigelii*) or bacteria of the *spp.* and *Capnocytophaga* genera.

In AIDS patients with suspected cryptococcal meningoencephalitis, the sensitiv ity of serum antigen testing is comparable to CSF testing and is a useful diagnosti modality in patients who cannot undergo lumbar puncture. Antigen titers generall correlate with organism burden. However, titers are not helpful in follow up of acu disease since changes in antigen titer can lag clinical response by months, or even year

DIMORPHIC FUNGI

Histoplasma

Histoplasma capsulatum is the most common endemic mycosis worldwide. Mos infections are asymptomatic or self-limited, but some can develop acute pulmonar

ctions or severe and progressive disseminated infection predominantly in patients
h T-cell deficiencies.

Disseminated infection usually presents with fever, fatigue, hepatospleno-
galy, and pancytopenia. Diarrhea and dyspnea occur less commonly. Patients
h AIDS or on immunosuppressive medications can present with overwhelm-
infection manifested by shock, respiratory distress, hepatic and renal failure,
undation, and coagulopathy. It is often confused with bacterial sepsis. A rare but
nificant complication to be monitored is adrenal insufficiency due to direct infil-
ion of the organism in the adrenal glands or Waterhouse–Friderichsen syndrome.
cases of fluid refractory shock in the setting of histoplasmosis, steroids should be
iated early.

The mortality in spite of amphotericin B treatment is 10% to 25% in the devel-
d world. In resource limited settings, mortality often reaches 50%.

For diagnosis, blood cultures along with urine and blood *Histoplasma* antigen
uld be performed in all patients suspected of having disseminated histoplasmosis
order to achieve the highest sensitivity. Serum serology can also be helpful in cases
acute pulmonary histoplasmosis. Elevated LDH, ferritin, alkaline phosphatase,
d an AST to ALT ratio greater than 2 are laboratory findings suggestive of his-
lasmosis. Biopsy of a skin lesion, mucous membrane lesion, bone marrow, CSF
uld be considered to confirm the diagnosis.

astomyces Spp.

used by *Blastomyces dermatitidis*, it is a systemic pyogranulomatous infection
t arises after inhalation of the conidia. Lungs are the most common site of infec-
n, followed by the skin, bones, brain, and genitourinary tract. Reported mor-
ity in disseminated blastomycosis with multiorgan involvement can range up to
%.

Acute pulmonary blastomycosis may be initially diagnosed as community-
quired bacterial or viral pneumonia, whereas chronic pulmonary blastomycosis
often initially thought to be malignancy or tuberculosis. Unlike other endemic
coses, blastomycosis is not heavily associated with immunodeficiencies, and is not
nificantly elevated in patients with HIV.

Rarely, patients may present with diffuse pneumonitis associated with acute
piratory distress syndrome (ARDS). In small case series, the mortality rate asso-
ted with ARDS due to blastomycosis was over 50% and most deaths occurred
ring the first few days of treatment. Blastomycosis should be considered in patients
o have lived or traveled to areas with high rates of blastomycosis and later present
h community-acquired ARDS.

Serology is not useful for the diagnosis of blastomycosis, however there is sig-
icant cross reactivity with the *Histoplasma* antigen, and is often positive in cases of
seminated histoplasmosis (Table 39.2).

ccidioides Spp.

ccidioides is endemic to the deserts in southwestern US, Central and South America.
e risk of endemic exposure to *Coccidioides spp.* is approximately 3% per year.

Primary *Coccidioides* infections manifest as community-acquired pneumo-
a that is usually self-limited but may be severe and require antifungal therapy.
ematogenous dissemination, predominantly in immunocompromised hosts, occurs
edominantly to skin, meninges and bones. Coccidioidal meningitis is suspected in
tients with persistent headache and fever after recent pneumonia.

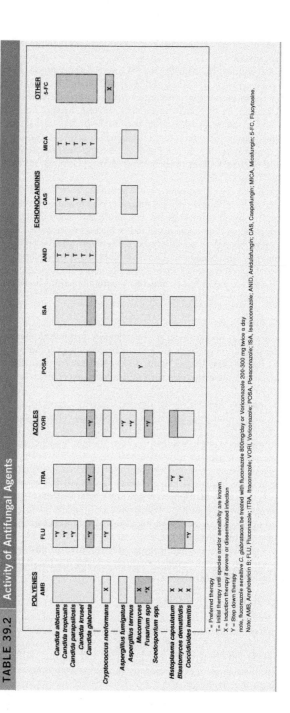

TABLE 39.2 Activity of Antifungal Agents

	POLYENES	AZOLES					ECHONOCANDINS			OTHER
	AMB	FLU	ITRA	VORI	POSA	ISA	ANID	CAS	MICA	5-FC
Candida albicans		*Y	*Y				T	T	T	
Candida tropicalis		*Y	*Y				T	T	T	
Candida parapsilosis		*Y					T	T	T	
Candida krusei	X	*Y		*Y			T	T	T	
Candida glabrata		*Y					T	T	T	X
Cryptococcus neoformans	X	*Y								
Aspergillus fumigatus			*Y	*Y						
Aspergillus terreus			*Y	*Y						
Mucormyces	X				Y					
Fusarium spp.	*X			*Y						
Scedosporium spp.										
Histoplasma capsulatum	X		*Y							
Blastomyces dematitidis	X		*Y							
Coccidioides immitis	X	*Y								

* = Preferred therapy

T = Initial therapy until species and/or sensitivity are known

X = Induction therapy if severe or disseminated infection

Y = Step down therapy

note, fluconazole sensitive *C. glabratacan* be treated with fluconazole 800mg/day or Voriconazole 200-300 mg twice a day

Note: AMB, Amphotericin B; FLU, Fluconazole; ITRA, Itraconazole; VORI, Voriconazole; POSA, Posaconazole; ISA, Isavuconazole; ANID, Anidulafungin; CAS, Caspofungin; MICA, Micafungin; 5-FC, Flucytosine.

Diagnoses are usually made using culture and histology, but serology is also lpful. Cases of meningitis may require a lifelong therapy, especially if the cause of munocompromise cannot be reversed.

enicillium

nicillium marneffei, endemic in Southeast Asia, is an important cause of morbid- and mortality in HIV-infected patients in that region. It presents as a syndrome nilar to disseminated histoplasmosis or tuberculosis, and may mimic bacterial osis.

OLDS

pergillus spp. are the most commonly isolated invasive molds. Only a few of the 200 so species are pathogenic to man, primarily *A. fumigatus, A. flavus,* and *A. niger.*

Other significant molds include *Fusarium spp.* and *Scedosporium spp.* (both of hich are hyalohyphomycoses like *Aspergillus spp.*) and *Rhizopus spp.* (a mucormycosis zygomycosis). They are capable of causing a wide variety of infections. Some of the olds are more prone to certain syndromes (e.g., *Fusarium* is the most likely to cause sseminated cutaneous lesions, but is able to do all of the syndromes listed below).

Most cases of disseminated infection occur in immunocompromised patients, rticularly in stem-cell and solid-organ recipients. Other risk factors include diabetes d renal failure.

The diagnosis of invasive aspergillosis is based upon both, isolating the organism r markers of the organism) and the pretest probability that it is the cause of disease able 39.3).

neumonia

vasive pulmonary aspergillosis is mostly seen in neutropenic patients with classic iad of fever, pleuritic chest pain, and dyspnea. Imaging may show single or multiple odules with or without cavitation, and a possible fungal ball creation.

Pathogenesis of invasive aspergillosis and respiratory failure includes vascular vasion of fungal cell with subsequent infarction followed by tissue necrosis distal to vaded arteries. Patients are most critically ill when fungus invades a large vessel and ay lead to massive hemoptysis which can be rapidly fatal. Such cases should have emergent evaluation by interventional radiology for embolization, and surgery for ossible definitive surgical therapy.

Invasive fusariosis involves the lung in 50% of cases.

TABLE 39.3	Risk Factors for Invasive Aspergillosis
Prolonged neutropenia (>10 days)	
Hematopoietic stem cell transplantation	
Solid organ transplantation	
Corticosteroid/other immunosuppressive therapy	
Advanced HIV	
Chronic granulomatous disease	

IV, human immunodeficiency virus.

TABLE 39.4	Indications/Dosing of Commonly Used Antifungal Agents	
Agent	Dose	Dosing Adjustment Necessary
	Invasive candidiasis	
Fluconazole	400–800 mg/day, IV or PO	Renal insufficiency
Voriconazole	IV: 6 mg/kg every 12 hr for 2 doses followed by 3–4 mg/kg every 12 hr	Hepatic dysfunction IV vehicle may accumulate in renal insufficiency
	PO: <40 kg: 100 mg every 12 hr. >40 Kg: 200 mg every 12 hr	
Caspofungin	70 mg loading dose followed by 50 mg/day, IV	Hepatic dysfunction
Anidulafungin	200 mg loading dose followed by 100 mg/day, IV	None
Amphotericin B deoxycholate[a]	0.6–1 mg/day, IV	None, careful monitoring renal and liver function
Amphotericin B lipid formulations[a] • Colloidal dispersion (Amphotec) • Lipid complex (Abelcet) • Liposomal (AmBisome)	3–5 mg/kg/day, IV	None, careful monitoring renal and liver function
	Invasive aspergillosis	
Itraconazole	IV: 200 mg every 12 hr for 4 doses followed by 200 mg/day	Multiple drug interactions IV not recommended for CrCl <30 mL/min
	PO: 200–400 mg/day	
Voriconazole	As listed above	As listed above
Isavuconazole	IV: 200 mg q8h × 6 (48 hrs), then 200 mg daily PO: 200 mg q8h × 6 (48 hrs), then 200 mg daily	
Amphotericin B deoxycholate[a]	1–1.5 mg/kg/day	As listed above
Amphotericin B lipid formulations[a]	5 mg/kg/day, IV	As listed above Higher doses sometimes used
Caspofungin	As listed above	As listed above
	Mucormycosis	
Amphotericin B deoxycholate[a]	1–1.5 mg/kg/day	As listed above
Amphotericin B lipid formulations[a]	≥5 mg/kg/day, IV[b]	As listed above Higher doses sometimes used
Isavuconazole	IV: 200 mg q8h × 6 (48 hrs), then 200 mg daily PO: 200 mg q8h × 6 (48 hrs), then 200 mg daily	

[a]Bolus infusion of normal saline with dose recommended to decrease incidence of nephrotoxicity. Premedication with acetaminophen and diphenhydramine may decrease infusion-related reactions. In severe cases, hydrocortisone 50 to 100 mg IV may also be administered.
[b]Recommended start dose. Higher doses of 7.5 to 10 mg/kg/day are sometimes used, although there are no prospective trials of efficacy in zygomycosis.
IV, intravenous; PO, by mouth; CrCl, creatine clearance.

inosinusitis

anasal sinus involvement is seen in *Aspergillus* and *Mucormyces* most commonly, can be caused by dozens of other species. *Fusarium* has propensity to paranasal paraorbital sinuses causing mucosal necrosis.

The infection can also extend locally into the vasculature and the brain, leading avernous sinus thrombosis and a variety of CNS manifestations. MRI will show al soft tissue lesions, focal bony erosions, or focal enhancement of the sinus lining. atment involves aggressive, early and repeated debridement as well as administra-a of Amphotericin B.

taneous Lesions

taneous lesions occur mostly due to direct inoculation from a trauma, from itiguous extension, or hematogenous spread. Cutaneous aspergillosis is more nmonly seen in burn, transplant and hematologic malignancy. Skin biopsy is the initive method for diagnosis.

Fusarium skin lesions, in immunocompromised patients, can present as either alized cellulitis or disseminated erythematous papular/nodular lesion with central rosis. Mortality is very high in cases of disseminated disease reaching up to 90% rtality in persistently neutropenic populations (Table 39.4).

JGGESTED READINGS

erg JA, Mundy LM, Powderly WG. Pulmonary cryptococcosis in patients without HIV infection. *Chest.* 1999;115(3):734–740.

erg JA, Watson J, Segal M, et al. Clinical utility of monitoring serum cryptococcal antigen (sCRAG) titers in patients with AIDS-related cryptococcal disease. *HIV Clin Trials.* 2000; 1(1):1–6.

des DR, Safdar N, Baddley JW, et al. Impact of treatment strategy on outcomes in patients with candidemia and other forms of invasive candidiasis: a patient-level quantitative review of randomized trials. *Clin Infect Dis.* 2012;54(8):1110–1122.

ady NE, Buckwalter SP, Hall L, et al. Detection of Blastomyces dermatitidis and Histoplasma capsulatum from culture isolates and clinical specimens by use of real-time PCR. *J Clin Microbiol.* 2011;49(9):3204–3208.

iola JR, Perry P, Pappas PG, et al. Blastomycosis of the central nervous system: a multicenter review of diagnosis and treatment in the modern era. *Clin Infect Dis.* 2010;50(6):797–804.

uwer AE, Rajanuwong A, Chierakul W, et al. Combination antifungal therapies for HIV-associated cryptococcal meningitis: a randomised trial. *Lancet.* 2004;363(9423): 1764–1767.

ang WC, Tzao C, Hsu HH, et al. Pulmonary cryptococcosis: comparison of clinical and radiographic characteristics in immunocompetent and immunocompromised patients. *Chest.* 2006;129(2):333–340.

apman SW, Dismukes WE, Proia LA, et al. Clinical practice guidelines for the management of blastomycosis: 2008 update by the Infectious Diseases Society of America. *Clin Infect Dis.* 2008;46(12):1801–1812.

y JN, Chau TT, Wolbers M, et al. Combination antifungal therapy for cryptococcal meningitis. *N Engl J Med.* 2013;368(14):1291–1302.

nning DW. Echinocandin antifungal drugs. *Lancet.* 2003;362(9390):1142–1151.

dkin SK. The changing face of fungal infections in health care settings. *Clin Infect Dis.* 2005; 41(10):1455–1460.

fter-Gvili A, Vidal L, Goldberg E, et al. Treatment of invasive candidal infections: systematic review and meta-analysis. *Mayo Clin Proc.* 2008;83(9):1011–1021.

Groll AH, Tragiannidis A. Recent advances in antifungal prevention and treatment. *Semin Hem* 2009;46(3):212–229.

Hage CA, Wheat LJ, Loyd J, et al. Pulmonary histoplasmosis. *Semin Respir Crit Care* 2008;29(2):151–165.

Jarvis JN, Harrison TS. HIV-associated cryptococcal meningitis. *AIDS*. 2007;21(16):2119–2

Kauffman CA. Histoplasmosis: a clinical and laboratory update. *Clin Microbiol Rev.* 2 20(1):115–132.

Leroy O, Gangneux JP, Montravers P, et al; AmarCand Study Group. Epidemiology, managem and risk factors for death of invasive candida infections in critical care: a multicenter, pros tive, observational study in France (2005–2006). *Crit Care Med.* 2009;37(5):1612–161

Manabe YC, Moore RD. Cryptococcal antigen screening and preemptive treatment in a cohort of patients with AIDS. *Clin Infect Dis.* 2015;61(10):1632–1634.

Marr KA, Schlamm HT, Herbrecht R, et al. Combination antifungal therapy for invasive as gillosis: a randomized trial. *Ann Intern Med.* 2015;162(2):81–89.

McKenney J, Bauman S, Neary B, et al. Prevalence, correlates, and outcomes of cryptococcal a gen positivity among patients with AIDS, United States, 1986–2012. *Clin Infect Dis.* 2 60(6):959–965.

Miceli MH, Kauffman CA. Isavuconazole: a new broad-spectrum triazole antifungal agent. *Infect Dis.* 2015;61(10):1558–1565.

Nguyen MH, Peacock JE Jr, Tanner DC, et al. Therapeutic approaches in patients with didemia. Evaluation in a multicenter, prospective, observational study. *Arch Intern I* 1995;155(22):2429–2435.

Nucci M, Colombo AL, Silveira F, et al. Risk factors for death in patients with candidemia. *I Control Hosp Epidemiol.* 1998;19(11):846–850.

Pappas PG, Kauffman CA, Andes DR, et al. Executive summary: clinical practice guideline the management of candidiasis: 2016 update by the Infectious Diseases Society of An ica. *Clin Infect Dis.* 2016;62(4):409–417.

Pappas PG, Perfect JR, Cloud GA, et al. Cryptococcosis in human immunodeficiency vi negative patients in the era of effective azole therapy. *Clin Infect Dis.* 2001;33(5):690–

Pappas PG, Rex JH, Lee J, et al; NIAID Mycoses Study Group. A prospective observatic study of candidemia: epidemiology, therapy, and influences on mortality in hospital adult and pediatric patients. *Clin Infect Dis.* 2003;37(5):634–643.

Perfect JR, Dismukes WE, Dromer F, et al. Clinical practice guidelines for the managem of cryptococcal disease: 2010 update by the Infectious Diseases Society of America. (*Infect Dis.* 2010;50(3):291–322.

Powderly WG, Saag MS, Cloud GA, et al. A controlled trial of fluconazole or amphotericin I prevent relapse of cryptococcal meningitis in patients with the acquired immunodeficie syndrome. The NIAID AIDS Clinical Trials Group and Mycoses Study Group. *N Er Med.* 1992;326(12):793–798.

Proia LA, Harnisch DO. Successful use of posaconazole for treatment of blastomycosis. *Antim Agents Chemother.* 2012;56(7):4029.

Saccente M, Woods GL. Clinical and laboratory update on blastomycosis. *Clin Microbiol* 2010;23(2):367–381.

Sarosi GA, Johnson PC. Disseminated histoplasmosis in patients infected with human immu deficiency virus. *Clin Infect Dis.* 1992;14(suppl 1):S60–S67.

Saubolle MA, McKellar PP, Sussland D. Epidemiologic, clinical, and diagnostic aspects of c cidioidomycosis. *J Clin Microbiol.* 2007;45(1):26–30.

Segal BH. Aspergillosis. *N Engl J Med.* 2009;360(18):1870–1884.

Segal BH, Walsh TJ. Current approaches to diagnosis and treatment of invasive aspergillosis. *J Respir Crit Care Med.* 2006;173(7):707–717.

Shelburne SA 3rd, Visnegarwala F, Adams C, et al. Unusual manifestations of disseminated his plasmosis in patients responding to antiretroviral therapy. *Am J Med.* 2005;118:1038–10

Shirley RM, Baddley JW. Cryptococcal lung disease. *Curr Opin Pulm Med.* 2009;15 254–260.

ingh N, Lortholary O, Alexander BD, et al. Antifungal management practices and evolution of infection in organ transplant recipients with cryptococcus neoformans infection. *Transplantation.* 2005;80(8):1033–1039.

an der Horst CM, Saag MS, Cloud GA, et al. Treatment of cryptococcal meningitis associated with the acquired immunodeficiency syndrome. National Institute of Allergy and Infectious Diseases Mycoses Study Group and AIDS Clinical Trials Group. *N Engl J Med.* 1997;337(1):15–21.

Walsh TJ, Anaissie EJ, Denning DW, et al; Infectious Diseases Society of America. Treatment of aspergillosis: clinical practice guidelines of the Infectious Diseases Society of America. *Clin Infect Dis.* 2008;46(3):327–360.

Wheat LJ. Approach to the diagnosis of the endemic mycoses. *Clin Chest Med.* 2009;30(2): 379–389.

Wheat LJ, Conces D, Allen SD, et al. Pulmonary histoplasmosis syndromes: recognition, diagnosis, and management. *Semin Respir Crit Care Med.* 2004;25(2):129–144.

Wheat LJ, Connolly-Stringfield PA, Baker RL, et al. Disseminated histoplasmosis in the acquired immune deficiency syndrome: clinical findings, diagnosis and treatment, and review of the literature. *Medicine.* 1990;69(6):361–374.

Wheat LJ, Freifeld AG, Kleiman MB, et al; Infectious Diseases Society of America. Clinical practice guidelines for the management of patients with histoplasmosis: 2007 update by the Infectious Diseases Society of America. *Clin Infect Dis.* 2007;45(7):807–825.

40 Infections in the Immunocompromised Host

Julianne S. Dean and Stephen Y. Liang

Infections in the critically ill immunocompromised patient carry significant morbidity and mortality. While empiric antimicrobial therapy is universally indicated the early stages of care, definitive diagnosis and therapy requires knowledge of the patient's level of immunosuppression, inherent or iatrogenic, upon which a broad differential of suspect pathogens can then be assembled. Immunocompromised patients are at risk for community-acquired infections as well as a myriad of opportunistic and nosocomial infections (Table 40.1). Clinical signs and symptoms of infection are frequently atypical and nonspecific. Muted inflammatory responses arising from neutropenia, corticosteroids, and other forms of immunosuppressive therapy may render identification of an infectious focus difficult. Multiple prior hospitalizations for infection and the outpatient use of prophylactic antimicrobials to prevent opportunistic infection may place patients at risk for acquiring multidrug-resistant organisms. The management of infections in an immunocompromised patient can be challenging and is often best accomplished in consultation with an infectious disease specialist.

NEUTROPENIC FEVER

Neutropenia is a common complication in patients receiving with primary hematologic malignancies or receiving chemotherapy. Prolonged duration and severity of neutropenia translate into an increased risk of bloodstream and other serious infections. Neutropenic fever is defined as an absolute neutrophil count (ANC) of <500 cells/mm³ or <1000 cells/mm³ with an anticipated decline below 500 cells/mm over the next 48 hours coupled with the presence of a single temperature of ≥38.3°C (101°F) or a persistent temperature of ≥38.0°C (100.4°F) for more than one hour. Neutropenia fever is an emergency and should always be assumed infectious in etiology until proven otherwise. More than half of all patients with neutropenic fever are ultimately found to have either an established or occult infection.

A number of conditions can predispose the neutropenic patient to developing neutropenic fevers. Mucositis secondary to chemotherapy increases the risk for infections of the sinuses, oropharynx, and the gastrointestinal tract. Invasive fungal sinusitis (mucormycosis) caused by zygomycetes can progress to severe rhino-orbital cerebral infections requiring extensive surgical debridement. Neutropenic enterocolitis, also known as typhlitis, manifests as a necrotizing infection of the cecum that can extend to the terminal ileum and ascending colon, leading to bowel perforation peritonitis, hemorrhage, and sepsis. *Clostridium difficile* infection (CDI) may present as abdominal pain with diarrhea (see Chapter 42 for more details). Translocation of

ABLE 40.1	Common and Important Pathogens in the Immunocompromised Host
Neutropenia	
A. Pneumonia	Bacteria, *Aspergillus* spp., CMV, respiratory viruses
B. CNS infection	Bacteria, *Listeria monocytogenes*, *Aspergillus* spp., *Cryptococcus neoformans*, HSV, CMV, HHV-6
Transplant	
A. Pneumonia	Bacteria, *Nocardia* spp., *Mycobacterium tuberculosis*, nontuberculous mycobacteria, *Pneumocystis jirovecii*, *Aspergillus* spp., CMV, respiratory viruses, *Strongyloides stercoralis*
B. CNS infection	*Nocardia* spp., *Listeria monocytogenes*, *Aspergillus* spp., *Cryptococcus neoformans*, endemic fungi, CMV, HHV-6, HSV, VZV, *Toxoplasma gondii*
HIV	
A. Pneumonia	
Any CD4+	Bacteria, *Mycobacterium tuberculosis*
CD4+ <200	Above + *Pneumocystis jirovecii*, endemic mycoses, *Toxoplasma gondii*
CD4+ <50	Above + *Mycobacterium avium complex*, CMV, VZV
B. CNS infection	
Any CD4+	Bacteria, *Listeria monocytogenes*, HSV
CD4+ <100	*Toxoplasma gondii*
CD4+ <50	*Cryptococcus neoformans*, CMV, EBV-associated lymphoma, VZV, JC polyomavirus (PML)

V, cytomegalovirus; CNS, central nervous system; EBV, Epstein–Barr virus; HHV, human pesvirus; HIV, human immunodeficiency virus; HSV, herpes simplex virus; PML, progressive ltifocal leukoencephalopathy; VZV, varicella zoster virus.

estinal bacteria across damaged mucosal membranes can precipitate serious blood-eam infections with *Enterococcus* species and gram-negative organisms. Pneumonia d urinary tract infections are common. Cutaneous and mucosal infections caused herpes viruses and fungi increase the risk of bacterial superinfection. Long-term scular access sites present avenues of infection from skin flora. Catheter-related fections associated with severe sepsis, suppurative thrombophlebitis, endocarditis, tic emboli, and bacteremia usually require catheter removal in order to clear the fection (see Chapter 38).

Similarly, the list of potential pathogens is long, and requires a broad differential ignosis to guide work-up and management. In the last two decades, the continuum of thogens implicated in neutropenic fever has shifted from gram-negative bacilli (*Pseudomas aeruginosa*, *Escherichia coli*, and *Klebsiella* species) toward gram-positive organisms *aphylococcus aureus*, *Staphylococcus epidermidis*, *Streptococcus* species, and *Enterococcus* ecies) and fungi. Patients with a prior history of tuberculosis are at increased risk for activation of disease. With protracted chemotherapy and neutropenia, *Nocardia* and ngal infections with *Aspergillus* (invasive pneumonia, sinusitis), *Fusarium*, *Cryptococcus neoformans*, and endemic mycoses (*Histoplasma capsulatum*, *Blastomyces dermatitis*, and *Coccidioides immitis*) may be encountered. Disseminated candidiasis is not common, and often presents with hepatic and splenic abscesses. Patients requiring prolonged high-dose corticosteroids without adequate antimicrobial prophylaxis m develop *Pneumocystis jirovecii* pneumonia. Viral infections secondary to herpes simp virus (HSV), cytomegalovirus (CMV), Epstein–Barr virus (EBV), varicella zoster vi (VZV), and human herpesvirus-6 (HHV-6) may assume a wide range of clinical ma ifestations including meningitis, encephalitis, esophagitis, hepatitis, and skin disease.

Despite the above-mentioned shift, broad spectrum antimicrobial covera continues to be the initial standard of care. Early (administered as soon as fever recognized) empiric antimicrobial therapy in neutropenic fever decreases mort ity and takes precedence once adequate blood cultures have been obtained. Bas on local antimicrobial resistance patterns, monotherapy with an antipseudom nal cephalosporin, beta-lactam, or carbapenem for broad gram-negative covera is initially recommended with or without vancomycin for gram-positive covera (Algorithm 40.1). If blood cultures remain negative and a fever persists for mc than 5 days, empiric antifungal therapy is usually warranted to cover mold infectio Empiric antiviral therapy is generally not recommended unless characteristic skin cutaneous lesions suggestive of HSV or VZV are identified or active influenza h been identified in the community.

SOLID-ORGAN TRANSPLANTATION

The spectrum of infectious diseases encountered in patients who have undergo solid-organ transplantation varies over time and with the degree of immunosuppr sion used to ensure graft survival (Table 40.2). The majority of infections in the fi month following a solid-organ transplant represent complications of surgery a prolonged hospitalization. Wound dehiscence, degradation of anatomic integri infected fluid collections (blood, urine, and bile), and other infectious complicatio may be encountered depending on the type of graft (Table 40.3). The importance early surgical debridement, early anatomic interrogation of the transplanted orga drainage of infected fluid collections, and antimicrobial therapy cannot be overe phasized. Health care–associated pneumonia, urinary tract infection, and infectio of vascular catheters, surgical drains, and other foreign objects are also comm during the postoperative period. Removal or exchange of any indwelling devic should be done in consultation with the surgical team when a device-related infecti is suspected. Reactivation of latent infections (HBV, HCV, HIV, tuberculosis, stro gyloidiasis) may be encountered. Infection by colonizing or nosocomial bacteria a fungi are not uncommon. Multidrug-resistant organisms (MRSA, VRE, extend spectrum beta lactamase gram-negative organisms, azole-resistant Candida speci must be considered. Although rare, infections transmitted to a transplant recipie through an infected donor organ must be considered in the setting of clinical det rioration during the first week after transplant if no other obvious explanations a plausible. *Toxoplasma gondii* can cause myocarditis in heart transplant recipien When treating any of the above infectious complications of organ transplantatio one must consider the effects of the chosen antibiotics on serum levels of antirejecti medications and adjust dosing accordingly.

Following the first month after transplant, immunosuppression to prevent acu rejection substantially increases the risk of opportunistic infection. In particula patients receiving high-dose corticosteroids and T-lymphocyte depleting agents (an thymocyte globulins, OKT3, alemtuzumab) may be especially vulnerable to seve viral (human herpesvirus) infections. CMV infection and reactivation are common

ALGORITHM 40.1 Management of Neutropenic Fever

Fever ≥38.3°C or persistently ≥38.0°C for at least 1 hr **AND** ANC ≤500/mm³ or ANC ≥500/mm³ with expected decline to ≤500/mm³

↓

- Blood cultures × 2, urinalysis and urine culture, chest radiograph, other testing as indicated (e.g., nasopharyngeal swab for influenza and other respiratory viruses; *Clostridium difficile* toxin)
- Empiric gram-negative antibiotics*
- Vancomycin 1 g q12hr × 72 hours if indicated**

If suspected intra-abdominal source or *Clostridium difficile* infection, consider adding Metronidazole 500 mg PO/IV q8hr

If *clinically unstable* consider adding double gram-negative coverage with aminoglycoside × 72 hours

Discontinue aminoglycoside if cultures negative after 72 hours

↓

New temp after afebrile ≥48 hours **OR** persistently febrile ≥72 hours and cultures negative

Clinically unstable
- Change gram-negative coverage
- Consider addition of vancomycin**

Clinically stable
- Culture negative: continue same regimen
- Culture positive: per culture and sensitivities

(**) Indications for Vancomycin
- Severe mucositis
- Clinical evidence of catheter-related infection
- Known colonization with resistant streptococci or staphylococci
- Sudden temperature spike of >40°C
- Hypotension

Discontinue Vancomycin after 72 hours if cultures negative for coagulase negative staphylococci, methicillin-resistant *Staphylococcus aureus*, or cephalosporin-resistant streptococci

Persistently febrile ≥5 days and cultures negative
- Consider infectious disease consult
- Consider addition of antifungal agent (voriconazole vs. liposomal amphotericin B)

ABBREVIATIONS
ANC: absolute neutrophil count
IV: intravenous

(*) Gram-negative coverage
Cefepime 1 g IV q8hr **OR**
Meropenem 500 mg IV q6hr **OR**
Piperacillin-tazobactam 3.375 g IV q6hr

Penicillin allergy
Ciprofloxacin 400 mg IV q12hr **OR**
Aztreonam 2 g IV q8hr

Adapted from Barnes-Jewish Hospital Stem Cell Transplant Unit Febrile Neutropenia Pathway.

TABLE 40.2 Timeline of Infections in the Solid-Organ Transplant Patient

≤1 mo	1–6 mo	≥6 mo
Postoperative complication and nosocomial infection	**Postoperative complication (less common)**	**Low-level immunosuppression**
• Surgical site infection	**Nosocomial infection**	• Community-acquired infection (pneumonia, UTI)
• Graft ischemia/ superinfection	**Opportunistic infection** (Depending upon antimi- crobial prophylaxis)	• *Nocardia* spp.
• Anastomotic leak	• *Listeria monocytogenes*	• *Rhodococcus*
• Abscess/infected fluid collection	• *Nocardia* spp.	• *Mycobacterium tuberculosis*
• Pneumonia	• *Mycobacterium tuberculosis*	• Nontuberculous mycobacteria
• Urinary tract infection	• Nontuberculous mycobacteria	• *Aspergillus* spp.
• Catheter-associated infection	• *Pneumocystis jirovecii*	• *Mucor* spp.
• *Clostridium difficile* infection	• *Aspergillus* spp.	• *Cryptococcus neoformans*
	• *Cryptococcus neoformans*	• Endemic fungi
Donor-derived infection	• Endemic fungi	• Herpesviruses (CMV, EBV, HSV, VZV), EBV-related PTLD
• *Aspergillus* spp., *Cryp- tococcus neoformans*, endemic fungi (*Histo- plasma capsulatum, Coccidioides immitis*)	• Herpesviruses (CMV, EBV, HSV, VZV, HHV-6/7/8)	• HBV, HCV
• Herpesviruses (CMV, EBV, HSV, VZV, HHV-6), HIV, HBV, HCV, WNV, LCMV, rhabdovirus (rabies)	• HBV, HCV	• JC polyomavirus (PML)
	• Adenovirus	• BK polyomavirus
• *Toxoplasma gondii, Try- panosoma cruzi* (Chagas)	• Influenza, RSV	**High-level immunosuppression**
• *Balamuthia mandrillaris, Strongyloides stercoralis*	• Parvovirus B19	• See Opportunistic Infection (1–6 mo)
	• BK polyomavirus (nephropathy)	
Recipient-derived infection	• *Toxoplasma gondii* (myocarditis)	
• *Mycobacterium tuberculosis*	• *Leishmania*	
• *Cryptococcus neoformans*, endemic fungi	• *Trypanosoma cruzi*	
• Herpesviruses, HIV, HBV, HCV	• Cryptosporidium	
	• Microsporidium	
• *Toxoplasma gondii, Strongyloides stercoralis* (hyperinfection)	• *Strongyloides stercora- lis* (hyperinfection)	

CMV, cytomegalovirus; EBV, Epstein–Barr virus; HBV, hepatitis B virus; HCV, hepatitis C virus; HHV, human herpesvirus; HIV, human immunodeficiency virus; HSV, herpes simplex virus; LCMV, lymphocytic choriomeningitis virus; PML, progressive multifocal leukoencephalopathy; PTLD, post-transplant lymphoproliferative disorder; RSV, respiratory syncytial virus; UTI, urinary tract infection; WNV, West Nile virus; VZV, varicella zoster virus.

Adapted from Fishman JA. Infection in solid-organ transplant recipients. *N Engl J Med*. 2007; 357(25):2601–2614.

TABLE 40.3	Graft Site–Specific Infections
Heart	Myocarditis (*Toxoplasma gondii* seropositive donor to seronegative recipient)
	Mediastinitis/sternal wound infection (*Staphylococcus aureus*, *Staphylococcus epidermidis*)
Lung	Pneumonia (*Pseudomonas aeruginosa*, *Escherichia coli*, *Klebsiella pneumoniae*, *Stenotrophomonas maltophilia*, *Staphylococcus aureus*, *Burkholderia cepacia*, *Mycobacterium tuberculosis*, CMV, *Candida* species, *Aspergillus* species)
	Mediastinitis (*Pseudomonas aeruginosa*, *Escherichia coli*, *Klebsiella pneumoniae*, *Staphylococcus epidermidis*)
Liver	Biloma/hepatic abscess/peritonitis (*Enterococcus*, *Klebsiella pneumoniae*, *Enterobacter cloacae*, *Candida* species)
Kidney	Urinary tract infection (*Escherichia coli*, *Enterobacter cloacae*, *Klebsiella* species, *Proteus mirabilis*, *Enterococcus* species)
	Nephropathy (BK polyomavirus)

patients not on prophylactic antiviral therapy. CMV donor–recipient mismatch leading to primary CMV infection carries the highest risk of invasive disease (pneumonitis, hepatitis, colitis). Coinfection with immunomodulating viruses (CMV, EBV, HHV-6, HBV, HCV) may further predispose a patient to serious bacterial and fungal infections. Information concerning a patient's antimicrobial prophylaxis regimen, geographic location, hobbies, and epidemiologic exposures may lend further insight into the types of opportunistic infections possible.

As the risk of acute graft rejection declines over time, the requirement for immunosuppression generally stabilizes and decreases. At 6 months posttransplant, most patients are more likely to suffer from community-acquired infections (e.g., pneumonia) than opportunistic ones. However, patients still on significant doses of immunosuppressive regimens remain prone to the latter.

HEMATOPOIETIC STEM CELL TRANSPLANTATION

The risk of infection after allogeneic hematopoietic stem cell transplant bears a resemblance to that of the neutropenic patient and can be separated into three general phases (Table 40.4). Patients undergoing autologous transplant share the same risks of infection during the pre-engraftment phase, but largely recover immune function thereafter. The differential diagnosis for infection can be narrowed by obtaining a focused history and physical examination assessing the type of transplant, amount of time since transplant, presence of chronic graft-versus-host disease (GVHD), immunosuppression, antimicrobial prophylaxis, travel history, occupation, and hobbies.

During the first three weeks after transplant, the pre-engraftment phase represents the period of greatest bone marrow suppression and is defined by neutropenia following conditioning chemotherapy. Recipients are at high risk for gram-negative infections as a result of chemotherapy-related mucositis and translocation of gut flora

TABLE 40.4	Timeline of Infections in the Hematopoietic Stem Cell Transplant Patient	
Pre-engraftment (<3 wks)	**Early Postengraftment (3 wks–3 mo)**	**Late Postengraftment (>3 mo)**
• Gram-negative bacteria (*Pseudomonas aerugi-nosa, Enterobacteriaceae, Stenotrophomonas maltophilia*) • Gram-positive bacteria (*Staphylococcus aureus,* coagulase-negative staph-ylococcus, *Streptococcus* spp., *Enterococcus*) • *Clostridium difficile* • *Candida* spp. • *Aspergillus* spp. • *Fusarium* spp • Zygomycetes • HSV (seropositive) • Respiratory viruses (RSV, parainfluenza, rhinovirus, influenza, adenovirus, human metapneumovirus)	• *Legionella pneumophila* • *Listeria monocytogenes* • *Nocardia* spp. • *Mycobacterium tuberculosis* • Nontuberculous mycobacteria • *Candida* spp. • *Aspergillus* spp. • *Fusarium* spp. • Zygomycetes • *Pneumocystis jirovecii* • CMV (seropositive) • EBV • HHV-6, -7 • VZV (seropositive) • Respiratory viruses • BK polyomavirus • *Toxoplasma gondii* • *Strongyloides stercoralis* • *Cryptosporidium*	• Encapsulated bacteria (*Streptococcus pneu-moniae, Haemophilus influenzae, Neisseria meningitidis*) • *Nocardia* spp. • Endemic mycoses • CMV • EBV • VZV (seropositive) • BK/JC polyomavirus • Parvovirus B19 • If chronic GVHD, then consider pre-engraftment and early postengraftment organisms as well

CMV, cytomegalovirus; EBV, Epstein–Barr virus; GVHD, graft-versus-host disease; HHV, human h pesvirus; HSV, herpes simplex virus; RSV, respiratory syncytial virus; VZV, varicella zoster virus. Adapted from Hiemenz JW. Management of infections complicating allogeneic hematopoietic stem cell transplantation. *Semin Hematol*. 2009;46(3):289–312.

as described above. Gram-positive infections from skin and oropharyngeal flora a also common. Infection with *Streptococcus viridans* can lead to a rapidly fatal sho syndrome. Bacteremia, pneumonia, and CDI figure prominently during this pha Localized and disseminated azole-resistant candidiasis as well as invasive mold inf tions (*Aspergillus, Fusarium, Zygomycetes*) presenting as pneumonia, sinusitis, cent nervous system infection, or skin lesions are also encountered. Seropositive recipie not taking antiviral prophylaxis are highly vulnerable to reactivation of HSV, whi can involve the skin, liver, and gastrointestinal tract. Finally, patients with a history delayed engraftment and prolonged neutropenia are at higher risk for invasive mc infections and *C. difficile* infections due to the use of broad spectrum antimicrobia

Bone marrow recovery marks the beginning of the immediate post-engraftme phase, which typically lasts from 3 weeks to 3 months after transplant. Cell-media and humoral deficiencies predominate. Acute GVHD, when present, requires hig dose immunosuppression that further increases the risk of infection. The risk many of the same fungal infections seen in the pre-engraftment phase persists. Re tivation of immunomodulating human herpesviruses, most importantly CMV, c result in life-threatening pneumonia, encephalitis, colitis, and marrow suppression. Reactivation of toxoplasmosis may also be seen during this phase.

Six months after transplantation, the recipient enters the late postengraftment phase. If a recipient has not developed GVHD, immune function may be largely restored within 1 to 2 years. Conversely, recipients who have chronic GVHD and receive additional immunosuppression remain at high risk for severe infection, particularly with encapsulated bacteria (*Streptococcus pneumoniae, Haemophilus influenzae, Neisseria meningitidis*), *Nocardia* species, fungi, and viruses (CMV, EBV, VZV, adenovirus).

HUMAN IMMUNODEFICIENCY VIRUS

The advent of antiretroviral therapy (ART) has revolutionized the care of patients with human immunodeficiency virus (HIV). ART-adherent patients are more likely to be admitted to the intensive care unit (ICU) with medical problems unrelated to their HIV infection or directly related to the antiretroviral regimens themselves. The decision to continue ART while in the ICU should be made in collaboration with an infectious disease specialist. Patients with a new diagnosis of HIV or lack of adherence to medications are more likely to present acutely ill requiring ICU admission. The CD4$^+$ lymphocyte cell count remains an accurate gauge of susceptibility to opportunistic infection in HIV patients. However, patients should be screened for coexisting chronic viral infections, as they may increase the risk of mortality (e.g., hepatitis C).

Pulmonary infection is common in this population and has a broad differential diagnosis. Community-acquired pneumonia due to *S. pneumoniae, H. influenzae,* and increasingly *S. aureus,* remains a common cause of pulmonary infection in this population, irrespective of CD4$^+$ cell count. *Mycobacterium tuberculosis* may present with pulmonary or extrapulmonary manifestations in HIV. The prevalence of *P. jirovecii* pneumonia increases dramatically once the CD4$^+$ cell count drops below 200 cells/mm^3; the use of prophylactic antimicrobials does not exclude the diagnosis. In severe cases (when PO$_2$ <60 and A-a gradient is >45), adjunctive steroids should be used to decrease mortality. Other fungal pneumonias such as *C. neoformans* and *H. capsulatum,* occur commonly below this CD4$^+$ cell threshold. Lower CD4$^+$ cell counts increase the risk for disseminated mycobacterial infection, fungal disease, and bacteremia associated with pneumonia. Pneumonia secondary to *Mycobacterium avium complex* (MAC), CMV, and VZV can occur below a CD4$^+$ cell count of 50 cells/mm^3. Adrenal insufficiency can complicate management and is associated with disseminated CMV, tuberculosis, Kaposi's sarcoma, lymphoma, and treatment with ketoconazole or pentamidine.

Central nervous system infections are more common when the CD4$^+$ cell count is severely depressed. *T. gondii* encephalitis generally manifests when the CD4$^+$ cell count falls below 100 cells/mm^3, and presents with fever, headache, altered mental status, neurologic deficits, and seizures. In most cases, ring-enhancing lesions are seen on contrasted head CT and/or MRI. Less common infections associated with ring-enhancing lesions may include bacterial brain abscess, cryptococcomas, and syphilitic gummas. Below a CD4$^+$ cell count of 50 cells/mm^3, meningoencephalitis secondary to *C. neoformans* may present with severe headache, photophobia, and possibly coma; and is associated with markedly elevated intracranial pressures. Herpesvirus encephalitis (HSV, CMV, VZV), primary CNS lymphoma (EBV), and progressive multifocal leukoencephalopathy (JC polyomavirus) must be considered in the patient with rapid neurologic deterioration and abnormalities on brain imaging.

Immune reconstitution inflammatory syndrome (IRIS) is a life-threatening complication of ART that can be indistinguishable from an acute opportunistic infection. Usually apparent within days to weeks of initiating ART, improvements in immune function lead to an exuberant inflammatory response against infectious agents that were previously clinically silent. *M. tuberculosis*, MAC, *P. jirovecii*, endemic fungi, and CMV infections are most commonly seen and may occur at previously known sites of infection or at new sites altogether. Corticosteroids may attenuate the inflammatory response and their use should be weighed against the risk of further immunosuppression.

ASPLENIA

Patients who have undergone splenectomy or who are functionally asplenic secondary to underlying disease (sickle cell disease, splenic artery thrombosis, malaria, infiltrative disease, complications of mononucleosis, or iatrogenic embolization for hemorrhage) or trauma are at increased risk for severe sepsis by encapsulated organisms including *S. pneumonia*, *H. influenza*, and *N. meningitidis*. It is important to inquire about prior immunizations and immunize appropriately as effective vaccines exist against each of these organisms.

BIOLOGIC AGENTS

Tumor necrosis factor (TNF) antagonists (e.g., etanercept, infliximab, adalimumab) have found increased use in the treatment of rheumatoid arthritis, Crohn's disease, and other inflammatory autoimmune disorders. Newer biologic agents such as rituximab, tocilizumab, abatacept, and tofacitinib are also growing in use. As TNF helps regulate cell-mediated immunity, its inhibition can increase the risk of infection due to a range of viruses, fungi, protozoa, and intracellular bacteria. Risk factors for systemic infection include increased age, comorbidities, steroid use, concurrent use of disease-modifying antirheumatic drugs (DMARDs), previous use of DMARDs, functional status, and previous history of systemic infections. Low-dose biologic agents do not increase the risk of infection compared to DMARDs alone. However, standard and high-dose biologics with or without DMARDs increase the risk of infection. The majority of the data on newer agents remains limited due to small study sample sizes. However, rituximab has received a black box warning for progressive multifocal leukoencephalopathy and tofacitinib has been associated with an increased risk of HSV infection when combined with other therapies. Of note, patients with untreated latent *M. tuberculosis* infection are susceptible to developing active disease after initiation of a TNF antagonist. Finally, infections due to opportunistic organisms (*T. gondii*, endemic fungi, *P. jirovecii*), *Legionella pneumophilia*, *Listeria monocytogenes*, *Nocardia*, Actinomyces, and nontuberculous mycobacteria are also possible.

SUGGESTED READINGS

Akgun KM, Miller RF. Critical care in human immunodeficiency virus-infected patients. *Semin Respir Crit Care Med.* 2016;37(2):303–317.

Corona A, Raimondi F. Caring for HIV-infected patients in the ICU in the highly active antiretroviral therapy era. *Curr HIV Res.* 2009;7(6):569–579.

man JA. Infection in solid-organ transplant recipients. *N Engl J Med.* 2007;357(25): 2601–2614.

man JA. Infections in immunocompromised hosts and organ transplant recipients: essentials. *Liver Transpl.* 2011;17:S34–S37.

menz JW. Management of infections complicating allogeneic hematopoietic stem cell transplantation. *Semin Hematol.* 2009;46(3):289–312.

iri M, Dixon W. Risk of infection with biologic antirheumatic therapies in patients with rheumatoid arthritis. *Best Pract Res Clin Rheumatol.* 2015;29(2):290–305.

den PK. Approach to the immunocompromised host with infection in the intensive care unit. *Infect Dis Clin North Am.* 2009;23(3):535–556.

alilavan G, Limaye A. Infections in transplant patients. *Med Clin North Am.* 2013:97: 581–600.

gh J, Cameron C, Noorbaloochi S, et al. Risk of serious infection in biologic treatment of patients with rheumatoid arthritis: a systematic review and meta-analysis. *Lancet.* 2015; 386:258–265.

41 Prevention of Infection in the Intensive Care Unit

Amy M. Hunter and Carol J. Sykora

Infections acquired in the intensive care unit (ICU) are a significant contributor morbidity and mortality. ICU-acquired infections increase patient length of s and lead to costs in excess of $45,000 per occurrence (*JAMA Intern Med.* 20 173(22):2039–2046). Multiple measures to prevent the transmission of organis within the ICU are necessary. Transmission-based precautions including conta droplet, and airborne should be instituted when necessary, and health care worl compliance should be monitored. Contact precautions (gown, gloves, and designa equipment) should be instituted for those with antibiotic-resistant organisms such methicillin-resistant *Staphylococcus aureus,* vancomycin-resistant *Enterococcus,* multip drug resistant gram-negative bacilli, and *Clostridium difficile.* Droplet precautic (surgical mask) are necessary for large droplet infectious agents such as influer and the meningococcus. Airborne precautions (N95 respirator and negative-press ventilation) are used for airborne infectious agents such as *Mycobacterium tubercule* and varicella. To prevent health care worker and patient exposure, transmission-bas precautions must be instituted on first clinical suspicion. Infection prevention shou be consulted in cases in which a patient or health care worker exposure may ha taken place.

Hospital-acquired infections that are device-associated, such as ventilatc associated pneumonia (VAP), catheter-associated urinary tract infections (CAUTI and central line–associated bloodstream infections (CLABSIs), pose the greatest ri to hospitalized patients. Clinical surveys suggest that 5% to 15% of ventilated patie develop nosocomial pneumonia. In 2011, CAUTI rates in adult ICUs reporting the National Healthcare Safety Network (NHSN) ranged from 1.2 to 4.5 per 10 urinary catheter-days. It is estimated that 70% to 80% of urinary tract infections attributable to an indwelling urethral catheter.

The Centers for Disease Control and Prevention (CDC) and Society of Heal care Epidemiology (SHEA)/Infectious Diseases Society of America (IDSA) have pu lished evidence-based guidelines for the prevention of device-associated infectio which are summarized in Tables 41.1 to 41.3.

GENERAL MEASURES

Foremost in prevention of infections is adequate hand hygiene prior to placing and/ handling an invasive device or examining a patient. Alcohol-based hand rubs plac at the bedside have been shown to increase compliance as well as maintain the sk integrity of health care workers' hands and should be encouraged. Alcohol hand ru

TABLE 41.1	Summary of Recommendations for the Prevention of Ventilator-Associated Pneumonia (VAP) and Other Ventilator-Associated Events (VAEs) in Adult Patients

Basic practices to prevent VAP and other VAEs:

Before intubation:

Use noninvasive positive pressure ventilation (NIPPV), if possible

After intubation is in place:

Minimize sedation
- Manage ventilated patients without sedation when feasible
- Interrupt sedation once a day using spontaneous awakening trials unless medically contraindicated

Assess ventilated patient for readiness to extubate once a day using spontaneous breathing trials unless medically contraindicated

Perform spontaneous breathing and awakening trials together to allow the patient the opportunity to pass the breathing trial and be extubated when they are maximally awake

Provide physical conditioning for the ventilated patient through exercise and mobilization as early as possible

- Avoid or eliminate pooling of secretions above the endotracheal tube (ET) with the use of subglottic drainage ports if intubation is expected to be required for longer than 48–72 hrs
- Elevate the head of the bed by 30–45 degrees
- Change the ventilator circuits when visibly soiled or if they are malfunctioning
- Follow the Centers for Disease Control and Prevention (CDC's) Healthcare Infection Control Practices Advisory Council (HICPAC) guidelines for sterilization and disinfection of the respiratory care equipment

Additional interventions for which there are insufficient data to determine their full impact include:
- Perform oral care using a chlorhexidine product
- Use ultrathin polyurethane ET cuffs
- Use an automated pressure control for ET cuff pressure
- Instill saline before tracheal suctioning
- Perform mechanical tooth brushing

Abbreviated and adapted from Klompas M, Branson R, Eichenwald EC, et al.; Society for Healthcare Epidemiology of America (SHEA). Strategies to prevent ventilator-associated pneumonia in acute care hospitals: 2014 update. *Infect Control Hosp Epidemiol.* 2014;35(8):915–936.

can be used whenever hands are not visibly soiled. Antimicrobial soaps should also be available in the ICU setting for use when hands are soiled or following a body substance exposure. Effective cleaning and disinfection of the ICU environment also plays a key role in reducing the transmission of microorganisms.

Additionally, commonly used invasive devices in the ICU allow organisms a portal of entry during a time when the patient is particularly susceptible to infection. Therefore, general prevention measures should include a daily review of the necessity of all invasive devices and removing them as soon as they are no longer clinically necessary. Additional prevention measures are aimed at the placement and maintenance of the device.

Finally, the NHSN provides standardized definitions for surveillance for ICU-acquired infections. Surveillance takes place on a routine basis in order to monitor

TABLE 41.2	Summary of Recommendations for the Prevention of Catheter-Associated Urinary Tract Infections (CAUTIs) in Acute Care Hospitals

Basic practices to prevent CAUTI:
- Follow written policies, protocols, or guidelines for the use, insertion, maintenance, and removal of the urinary catheter
- Require only trained staff be allowed to insert urinary catheters using aseptic technique and that the necessary sterile supplies, including: sterile gloves, drape, sponges, antiseptic solution, and single-use lubricant, be readily available for use
- Perform hand hygiene before donning sterile gloves for inserting the urinary catheter; and before or after manipulating the catheter or site
- Use the smallest-sized urinary catheter as is feasible to minimize urethral trauma
- Secure indwelling urinary catheters
- Maintain a sterile, closed drainage system; replace the urinary catheter and drainage system if sterility has been compromised (e.g., system contaminated, seal broken, or there is leakage)
- Maintain unobstructed urine flow
- Document the insertion, care, and removal of the urinary catheter; daily assessment should include reason for continued use; or document removal criteria that was met
- Provide education for staff on proper insertion, care and removal of the urinary catheter to prevent CAUTIs
- Assess staff competency in performing insertion, maintenance and removal of the urinary catheter
- Insert urinary catheters only when necessary and remove as soon as assessment indicates there is no reason for continued use
- Use intermittent catheterization instead of indwelling catheters, whenever possible

Perform CAUTI surveillance per hospital risk assessment and regulatory requirements
- Determine patient population at risk of CAUTI
- Using National Healthcare Safety Network (NHSN) criteria, calculate CAUTI rates and/or the standardized infection ratio (SIR) for at risk patient populations
- Provide feedback of CAUTI data to the patient-based unit and hospital leadership

Abbreviated and adapted from Lo E, Nicolle LE, Coffin SE, et al. Strategies to prevent catheter-associated urinary tract infections in acute care hospitals: 2014 update. *Infect Control Hosp Epidemiol.* 2014;35(5):464–479.

patient outcomes of care. Infection rates should be provided to ICU medical an nursing staff for review, and immediate action taken in times of increased rates. Addi tionally, prevention measures should be monitored regularly for consistency of appli cation. For optimal reduction in the transmission of infections, all evidence-base prevention methods for each infection must be applied together.

CATHETER-ASSOCIATED URINARY TRACT INFECTION

Basic practices outlined in the SHEA and IDSA updated strategies for reducin CAUTIs include recommendations that should be adopted by all acute care hos pitals. Appropriate use of urinary catheters is paramount in preventing infection

ABLE 41.3	Summary of Recommendations for the Prevention of Central Line-Associated Bloodstream Infections (CLABSIs) in Acute Care Hospitals

ior to Insertion

Provide an evidence-based indication for placement of central venous catheter (CVC)

Educate health care workers involved in placement and care of CVC

Bathe patients with chlorhexidine daily

Insertion

Establish a process, such as a checklist to ensure adherence to infection prevention practices

Perform hand hygiene prior to manipulating or inserting CVC

Avoid placing CVC in the femoral vein in obese patients when placing under planned and controlled conditions

Utilize a cart or kit containing all supplies necessary for aseptic CVC insertion

Use ultrasound guidance when placing CVC in the internal jugular vein

Use maximum sterile barrier precautions during placement including mask, sterile gown and gloves for the health care workers involved in the CVC insertion, as well as, the draping of the patient with a full body drape

Prepare insertion site with a 0.5% chlorhexidine and alcohol skin preparation

ter Insertion

Provide appropriate nurse-to-patient ratio and limit use of float nurses

Disinfect injection ports and catheter hubs prior to accessing the catheter utilizing an antiseptic (chlorhexidine/alcohol, 70% alcohol or povidone-iodine) and mechanical friction

Remove catheters that are no longer essential to the patient's care

Change transparent dressings on nontunneled CVCs and perform site care with a chlorhexidine based antiseptic every 5–7 days and when soiled or loose

Replace administration sets not used for blood products, blood or lipids within 96 hrs of use

Apply antimicrobial ointments to hemodialysis catheter insertion sites (mupirocin ointment is not recommended due to potential for resistance; catheter manufacturer recommendations should be consulted to assess for ointment compatibility)

Perform surveillance for central line-associated bloodstream infections (CLABSI)

A CLABSI risk assessment should be conducted in areas with unacceptably high rates to ensure compliance with the above prevention strategies prior to implementing approaches such as antimicrobial impregnated catheters and dressings

breviated and adapted from Marschall, J, Mermel LA, Fakih, M, et al. Strategies to prevent ntral line associated bloodstream infections in acute care hospitals: 2014 update. *Infect Contrl sp Epidemiol.* 2014;35(suppl 2):S89–S107.

utine use of urinary catheters for incontinence or postoperative use without specific dications is not recommended. Placement should be performed after adequate hand giene, by a trained professional, and under aseptic technique and conditions. Care the catheter should include maintenance of a closed drainage system and an unobucted flow of urine. Should the integrity of the system be interrupted, the entire stem should be replaced. All specimen collections should be performed aseptically.

VENTILATOR-ASSOCIATED PNEUMONIA

Recommendations to prevent VAP include measures to prevent aspiration of se tions, prevent contamination of the ventilator circuit, and minimize sedation, e mobilization, and daily assessment of readiness to extubate. Maintaining the hea the patient's bed at a minimum of 30 degrees assists with prevention of aspirat The CDC recommends oropharyngeal cleaning and decontamination for patien risk for VAP. There is no longer a recommendation to routinely change the ventil circuit unless it is visibly soiled. Adult patients on mechanical ventilation are at for serious complications, in addition to pneumonia. Serious complications incl sepsis, barotrauma, acute respiratory distress syndrome, pneumothorax, pulmoi embolism, and pulmonary edema. These are classified as ventilator-associated ev (VAEs). The CDC developed surveillance definitions for VAEs that include crit for ventilator-associated conditions (VACs), infection-related ventilator-associ complications (IVACs), and possible ventilator-associated pneumonia (PVAP).

CENTRAL LINE–ASSOCIATED BLOOD STREAM INFECTIC

The risk for CLABSI in the ICU is high due to the prolonged use of mult catheters that are frequently accessed. Recommendations to prevent bloodstre infections (BSI) include placing the central venous catheter (CVC) using asep technique with maximal sterile barriers including sterile gown, sterile glo mask, and a full drape. A chlorhexidine and alcohol tincture is the prefer agent for skin antisepsis prior to CVC placement, as well as preparation dur dressing changes. When selecting a site for insertion, the femoral vein should avoided. The subclavian vein has the least instance of infection, however the and benefits of infections and noninfectious complications should be weighed an individual basis. The use of a catheter insertion checklist and a standardi insertion kit to promote best practices is also recommended. The decision to antimicrobial or antiseptic impregnated catheters, devices, dressings, or spor should be made by the critical care and infection prevention team and based on evaluation of current infection rates and compliance with evidence-based practi Daily chlorhexidine bathing has also been shown effective to prevent CLA in the ICU. Care should be taken to avoid CLABSI because the blood stre infection can lead to other infectious complications such as endocarditis, sep thrombophlebitis, and osteomyelitis.

SUGGESTED READINGS

Gould C, Umscheid C, Agarwal RK, et al; Healthcare Infection Control Practices Advis
    Committee. Guidelines for prevention of catheter-associated urinary tract infections 20
    https://www.cdc.gov/hicpac/cauti/001_cauti.html. Checked July 20, 2016.
    HICPAC Guideline for the prevention of catheter-associated urinary tract infections, inc.
      ing specific recommendations for implementation, performance measurement,
      surveillance.
Klompas M, Branson R, Eichenwald EC, et al; Society for Healthcare Epidemiology of Ame
    (SHEA). Strategies to prevent ventilator-associated pneumonia in acute care hospi
    2014 update. *Infect Control Hosp Epidemiol.* 2014;35(8):915–936.
    Update presenting strategies for preventing ventilator-associated events, including ventila
      associated pneumonia.

o E, Nicolle LE, Coffin SE, et al. Strategies to prevent catheter-associated urinary tract infections in acute care hospitals: 2014 update. *Infect Contrl Hosp Epidemiol.* 2014;35(suppl 2): S32–S47.

> *Update on strategies for preventing catheter-associated urinary catheter infections, including documentation of daily presence of catheter, and aseptic insertion technique by trained personnel.*

larschall, J, Mermel LA, Fakih, M, et al. Strategies to prevent central line associated bloodstream infections in acute care hospitals: 2014 update. *Infect Contrl Hosp Epidemiol.* 2014;35(suppl 2):S89–S107.

egel J, Rhinehart E, Jackson M, et al; Health Care Infection Control Practices Advisory Committee. 2007 Guideline for isolation precautions: preventing transmission of infectious agents in health care settings. *Am J Infect Control.* 2007;35(10 suppl 2):S65–S164.

42 Clostridium difficile and Other Infectious Causes of Diarrhea

Ian R. Ross and Erik R. Dubberke

The most commonly encountered etiologies of infectious diarrhea in hospitalized adults in industrialized countries are *Clostridium difficile*, with *Salmonella* sp., Noro virus, and Rotavirus, and *Cryptosporidium* in the immunocompromised host bein less common.

NON-*CLOSTRIDIUM DIFFICILE* INFECTIOUS DIARRHEA

Diarrhea adversely impacts critically ill patients by contributing to dehydratio electrolyte imbalances, hemodynamic instability, malnutrition, and skin breakdow Most diarrhea in hospitalized patients is noninfectious. However, it is essential t consider an infectious etiology in an ICU patient when they have three or mo watery bowel movements per day, blood or mucus in the stool, vomiting, seve abdominal pain, and fever. Non-*C. difficile* enteropathogenic bacteria and parasite are detected in <1% of patients hospitalized for greater than 3 days with diarrhe A modified "3-day rule" has therefore been proposed to aid in when to cultu stool for enteropathogenic bacteria other than *C. difficile*. The rule states that sto cultures sent more than 72 hours after admission for diarrhea should be rejecte unless one of the following are present: neutropenia (<0.5 × 10^6 cells/mL), huma immunodeficiency virus (HIV) infection, suspected nondiarrheal manifestatio of enteric infection (erythema nodosum, mesenteric lymphadenitis, polyarthriti or fever of unknown origin), patient age of >65 years with comorbidities causin end-organ damage, or a suspected hospital-acquired outbreak. This rule is a safe an cost-effective cut-off for rejecting stool samples of adult patients.

Establishing the etiology of diarrhea if an infectious cause is suspected is import ant so pathogen-specific treatment can be initiated (if available), and the appropriat precautions can be taken to prevent transmission to other patients. It is important t obtain history of potential risk factors including recent antibiotic use, type of foo consumed, ingestion of untreated water, recent travel, contact with animals and il family members, immunosuppression due to HIV or chemotherapy, asplenia, sickl cell disease, and residence in a nursing home in the past 30 days. It is also importan to be cognizant that some etiologies of infectious diarrhea occur seasonally, such a norovirus, because hospital outbreaks can be coincident with those in the community The fecal–oral route is the usual mode of infection, and person-to-person spread is th most common form of transmission. It is important to work with Infectious Disease and Infection Prevention and Control personnel to implement appropriate measure to halt the spread of the causative organism to other patients and staff in the ICU.

CLOSTRIDIUM DIFFICILE INFECTION

Background

C. difficile is the leading cause of hospital-associated infectious diarrhea. It has also surpassed methicillin-resistant *Staphylococcus aureus* as the leading cause of hospital-associated infections. Beginning in 2001, there was a dramatic increase in incidence and severity of C. difficile infection (CDI) as well as an increased recognition of its role in community-acquired infection. These increases were associated in part with the emergence of a new prevalent strain of C. difficile, the BI/NAP1/027 strain. This strain is highly fluoroquinolone resistant, produces more toxin A and B in vitro than typical strains that cause disease in humans, and produces a third toxin, binary toxin. More recent data indicate that the number of diagnoses of CDI has plateaued.

C. difficile is a spore-forming anaerobic bacillus that produces two exotoxins, A and B, which cause intestinal pathology. Most patients who acquire C. difficile remain asymptomatic. When C. difficile does cause symptomatic infection, this is referred to as CDI. Most strains produce both toxin A and B, although some strains produce only toxin B. Strains that produce only toxin B can cause the same spectrum of illness as strains that produce both toxins and have caused hospital-associated outbreaks. Nontoxigenic strains are nonpathogenic. The differences in ability to produce toxin are important from a diagnostic standpoint, as some diagnostics detect C. difficile whether or not it produces toxin. This is discussed in more detail below.

Antimicrobial exposure is the most common and potentially modifiable risk factor for CDI, especially in the ICU where patients are frequently on several antibiotic classes concurrently. Historically, the most common antibiotics associated with CDI have been clindamycin, broad-spectrum cephalosporins, and ampicillin/amoxicillin, but nearly all antibacterial agents can predispose to CDI. Specifically, the fluoroquinolones have been increasingly associated with CDI, due in part to the emerging epidemic BI/NAP1/027 strain that is highly fluoroquinolone resistant. Patients can become symptomatic during treatment or several weeks after antibiotics have been stopped. Other risk factors include increasing age and severity of underlying illness. Although the mechanism is unclear, gastric acid suppressants such as H_2 antagonists and proton pump inhibitors are also associated with increased risk of CDI. CDI pressure, or the number of other patients with CDI in the same patient care area as the patient at risk, was found to be one of the factors most strongly associated with CDI. This provides additional evidence that CDI is caused from acquisition of C. difficile within the hospital setting, and stresses the importance of preventing patient-to-patient transmission of C. difficile.

Assessment

Symptoms of CDI range from mild self-limited diarrhea to life-threatening colitis. Distal ileitis has also been recognized but is uncommon and typically occurs in patients with a remote colectomy. Common symptoms of CDI include a watery diarrhea, nausea, and abdominal pain or cramping. About 30% of patients with CDI are febrile and 50% have a leukocytosis. A WBC >20,000 may herald a patient at risk for rapid progression to fulminant colitis and septic shock. Although diarrhea is the hallmark for symptomatic CDI, severe abdominal pain and lack of diarrhea could indicate the patient has ileus with toxic megacolon.

Diagnosis

CDI is a clinical diagnosis with laboratory confirmation. *C. difficile* should be suspected in adults and children more than 2 years old with unexplained clinically significant diarrhea or if ileus is present in association with recent antibiotic use. Patients with pseudomembranes at endoscopy should be presumed to have CDI, but this finding is neither sensitive nor specific (pseudomembranes are present in only 50% of patients with CDI, and ischemic colitis and CMV colitis can also cause pseudomembranes). Diagnosis of CDI is most commonly established with detection of *C. difficile* and/or its toxins in patients with diarrhea. The most sensitive method to detect toxigenic *C. difficile*, when performed correctly, is toxigenic culture. Anaerobic culture of stool using selective methods is used to isolate *C. difficile*, and toxin production is confirmed in vitro. However, this method is not typically clinically feasible due to cost, labor, and minimum of 72- to 96-hour turnaround time. The cell culture cytotoxicity neutralization assay, which detects biologically active toxin in stool, is the most sensitive toxin detection test. This test requires a tissue culture facility, is labor intensive, is operator dependent, and takes at least 24 to 48 hours for results.

Enzyme immunoassays (EIAs) detecting either toxin A or both toxin A and B replaced this method in routine clinical testing. Concerns over the sensitivity of toxin EIAs historically have mostly been resolved. For one, assays that detect only toxin A and, therefore, miss CDI due to toxin B–only producing *C. difficile* strains are no longer commercially available in the United States. Additionally, *C. difficile* assay comparisons are not designed to distinguish between asymptomatic *C. difficile* colonization and true CDI. Toxin EIAs lack sensitivity to detect asymptomatic colonization but have a negative predictive value of >95% for CDI.

An EIA for *C. difficile* glutamate dehydrogenase (GDH) is advocated by some in an algorithmic approach as a screening test. The GDH EIA is highly sensitive in general, but it is not specific for toxigenic *C. difficile*. It will detect nontoxigenic *C. difficile* and some non-*C. difficile* strains that also produce GDH and, therefore, must be combined with another test, usually one that detects toxin. In the algorithmic approach, stools submitted for *C. difficile* testing are first screened with the GDH EIA. GDH-negative results are reported out as negative. GDH-positive specimens are tested with a confirmatory assay, typically a toxin EIA or PCR. When the GDH testing is combined with a toxin EIA, the number of false-positive test results with use of a toxin EIA alone is reduced. If the toxin EIA is negative, then the patient does not have CDI. If positive, then the patient is considered to have CDI.

Available PCR-based assays for *C. difficile* typically detect toxin genes. These tests are rapid and have increased sensitivity compared to toxin EIAs. One concern that has become apparent with PCR-based assays is they are much more likely to detect asymptomatic *C. difficile* carriage than toxin EIAs. As most patients in the hospital with diarrhea do not have CDI, PCR-based assays have been demonstrated to detect asymptomatic *C. difficile* carriage among people with diarrhea due to other reasons. One way to improve the performance of PCR-based assays and reduce false-positive tests would be to improve patient selection for *C. difficile* testing.

In summary, in the absence of clinical data, it is impossible to determine if a positive *C. difficile* diagnostic assay represents asymptomatic *C. difficile* colonization or CDI. The best test to diagnose CDI is not known. There are advantages and disadvantages to all available diagnostic assays, and results must be correlated with the clinical picture. The clinician must be familiar with what testing is used at his or her facility and how best to interpret the results that are generated by those tests.

eatment

pportive therapy with fluid and electrolyte repletion should always be provided. In dition, it is recommended to discontinue the offending antibiotic if possible, as this ay reduce the risk of CDI recurrence. Empiric CDI treatment without confirmed agnosis should only occur in the setting of fulminant infection, characterized by ock, ileus, or toxic megacolon. Previously published Infectious Disease Society of nerica (IDSA) guidelines recommended specific anti-*C. difficile* treatment should based on CDI severity and whether the infection is recurrent (Table 42.1). Met-nidazole at 500 mg three times a day orally is used for mild or moderate CDI and al vancomycin at 125 mg four times a day is recommended for severe or multiply current CDI. However, recommendations on optimal treatment of CDI will likely olve with new data on these established agents and introduction of a new, U.S.)A-approved drug, fidaxomicin. Several double-blinded, randomized controlled als have shown the superiority of oral vancomycin over oral metronidazole for itial treatment response. Metronidazole response rates vary from 72% to 84%, •mpared to 81% to 97% for vancomycin. The pharmacokinetics of the two drugs ay explain the difference in clinical outcomes. When metronidazole is administered ally, it is absorbed rapidly with only 6% to 15% of the drug excreted in stool hile the colon is inflamed. As the inflammation improves, the measured amount in ool decreases as the consistency changes from watery to formed. Oral vancomycin poorly absorbed and fecal concentrations at the recommended treatment dose e very high. These fecal concentrations are maintained throughout the treatment urse, despite changes in stool consistency. There is no difference in risk of recurrent DI between metronidazole and oral vancomycin.

Fidaxomicin is a new macrolide antibiotic that was U.S. FDA approved in lay 2011 for treatment of CDI. It is minimally absorbed and highly excreted in feces. daxomicin has a narrow spectrum of activity and may be less disruptive to nor-al flora and less likely to promote bacterial resistance. In two randomized con-olled trials, oral fidaxomicin resulted in similar rates of diarrhea resolution when ompared to oral vancomycin (88% vs. 86%, respectively; RR: 1.0; 95% CI: 0.98 1.1). In a subsequent meta-analysis, the two studies investigated a composite idpoint of persistent diarrhea or CDI recurrence or death over 40 days in patients ven fidaxomicin or vancomycin. Fidaxomicin reduced the incidence of all primary itcomes by 40% compared to vancomycin (95% CI: 26% to 51%, $p <0.001$). ased on these results, fidaxomicin should be considered for initial treatment for DI, especially in patients with contraindications to other treatments, and for first DI recurrences. Patients with more than one recurrence of CDI were excluded om the phase 3 trials.

Several other therapeutic options are available for CDI but have not yet received .S. FDA approval. Antitoxin antibodies are present in intravenous immunoglobu-n (IVIG) and are thus a theoretically attractive option for adjunctive treatment of :DI, which is a toxin-mediated infection. IVIG has been used as a salvage therapy a small retrospective studies and case reports in incidences of severe or recurrent :DI. Success rates of treatment have been variable across studies, which are limited y small sample sizes, differing treatment regimens, and potential confounding fac-ors. Tigecycline, a glycylcycline antibiotic, has shown some in vitro activity against *. difficile* and is delivered intravenously, which is an advantage for use in patients ith decreased intestinal motility. However, evidence for clinical efficacy is limited to ase reports and case series with a lack of randomized clinical trials.

TABLE 42.1	Treatment Guidelines Based on Clinical Severity and Number of Recurrences	
Presentation	2010 IDSA/SHEA Guidelines	Expert Opinion Based on More Recent Data
Initial infection with mild-to-moderate infection	Metronidazole 500 mg PO q8h, 10–14 days; multiple and prolonged courses can cause irreversible peripheral neuropathy	Vancomycin 125 mg PO q6h, 10–14 days OR Fidaxomicin 200 mg PO q12h, 10 days Second line: Metronidazole 500 mg PO q8h, 10–14 days
Severe infection without complications	Vancomycin 125 mg PO q6h, 10–14 days	Vancomycin 125 mg PO q6h, 10–14 days OR Fidaxomicin 200 mg PO q12h, 10 days
Severe infection with complications	Vancomycin 500 mg q6h PO or by NG tube plus metronidazole 500 mg IV q8h Vancomycin 250 mg q6h per rectal retention enema for ileus Surgical consult for possible subtotal colectomy	No change
First recurrence	Same as initial infection based on disease severity	Fidaxomicin 200 mg PO q12h, 10 days OR Vancomycin 125 mg PO q6h, 10–14 days followed by taper
After a second relapse within 30–90 days or if the patient significantly worsens after treatment cessation	Vancomycin taper or pulse dosing Taper: Week 1: 125 mg PO q6h; week 2: 125 mg q12h; week 3: 125 mg daily; week 4: 125 mg every other day; week 5–6: 125 mg every 3 days. Pulse dosing: up to 125–500 mg PO every 2–3 days for 3 wks	Vancomycin 125 mg PO q6h, 10–14 days followed by taper OR Fidaxomicin 200 mg PO q12h, 10 days followed by taper OR Fecal microbiota transplant (FMT)

Actoxumab and bezlotoxumab are fully human monoclonal antibodies which
1 *C. difficile* toxins A and B, respectively. Two recently completed phase 3 studies,
)DIFY I and MODIFY II, demonstrated the effectiveness of bezlotoxumab in
venting recurrent disease after initial treatment. MODIFY I and MODIFY II
uited 1412 and 1168 adult patients, respectively, being treated for CDI. Patients
ived standard-of-care antibiotic treatment and were then randomized to receive
ngle infusion of both monoclonal antibodies, actoxumab alone, bezlotoxumab
e, or placebo. At 12-week follow-up, patients treated with bezlotoxumab were
ificantly less likely to have CDI recurrence than the placebo group (17.4% vs.
5%, $p = 0.0003$ for MODIFY I; 15.7% vs. 25.7%, $p = 0.0003$ for MODIFY II).
prisingly, the combination of actoxumab and bezlotoxumab provided no added
efit beyond treatment with bezlotoxumab alone, and actoxumab was no more
ctive than placebo. Adverse events were minor and occurred at similar rates
he bezlotoxumab group and the placebo group. Bezlotoxumab was approved
he FDA in October 2016 for the prevention of CDI recurrence in patients aged
years or older.

It is recommended to administer both intravenous metronidazole and a higher
e of oral vancomycin for patients with CDI who are hemodynamically unstable
vho have fulminant CDI. There are no data to indicate there is synergy between
:ronidazole and vancomycin or data to suggest a higher dose of vancomycin is any
ter than the standard 125-mg dose (which achieves levels of vancomycin 500 to
0 times the MIC_{90} of *C. difficile* in stool). Rather, the rationale behind this rec-
mendation is an attempt to get therapeutic antibiotics to the colon as quickly as
sible in these acutely ill patients. Vancomycin retention enemas of 250 mg in
mL of normal saline four times daily should be considered if the patient has an
s. It is also recommended that a surgical consult be obtained for these patients as
y may require a therapeutic subtotal colectomy, which is the established treatment
patients with septic shock, organ failure, megacolon, or organ perforation. Surgical
:rventions can benefit select patients, which may be identified by a rising white
od cell count (≥25,000) or a rising lactate (≥5 mmol/L). There is recent evidence
t a diverting loop ileostomy and colonic vancomycin lavage may be a less invasive
gical option. In a study of 84 patients with CDI who were critically ill, mortality
; lower in patients treated with ileostomy versus historical controls (colectomy)
42 (19%) in the ileostomy group versus 21/42 (50%) in the colectomy group,
0.006). Further studies are needed to demonstrate a consistent benefit in mortal-
but the procedure has proven benefit in sparing the colon as 79% of the ileosto-
:s were reversed at 6 months.

currence

general, about 20% of patients with an initial episode of CDI will have a recur-
ce, 45% of patients with one recurrence will have another recurrence, and more
n 60% with at least two recurrences will have another recurrence. The recom-
nded treatment for multiply recurrent CDI (defined as at least a third episode of
)I) is tapered oral vancomycin. Vancomycin is initially administered four times a
for 10 to 14 days, and then a dose per day is removed a week at a time until the
ient is taking one dose every 2 to 3 days. The rationale for this regimen is as the
ses are spaced out it provides the colonic microbiota an opportunity to regenerate.
laxomicin, as previously described, may also be used for a first recurrence and may
:rease incidence of further recurrences. Probiotics are not effective to prevent CDI

recurrences. Caution should also be used when administering probiotics to pati with central venous catheters and immunocompromised patients, as they a increased risk for infections due to the organisms in the probiotic.

For patients who have recurrent CDI despite multiple attempts at treatm fecal microbiota transplant (FMT) has emerged as a viable and effective option. F can restore a normal microbiome to patients who have suffered significant disrup to their normal flora via multiple courses of antibiotics and repeated episode CDI. There have been a large number of case reports and case series documen the success of FMT. To date, there has been one unblinded clinical trial compa FMT to a prolonged 2-week course of oral vancomycin and vancomycin with be lavage. The FMT group also received a 4-day course of oral vancomycin follo by bowel lavage. At 10 weeks after completion of therapy, 81% of the FMT gr had a sustained resolution of diarrhea compared to 27% of the vancomycin gr (p <0.001). FMT should be considered in any patient with multiple recurrence CDI but should be performed by an experienced treatment center.

Infection Prevention and Control

The approaches to prevent CDI in the hospital are to decrease risk of infectio *C. difficile* exposure occurs and to prevent *C. difficile* transmission to other patic The first line of defense against CDI is healthy intestinal microbiota, and anti crobial stewardship is therefore the mainstay of decreasing CDI. By decreasing numbers of patients on antimicrobials and/or decreasing high-risk antimicro exposures, the number of patients at risk for CDI is decreased. Up to 25% of ant otic usage is not needed and this is true even in the ICU setting. Some studies indi probiotics may be effective for primary prevention of CDI; several meta-analyses f shown a possible benefit in reducing incidence of CDI. However, many of the stu in the meta-analyses had a CDI incidence much higher than would be expected ba on the patient population in the placebo arms, which may bias the results of th studies, and as previously noted, caution should be used when administering pr otics to patients with central venous catheters and immunocompromised patients to increased rates of bloodstream infections.

C. difficile transmission is through the fecal–oral route. Infected patients excrete large numbers of spores in feces. The resistant spores contaminate the ha of health care workers, bedding, medical equipment, and other structures in patient's room and unit. Hand contamination can occur even when the patient is touched. Strategies to interrupt transmission involve using contact precautions, nage, and environmental cleaning. Quaternary detergents used to clean patient roc are not sporicidal, so using sporicidal hypochlorite-based disinfectants on surfa (1000 to 5000 ppm) is recommended in outbreak settings. Routine use of sporici agents to clean the environment is not routinely recommended in nonoutbreak tings, as they do not appear to be associated with reductions in CDI. Despite the that alcohol does not kill *C. difficile* spores and alcohol-based hand hygiene prode are less effective than hand washing at removing spores from hands of volunteers is not recommended to preferentially perform hand washing with soap and wa over alcohol-based foams/gels after caring for a patient with CDI in nonoutbr settings. Numerous studies have failed to demonstrate an increase in CDI with use of alcohol-based hand hygiene products. Potential explanations for these findi are extremely poor adherence to hand hygiene when soap and water is the prefer method, the efficacy of gloves at preventing contamination of hands, and poten or contamination of hands after removing gloves if the sink used to wash hands is the same sink used by the patient.

OTHER INFECTIOUS AGENTS

Many bacteria, viruses, and parasites have similar clinical presentations. The most commonly encountered in industrialized countries are *Salmonella* sp., norovirus, rotavirus, and *Cryptosporidium* (Table 42.2). Excluding *C. difficile*, these four organisms have a higher reported incidence of infection in the healthcare setting than other bacterial, viral, or parasitic pathogens. They may occur concurrently with community or institutional outbreaks. When associated with large institutional outbreaks, these organisms have caused substantial economic loss due to the need for extensive disinfection, unit closures, and the furloughing or cohorting of staff.

Recognition of *Salmonella* outbreaks can be difficult due to its longer incubation period and because this organism can cause extraintestinal infection. Antibiotics are usually not used because the gastroenteritis is typically self-limited, and antibiotics will prolong shedding in the stool after symptoms resolve. The exceptions are moderate or severe disease, bacteremia, sickle cell disease or prosthetic grafts, extraintestinal disease, and disease in immunocompromised hosts. Stool cultures are the mainstay of diagnosis, and blood cultures are indicated if persistent fever or signs of sepsis are present. Salmonella is a reportable disease, and local reporting requirements should be followed. It is frequently associated with contaminated food, and one case should prompt an investigation of whether it is health care associated. Because the hospital case/outbreak could be part of a larger epidemic, it is important that the ICU works closely with infectious disease specialists, infection prevention and control personnel, and public health officials. Standard disinfectants and alcohol-based hand hygiene products are effective against *Salmonella* sp. Contact precautions are reserved for incontinent or diapered patients to control institutional spread.

Norovirus is disseminated by transfer of infective feces and/or vomitus. A specific diagnosis requires laboratory confirmation because the signs and symptoms of norovirus are not specific. There are now commercially available PCR-based diagnostics for norovirus. Norovirus has been associated with pseudo-outbreaks of *C. difficile* due to more frequent testing for *C. difficile* and detection of asymptomatic *C. difficile* colonization in patients with diarrhea due to norovirus. Treatment is supportive in nature. Early recognition of norovirus is important because it has a short incubation period of 24 hours and can disseminate rapidly in the hospital causing large economic loss and morbidity. Patients who are incontinent or diapered should remain in contact precautions for the duration of their illness. Special attention to environmental cleaning is needed even if surfaces do not appear to be soiled. It may be necessary to use bleach (500 ppm available chlorine) to clean the environment during an outbreak. Aerosolization as a mode of infection may occur, so those engaged in cleaning heavily infected areas should wear masks. Although norovirus is relatively resistant to alcohol, there is no evidence that alcohol-based hand hygiene products are ineffective for hand decontamination.

Rotavirus is spread by fecal–oral route. Infection is more prevalent in children, but the incidence has come down with more widespread use of the vaccine. Profuse watery diarrhea with dehydration and electrolyte abnormalities is generally more severe in infants and children than diarrhea with other common enteric pathogens. In immunocompromised children, rotavirus can be associated with chronic diarrhea,

TABLE 42.2 Other Common Causes of Bacterial, Viral, and Parasitic Diarrhea Found in the Hospital

Organism	Transmission	Incubation Period	Symptom Duration	Laboratory Diagnosis	Treatment	Control Measures
Salmonella spp	Food, water, fecal contact	6–48 hrs	3–7 days	Culture	Non-typhi: supportive; ciprofloxacin 500 mg PO daily 5–7 days; bacteremia—ciprofloxacin 400 mg IV q12h × 14 days (switching to 750 mg bid when possible) or ceftriaxone 2 g IV q24h × 14 days (switch to PO cipro)	Review food handling; contact precautions
Norovirus	Fecal, vomitus contact, aerosol?	24 hrs	2–3 days	PCR	Supportive	Contact precautions; consistent environment cleaning, disinfection; hypochlorite if continued transmission; consider cohorting affected patients to separate airspaces, toilet facilities
Rotavirus	Fecal contact	24–72 hrs	1–4 days	PCR, EIA, EM	Supportive	Contact precautions; consistent environmental cleaning, disinfection, frequent diapering
Cryptosporidium	Fecal contact, food, water	1–30 days	5–10 days or chronic	Smear, EIA, PCR	Supportive; immunocompetent—no HIV: nitazoxanide 500 mg PO bid × 3 days; HIV—effective antiretrovirals; nitazoxanide not licensed for immunodeficient patients	Contact precautions

longed shedding, and extraintestinal infection. Confirmation of rotavirus is important in complicated cases, in immunocompromised patients, and for epidemiologic infection control purposes. Rotavirus can be detected by EIA for VP2 and VP6 viral proteins in stool, but PCR is now the major diagnostic test. Treatment is primarily supportive. All patients with rotavirus infection should be placed on contact precautions for the duration of their illness. Rotavirus is generally a hardy virus that resists inactivation by chlorination in sewage effluents and drinking water. It can be inactivated by antiseptics with >40% alcohol, free chlorine >20,000 ppm, and phenol-based compounds.

Cryptosporidium is a protozoan parasite, which is infectious by way of feces contaminated with the oocyst. Symptoms vary from mild, self-limited to extremely severe. Relapses can occur following a diarrhea-free period of days to weeks. It can also cause chronic diarrhea, especially in HIV patients with low CD4 counts who have had inadequate antiretroviral therapy (ART). Chronic diarrhea is characterized by frequent, foul-smelling bulky stools with development of malabsorption or, less frequently, voluminous watery diarrhea. In HIV-AIDS patients, *Cryptosporidium* can also cause extraintestinal infection. For laboratory diagnosis, sensitivity and specificity of the acid-fast stain of the oocyst is poor, and antigen EIA gives variable sensitivity and specificity. PCR has the best sensitivity and specificity for detection of the organism in stool. Treatment for immunocompetent patients is primarily supportive. For HIV patients, ART is their best option, and nitazoxanide has had variable results. Large community outbreaks have occurred due to contamination of surface water. Hospital-associated infections are uncommon, and this organism has been shown to have low infection transmission in the hospital setting. Patients with bowel incontinence or who are diapered should be placed in contact precautions for the duration of their illness. The oocyst is relatively resistant to a variety of environmental cleaners, but a 1000-fold decrease in infectivity occurs with a 4-minute exposure to 6% to 8% hydrogen peroxide. Despite the resistance of *Cryptosporidium* oocysts to multiple agents, standard hospital disinfectants can be used in the absence of an institutional outbreak.

SUGGESTED READINGS

Agency for Healthcare Research and Quality. Healthcare Cost and Utilization Project (HCUP). 2016. Available at: http://hcupnet.ahrq.gov/. Accessed September 1, 2016.

Bauer TM, Lalvani A, Fehrenbach J, et al. Derivation and validation of guidelines for stool cultures for enteropathogenic bacteria other than Clostridium difficile in hospitalized patients. *JAMA*. 2001;285:313–319.

Crobo LD, Dubberke ER. Recognition and prevention of hospital-associated enteric infections in the intensive care unit. *Crit Care Med*. 2010;38(Suppl):S324–S334.

Cohen SH, Gerding DN, Johnson S, et al. Clinical practice guidelines for Clostridium difficile infection in adults: 2010 update by the society for healthcare epidemiology of America (SHEA) and the infectious diseases society of America (IDSA). *Infect Control Hosp Epidemiol*. 2010;31(5):431–455.

Cornely OA, Crook DW, Esposito R, et al. Fidaxomicin versus vancomycin for infection with Clostridium difficile in Europe, Canada, and the USA: a double-blind, non-inferiority, randomised controlled trial. *Lancet Infect Dis*. 2012;12(4):281–289.

Crook DW, Walker AS, Kean Y, et al. Fidaxomicin versus vancomycin for Clostridium difficile infection: meta-analysis of pivotal randomized controlled trials. *Clin Infect Dis*. 2012; 55(Suppl 2):S93–103.

Deshpande A, Hurless K, Cadnum JL, et al. Effect of fidaxomicin versus vancomycin on s ceptibility to intestinal colonization with vancomycin-resistant enterococci and Klebsi pneumoniae in mice. *Antimicrob Agents Chemother.* 2016;60(7):3988–3993.

Dubberke ER, Burnham CA. Diagnosis of Clostridium difficile infection: treat the patient, the test. *JAMA Intern Med.* 2015;175(11):1801–1802.

Eren Z, Gurol Y, Sonmezoglu M, et al. Saccharomyces cerevisiae fungemia in an elderly pati following probiotic treatment. *Mikrobiyol Bul.* 2014;48(2):351–355.

Fan K, Morris AJ, Reller LB. Application of rejection criteria for stool cultures for bacte enteric pathogens. *J Clin Microbiol.* 1993;31:2233–2235.

Goldenberg JZ, Ma SS, Saxton JD, et al. Probiotics for the prevention of Clostridium diffic associated diarrhea in adults and children. *Cochrane Database Syst Rev.* 2013;5:Cd0060

Gouriet F, Million M, Henri M, et al. Lactobacillus rhamnosus bacteremia: an emerging clin entity. *Eur J Clin Microbiol Infect Dis.* 2012;31(9):2469–2480.

Johnson S, Louie TJ, Gerding DN, et al. Vancomycin, metronidazole, or tolevamer for Clostr ium difficile infection: results from two multinational, randomized, controlled trials. C *Infect Dis.* 2014;59(3):345–354.

Johnson S, Maziade PJ, McFarland LV, et al. Is primary prevention of Clostridium difficile inf tion possible with specific probiotics? *Int J Infect Dis.* 2012;16(11):e786–792.

Lamontagne F, Labbe AC, Haeck O, et al. Impact of emergency colectomy on survival of patie with fulminant Clostridium difficile colitis during an epidemic caused by a hypervirul strain. *Ann Surg.* 2007;245(2):267–272.

Lau CS, Chamberlain RS. Probiotics are effective at preventing Clostridium difficile-associa diarrhea: a systematic review and meta-analysis. *Int J Gen Med.* 2016;9:27–37.

Longo WE, Mazuski JE, Virgo KS, et al. Outcome after colectomy for Clostridium diffi colitis. *Dis Colon Rectum.* 2004;47(10):1620–1626.

Louie TJ, Miller MA, Mullane KM, et al. Fidaxomicin versus vancomycin for Clostridium di cile infection. *New Engl J Med.* 2011;364(5):422–431.

Magill S, Edwards J, Bamberg W, et al. Multistate point-prevalence survey of hea care-associated infections. *N Engl J Med.* 2014;370:1198–1208.

McConnell J. ICAAC/ICC 2015. *Lancet Infect Dis.* 2015;15:1267.

Mullane KM, Miller MA, Weiss K, et al. Efficacy of fidaxomicin versus vancomycin as thera for Clostridium difficile infection in individuals taking concomitant antibiotics for oth concurrent infections. *Clin Infect Dis.* 2011;53(5):440–447.

Neal MD, Alverdy JC, Hall DE, et al. Diverting loop ileostomy and colonic lavage: an altern tive to total abdominal colectomy for the treatment of severe, complicated Clostridiu difficile associated disease. *Ann Surg.* 2011;254(3):423–7; discussion 7–9.

Pattani R, Palda VA, Hwang SW, et al. Probiotics for the prevention of antibiotic-associa diarrhea and Clostridium difficile infection among hospitalized patients: systematic revi and meta-analysis. *Open Med.* 2013;7(2):e56–67.

Santino I, Alari A, Bono S, et al. Saccharomyces cerevisiae fungemia, a possible consequer of the treatment of Clostridium difficile colitis with a probioticum. *Int J Immunopat Pharmacol.* 2014;27(1):143–146.

Tart SB. The role of vancomycin and metronidazole for the treatment of Clostridium diffic associated diarrhea. *J Pharm Pract.* 2013;26(5):488–490.

Thygesen JB, Glerup H, Tarp B. Saccharomyces boulardii fungemia caused by treatment wit probioticum. *BMJ Case Rep.* 2012;2012. pii: bcr0620114412.

Valenstein P Pfaller M, Yungbluth M: The use and abuse of routine stool microbiology: a colle of American pathologists q-probes study of 601 institutions. *Arch Pathol Lab Med.* 19 120:206–211.

van Nood E, Vrieze A, Nieuwdorp M, et al. Duodenal infusion of donor feces for recurre Clostridium difficile. *New Engl J Med.* 2013;368(5):407–415.

Zar FA, Bakkanagari SR, Moorthi KM, et al. A comparison of vancomycin and metronidaz for the treatment of Clostridium difficile-associated diarrhea, stratified by disease severi *Clin Infect Dis.* 2007;45(3):302–307.

43

Acute Kidney Injury
Fahad Edrees and Anitha Vijayan

cute kidney injury (AKI), previously known as acute renal failure, is manifested by
rapid decline in renal function, usually with decreased urine output, and resultant
ccumulation of end products of nitrogen metabolism. It is a common clinical prob-
m encountered in critically ill patients, frequently in the setting of multiple organ
ilure, and is an independent risk factor for increased in-hospital and long-term
ortality. In a recent multicenter study, the incidence of AKI in the intensive care
it (ICU) was noted to be 57%, with sepsis being attributed as the etiology in 41%
the cases.

EFINITION

he lack of consensus definition for AKI confounds the comparisons between stud-
s of prevention, therapy, and outcome. The RIFLE (risk, injury, failure, loss of
dney function, and end-stage kidney disease) criteria and the Acute Kidney Injury
etwork (AKIN) criteria have been replaced now by the Kidney Disease: Improving
lobal Outcomes (KDIGO) staging of AKI (Table 43.1), which provides a single
efinition for practice, research, and public health purposes.

The KDIGO clinical practice guidelines for AKI included a revision to the
efinition of AKI while retaining the AKIN staging criteria. The timeframe for an
icrease in serum creatinine of ≥0.3 mg/dL is retained, while the timeframe for a ≥1.5
mes increase in serum creatinine is changed to 7 days.

Patients with AKI are frequently classified as being nonoliguric (urine output
400 mL/day), oliguric (urine output <400 mL/day), or anuric (urine output
100 mL/day). Lower urine output suggests more severe renal injury, and is asso-
ated with a worse outcome. Prognosis is also worse in patients who require renal
placement therapy. Therefore, a timely diagnosis is critical, as identification and
rompt treatment of the cause of renal injury may hasten recovery and avoid the
eed for dialysis.

IAGNOSTIC APPROACH TO THE PATIENT WITH AKI

KI is a syndrome of multiple etiologies. In using an algorithmic approach in the
valuation of AKI, a key step early in the process is to delineate whether the insult is
rerenal, intrinsic, or postrenal (Algorithm 43.1). In many cases, the patient's history,
hysical examination, laboratory/radiographic data, and meticulous review of med-
al records will provide the necessary information in making such a determination.

TABLE 43.1	KDIGO Staging of AKI	
Stage	Serum Creatinine	Urine Output
1	1.5–1.9 times baseline OR ≥0.3 mg/dL increase	<0.5 mL/kg/hr for 6–12 hrs
2	2.0–2.9 times baseline	<0.5 mL/kg/hr for ≥12 hrs
3	3.0 times baseline OR Increase in serum creatinine to ≥4.0 mg/dL OR Initiation of renal replacement therapy	<0.3 mL/kg/hr for ≥24 hrs OR Anuria for ≥12 hrs

Only one criterion (creatinine or urine output) has to be fulfilled to qualify for a stage.
KDIGO, Kidney Disease: Improving Global Outcomes.

However, the most common cause of AKI in the ICU is ischemic or toxic injury usually referred to acute tubular necrosis (ATN).

The history should focus on recent events that might have led to renal hypoperfusion, or recent exposure to nephrotoxins, both endogenous and exogenous. Causes of renal hypoperfusion must be investigated (e.g., intravascular volume depletion, decreased cardiac output, shock, cirrhosis, and renal vasoconstriction of various causes). Recent trauma should raise the suspicion for myoglobin-induced ATN. Pulmonary manifestations such as dyspnea and hemoptysis may raise the possibility of a pulmonary–renal syndrome such as Goodpasture's disease and granulomatosis with polyangitis (GPA). A history of fever, rash, and arthralgia may suggest vasculitides or an infectious etiology (e.g., endocarditis). Flank pain can be seen in nephrolithiasis, urinary obstruction, renal vein thrombosis, or renal infarct. The presence or absence of anuria and hematuria is an important clue as well. A detailed examination of medical history and of recent medications (e.g., antibiotics, nonsteroidal antiinflammatory drugs [NSAIDs], diuretics, and chemotherapeutic agents), including over-the-counter drugs and radiocontrast agents, should be conducted. In the setting of postoperative AKI, careful review of intraoperative records may reveal episodes of hypotension or use of nephrotoxic drugs. In the in-patient setting, an ischemic or nephrotoxic event should be sought. In patients with mental status changes, obtaining history from a family member or friend is crucial as it can provide clues regarding overdose (e.g., acetaminophen or other medications) or accidental or deliberate ingestion (e.g., ethylene glycol and methanol).

On examination, a careful assessment of the patient's volume status often yields valuable clues as to the nature and degree of renal dysfunction. Systemic signs such as arthritis, rash, and mental status changes also give valuable clues as these can be associated with systemic illnesses such as infection, vasculitides, atheroembolic disease, or thrombotic microangiopathy. The finding of lower abdominal distention makes bladder outlet obstruction highly likely as the cause of AKI. A very tense and distended abdomen in the setting of ascites or recent abdominal surgery raises the suspicion for abdominal compartment syndrome.

Objective laboratory and radiologic tests that are essential include complete blood count, renal function panel, urinalysis, microscopy of the fresh spun urine

LGORITHM 43.1 **Features to Distinguish Among the Three Categories of Acute Kidney Injury**

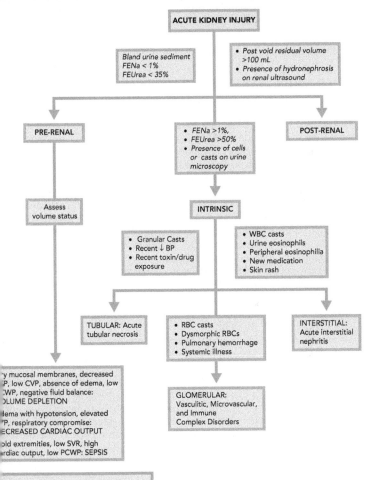

ACUTE KIDNEY INJURY

Bland urine sediment
FENa < 1%
FEUrea < 35%

• Post void residual volume >100 mL
• Presence of hydronephrosis on renal ultrasound

PRE-RENAL

• FENa >1%,
• FEUrea >50%
• Presence of cells or casts on urine microscopy

POST-RENAL

Assess volume status

INTRINSIC

• Granular Casts
• Recent ↓ BP
• Recent toxin/drug exposure

• WBC casts
• Urine eosinophils
• Peripheral eosinophilia
• New medication
• Skin rash

TUBULAR: Acute tubular necrosis

• RBC casts
• Dysmorphic RBCs
• Pulmonary hemorrhage
• Systemic illness

INTERSTITIAL: Acute interstitial nephritis

GLOMERULAR: Vasculitic, Microvascular, and Immune Complex Disorders

y mucosal membranes, decreased
P, low CVP, absence of edema, low
WP, negative fluid balance:
OLUME DEPLETION

dema with hypotension, elevated
P, respiratory compromise:
ECREASED CARDIAC OUTPUT

old extremities, low SVR, high
rdiac output, low PCWP: SEPSIS

BBREVIATIONS

VP:	central venous pressure
ENa:	fractional excretion of sodium
EUrea:	fractional excretion of urea
VP:	jugular venous pressure
CWP:	pulmonary capillary wedge pressure
VR:	systemic vascular resistance
P:	blood pressure
BC:	red blood cell
VBC:	white blood cell

sediment, calculated fractional excretion of sodium (FENa) and urea (FEUrea), a when obstruction is suspected, a renal ultrasound. Based on the initial suspic additional diagnostic tests such as serologic studies or renal ultrasound with Dop can be obtained. Renal biopsy is necessary to make a diagnosis when glomer nephritis is suspected and is also used to make a definitive diagnosis of interst nephritis. The diagnosis of ATN should be based on clinical findings and suppor laboratory data.

URINE CHEMISTRIES

Fractional Excretion of Sodium

FENa is based on the premise that intact tubules will reasbsorb sodium in the renal setting whereas injured tubules like in ATN will not. It is important to k in mind that FENa is helpful in specific patients and in certain clinical scenar particularly oliguric AKI in patients who are not on diuretics or intravenous containing fluids and without underlying chronic kidney disease (CKD), glucos or bicarbonaturia. It is important to appreciate that FENa of <1% can be seen several other renal conditions, including acute glomerulonephritis, contrast neph athy, pigment-induced ATN, transplant rejection, and in early urinary obstructi In patients with impaired urinary concentrating ability (CKD or elderly patien FENa can be >1% in the prerenal state. In general any disease that can disturb typical tubular response to sodium reabsorption can make FENa poorly reflectiv the actual cause of AKI. However, FENa has not proven to be useful in establishin diagnosis or prognosis in critically ill patients and should be interpreted with caut in the ICU.

Fractional Excretion of Urea

Urea reabsorption is less affected by diuretics, which act distally to the proxi tubule. FEUrea <35% reflects prerenal AKI, whereas >50% reflects loss of tub function from ATN. Multiple studies showed different sensitivity (68% to 90%) a specificity (48% to 96%). Same factors like older, sicker, comorbid conditions t affect FENa also affect FEUrea. A study used FEUrea <40% as cutoff for prere AKI in oliguric patients with AKI. FEUrea <40% tested well in detecting prere AKI even in the presence of diuretics (98% overall accuracy). Similar to FE FEUrea should not be used in isolation, but should be incorporated with the clin scenario before making a diagnosis.

Urine Microscopy

Physician examination of the urinary sediment is essential as abnormal urinary sedim is strongly suggestive of an intrarenal process. "Muddy" granular casts and renal tubu epithelial cell (RTEC) casts are most often seen in ATN. Red blood cell casts and d morphic red blood cells suggest a glomerular origin, and white blood cell casts are fou when inflammation is present in the interstitium as in acute interstitial nephritis (AI and pyelonephritis. It is important to note that red and white blood cell casts are frag and that their absence alone does not necessarily eliminate their associated disorders fr the differential diagnosis. Bland sediment and hyaline casts are consistent with prere AKI. Since it is believed that prerenal AKI and ATN are a spectrum and may coex it would be helpful to assess the urine findings quantitatively (numbers of cells or c per low- or high-power field). Different scoring systems have been developed showing correlation with increased number of RTECs or granular casts with poor renal recovery. Urine microscopy by a trained physician has significant diagnostic and prognostic value in the critically ill patient and should be strongly encouraged.

Urine Biomarkers

Several urine biomarkers are approved for clinical use for prediction of AKI. These include neutrophil gelatinase-associated lipocalin (NGAL), interleukin 18 (IL-18), kidney injury molecule 1 (KIM-1), tissue inhibitor of metalloprotease 2 (TIMP-2), and insulin-like growth factor binding protein 7 (IGFBP7). In 2014, the Food and Drug Administration (FDA) allowed the marketing of (TIMP-2) × (IGFBP7) under the brand name NephroCheck to be the first and only biomarker for AKI risk stratification for use in the United States. It is to be used in ICU patients older than 21 years with cardiovascular and/or respiratory compromise within the prior 24 hours. It is an aid in the risk assessment for moderate or severe AKI. A positive test (value >0.3) means high risk for AKI within 12 hours and might lead to a nephrology consultation and implementation of preventive strategies like optimizing volume status and avoiding nephrotoxic drugs.

ETIOLOGY OF AKI

Prerenal AKI

Etiology

In the prerenal process, the integrity of renal parenchyma is preserved. The decreased glomerular filtration rate is a physiologic response to renal hypoperfusion that is due to either true or "effective" volume depletion. Examples include true hypovolemia of various causes, decreased cardiac output, liver failure, anaphylaxis, and sepsis. Renal vasoconstriction (e.g., hypercalcemia, sepsis, liver failure, calcineurin inhibitors, and norepinephrine) and impairment of renal autoregulation (e.g., NSAIDs, angiotensin-converting enzyme inhibitor [ACEI], and angiotensin II receptor blockers [ARBs]) are common scenarios leading to prerenal azotemia. Hypoperfusion may also result from sustained intra-abdominal pressure >20 mm Hg, leading to abdominal compartment syndrome. This syndrome can be seen in intra-abdominal hemorrhage, massive ascites, bowel distension, abdominal surgery, and post-liver transplantation.

Diagnosis

The diagnosis is suspected from the history and physical examination. In prerenal AKI, the urine sediment is typically bland, lacking cells, crystals, and cellular casts. The urine chemistry reflects the appropriate tubular response to hypoperfusion, with avid sodium reabsorption. The calculated FENa is <1% and the urine sodium is usually <10 mmol/L. The urine is markedly concentrated and urine osmolality is usually >500 mOsm/kg. FENa and FEUrea are most useful in oliguric patients as discussed before.

Management

Rapid reversal of the cause of renal hypoperfusion is critical because prolonged renal ischemia leads to renal tubular injury (Algorithm 43.2). All offending drugs/agents

ALGORITHM 43.2 Management of Prerenal Causes of Acute Kidney Injury

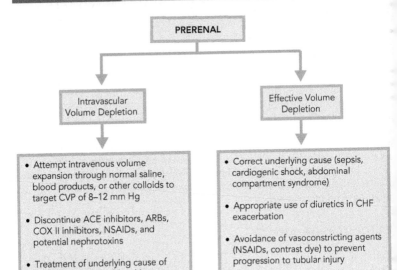

PRERENAL

Intravascular Volume Depletion

- Attempt intravenous volume expansion through normal saline, blood products, or other colloids to target CVP of 8–12 mm Hg
- Discontinue ACE inhibitors, ARBs, COX II inhibitors, NSAIDs, and potential nephrotoxins
- Treatment of underlying cause of volume depletion – blood loss, gastrointestinal losses, extensive burns, extravasation into extravascular compartments (e.g., peritonitis, intestinal obstruction)

Effective Volume Depletion

- Correct underlying cause (sepsis, cardiogenic shock, abdominal compartment syndrome)
- Appropriate use of diuretics in CHF exacerbation
- Avoidance of vasoconstricting agents (NSAIDs, contrast dye) to prevent progression to tubular injury

ABBREVIATIONS
ACE: angiotensin-converting enzyme
ARBs: angiotensin II receptor blockers
CHF: congestive heart failure
COX: cyclo-oxygenase
CVP: central venous pressure
NSAIDs: nonsteroidal anti-inflammatory drugs

should be discontinued immediately. In cases of hypovolemia, depending on the source of fluid loss, volume resuscitation with normal saline or blood products should be administered without delay. In conditions associated with overfill situations, such as congestive heart failure or cardiogenic shock, treatment is directed at maximizing cardiac function, particularly with diuretics, positive inotropes, afterload reduction, and possibly mechanical circulatory assist devices. Invasive hemodynamic monitoring can guide management when intravascular volume status is difficult to determine based on noninvasive assessment.

Management of hepatorenal syndrome (HRS) remains a clinical challenge. HRS is a serious but potentially reversible complication of end-stage liver disease as well as fulminant hepatic failure of any cause (e.g., tumor infiltration and acetaminophen

TABLE 43.2	Diagnostic Criteria of Hepatorenal Syndrome

- Cirrhosis with presence of ascites
- Worsening renal function over days to weeks with serum creatinine at least 1.5 mg/dL
- Absence of intrinsic renal disease as indicated by proteinuria (>500 mg/day), microscopic hematuria (>50 red blood cells per high-power field), and/or structural abnormalities detected by imaging studies.
- Absence of shock
- Absence of concurrent or recent use of nephrotoxic medications
- No improvement of renal function after diuretic withdrawal and volume expansion with albumin for at least 2 days. Albumin should be dosed 1 g/kg of body weight per day up to a maximum of 100 g/day.

SUBTYPES	**Type 1:** Rapidly progressive form, with doubling of serum creatinine to a level >2.5 mg/dL in <2 wks
	Type 2: Moderate renal failure, with a slowly progressive course. Serum creatinine 1.5–2.5 mg/dL. Typically associated with refractory ascites

Diagnostic criteria of hepatorenal syndrome are adapted from Salerno F, Gerbes A, Ginès P, et al. Diagnosis, prevention, and treatment of hepatorenal syndrome in cirrhosis.

toxicity). It is a result of severe intrarenal vasoconstriction in the setting of splanchnic vasodilatation and effective hypovolemia. It can occur spontaneously in advanced liver disease, or develop after a precipitating event such as infection (e.g., spontaneous bacterial peritonitis), gastrointestinal bleeding, or large-volume paracentesis without albumin. In patients with spontaneous bacterial peritonitis, albumin infusion may prevent development of HRS.

HRS is a diagnosis of exclusion (see Table 43.2 for diagnostic criteria of HRS). The prognosis of HRS is very poor (type 1 worse than type 2) as there are very few therapeutic strategies in HRS and liver transplantation is the only definitive treatment (Table 43.3). Resolution of HRS can occur with improvement in hepatic function in the cases of acute liver injury and alcoholic hepatitis. Renal replacement therapy should primarily be reserved for those whose liver function is expected to recover or those who are candidates for liver transplantation.

POSTRENAL AKI

A postrenal process occurs when the glomerular filtration rate is decreased secondarily to an impediment to urine outflow as a result of structural or functional changes in the urinary tract. This is a very rare cause of AKI in the ICU. The increased pressure in the urinary tract is conveyed proximally from the obstruction, resulting in a rise in tubular pressure and an eventual decrease in the hydraulic pressure gradient across the glomerular capillaries, leading to a decline in glomerular filtration rate as well as changes in tubular function (decreased concentrating ability, distal renal tubular acidosis).

Urinary obstruction can be unilateral or bilateral, acute or chronic, partial or complete, intrarenal (tubular obstruction from crystals, casts) or extrarenal. Clinical symptoms vary according to the duration, degree, and site of obstruction. Unilateral

TABLE 43.3	Treatment of Type 1 Hepatorenal Syndrome

Vasoconstrictors and albumin
- Terlipressin: not available in the United States
- Midodrine (systemic vasoconstrictor) + octreotide (inhibitor of endogenous vasodilator release)
  - Midodrine 5–15 mg orally three times a day
  - Octreotide 100–200 µg subcutaneously three times a day
- Norepinephrine: limited data

Transjugular intrahepatic portosystemic shunt
- Treatment of refractory ascites
- May provide gradual improvement in renal function
- Data very limited
- Effect on survival unclear

Renal replacement therapy
- Bridge to liver transplantation OR
- Awaiting recovery of hepatic function

Liver transplantation

obstruction does not typically lead to renal failure. Urine output is nondiagnos except in the case of anuria that suggests complete obstruction.

The diagnosis is initially suspected based on the history and physical examina tion, and confirmed by findings of hydronephrosis on renal ultrasound or comput tomography (CT). Absence of hydronephrosis on radiologic testing does not co pletely exclude obstruction. In the setting of severe volume depletion, retroperiton fibrosis, and in the very early phase of obstruction, dilatation of the calyces may n occur and ultrasound may be falsely negative. A simple method to evaluate for dis obstruction is to measure the postvoid residual that, if >100 mL, is consistent w bladder outlet obstruction. Obstruction of the Foley catheter with clots should a be considered, and this is ruled out either by flushing the catheter or by replacing with a new one. In the intensive care setting, unless there is high index of suspici based on the clinical picture (e.g., recent abdominal surgery, history of malignan and anticholinergic medications), the yield from renal ultrasound is low.

Once the diagnosis of urinary obstruction/obstructive nephropathy is mac prompt intervention is necessary to minimize long-term renal impairment. T method of intervention is dictated by the location and cause of the obstructic Postobstructive diuresis with marked polyuria is often seen after relief of comple obstruction. Although this is considered an appropriate response in many cases, v ume depletion and electrolyte imbalances can occur and require close monitori and intervention.

INTRINSIC AKI

Intrinsic renal disease is present when the injury is at the level of the kidney pare chyma. Further classification depends on the area of involvement: glomeruli, vasc lature, tubules, or interstitium. Such differentiation can frequently be achieved careful analysis of the urine sediment as mentioned before. In the critical care setting, ischemic and nephrotoxic ATN account for up to 90% of intrinsic AKI.

Acute Tubular Necrosis

Etiology

ATN can result from prolonged prerenal states (e.g., volume depletion and hypotension) or toxins (e.g., intravenous contrast, aminoglycosides, antiviral and antifungal medications, and myoglobin). In the critical care setting, the insults are usually simultaneous or sequential and no single precipitating factor can be identified (Table 43.4 contains a list of common causes of ATN). In severe cases, renal hypoperfusion can result in bilateral cortical necrosis, which may lead to prolonged need for renal replacement therapy and sometimes irreversible renal damage.

Diagnosis

With severe or prolonged injury, the renal tubules lose their ability to retain sodium and concentrate urine. The FENa is usually above 1% and the FEUrea is >50% with a serum blood urea nitrogen to creatinine <20:1. Examination of the urine sediment can reveal RTECs and muddy brown granular casts in a majority of the patients. Because the glomeruli and interstitium are typically spared, other urinary findings such as heavy proteinuria and hematuria are absent.

Although the FENa is a useful indicator to differentiate between prerenal states and ATN, as noted before, there are some exceptions to the rule. Certain conditions that result in ATN can demonstrate a low FENa. Contrast-induced nephropathy (CIN) typically manifests as nonoliguric AKI, occurring 3 to 5 days after radiocontrast exposure. Early in the course of the renal injury, the FENa is low (<1%) despite the absence of systemic volume depletion. This is a result of the profound renal vasoconstriction caused by release of endothelin induced by intravenous contrast. Rhabdomyolysis and severe hemolysis release pigments (myoglobin and hemoglobin, respectively) that are toxic to the tubules, but may also present early in the course with a low FENa secondary to renal vasoconstriction.

Prevention

Close monitoring of intravascular volume status and cautious use of nephrotoxic agents can dramatically reduce the incidence of AKI secondary to ATN. The majority of the preventive techniques have been studied in the area of CIN. Various intravenous hydration regimens have been shown to reduce the risk of renal injury in patients undergoing radiocontrast procedures, with regimens consisting of normal saline or sodium bicarbonate-based intravenous fluids being most effective. "Renal-dose" dopamine infusions have *not* shown to be beneficial in prevention nor aid in recovery from renal injury. In fact, some studies have suggested increased risk for AKI, and thus there is *no* role for this agent in the prevention or treatment of AKI. N-acetylcysteine has been studied in small randomized trials, and its combination with intravenous hydration may result in a lower incidence of CIN. Although this advantage has not been clearly defined, N-acetylcysteine can be considered for use in high-risk patients undergoing contrast administration, given its low cost, safety, and potential benefit. The Renal Guard System is a new device that is being investigated for prevention of CIN. It entails the use of a physician-prescribed loop diuretic that may induce the required high urine output. The system measures urine output and

TABLE 43.4	Common Causes of Acute Tubular Necrosis
Cause	Description
Ischemia	Results from prolonged prerenal state (hypovolemia, sepsis, cardiogenic shock) Treat by addressing underlying cause and maximizing renal perfusion
Intravascular iodinated contrast	Characterized by both renal vasoconstriction and tubular injury Risk factors: pre-existing renal dysfunction, heart failure, diabetes, volume depletion, multiple myeloma, large volume of contrast, and high-osmolarity contrast FENa <1% Hydration with intravenous sodium chloride or sodium bicarbonate shown to be beneficial N-acetylcysteine orally or intravenously may help in prevention Most patients recover renal function
Rhabdomyolysis	May result from crush injury, prolonged immobilization, status epilepticus, hyperthermia, statin medication, cocaine use, hypophosphatemia, hypokalemia, snake venom, or inherited metabolic disorders Degree of muscle enzyme elevation does not always correlate with severity of renal injury Mechanisms of AKI: renal vasoconstriction, proximal tubular injury, and tubular obstruction by pigment casts Hyperkalemia, hyperphosphatemia, hypocalcemia, hyperuricemia Urine dipstick may show heme pigment in absence of RBCs on urine sediment Urine supernatant red to brown in color FENa <1% Treat with vigorous hydration (may require up to 10 L of normal saline during 24 hr) to replete volume and increase urinary flow rate
Hemoglobinuria	Result from intravascular hemolytic processes Urine dipstick may show heme pigment in absence of RBCs on urine sediment FENa <1% Lactate dehydrogenase elevated, haptoglobin decreased, and unconjugated bilirubin elevated Treatment similar to rhabdomyolysis and focus on underlying cause
Cast nephropathy	Casts composed of light chain (myeloma) and Tamm–Horsfall protein can lead to direct tubular injury and intratubular obstruction Risk factors: volume depletion, loop diuretics, hypercalcemia, IV contrast Role of plasmapheresis unclear

TABLE 43.4	Common Causes of Acute Tubular Necrosis (*Continued*)
Cause	Description
Aminoglycosides	Typically presents 5–7 days after initiating drug Length of treatment correlates with increased incidence of nephrotoxicity FENa >1% in most cases Usually nonoliguric Significant urinary loss of magnesium, potassium, and calcium Recovery may take several weeks, even if drug is promptly discontinued
Amphotericin B	Effect is cumulative Causes intense renal vasoconstriction as well as direct toxicity to tubules by disrupting cell membrane Liposomal preparations have lower incidence of nephrotoxicity
Intravenous acyclovir	Insoluble precipitation in renal tubules resulting in obstruction Needle-shaped crystals may be seen on urine sediment Discontinuation of medicine usually reverses renal injury
Cisplatin	Dose-related and cumulative effect Profound renal magnesium wasting; hypokalemia can be seen Vigorous fluid hydration should be given prior to medication to increase urine flow
Ethylene glycol/ methanol	Toxicity can result from ingestion of wood alcohol (methanol) or antifreeze radiator fluid (ethylene glycol) Elevated osmol gap Anion gap metabolic acidosis presents later in course Oxalate crystals (envelope-shaped) are present in the urine sediment with ethylene glycol but not with methanol intoxication Fomepizole antidote is loaded as 15 mg/kg over 30 min, then 15 mg/kg every 12 hr Hemodialysis may be required to treat refractory metabolic acidosis/AKI
Tumor lysis syndrome	Results after large numbers of neoplastic cells are rapidly killed after cancer treatment or tumor autolysis Intracellular contents are released into the circulation, including potassium, phosphate, and uric acid Most often seen 48–72 hrs after cancer treatment Renal injury is through uric acid precipitation in the acidic environment of the tubules Hyperphosphatemia can lead to calcium–phosphate crystal formation and nephrocalcinosis Patients are typically oliguric; may require temporary dialysis, although usually reversible if addressed early Treatment is with aggressive hydration, allopurinol, and rasburicase

Na, fractional excretion of sodium; RBCs, red blood cells.

replaces it in real time with an equal volume of sterile saline. This leads to more r
transit of contrast through the kidney and less overall exposure to contrast.

Management and Prognosis

There is no specific treatment of ATN once it has occurred. Therapy is gene
supportive and includes the use of renal replacement therapy if necessary. Attemp
reverse the initial insult should be made. Management should also focus on avoi
additional nephrotoxic insults and adjusting drug doses appropriately for the
of renal function. Depending on the cause and severity, as well as the baseline r
function, renal recovery takes days, weeks, or even months, if at all. Generally, r
recovery can be expected in about 75% of patients who previously had normal b
line function, provided they survive the hospitalization.

Glomerular and Microvascular Processes

Glomerular causes of renal injury are much less common in an acute inten
care setting (Table 43.5). However, the pulmonary–renal syndromes of GPA
Goodpasture's disease should be considered in anyone presenting with simultane

TABLE 43.5	Selected Glomerular and Microvascular Disorders in the IC	
Cause	Characteristics	Treatment
Immune complex	Hypocomplementemia seen with postinfectious GN, MPGN, SLE, endocarditis, and cryoglobulinemia	Treat the underlying cause
Pauci-immune and anti-GBM disease	Pulmonary hemorrhage syndromes may have positive serum c-ANCA or p-ANCA or anti-GBM antibody (Goodpasture's) Dysmorphic RBCs in urine suggest glomerular origin	Supportive therapy for pulmo nary compromise, mechani- cal ventilation if necessary Corticosteroids and cytotoxic agents Plasma exchange for Good- pasture's or vasculitis with pulmonary hemorrhage or advanced renal failure
Microvascular	HUS and TTP with low platelets, hemolytic anemia, and schisto- cytes on peripheral smear Atheroembolic disease Subacute renal failure, days to weeks after invasive vascular procedure, with livedo reticu- laris and transient peripheral eosinophilia	TTP requires emergent plasm exchange Supportive care for HUS Refractory TTP may benefit from immunosuppression with prednisone and/or rituximab Avoid anticoagulation and fur ther vascular procedures

GN, glomerulonephritis; MPGN, membranoproliferative glomerulonephritis; SLE, systemic lupus erythematosus; c-ANCA, cytoplasmic antineutrophilic cytoplasmic antibody; p-ANCA, perinuclea antineutrophilic cytoplasmic antibody; GBM, glomerular basement membrane; RBCs, red blood cells; HUS, hemolytic–uremic syndrome; TTP, thrombotic thrombocytopenic purpura.

spiratory and renal dysfunction, as they are universally fatal if not recognized and eated in a timely manner. The presence of red blood cell casts specifically suggests glomerular origin. In the appropriate clinical setting, such findings should trigger a arch for vasculitic and nephritic disorders. Serologic tests are helpful in these cases, though kidney biopsy may ultimately be necessary for a definitive diagnosis.

The antiglomerular basement membrane antibody is a highly sensitive (95%) d specific test (99%) for Goodpasture's disease. In GPA, the serine proteinase 3 tibody (c-ANCA, cytoplasmic antineutrophil cytoplasmic antibody) is elevated >75% of cases; approximately 20% have an elevated myeloperoxidase antibody -ANCA) and <5% are ANCA-negative. Treatment of these syndromes is with imediate intravenous corticosteroids (methylprednisolone at 7 to 15 mg/kg/day, d/or up to 1 g/day for 3 days followed by oral prednisone at 1 mg/kg/day up 60 to 80 mg) and with cytotoxic immunosuppressants (oral cyclophosphamide 2 to 3 mg/kg/day, intravenous cyclophosphamide at 15 mg/kg or 750 mg/m^2). herapeutic plasma exchange is also employed in the treatment of Goodpasture's isease. In ANCA-positive vasculitis with advanced renal failure, one study demon-rated that the single predictive factor associated with long-term independence from ialysis was the use of therapeutic plasma exchange. Therapeutic plasma exchange is so recommended for the management of pulmonary hemorrhage associated with NCA-positive vasculitis. The differential diagnoses of pulmonary–renal syndromes clude community-acquired pneumonia with sepsis and ATN, systemic lupus ery-ematosus with lung involvement and lupus nephritis, sarcoidosis, infections such as ptospirosis, legionella, ehrlichiosis (pneumonia with AIN or ATN), and pancreatitis ith pneumonia and ATN.

Hemolytic–uremic syndrome (HUS) and thrombotic thrombocytopenic pur-ura (TTP) are two distinct thrombotic microangiopathies that can result in renal jury. Although distinct clinical entities, they share several common precipitating ctors such as HIV infection, malignancy, calcineurin inhibitors, pregnancy, and hemotherapeutic agents. Ticlopidine and, less commonly, clopidogrel are more osely associated with TTP. In the diarrheal form of HUS, a Shiga-like toxin enters e circulation through compromised colonic epithelium and results in inflamma-on, endothelial injury, and thrombosis in the renal microvasculature. Therapy is ipportive for Shiga toxin-associated HUS, with no proven efficacy of antibiotics, nticoagulation, immunoglobulin, or plasmapheresis. However in atypical HUS, umanized monoclonal antibody inhibiting the action of complement factor C5 Eculizumab) has been shown to be beneficial. In the case of TTP, daily plasma olume exchange is a life-saving therapy and thus must not be delayed. In resistant ases, immunosuppression with high-dose prednisone and rituximab can be used. plenectomy has been attempted in refractory cases, but is of unproven benefit.

Another microvascular process affecting the kidneys is atheroembolic disease. As ospitalized patients frequently undergo invasive vascular procedures, a high index of uspicion for atheroembolic disease should be maintained in the appropriate clinical etting. These patients demonstrate renal dysfunction days to weeks after manipula-ion of aorta or other large arteries, and follow a slowly progressive course. Transient eripheral eosinophilia may be present in >65% of cases. Hypocomplementemia can e seen in the initial phase of the disease. Skin findings are highly variable and may nclude livedo reticularis of the extremities or digital necrosis with gangrene (blue toe yndrome). Distal pulses are typically present as the occlusion is at the level of smaller rteries and arterioles. The general rule from the renal standpoint is a slow decline

TABLE 43.6 Selected Causes of Acute Interstitial Nephritis

Agent	Diagnosis	Course
Methicillin	Hypersensitivity symptoms predominate with fever in 85% Urinary findings also very common, as >80% of patients with hematuria, pyuria, eosinophiluria, or nonnephrotic proteinuria	Most patients recover renal function within 2 months, although nearly one-fifth require temporary dialysis CKD remains in only 10%
Rifampin	Gastrointestinal symptoms (nausea, vomiting, abdominal pain) Oligoanuria in nearly all patients Eosinophilia uncommon, although other hematologic abnormalities such as hemolysis (25%) and thrombocytopenia (50%) may occur Elevation of liver enzymes seen in one-quarter of patients Anti-rifampin antibodies in almost all patients Renal biopsy rarely shows immune complex deposition at tubular basement membrane	Occurs 24 hrs following dose with prior exposure (up to 1 yr prior) Temporary dialysis required in almost all cases CKD remains in only 3%
Other antibiotics (sulfonamides, fluoroquinolones, beta-lactams)	Fever less common than with methicillin (45%), but with rash and flank pain in almost 50%; oliguria in 40% Urinary findings less common than with methicillin	Mean exposure to antibiotic is 10 days CKD remains in approximately 40%
NSAIDs	Hypersensitivity symptoms uncommon More than one-third with nephrotic range proteinuria Renal biopsy may show minimal change disease	Exposure is frequently months before presentation CKD remains in half of patients
Allopurinol	Hypersensitivity symptoms very common and robust with accumulation of metabolite oxypurinol Eosinophilia and hepatitis are common Renal biopsy may show immune complex deposition at	Mortality may be as high as 25%

Proton pump inhibitors	...ous onset
Initial signs and symptoms are nonspecific
Requires high level of clinical suspicion	Prognosis generally good once PPIs discontinued
Steroids may be tried
Leptospiral nephropathy	Fever and jaundice are very common
Other findings may include hepatomegaly, gingival and gastrointestinal bleeding, macroscopic hematuria, conjunctival suffusion, altered mental status; oligoanuria in nearly all patients
Rhabdomyolysis, cholestatic hepatitis, hemolytic anemia, and thrombocytopenia are common findings
Confirm with positive blood/urine culture or serology
Renal biopsy shows inflammation predominantly at proximal tubules, and may also show interstitial hemorrhage	Nephropathy occurs in 40% of leptospirosis
Mortality is ~25%
CKD remains in only 10%
Sarcoidosis	Extrarenal symptoms predominate, most commonly affecting lungs, eyes, and skin
Eosinophilia seen in one-quarter of patients
Hypercalcemia common despite advanced renal failure
Hilar adenopathy on chest radiograph
ACE levels not reliable with renal involvement
Renal biopsy can show noncaseating granulomas and giant cells	Often remitting and relapsing course
CKD remains in 90%

CKD, chronic kidney disease; NSAIDs, nonsteroidal anti-inflammatory drugs; ACE, angiotensin-converting enzyme.

in renal function during months, with a third of the patients requiring dialysis. multivisceral atheroembolic disease, manifested by intestinal ischemia, pancreat and other systemic manifestations, 1-year mortality can be as high as 70%. Ther no effective medical treatment. Avoidance of further vascular procedures along v judicious control of blood pressure, use of ACEIs, and nutritional support have been associated with better prognosis. A case series has noted a possible benefit fi statin therapy in improving the long-term renal outcome.

Interstitial Processes

AIN is an inflammatory process caused by medications or by infections. The cla triad of rash, eosinophilia, and fever is not commonly seen. Urinary findings s gestive of AIN include white blood cells, white blood cell casts, and eosinop Occasionally, the urine sediment can be bland. Detection of eosinophiluria sho be done with the Hansel's stain. However, eosinophiluria is a nonspecific finding has a relatively low sensitivity and specificity. Renal biopsy may be necessary to est lish a definitive diagnosis. Beta-lactam antibiotics are common culprits, altho nearly every antibiotic and many nonantibiotic medications have been implicat Table 43.6 lists some of the more common causes of AIN in the ICU.

Removal of the offending agent or treatment of the underlying infectious ease is the mainstay of therapy. Recovery of renal function may not occur for d to weeks, and sometimes several months. The role of corticosteroid therapy rema controversial. Some studies suggest a better outcome in patients who are trea with steroids. Cyclophosphamide, mycophenolate mofetil, or other immunos pressants have also been used in corticosteroid nonresponders after 2 to 3 we of therapy.

SUMMARY

An algorithmic approach to AKI can help uncover the etiology and devise a treatm plan. Early in the investigation, it is important to determine if the insult is prerer intrinsic, or postrenal in nature, using the history, physical examination, laborate data, and imaging studies. Microscopic examination of the urine sediment is of h value in identifying the underlying renal disorder and may help in further classify some disorders. In the cases of glomerular injury and interstitial nephritis, immur suppression may be required to reverse the disease process. However, the majority the AKI in the ICU is due to tubular injury (ATN), and specific therapies are available for reversing or even preventing further progression of the injury. Treatm remains supportive, primarily with renal replacement therapy that will be discus: in the next chapter.

SUGGESTED READINGS

Bellomo R, Kellum JA, Ronco C. Acute kidney injury. *Lancet.* 2012;380:756–766.

Durand F, Graupera I, Gines P, et al. Pathogenesis of hepatorenal syndrome: implications therapy. *Am J Kidney Dis.* 2016;67(2):318–328.

Faubel S, Patel NU, Cadnapaphornchar MA. Renal relevant radiology: use of ultrasonograp in patients with AKI. *Clin J Am Soc Nephrol.* 2014;9(2):382–394.

George JN, Nester CM. Syndromes of thrombotic microangiopathy. *N Engl J Med.* 2014;3 654–666.

ste EA, Bagshaw SM, Bellomo R, et al. Epidemiology of acute kidney injury in critically ill patients: the multinational AKI-EPI study. *Intensive Care Med.* 2015;41:1411–1423.

dney Disease: Improving Global Outcomes (KDIGO). Acute Kidney Injury Work Group. KDIGO clinical practice guideline for acute kidney injury. *Kidney Int Suppl.* 2012;2: 1–138.

arenzi G, Assanelli E, Marana I, et al. N-acetylcysteine and contrast-induced nephropathy in primary angioplasty. *N Engl J Med.* 2006;354:2773–2782.
Randomized controlled trial comparing high and low doses of N-acetylcysteine in preventing contrast-induced nephropathy.

arkowitz GS, Perazella MA. Drug-induced renal failure: a focus on tubulointerstitial disease. *Clin Chim Acta.* 2005;351:31–47.
Review of pattern of drug-induced renal injury.

erten GJ, Burgess WP, Gray LV, et al. Prevention of contrast-induced nephropathy with sodium bicarbonate: a randomized controlled trial. *JAMA.* 2004;291:2328–2334.
Randomized study evaluating efficacy of sodium bicarbonate in preventing renal injury.

razella MA, Coca SG. Traditional urinary biomarkers in the assessment of hospital-acquired AKI. *Clin J Am Soc Nephrol.* 2012;7(1):167–174.

aga M, González E. Acute interstitial nephritis. *Kidney Int.* 2010;77:956–961.

razella MA. The urine sediment as a biomarker of kidney disease. *Am J Kidney Dis.* 2015;66(5): 748–755.

lerno F, Gerbes A, Ginès P, et al. Diagnosis, prevention and treatment of hepatorenal syndrome in cirrhosis. *Gut.* 2007;56:1310–1318.

jayan A, Faubel S, Askenazi DJ, et al.; American Society of Nephrology Acute Kidney Injury Advisory Group. Clinical use of the urine biomarker [TIMP-2] × [IGFBP7] for acute kidney injury risk assessment. *Am J Kidney Dis.* 2016;68(1):19–28.

44 Renal Replacement Therapy

Fahad Edrees and Anitha Vijayan

The principal strategy regarding acute kidney injury (AKI), particularly in the intensive care setting, is prevention. Once AKI occurs, the presentation and course a variable and treatment is generally supportive. The optimal time to initiate ren replacement therapy (RRT) remains unknown.

INDICATIONS

Conventional indications for RRT include metabolic acidosis, hyperkalemia, volum overload, and severe uremic symptoms refractory to medical management. Oth indications include certain intoxications of certain substances (ethylene glycol, met anol, lithium, etc.), where either the substance or the toxic metabolite will be cleare with dialysis. Patient with chronic kidney disease (CKD) stage 3 or higher, have substantial increase in risk of developing AKI requiring dialysis.

Acidosis

Refractory metabolic acidosis is an acute indication for dialytic therapy in the severel ill patient. Progressive acidemia can develop as the kidneys lose their ability to reclain bicarbonate and excrete organic acids. More commonly in the intensive care setting tissue hypoperfusion with multiorgan system failure results in severe lactic acidosi Aggressive alkali therapy can encounter problems with volume overload, metabol alkalosis, and hypocalcemia. Initiation of RRT would obviate the concern over vo ume overload and could restore the blood pH to its physiologic range.

Hyperkalemia

Hyperkalemia can be rapidly fatal and need to be addressed promptly. Temporizin measures include intravenous calcium to stabilize the myocardial cell membrane, a well as insulin (with dextrose 50% in water), sodium bicarbonate, and inhaled bet agonists to promote an intracellular shift in potassium. Elimination of potassiur from the body can be achieved with ion-exchange resins, but this effect is unpredict able and inefficient. In the volume-depleted patient, aggressive fluid resuscitation ca enhance sodium delivery to the distal nephron. The reabsorption of sodium make the lumen electronegative, promoting secretion of potassium via the potassiur channel.

When these efforts are unsuccessful, urgent RRT becomes necessary. Intermit tent hemodialysis (IHD) with higher blood flow and dialysate flow rates is ver effective in lowering potassium rapidly and is the preferred modality of choice. Th

ents are dialyzed using a 0 or 1 mEq/L potassium concentration in the dialysate. wever, in a critically ill hypotensive patient with or without pressors, continuous al replacement therapy (CRRT) with high flow rates (>35 mL/kg/hr) of replace-nt fluid and dialysate with 0 potassium concentration can also be utilized to lower assium levels.

ume Overload

ume overload is another frequently encountered problem in the critical care set-g. There is evidence that in patients with AKI, fluid overload is an independent : factor for mortality. Although randomized trials studying the use of diuretics in I have not demonstrated any survival advantage, improvement in renal recovery, avoidance of dialytic therapy, it is not unreasonable to offer a trial of intravenous h-dose loop diuretic (e.g., 160 to 200 mg of furosemide or 4 to 5 mg of bumeta-e) in the setting of fluid overload. Respiratory compromise with pulmonary ·ma and/or significant soft tissue edema that impairs the barrier defense of the n is the most common subjective criteria for initiating renal replacement in oliguric patient.

emia

ch progressive renal dysfunction, there is an impaired ability to excrete nitrogenous stes and glycosylated end products. Blood urea nitrogen (BUN) level is generally ·d as a surrogate marker for uremic toxin accumulation. Unfortunately, many signs l symptoms commonly found in the uremic syndrome do not always correlate h BUN levels, and therefore there is no established objective cutoff beyond which lytic therapy is recommended. Rather, acute indications for initiating urgent RRT ·ter on the presence of specific clinical findings, namely uremic encephalopathy l uremic pericarditis. The latter possesses a high risk of converting into hem-hagic pericarditis with cardiac tamponade. Systemic anticoagulation should be ·ided in such patients.

MING OF INITIATION OF RRT

e optimal timing for initiation of RRT is undefined at this time. A few studies have)wn a survival advantage with early initiation (definition varies greatly among stud-, most used BUN <60 vs. >60). However, all the studies have significant design flaws l no definitive conclusions can be drawn. Two small randomized control studies ich evaluated the timing of initiation of RRT on outcome have not shown a benefit :h early initiation of RRT. The Kidney Disease Improving Global Outcomes DIGO) guidelines recommend initiating RRT emergently when life-threatening anges in fluid, electrolyte, and acid–base balance exist). The ongoing multinational indard versus Accelerated Initiation of RRT in AKI (STARRT-AKI) trial will be trumental in providing answers regarding the optimal time for starting RRT in <I patients.

ODALITIES

nce the decision has been made to initiate RRT, one needs to select a modality. ie available modalities are IHD, CRRT, prolonged intermittent renal replacement therapy (PIRRT), or peritoneal dialysis. The choice depends on the availabilit therapies at the institution, physician preference, the patient's hemodynamic sta and the presence of comorbid conditions. Intermittent modalities generally c greater fluctuations in blood pressure and produce greater fluid shifts in a sl amount of time. Continuous modalities allow for the same solute clearance and f removal, but spread out during a 24-hour period, and thus are favored in hemc namically unstable patients such as those with sepsis or fulminant hepatic failure

In the United States, CRRT is performed in approximately 30% of adult pati with AKI and has almost completely replaced peritoneal dialysis in the intensive unit (ICU) setting. However, although CRRT has some potential benefits over IF as seen in randomized trials, CRRT has not shown improved survival over IHL critically ill patients. Likewise, randomized trials have not shown a difference in t to renal recovery or length of ICU or hospital stay between groups treated with I versus CRRT.

In the recent years, the use of PIRRT or sustained low-efficiency dialysis (SL has increased and is mainly driven by its convenience and lower cost compare CRRT. Treatments are intermittent but with longer duration (8 to 12 hours/sessi and with lower blood and dialysate flow rates, compared to IHD. Compare CRRT, PIRRT is performed with higher blood flow and dialysate flow rates. PIR is often performed five to six times per week, usually during the night at some in tutions including ours. It is an excellent modality for those patients who are pron hemodynamic instability. It also provides "down time" for procedures and at the sa time does not compromise the dialysis dose. PIRRT requires less anticoagulation t CRRT, demands less nursing care, and is a good alternative to CRRT in the IC Randomized, controlled studies have suggested similar safety and efficacy compa to CRRT and IHD.

Table 44.1 lists the advantages and disadvantages of the different modalitie dialysis.

DIALYSIS DOSE

The ideal dose of dialytic therapy in critically ill patients has not yet been conclusi determined. Evidence from end-stage, dialysis-dependent patients suggests tha thrice-weekly regimen should be performed with a urea reduction of approxima 70% per session. However, in the acutely ill intensive care population, these ca lations are not always equivalent. The actual urea clearances are approximately 2 lower than what would be expected in a stable chronic dialysis patient, and thus it been proposed that additional benefit may be derived from higher treatment do more frequent treatments, or greater hemofiltration.

In IHD, a few small studies had shown a survival advantage in critically patients who receive either a higher delivered dialysis dose three times per w or undergo daily dialysis. In contrast, the VA/NIH Acute Renal Failure Trial N work (ATN) study, a large multicenter, prospective, randomized trial, did not f a decrease in mortality or increase in renal recovery with more frequent dialysis times per week vs. three times). We recommend IHD be provided three times a we targeting the urea reduction ratio of >70%, or Kt/V of 1.2 to 1.4 per treatment.

Similarly, in CRRT, small randomized controlled trials had shown a survival b efit with high-intensity dialysis. Subsequent trials have shown conflicting results. T largest trials to date, the ATN study (effluent rate of 35 mL/kg/hr vs. 20 mL/kg/

TABLE 44.1 Renal Replacement Modalities

Modality	Advantages	Disadvantages
IHD	High-efficiency transport of solutes when rapid clearance of toxins or electrolytes is required Allows time for off-unit testing	Hemodynamic intolerance secondary to fluid shifts "Saw-tooth" pattern of metabolic control between sessions
CRRT	Gentler hemodynamic shifts than IHD Steady solute control	Continuous need for specialized nursing Requires continuous anticoagulation (heparin vs. citrate)
PIRRT	All of the advantages of CRRT Provides "down time" for off-unit testing Less nursing care than CRRT Less expensive than CRRT Anticoagulation generally not necessary	Requires almost daily treatments Less "middle molecule" removal than CRRT
Peritoneal dialysis	Gentler hemodynamic shifts than IHD	Requires invasion of peritoneal cavity, which may not be possible in postoperative patients Less predictable fluid removal rates

CRRT, continuous renal replacement therapy; IHD, intermittent hemodialysis; PIRRT, prolonged intermittent renal replacement therapy.

and the study from the RENAL Replacement Therapy Study Investigators (effluent rate of 40 mL/kg/hr vs. 25 mL/kg/hr), did not demonstrate a survival advantage with higher-intensity dialysis at day 60. In the ATN study, higher-intensity dialysis did not improve recovery of renal function or reduce the rate of nonrenal organ failure. Subsequent meta-analysis showed similar results. If continuous venovenous hemodiafiltration (CVVHDF) is the preferred modality at the institution, we recommend using flow rates of 20 mL/kg/hr, divided equally between the replacement flow rate and dialysate flow rate. With this dosing we recommend that patients remain on therapy for a minimum of 20 hours per day. If the patient is not receiving at least 18 to 20 hours of CRRT in a 24-hour period, because of diagnostic testing, surgical procedures, clotting of the circuit or other factors, then prescribed dose can be increased by 15% to 20% to ensure that delivered dose will be about 20 mL/kg/hr. Also, in patients who need higher clearances for severe acidosis or hyperkalemia, then higher flow rates should be used.

DRUG DOSING DURING CRRT

Various factors affect the dosing of medications in the setting of CRRT. The pharmacokinetics of drug removal during CRRT can be highly complex, depending on the drug's molecular size, protein binding, volume of distribution, dialyzer membrane permeability, the dose of dialysis, and the modality of CRRT (continuous venovenous hemodialysis [CVVHD] vs. continuous venovenous hemofiltration [CVVH] v CVVHDF). The clearance of a drug can also be affected by its elimination by nonr nal routes or by the degree of residual renal function. Generally, the nonrenal clea ance is taken to be constant, although in critically ill patients with multiorgan syste failure, this component may be less than predicted. In sepsis, certain variables such volume of distribution and protein binding can be altered. There is a paucity of da about drug dosing during CRRT in critically ill patients. One important princip to remember is that elimination is continuous; therefore, most drugs will need to I given twice or thrice daily. Drug levels, when available, should be measured dai The recommended doses for some of the more commonly prescribed antibiotics a listed in Table 44.2. These recommendations should not replace clinical judgment clinical situations vary greatly.

TABLE 44.2	Dosing of Common Antimicrobial Agents During Continuous Renal Replacement Therapy (CRRT)	
Drug	Dosing in CVVH	Dosing in CVVHD or CVVHDF
Vancomycin	LD 15–20 mg/kg, then 1 g q48h	LD 15–20 mg/kg, then 1 g q24h
Cefepime	1–2 g q12h	2 g q12h or 1 g q8h
Ceftazidime	1–2 g q12h	2 g q12h or 1 g q8h
Cefotaxime	1–2 g q12h	2 g q12h
Ceftriaxone	1–2 g q12–24h	2 g q12–24h
Imipenem–cilastatin	250 mg q6h or 500 mg q8h	250 mg q6h, 500 mg q6h, or 500 mg q8h
Meropenem	1 g q12h	1 g q12h
Ciprofloxacin	200 mg q12h	200–400 mg q12h
Metronidazole	500 mg q8h	500 mg q8h
Piperacillin–tazobactam	2.25 g q6h	3.375 g q6h
Amikacin	LD 10 mg/kg, then 7.5 mg/kg q24–48h	LD 10 mg/kg, then 7.5 mg/kg q24–48h
Tobramycin	LD 3 mg/kg, then 2 mg/kg q24–48h	LD 3 mg/kg, then 2 mg/kg q24–48h
Gentamicin	LD 3 mg/kg, then 2 mg/kg q24–48h	LD 3 mg/kg, then 2 mg/kg q24–48h
Daptomycin	4 or 6 mg/kg q48h	4 or 6 mg/kg q48h
Linezolid	600 mg q12h	600 mg q12h
Fluconazole	200–400 mg q24h	400–800 mg q24h
Acyclovir	5–7.5 mg/kg q24h	5–7.5 mg/kg q24h

CVVH, continuous venovenous hemofiltration; CVVHD, continuous venovenous hemodialysis; CVVHDF, continuous venovenous hemodiafiltration; LD, loading dose.

UG DOSING DURING PIRRT

re is limited data on drug clearance and appropriate drug dosing in patients
ergoing PIRRT. The same factors affecting drug dosing in CRRT are applied
. However, drug clearance is more unpredictable due to the intermittent nature
'IRRT. It is also difficult to make general dosing recommendations for a particular
g as the half-life can be quite variable during PIRRT, due to lack of uniformity in
yzer membrane, blood, and dialysate flow rates (machine and center dependent).
once a day medications, the dose should be given post-PIRRT. For twice a day
lications, the first dose should be given post-PIRRT and the second dose 12 hours
r. Ideally, the PIRRT treatment should be initiated around the same time every
, Close communication between the nephrology team, pharmacist, and the ICU
n is essential to ensure adequate drug dosing.

MPLICATIONS OF RRT

with any procedure, there are certain complications and adverse events that can
associated with renal replacement therapies. Vigilance for such complications and
ir immediate rectification are essential to prevent life-threatening situations, espe-
ly in the vulnerable population of the ICU. In addition, the necessity for a central
ous catheter places the patient at risk for infectious complications.

potension

radialytic hypotension can occur in all clinical settings with all modalities,
ough it is more commonly seen with IHD. Volume-depleted and septic patients
at heightened risk, and careful attention to the physical examination and invasive
nodynamic monitoring when indicated can help ensure adequate volume resus-
ition prior to initiating the dialysis session. A target central venous pressure of
12 mm Hg can be used in these settings and may dictate a reduction or stop-
e of fluid ultrafiltration. Other factors can also result in intradialytic hypotension.
e rapid clearance of uremic solutes can lower the serum osmolality and lead to
uid shift toward the intracellular space, depleting the intravascular volume. A
rmal saline bolus of 250 mL or administration of 25% albumin in 100 mL can be
d as initial management steps in the treatment of intradialytic hypotension, and
rafiltration may need to be turned off. The dialysate temperature can be decreased
promote vasoconstriction. Patients who are persistently hypotensive may need to
tch to a continuous modality. Air embolism is a very rare complication of dialysis
at can lead to hemodynamic instability. Other differential diagnoses to consider
lude internal hemorrhage, pericardial tamponade, and myocardial infarction.

rhythmias

rdiac arrhythmias can occur in the setting of rapid electrolyte shifts in acute hemolysis. The removal of certain antiarrhythmic drugs during dialysis is also a risk
tor. In chronic dialysis, a bath with a potassium concentration of 2 to 3 mEq/L is
quently used. However, when hyperkalemia necessitates a dialysate with a potas-
m concentration of 0 to 1 mEq/L, it is important to monitor hourly potassium
els. A low-potassium dialysate should not be used longer than 1 hour unless the
um potassium remains critically elevated. Patients on digitalis are especially sen-
ve to hypokalemia. Supraventricular arrhythmias can also be triggered during the

placement of the dialysis catheter, by a malpositioned dialysis catheter, and sometin during dialysis. If the arrhythmia is resulting in hemodynamic compromise, t therapy is discontinued immediately and cardioversion should be attempted.

Dialyzer Reactions

Dialyzer reactions are rare during hemodialysis. Type A, or anaphylactic, reacti are estimated to occur in 4 of every 100,000 sessions and present in the first minutes once the blood in the circuit returns to the patient. Symptoms are varied a may include urticaria, flushing, chest pain, back pain, dyspnea, vomiting, and ch Severe cases can progress to hypotension, cardiac arrest, and death. The cause for reaction is believed to be related to residual amounts of ethylene oxide, which is u to sterilize dialyzers. Type A reactions are treated by immediately discontinuing dialysis session and discarding the blood in the circuit. Further therapy with epine rine or bronchodilators depends on the severity of the reaction.

Type B reactions are more common, and are distinguished from type A reacti in that they are usually less severe and present later, usually after the first 15 minu of dialysis. They are thought to be due to the use of unsubstituted cellulose dialy membranes and complement activation. They occur in 3% to 4% of sessions a also present with chest pain, back pain, dyspnea, or gastrointestinal symptoms. If symptoms are not severe, then dialysis is continued and the symptoms slowly resol Treatment is supportive, with appropriate use of intravenous saline, analgesics, a antihistamines.

Dialysis Catheter-Related Problems

The dialysis catheter itself can also pose problems. When needed acutely, a nontu neled catheter can be inserted into a central vein at the bedside. When infection a bacteremia occur, prompt catheter removal is generally recommended unless vascu access is especially difficult. Thrombus or fibrin sheaths can form around or inside catheters causing inadequate blood flows for dialysis. Even though heparin is usu instilled into the hub of the catheter after each dialysis, this does not necessary p vent the clot formation. An attempt at clot lysis can be made by instilling 1 to 2 of alteplase into each catheter lumen. The catheter is then capped for 2 to 3 hours a the medication is aspirated before dialysis is again attempted. Alteplase should not administered systemically for this purpose. If the catheter continues to malfunctic it may be changed over a guidewire or replaced completely.

In patients with CKD, subclavian veins are not used for dialysis cathete as there is a high risk of subclavian venous stenosis, which can prevent the futu placement of an arteriovenous fistula or graft in that extremity for dialysis. The are no data to suggest that tunneled catheters are more beneficial regarding infecti rates or adequacy of dialysis in intensive care patients with AKI. Tunneled cathet are typically used in patients with multiple malfunctioning temporary cathete poor chance for early renal recovery, or for those being transferred out of the IC to a different facility. For clotted tunneled catheters, interventional radiology co sultation is required to perform endoluminal brushing to dislodge thrombi a fibrin sheaths.

Problems Associated With CRRT

One of the advantages of CRRT over IHD is that the slower blood flow rates pla a gentler hemodynamic burden on unstable patients. However, hypotension can st

cur in this group, especially when high ultrafiltration rates are attempted. Some
verse events are specific to continuous modalities, mostly related to electrolyte
normalities. Uninterrupted high-flow CRRT can cause dramatic hypophosphate-
a, hypokalemia, and hypomagnesemia. Serum electrolytes need to be monitored at
st daily. Hypokalemia can be corrected by increasing the potassium concentration
the replacement fluid and dialysate. Hypophosphatemia and hypomagnesemia can
corrected by supplementation.

Given its lower flow rates, CRRT usually requires some form of anticoagu-
ion to prevent clotting in the extracorporeal circuit. Heparin is the preferred
ticoagulant at many institutions. In cases of heparin-induced thrombocytopenia,
direct thrombin inhibitor, argatroban or bivalirudin, can be used. When systemic
ticoagulation is contraindicated, citrate can be used regionally in the dialysis cirit. Citrate chelates calcium in the serum and inhibits activation of the coagulation
scade. Citrate is quickly metabolized to bicarbonate in the liver and thus does not
sult in systemic anticoagulation. Calcium is replaced through a separate central
nous line and this process requires close monitoring of serum-ionized calcium
els. With the breakdown of citrate to bicarbonate, the development of a metabolic
calosis is another concern with this form of anticoagulation. Metabolic alkalosis can
treated by changing the replacement fluid to normal saline from a bicarbonate-
sed product.

Hypothermia is a well-known complication of CRRT and is common at high
w rates. Significant amounts of heat are lost from the slow-flowing extracorporeal
rcuit and can cause drops in body temperature of 2° to 5°C. This can be addressed
ensuring the use of warmers on CRRT devices, which either warms the dialysate or
placement fluid or warms the venous return tubing. However, this poses a problem
garding the detection of fever. Unpublished reports have shown no advantage to
ecking routine cultures; therefore, reliance on the other clinical signs of infection is
eded.

ISCONTINUATION OF RRT

RT should be continued until patients show evidence of renal recovery. This can
assessed by a decrease in the creatinine after a steady state in an oliguric patient or
crease in urine output in a nonoliguric patient. If there is uncertainty regarding the
tent of renal recovery, a 24-hour urine collection for creatinine clearance (CrCl)
n be obtained. In most patients RRT can be discontinued if CrCl is above 15 to
) mL/min.

UMMARY

RT is initiated when more conservative medical management has failed to con-
ol the fluid, electrolyte, and metabolic complications of AKI. Several modalities
e available to the clinician, and selection between intermittent and continuous
orms depends on the availability at the institution, the patient's hemodynamic
ability, and comorbid illnesses. Despite the overall safety of these procedures,
mplications and adverse events can occur, requiring meticulous attention and,
some cases, frequent laboratory monitoring to anticipate and prevent their
ccurrence.

SUGGESTED READINGS

Bagshaw SM, Berthiaume LR, Delaney A, et al. Continuous versus intermittent renal replace ment therapy for critically ill patients with acute kidney injury: a meta-analysis. *Crit C. Med.* 2008;36(2):610–617.

Brause M, Neumann A, Schumacher T, et al. Effect of filtration volume of continuous venov nous hemofiltration in the treatment of patients with acute renal failure in intensive ca units. *Crit Care Med.* 2003;31(3):841–846.
Prospective pilot study comparing patients dialyzed with different target Kt/V.

Cho KC, Himmelfarb J, Paganini E, et al. Survival by dialysis modality in critically ill patier with acute kidney injury. *J Am Soc Nephrol.* 2006;17(11):3132–3138.
Multicenter observational study comparing continuous and intermittent dialysis.

Jun M, Lambers Heerspink HJ, Ninomiya T, et al. Intensities of renal replacement therapy acute kidney injury: a systemic review and meta-analysis. *Clin J Am Soc Nephrol.* 2010;5(4 956–963.

Kidney Disease: Improving Global Outcomes (KDIGO) Acute Kidney Injury Work Grou KDIGO Clinical practice guideline for acute kidney injury. *Kidney Int.* 2012;(suppl 2 1–138.

Kroh UF, Holl TJ, Steinhauber W. Management of drug dosing in continuous renal replaceme therapy. *Semin Dial.* 1996;9(2):161–165.
Review of factors determining drug dosing in CRRT.

Mushatt DM, Mihm LB, Dreisbach AW, et al. Antibiotic dosing in slow extended daily dialys *Clin Infect Dis.* 2009;49(3):433–437.

O'Reilly P, Tolwani A. Renal replacement therapy III: IHD, CRRT, SLED. *Crit Care Clin.* 2005;21(2 367–378.
Review of replacement options.

Palevsky PM. Renal replacement therapy I: indications and timing. *Crit Care Clin.* 2005;21(2 347–356.
Review of dialytic indications.

Palevsky PM, Liu KD, Brophy PD, et al. KDOQI US commentary on the 2012 KDIGO clin ical practice guideline for acute kidney injury. *Am J Kidney Dis.* 2013;61(5):649–672.

Ricci Z, Ronco C. Renal replacement therapy II: dialysis dose. *Crit Care Clin.* 2005;21:357–36 *Review of dialysis dosing.*

Ronco C, Bellomo R, Homel P, et al. Effects of different doses in continuous veno-venou haemofiltration on outcomes of acute renal failure: a prospective randomised trial. *Lanc* 2000;356(9223):26–30.
Randomized study comparing patients assigned to different ultrafiltration doses.

Schiffl H, Lang SM, Fischer R. Daily hemodialysis and the outcome of acute renal failur *N Engl J Med.* 2002;346(5):305–310.
Randomized study comparing daily and intermittent conventional dialysis.

The RENAL Replacement Therapy Study Investigators, Bellomo R, Cass A. Intensity of continuou renal-replacement therapy in critically ill patients. *N Engl J Med.* 2009;361(17):1627–1638

The VA/NIH Acute Renal Failure Trial Network. Intensity of renal support in critically i patients with acute kidney injury. *N Engl J Med.* 2008;359(1):7–20.

Trotman RL, Williamson JC, Shoemaker DM, et al. Antibiotic dosing in critically ill adult patien receiving continuous renal replacement therapy. *Clin Infect Dis.* 2005;41(8):1159–1166.

Vinsonneau C, Camus C, Combes A, et al; Hemodiafe Study Group. Continuous venovenou haemodiafiltration versus intermittent haemodialysis for acute renal failure in patien with multiple-organ dysfunction syndrome: a multicentre randomised trial. *Lancet.* 200(368(9533):379–385.
Multicenter randomized study comparing continuous and intermittent dialysis.

45

Acute Liver Failure

Claire Meyer and Jeffrey S. Crippin

_te liver failure (ALF) is characterized by coagulopathy, encephalopathy, and severe
_atic injury in patients without chronic liver disease (Table 45.1). Exceptions to the
_nce of pre-existing liver disease include autoimmune hepatitis and Wilson's dis-
_, if the disease has only been recognized within the last 26 weeks. Approximately
_0 cases of ALF are reported per year in the United States.

_USES AND DIAGNOSIS

_ermining the cause of ALF is imperative, since some etiologies dictate specific
_tments. In a prospective multicenter study of 308 patients (1998 to 2001) by the
_te Liver Failure Study Group, the following causes were most frequently identified:
_aminophen overdose (39%), indeterminate (17%), idiosyncratic drug reactions
_%), and viral hepatitis (hepatitis A virus or hepatitis B) (11%). Table 45.1 outlines
_possible causes of ALF, as well as the studies needed to evaluate patients for each
_logy. On presentation, initial laboratory analysis should include a complete blood
_nt, basic metabolic panel, liver chemistries, magnesium, phosphate, prothrombin
_e, lactic acid, arterial blood gas, ammonia, acetaminophen level, acute viral hepa-
_s panel, toxicology screen, ceruloplasmin level, antinuclear antibodies, antismooth
_scle antibodies, HIV status, and a pregnancy test (if applicable).

_IOLOGY-SPECIFIC MANAGEMENT OF ACUTE
_VER FAILURE (See Algorithm 45.1)

_etaminophen Toxicity

_acetaminophen toxicity is the leading cause of ALF in the United States, clinicians
_uld have a high index of suspicion for acetaminophen overdose, particularly when
_re is inadequate knowledge of the circumstances preceding a patient's presentation
_the hospital. N-acetylcysteine (NAC) therapy is indicated when acetaminophen-
_ted ALF is known or suspected, regardless of the grade of encephalopathy, and
_uld be initiated as soon after acetaminophen ingestion as possible. The nomogram
_wn in Figure 45.1 helps to guide treatment based on the serum acetaminophen
_el when a single ingestion occurred at a known time. However, in the setting of
_F, treatment with NAC should be initiated if the serum acetaminophen is elevated
_any level, as significant liver injury can result from multiple relatively small doses
_er time. If ingestion is known to have occurred within 4 hours of presentation,
_ivated charcoal lowers the plasma acetaminophen level more effectively than

TABLE 45.1	Diagnosis and Causes of Acute Liver Failure

1. Acute hepatic injury <26 wks without evidence of pre-existing liver disease
2. Encephalopathy
3. Coagulopathy (INR ≥1.5)

↓

Etiology	History and Physical Examination	Diagnostic Evaluation
Acetaminophen	History of ingestion	Acetaminophen level (short half-life, low serum level does not rule out ingestion), use nomogram when time of ingestion known
Drug toxicity	New medications, antibiotics, NSAIDs, anticonvulsants, psychiatric history, herbals; unlikely if >1 yr on medication	Serum drug levels
Other toxins	Mushroom ingestion, cocaine or MDMA use	Urine drug screen
Viral	Viral syndrome, pregnancy, recent travel, skin lesions, immunocompromised state	Hepatitis B surface antigen, hepatitis B core IgM, Hepatitis A IgM, hepatitis E antibody, hepatitis C antibody, hepatitis C RNA, HIV antibody, HSV antibodies and DNA, VZV DNA; consider evaluation for rare viral causes including parvovirus B19, adenovirus, and EBV
Shock liver	History of heart failure, cardiac arrest, volume depletion, or substance abuse	BNP, lactate dehydrogenase, lactate, echocardiogram
Infiltrative malignancy	History of malignancy, hepatomegaly	If suspected, cross-sectional abdominal imaging and liver biopsy (if feasible)
Budd–Chiari syndrome	History of malignancy or other prothrombotic condition, including recent pregnancy or exogenous estrogens; personal or family history of venous thromboembolism; lymphadenopathy	Abdominal ultrasound with Doppler
Wilson's disease	Patient <40 yrs old, history of neuropsychiatric symptoms; Kayser–Fleischer rings on slit lamp exam	Serum ceruloplasmin and copper, 24-hr urine copper, uric acid, hemolysis labs; if suspected, liver biopsy (if feasible) for quantitative copper measurement
Acute fatty liver of pregnancy, HELLP	Pregnancy	B-HCG in women of childbearing potential; if suspected, urinalysis to evaluate for proteinuria. If liver biopsy performed, frozen section needed for *oil red O* stain (AFLP)
Autoimmune Hepatitis	History of other autoimmune diseases	Antinuclear antibody, antismooth muscle antibody, anti-LKM1, serum immunoglobulins; if suspected, liver biopsy (if feasible)

ALGORITHM 45.1 Treatment Algorithm for Acute Liver Failure

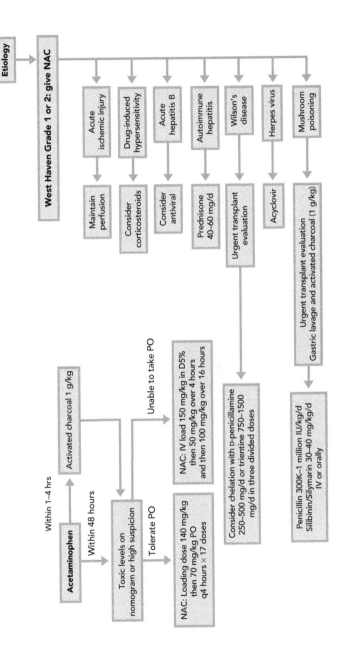

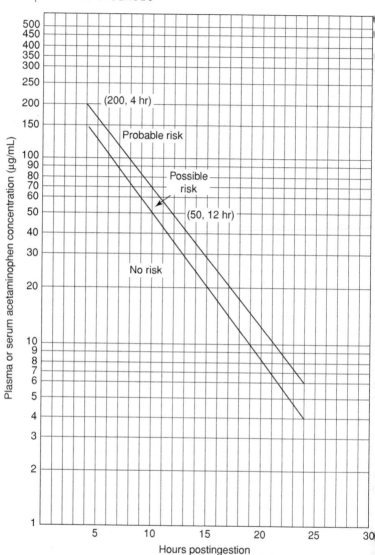

Figure 45.1. Acetaminophen toxicity nomogram. (Adapted from Rumack BH, Peterson RC, Koch GG et al. Acetaminophen overdose: 662 cases with evaluation of oral acetylcysteine treatment. *Arch Intern Med* 1981;141:380.)

s gastric lavage or ipecac, and is typically given as a single dose (1 g/kg). The
:acy of NAC is not reduced by prior treatment with activated charcoal. Patients
ι acetaminophen toxicity should be treated with NAC even if they present to
lical care after a significant delay. A retrospective study including patients who
an NAC 10 to 36 hours after overdose showed improved outcomes in this group,
ιpared to those receiving no antidote. Refer to Algorithm 45.1 for PO and IV
C dosing. The route of administration (oral or intravenous) has not been shown
ιffect outcomes. Cochrane analysis of one prospective, controlled trial of NAC
acetaminophen-related ALF showed reduced mortality (Peto odds ratio 0.29) in
ιents treated with NAC.

ιn-Acetaminophen Etiologies

ε benefit of NAC in acetaminophen toxicity has been demonstrated for decades,
its role in non-acetaminophen–related ALF has only recently been established.
ιandomized placebo-controlled trial including 173 patients with non-acetamino-
ι–related ALF, demonstrated improved transplant-free survival at 3 weeks and
ear in patients who received 72 hours of NAC therapy. This benefit was seen only
ιatients with grade 1 to 2 encephalopathy, but not in those with more advanced
des. Given its minimal adverse reaction profile, NAC therapy should be initiated
all patients with ALF presenting with grade 1 to 2 encephalopathy. Treatment
ι NAC should not delay transfer to a transplant facility.

For non-acetaminophen–related causes of liver damage, etiology-specific inter-
ιtions are unlikely to be life-saving in the setting of ALF; rather, the decision
ιarding need and eligibility for liver transplant is crucial. Nonetheless, when a spe-
ε etiology is identified, initiation of directed therapy can be considered as outlined
ιlgorithm 45.1. Hepatitis B, with or without hepatitis D, accounts for more than
f of viral causes of ALF. Treatment with a nucleotide or nucleoside analog is gen-
ιly recommended, though evidence is mixed with regard to its impact on clinical
ιcomes in this setting; lamivudine (100 mg/day) has been used in the majority of
orts. Hepatitis E is a more common viral cause of ALF in endemic countries and
ιuld be considered in returning travelers or recent immigrants from these regions.
ιatment for acute hepatitis A and E is supportive. Hepatitis C alone rarely causes
F; however, other viruses such as HSV, EBV, adenovirus, and parvovirus B19 have
ιn reported.

ΛNAGEMENT OF SYSTEMIC COMPLICATIONS

ιntral Nervous System

ιrebral edema and increased intracranial pressure (ICP) are serious complications of
F. The risk of cerebral edema increases with progression of encephalopathy, with a
5% incidence in patients with grade 4 encephalopathy. Advanced cerebral edema
ι lead to uncal herniation and death.

Management of neurologic complications is outlined in Algorithm 45.2.
ιients with any degree of encephalopathy should be transferred to a liver transplant
ιter. Patients with grade 3 to 4 encephalopathy should be intubated for airway
ιtection. Peri-intubation, attempts should be made to avoid coughing and paralysis
ιften used as part of the induction regimen. Frequent neurologic examinations are
ιperative, and findings such as systemic hypertension, bradycardia, posturing, and
ιreased pupillary reflexes can suggest impending herniation.

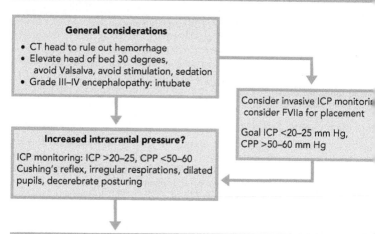

ALGORITHM 45.2 CNS Complications of Acute Liver Failure

General considerations

- CT head to rule out hemorrhage
- Elevate head of bed 30 degrees, avoid Valsalva, avoid stimulation, sedation
- Grade III–IV encephalopathy: intubate

Consider invasive ICP monitoring; consider FVIIa for placement

Goal ICP <20–25 mm Hg, CPP >50–60 mm Hg

Increased intracranial pressure?

ICP monitoring: ICP >20–25, CPP <50–60
Cushing's reflex, irregular respirations, dilated pupils, decerebrate posturing

Intervention	Administration	Comments
Mannitol	Bolus 0.5–1 g/kg; can repeat twice at 4–6 hour intervals.	No proven role in prophylaxis Keep serum osmolality <320 mOsm/kg Side effects: hypernatremia, volume overload
Hypertonic saline	30% NaCl 5–20 mL/hour (titrated to achieve serum sodium 145–155 mmol/L)	May only apply to patients on renal replacement therapy
Sedation	Propofol infusion *Alternatives*: thiopental, pentobarbital	Side effects of barbiturates: severe hypotension, prolonged sedation
Hyperventilation	Titrate respiratory rate to pCO$_2$ 25–30 mm Hg for acute management of refractory ICH	Temporary measure; no proven role in prophylaxis
Management of body temperature	Treat fever; permit spontaneous core body temperatures 35–36°C	No proven benefit of induced hypothermia

ABBREVIATIONS
CPP: central perfusion pressure
ICH: intracranial hypertension
ICP: intracranial pressure

ICP monitoring should be considered for patients with rapidly progressing encephalopathy and those listed for liver transplantation. In the absence of definitive evidence of a mortality benefit, the frequency with which ICP monitoring is used varies widely among liver transplant programs. ICP can be measured with epidural, subdural, parenchymal, or ventricular catheter. Epidural catheters generally have a lower complication rate, but are less reliable. The most common complications include bleeding in the setting of coagulopathy, infection, and volume overload resulting from correction of coagulopathy. Recombinant factor VIIa has been used

small trial to aid with placement of ICP transducers with favorable results. The role noninvasive ICP monitoring (using transcranial Doppler) is not yet established. ICP should be maintained at a level <20 mm Hg, with a cerebral perfusion pressure mean arterial pressure [MAP] minus ICP) >50 mm Hg.

Once increased ICP or cerebral edema is present, aggressive measures should be undertaken to prevent herniation. Propofol sedation, avoidance of sensory stimulation, and raising the head of the bed can be helpful. Therapies focused on decreasing cerebral edema include osmotic agents (mannitol or hypertonic saline) or decreasing cerebral blood flow (hyperventilation or hypothermia).

Mannitol is administered as a bolus dose (0.5 to 1 g/kg of a 20% solution). The dose can be repeated twice, however, administration is limited by maintaining a serum osmolality <320 mOsm/kg. If patients have concomitant renal failure, hemofiltration should be considered. Hyperventilation has only a short-term benefit, but can be used with the goal of reducing $PaCO_2$ to 25 mm Hg. An RCT demonstrated no benefit of prophylactic continuous hyperventilation in ALF. A study of 30 patients with ICP monitoring randomized to 3% hypertonic saline with a goal serum sodium concentration of 145 to 155 mmol/L, showed a significant decrease in average ICP and episodes of increased ICP, but no survival benefit. Hypothermia (32° to 34°C) has been associated with a beneficial effect in uncontrolled trials. Patients with ALF may have seizure activity, but prophylactic phenytoin has not proven to be effective in improving survival. Despite an association between an arterial ammonia level of 200 mcmol/L and herniation, no benefit of gut decontamination or lactulose has been demonstrated in ALF. Hemofiltration via CRRT can reduce ammonia levels, though its effect on ICP has not been studied. Barbiturate coma can be attempted for refractory increased ICP, but requires close monitoring of MAP due to its association with hypotension. Dexamethasone is not effective at prolonging survival.

Coagulopathy

The management of coagulopathy is outlined in Algorithm 45.3. Synthesis of coagulation factors I, II, V, VII, IX, and X is depressed in patients with ALF. Sources of bleeding include procedure sites, stress ulcers, lungs, and the oropharynx. Proton pump inhibitors should be used for stress ulcer prophylaxis. Platelets should only be transfused for counts <10,000/μL or in the face of active bleeding. Vitamin K is routinely given, but fresh-frozen plasma should not be transfused unless there is active bleeding or a planned procedure. Packed red blood cells can be transfused for symptomatic anemia or to replace blood loss secondary to hemorrhage.

The role of recombinant factor VIIa has been evaluated during the placement of ICP monitors. In an unblinded study comparing patients with ALF given recombinant factor VIIa with a cohort of historic controls, patients receiving recombinant factor VIIa all had successful placement (7/7 vs. 3/8). Patients receiving recombinant factor VIIa also had a significant decrease in mortality and anasarca from fluid overload.

Hypotension

Hypotension is multifactorial in patients with ALF, resulting from volume depletion, third spacing, infection, gastrointestinal bleeding, or as a result of overall low systemic vascular resistance and a hyperkinetic cardiovascular state. Fluid resuscitation should be balanced with avoidance of volume overload and the theoretical risk of increasing ICP. Maintenance fluid should be glucose based due to the hypoglycemia associated with liver failure. Although not compared directly in trials, dopamine or norepinephrine can be used for vasopressor support with a MAP goal of 65 to 75 mm Hg. In a

ALGORITHM 45.3 Management of the Complications of Fulminant Hepatic Failure

Management of Complications

Hypotension

Albumin or saline

MAP <55–60 mm Hg

Norepinephrine (preferred) or dopamine; can add vasopressin if needed

Maintenance

D5% based

Coagulopathy

Bleeding?

Local measures; vitamin K 5–10 mg SC × 3 d; transfuse FFP and platelets, as indicated

Prophylaxis

Proton pump inh
Do not give plts until plts <10 k

Planned procedure?

• Give plts to >50 k
• Consider FVIIa if renal insufficiency/volume overload

Infection

Obtain surveillance Cx; low threshold for prophylactic broad-spectrum antibiotics
No role for bowel decontamination

Ascites?

PMN >250/mm³

Cefotaxime 2 g q8 hr
Albumin 1.5 g/kg day 1 and 1 g/kg day 3

Renal

Fluid challenge; avoid nephrotoxins

Worsening failure?

CVVHD better than HD

Metabolic

Initiate early enteral or parenteral nutrition; replete electrolytes; replete glucose

CNS

See Algorithm 45.2

ABBREVIATIONS
SC: subcutaneously
FFP: fresh-frozen plasma
Cx: cultures
MAP: mean arterial pressure
inh: inhibitors
plts: platelets
PMN: polymorphonuclear leukocyte
CVVHD: continuous venovenous hemodialysis
HD: hemodialysis
CNS: central nervous system
D5%:   5% dextrose
CRRT: continuous renal replacement therapy
IHD: intermittent hemodialysis FVII, factor VII

ll study, dopamine led to a significant increase in cardiac output, systemic oxygen
very, and hepatic and splanchnic blood flow when used to increase MAP by
mm Hg. Although systemic oxygen consumption was increased, splanchnic oxy-
consumption was decreased. A small trial evaluating the role of norepinephrine
LF noted an increase in MAP, although it was not associated with an increase
ardiac index and actually resulted in a decrease in systemic oxygen consumption.
uscitation with colloid is theoretically better than crystalloid, given that albumin
ces a more effective expansion of the central blood volume, but no mortality
efit has been shown.

ection

ctions are found in 80% of patients with ALF, with 25% of patients developing
umented bacteremia and 33% developing systemic fungal infections. Periodic
veillance cultures should be obtained to detect infections as early as possible.
hough prophylactic antibiotics do not provide a survival advantage, a low thresh-
for initiation of broad-spectrum coverage should be maintained. Infections and
erthermia increase the risk of hepatic encephalopathy, therefore a theoretical ben-
of empiric antibiotic therapy exists for patients with worsening encephalopathy.

nal Failure

nal failure is multifactorial in patients with ALF because of the direct toxic effect
ingested substances, volume depletion, hypotension, acute tubular necrosis, and/
the hepatorenal syndrome. In contrast to acute tubular necrosis, renal failure due
the hepatorenal syndrome is characterized by low urinary sodium (<10 mEq/L),
gressive hyponatremia, and a lack of improvement with volume expansion. Neph-
oxic agents such as aminoglycosides and NSAIDs should be avoided and NAC
uld be used prior to intravenous contrast studies. When dialysis is needed, contin-
us renal replacement therapy should be used over daily intermittent hemodialysis,
e to its association with improved cardiovascular dynamics.

tabolic Complications

tabolic complications include hypoglycemia resulting from diminished glucose
thesis and lactic acidosis due to anaerobic glucose metabolism. Patients benefit from
cose monitoring and treatment of hypoglycemia with dextrose-based solutions.
ctrolytes such as phosphorus, potassium, and magnesium are usually abnormal, and
uld be repleted as indicated. Enteral or parenteral nutrition should be initiated
ly and protein should not be restricted. A recent Cochrane database review did not
d convincing evidence of a beneficial role of branched chain amino acids in the
atment of patients with hepatic encephalopathy.

ROGNOSTIC INDICATORS

e most important prognostic indicator in ALF is the etiology of hepatic damage.
etaminophen toxicity, hepatitis A, ischemic liver injury, and pregnancy-related liver
lure portend a transplant-free survival of >50% while idiosyncratic drug reactions,
patitis B, autoimmune hepatitis, Wilson's disease, and Budd–Chiari Syndrome
rry a survival rate of <25% without transplantation. The timing of disease onset is
o important, but this data may be confounded by the etiology of ALF. An illness
<1 week in duration suggests ischemic hepatopathy or acetaminophen overdose

TABLE 45.2	West Haven Criteria for Semiquantitative Grading of Mental State
Grade 1	Trivial lack of awareness Euphoria or anxiety Shortened attention span Impaired performance of addition
Grade 2	Lethargy or apathy Minimal disorientation for time or place Subtle personality change Inappropriate behavior Impaired performance of subtraction
Grade 3	Somnolence to semistupor, but responsive to verbal stimuli Confusion Gross disorientation
Grade 4	Coma (unresponsive to verbal or noxious stimuli)

Atterbury CE, Maddrey WC, Conn HO. Neomycin-sorbitol and lactulose in the treatment of acute portal-systemic encephalopathy. A controlled, double-blind clinical trial. *Am J Dig Dis.* 1978;23(398–406.

and is associated with improved survival, while an illness >4 weeks in duration s gests an indeterminate or viral etiology and indicates a poor transplant-free surviv The degree of encephalopathy is another strong predictor of outcome (Table 45. Patients with grade 2 encephalopathy have a 65% to 70% chance of survival, whe patients with grade 3 or 4 have a 30% to 50% and a 20% chance of survival, resp tively. The King's College Criteria (Table 45.3) are important indicators of outco

TABLE 45.3	King's College Hospital Criteria for Liver Transplantation in FHF
Acetaminophen-induced disease	Arterial pH <7.30 OR Prothrombin time >100 s AND Creatinine >3.4 mg/dL AND Grade III or IV encephalopathy
Nonacetaminophen-induced disease	Prothrombin time >100 s (regardless of encephalopathy grade OR Any three of the following (regardless of encephalopathy grade): Age <10 yrs or >40 yrs Etiology: non-A, non-B hepatitis, halothane hepatitis, or idiosyncratic drug reaction Duration of jaundice before onset of encephalopathy >7 day Prothrombin time >50 s Serum bilirubin >18 mg/dL

O'Grady JG, Alexander GJ, Kayllar KM, et al. Early indicators of prognosis in fulminant hepatic failure. *Gastroenterology.* 1989;97(2):439–445.

patients with non-acetaminophen–associated ALF, the presence of a single factor associated with a mortality rate of 80%, while the presence of all three factors is associated with 95% mortality. In patients with acetaminophen hepatotoxicity and ALF, a single risk factor is associated with a mortality of 55%, and the presence of severe acidosis confers 95% mortality.

LIVER TRANSPLANTATION

Liver transplantation is a proven treatment for ALF, although limited by the prompt availability of donors. Posttransplant survival rates are as high as 80% to 90%. The decision to pursue transplantation versus continuing medical therapy (such as NAC) is difficult. Factors to consider include the possibility of spontaneous recovery, the feasibility of transplantation, and assessment of contraindications to transplantation. Prognostic models such as the King's College Criteria (Table 45.3) and the Acute Physiology and Chronic Health Evaluation (APACHE) II score help in determining the need for liver transplantation. For patients with acetaminophen-associated ALF, a recent meta-analysis reported that the King's College Criteria had a sensitivity of 0.59 and specificity of 0.92 in determining the need for transplantation. An APACHE II score of >15 was associated with a specificity of 0.81 and sensitivity of 0.92 in determining the need for transplantation. The APACHE II score had a higher positive likelihood ratio of 16.4 and negative likelihood ratio of 0.19 (one study) versus the King's criteria, with a positive and negative likelihood ratio of 12.33 and 0.29, respectively, based on six pooled studies.

SUGGESTED READINGS

Brok J, Buckley N, Gluud C. Interventions for paracetamol (acetaminophen) overdose. Cochrane Database Syst Rev. 2006;CD003328.
This meta-analysis provides a comprehensive review of proven and unproven therapies for the leading cause of fulminant hepatic failure.

Hoofnagle JH, Carithers RL, Shapiro C, et al. Fulminant hepatic failure: summary of a workshop. Hepatology. 1995;21(11):240–252.
This paper summarizes issues in the management of fulminant hepatic failure.

Kulkarni S, Cronin DC. Fulminant hepatic failure. In: Hall JB, Schidt GA, Wood LD, eds. Principles of Critical Care. 3rd ed. New York: McGraw-Hill Professional; 2005:1279–1288.
This chapter provides an excellent overview of the pathophysiology and management issues in fulminant hepatic failure.

Lee WM, Larson AM, Stravitz RT. AASLD position paper: the management of acute liver failure: update 2011.http://www.aasld.org/practiceguidelines/Documents/AcuteLiverFailureUpdate2011.pdf.
This paper provides guidelines by the American Association for the Study of Liver Diseases on the management of fulminant hepatic failure.

O'Grady J. Acute liver failure. In: Feldman M, Friedman LS, Brandt LJ, eds. Sleisenger & Fordtran's Gastrointestinal and Liver Disease. 10th ed. Philadelphia, PA: Saunders; 2016:1591–1602.
This chapter provides an excellent overview of the pathophysiology and management issues in fulminant hepatic failure.

Raghavan M, Marik PE. Therapy of intracranial hypertension in patients with fulminant hepatic failure. Neurocrit Care. 2006;4(2):179–189.
This paper provides an excellent overview of treatment for intracranial hypertension and reviews the current understanding of the mechanisms leading to this life threatening complication.

46 Hyperbilirubinemia

Yeshika Sharma and Jeffrey S. Crippin

PHYSIOLOGY

Heme is a breakdown constituent of senescent erythrocytes. It is converted to bili erdin by heme oxygenase and further reduced by biliverdin reductase to bilirubin the reticuloendothelial system. Bilirubin, unconjugated and water insoluble at th point, is tightly bound to albumin and delivered to the liver. It is transported in the hepatocytes by carrier-mediated mechanisms, transferred to the endoplasm reticulum bound by cytosolic proteins, and converted to a water soluble form wi the addition of uridine diphosphate glucuronic acid, the conjugated form of bilir bin. An ATP-dependent export pump, the rate limiting step in bilirubin transpo transfers conjugated bilirubin into the biliary canaliculi, where it is added to bile. Bi eventually drains into the small intestine and is subsequently metabolized by ileal a colonic bacteria to urobilinogen. Eighty per cent of urobilinogen is excreted in stoc while approximately 20% is reabsorbed in the small intestine and enters the port circulation. The reabsorbed urobilinogen is subsequently excreted in stool and urin

Based on the above physiology, the bilirubin pathway can be divided into fo steps: (1) bilirubin production, (2) hepatic bilirubin uptake, (3) bilirubin conj gation, and (4) bilirubin excretion. Hyperbilirubinemia is classically divided in unconjugated and conjugated forms with disruption at steps 1, 2, and 3, leading unconjugated hyperbilirubinemia and disruption of step 4 causing conjugated hype bilirubinemia. However, this division is rarely absolute and clinicians may encount a mixed picture.

Indirect Hyperbilirubinemia

Unconjugated hyperbilirubinemia occurs when indirect bilirubin is >80% of th total bilirubin. This may be caused by increased bilirubin production or decrease hepatocyte uptake and conjugation. Hemolysis, extravasation of blood into tissu (resorption of internal bleeding or hematoma), dyserythropoiesis (thalassemi myelodysplasia, aplastic anemia, vitamin B12 and folate deficiency), and sepsis a frequent causes of unconjugated hyperbilirubinemia. Hemolysis is frequently cha acterized by an elevated reticulocyte count, schistocytes or spherocytes on peripher smear, a positive Coombs test, an increased lactate dehydrogenase, and a decrease haptoglobin level. Physical examination may reveal splenomegaly. Unconjugate hyperbilirubinemia can lead to formation of pigmented gallstones. A decrease i hepatocyte uptake and conjugation is the result of inhibition of uptake mechanism inhibition of glucoronidation, or defects in conjugation. Competitive inhibition ilirubin uptake may be caused by medications such as rifampin and probenecid, while inhibition of glucuronidation can occur with hyperthyroidism and estradiol therapy. A common enzymatic defect, decreased activity of bilirubin UDP-glucuronyl transferase, results in asymptomatic unconjugated hyperbilirubinemia, better known as Gilbert's Syndrome. A more severe quantitative defect in UDP-glucuronyl transferase leads to Crigler-Najjar types I and II. In addition, cardio-pulmonary failure can lead to congestive hepatopathy that presents as indirect hyperbilirubinemia.

Direct Hyperbilirubinemia

Conjugated or direct hyperbilirubinemia is usually secondary to hepatocellular dysfunction, biliary obstruction, or biliary injury. Hepatocellular dysfunction, whether acute or chronic, can cause reflux of conjugated bilirubin into the circulation. This is dependent largely on the fact that active canalicular excretion of conjugated bilirubin is the rate-limiting step in the bilirubin pathway and extremely sensitive to liver dysfunction. Acute hepatocellular dysfunction is characterized by an elevated bilirubin in association with elevated aminotransferases. Chronic dysfunction results in lower aminotransferase levels, common causes including chronic viral hepatitis, alcoholic liver disease, and nonalcoholic steatohepatitis (NASH). Both acute and chronic liver dysfunction may give rise to a mixed hyperbilirubinemia if a disease process causing unconjugated hyperbilirubinemia is superimposed on hepatic dysfunction.

Biliary dysfunction may result from obstruction of the extrahepatic biliary ducts or nonobstructive injury of the intra- or extra-hepatic ducts. A direct bilirubin fraction >50% of the total bilirubin suggests a hepatobiliary etiology and, if accompanied by an elevated alkaline phosphatase and gamma-glutamyl transpeptidase (GGTP), favors biliary obstruction. Causes of intrinsic obstruction include choledocholithiasis, biliary strictures, cholangiocarcinoma, primary sclerosing cholangitis, AIDS cholangiopathy, and parasitic infection (e.g., cryptosporidium). Extrinsic compression can be secondary to pancreatic masses (tumor, fibrosis, pseudocyst, or abscess), or lymphadenopathy. Nonobstructive biliary disease also presents with an elevated alkaline phosphatase, an elevated GGTP, and direct hyperbilirubinemia, but without imaging evidence of obstruction. Potential etiologies include acute viral hepatitis, primary biliary cirrhosis, infiltrative diseases such as amyloidosis and sarcoidosis, drug toxicity, sepsis, total parenteral nutrition, and paraneoplastic syndrome secondary to renal cell carcinoma. Other diseases such as Dubin-Johnson and Rotor syndrome can also cause direct hyperbilirubinemia.

Diagnosis and Therapy

Imaging is required for diagnosis and guides therapy. Imaging modalities include ultrasound, computed tomography (CT), endoscopic retrograde cholangiopancreatography (ERCP), percutaneous transhepatic cholangiography (PTC), and magnetic resonance cholangiopancreatography (MRCP) (Algorithm 46.1). An abdominal ultrasound or CT, both with high specificity, can confirm an obstructive process. Ultrasound is a more sensitive technique for detecting stones within the gallbladder, whereas both techniques are less apt to identify choledocholithiasis. An ultrasound is less helpful in obese patients and when overlying bowel gas is present. If these studies fail to reveal the cause of biliary obstruction, an MRCP gives better visualization of the intrahepatic ducts. If an obstructive process is confirmed, cholangiography can provide direct access to the biliary tree. An ERCP gains access to the proximal biliary tree while PTC, starting at the peripheral bile ducts, allows visualization of the biliary

ALGORITHM 46.1 Evaluation and Management of Hyperbilirubinemia

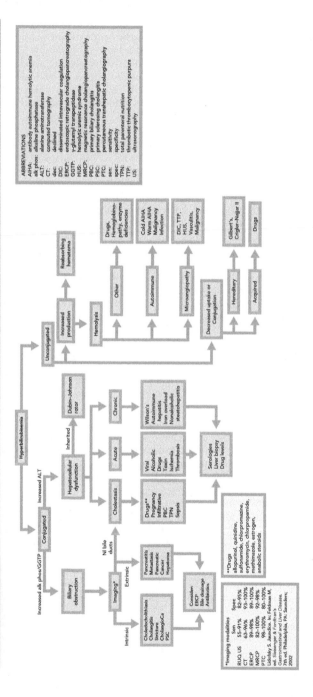

ABBREVIATIONS
AIHA: antibody autoimmune hemolytic anemia
alk phos: alkaline phosphatase
ALT: alanine aminotransferase
CT: computed tomography
dec: declined
DIC: disseminated intravascular coagulation
ERCP: endoscopic retrograde cholangiopancreatography
GGTP: γ-glutamyl transpeptidase
HUS: hemolytic uremic syndrome
MRCP: magnetic resonance cholangiopancreatography
PBC: primary biliary cholangitis
PSC: primary sclerosing cholangitis
PTC: percutaneous transhepatic cholangiography
sen: sensitivity
spec: specificity
TPN: total parenteral nutrition
TTP: thrombotic thrombocytopenic purpura
US: ultrasonography

Hyperbilirubinemia

Conjugated — Increased alk phos/GGTP

Unconjugated — Increased ALT

Biliary obstruction

Imaging*

Intrinsic
- Choledocholithiasis
- Cholangitis
- Stricture
- CholangioCa
- PSC

Extrinsic
- Pancreatitis
- Metastasis
- Pancreatic Cancer
- Hepatoma

Consider:
ERCP
Bile drainage
Antibiotics

Nl bile ducts

Hepatocellular dysfunction

Inherited
- Dubin–Johnson
- rotor

Cholestasis
- Drugs**
- Pregnancy
- Infiltrative
- PBC
- TPN
- Sepsis

Acute
- Viral
- Alcoholic
- Drugs
- Toxin
- Ischemia
- Thrombosis

Chronic
- Wilson's
- Autoimmune hepatitis
- Iron overload
- Nonalcoholic steatohepatitis

Serologies
Liver biopsy
Drug levels

Unconjugated

Increased production

Reabsorbing hematoma

Hemolysis

Other
- Drugs,
- Hemoglobino-pathy, enzyme deficiencies

Autoimmune
- Cold AIHA
- Warm AIHA
- Malignancy
- Infection

Microangiopathy
- DIC, TTP,
- HUS,
- Vasculitis,
- Malignancy

Decreased uptake or conjugation

Hereditary
- Gilbert's,
- Crigler–Najjar II

Acquired
- Drugs

*Imaging modalities

	Sen	Spec
RUQ US	55–91%	82–95%
CT	63–96%	93–100%
ERCP	89–98%	89–100%
MRCP	82–100%	92–98%
PTC	98–100%	80–100%

Lidofsky S. Jaundice. In: Feldman M, ed. Sleisenger & Fortran's
Gastrointestinal and Liver Diseases.
7th ed. Philadelphia, PA: Saunders;
2002

**Drugs
allopurinol, quinidine,
sulfonamide, chlorpromazine,
erythromycin, chlorpropamide,
methimazole, estrogen,
anabolic steroids

e. Either study allows decompression of obstructive processes via sphincterotomy d stone retrieval, stricture dilation, or stent placement. Superimposed infection of an structed biliary tract must promptly be treated with broad spectrum antibiotics and ompt decompression of the biliary tree. If no obstruction is found and a cholestatic ttern still persists, cholangiography may be useful to delineate biliary anatomy. CT aging can reveal infiltrative disease, and a liver biopsy may be required to further fine the amount and type of liver injury.

UGGESTED READINGS

eenberger NJ, Paumgartner G. Diseases of the gallbladder and bile ducts. In: Kasper D, et al., eds. *Harrison's Principles of Internal Medicine*. 16th ed. New York: McGraw-Hill; 2005.

This chapter discusses common causes of biliary dysfunction and provides an approach to diagnosing biliary disease.

lofsky S. Jaundice. In: Feldman M, ed. *Sleisenger & Fordtran's Gastrointestinal and Liver Disease*. 7th ed. Philadelphia, PA: Saunders; 2002.

This chapter provides a systematic approach to evaluating a patient with jaundice and compares the various imaging modalities to evaluate biliary disease.

att DS, Kaplan MM. Jaundice. In: Kasper D, et al., eds. *Harrison's Principles of Internal Medicine*. 16th ed. New York: McGraw-Hill; 2005.

This chapter also provides a systematic approach to evaluating a patient with jaundice.

oche SP, Kobos R. Jaundice in the adult patient. *Am Fam Physician*. 2004;69(2):299–304.

mmerfield JA. Diseases of the gallbladder and biliary tree. In: Warrell DA, Cox TM, Firth JD, et al., eds. *Oxford Textbook of Medicine*. 4th ed. Oxford: Oxford University Press; 2003.

This source provides an excellent overview of investigations in biliary disease.

olkoff A. The hyperbilirubinemias. Kasper D, et al., eds. *Harrison's Principles of Internal Medicine*. 16th ed. New York: McGraw-Hill; 2005.

This chapter provides a great review of the pathophysiology and disorders of the biliary system.

47

End-Stage Liver Disease

Kevin M. Korenblat

The shared outcome of most untreated, chronic liver diseases is the development of cirrhosis. The resulting liver disease is commonly referred to as decompensated cirrhosis and is characterized by the signs and symptoms of both portal hypertension and hepatic synthetic dysfunction. These complications typically coexist in patients with cirrhosis and are the major cause of liver disease-related morbidity and mortality. Common complications of portal hypertension are ascites, portal hypertensive-related bleeding, hepatic encephalopathy, and acute kidney injury (AKI). Intensive care unit (ICU) admissions for these complications are a frequent occurrence, and successful management depends on prompt diagnosis and treatment.

ASCITES

Ascites describes the pathologic accumulation of serous fluid in the peritoneal cavity. It is the most frequent manifestation of decompensated cirrhosis and is associated with a median 2-year mortality rate of 50%. Cirrhotic ascites is identified by its low albumin content and >1.1 g/dL difference between serum and ascites albumin concentrations (serum ascites-albumin gradient).

Paracentesis for sampling of the ascites is required in all patients with new-onset ascites or in those with a change in their clinical condition, such as confusion, renal dysfunction, or gastrointestinal bleeding. Paracentesis (Fig. 47.1) is a safe procedure that can be done even in patients with coagulopathy and thrombocytopenia. The right and left lower quadrants are the preferred site for paracentesis, and complications are unusual and mostly limited to abdominal wall hematomas. The ascites should be analyzed for albumin, cell count with differential and the fluid inoculated directly into blood culture media.

Although ascites is best managed with oral furosemide and spironolactone, diuretics may need to be withheld in ICU patients who frequently have renal dysfunction, hypovolemia, or electrolyte disturbances. Intravenous (IV) diuretics for treatment of ascites and edema should be avoided in patients with cirrhosis as they can precipitate renal failure. Repeated large-volume paracentesis is a valid strategy for the management of ascites refractory to medical therapy. The administration of albumin at the time of paracentesis has been advocated to ameliorate the risk of post-paracentesis circulatory dysfunction. In practice, 12.5 g of 25% albumin can be infused for every 2 L of ascites removed. The timing of administration has not been rigorously studied, but owing to the long half-life of albumin in the circulation, the administration after completion of the paracentesis is likely to be sufficient.

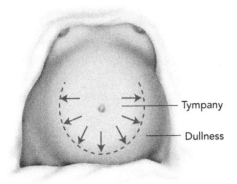

re 47.1. Areas of dullness in both right and left lower abdominal quadrants are ideal sites for diagnostic centesis.

e principle benefit of large-volume paracentesis is relief of symptoms; there is no lence that those with large-volume cirrhotic ascites are at risk for the abdominal npartment syndrome and, thus, paracentesis should not be expected to improve al function.

Hepatic hydrothorax occurs in as many as 13% of patients with ascites, is typ-ly right-sided, and occurs as a result of defects in the diaphragm that permit sage of ascites into the pleural space. This complication can be managed by thora-tesis, diuretics, and, when refractory to medical therapy, transjugular intrahepatic nt (TIPS). Tube thoracostomy should be avoided because volume losses can be stantial and precipitate renal dysfunction.

ONTANEOUS BACTERIAL PERITONITIS

e most common infectious complication of ascites is the development of spon-eous bacterial peritonitis (SBP). Infections, including SBP, are associated with a rfold increase in in-hospital mortality. Between 10% and 27% of those with cir-tic ascites will have SBP at the time of hospitalization. There is no typical presen-ion of SBP, and signs such as abdominal pain, fever, or leukocytosis are frequently ent. The diagnosis is established by the finding of >250/mL polymorphonuclear ls in the ascites or the growth of organisms in a culture of ascites fluid. SBP should differentiated from secondary bacterial peritonitis as a consequence of bowel per-ation or intra-abdominal abscess (Algorithm 47.1).

SBP should be treated with IV antibiotics. Second- and third-generation cepha-porins (cefotaxime 1 g IV q8h or ceftriaxone 1 g q24h) have proven effective in the nagement of SBP; however, these antibiotics may not always be adequate. Infec-ns with multidrug resistant (MDR) bacteria are increasing. The rates of infection h MDR organisms, primarily SBP and urinary tract infections, can be as high as % in hospitalized patients with ascites. Risk factors for MDR infections include socomial infections and exposure to systemic antibiotics within 30 days prior to infection. Exposure to oral, nonabsorbed antibiotics used in the management of cephalopathy has not been shown to be a risk factor.

ALGORITHM 47.1 Algorithm of the Assessment of Cirrhotic Ascites

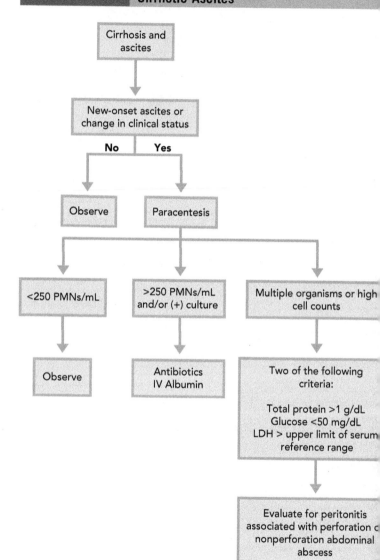

Renal dysfunction occurs in as many as one-third of patients with SBP despite adequate antibiotic treatment. Discontinuation of diuretics and the administration of IV albumin (25%) given at a dose of 1.5 g/kg body weight (day 1) and 1 g/kg (day 3) reduces rates of renal dysfunction. This intervention should be strongly considered in all patients with SBP and particularly those with jaundice and renal insufficiency.

Antibiotic prophylaxis has been advocated in cirrhotic patients at high risk for bacterial complications. These include patients with variceal hemorrhage, primary prevention of SBP in those with ascitic fluid protein <1.5 g/dL, and at least one of the following criteria: serum creatinine >1.2 mg/dL, BUN >25 mg/dL, Na <130 mEq/L, or bilirubin >3 mg/dL or secondary prevention in those with a prior episode of SBP. Balancing the benefits of prophylactic antibiotics with the inevitable risks of selecting for antimicrobial resistance remains the central concern with antibiotic prophylaxis, and additional studies will be required to define their optimal use.

ACUTE KIDNEY INJURY

AKI in decompensated cirrhosis can arise from changes in intravascular volume, parenchymal renal disease, medication-related injuries, and disturbance to renal perfusion from the vascular dilation in mesenteric and systemic circulation that is the hallmark of decompensated cirrhosis.

A consensus definition of AKI in cirrhosis is an increase in serum creatinine (sCR) ≥0.3 mg/dL or increase in sCR ≥50% from baseline levels within the past 7 days. The stage of AKI is defined by the magnitude of the change in sCR from baseline (Table 47.1).

Patients with stage 2 or 3 AKI who fail to respond to therapeutic interventions and who meet other consensus criteria (Table 47.2) are considered to have the hepatorenal syndrome (HRS). The syndrome can be subdivided into a rapidly progressive (type 1) and a slower (type 2) form.

TABLE 47.1	AKI in Patients With Cirrhosis
Definition	Increase in sCR ≥0.3 mg/dL within 48 hours or increase in sCR ≥50% from baseline within the prior 7 days
Staging	
Stage 1	Increase in sCR ≥0.3 mg/dL or increase in sCR ≥1.5–2-fold from baseline
Stage 2	Increase in sCR ≥2–3-fold from baseline
Stage 3	Increase in sCR >3-fold from baseline or sCR ≥4.0 mg/dL with an acute increase ≥0.3 mg/dL or initiation of renal replacement therapy
Treatment Response	
Partial response	Regression of AKI stage with a reduction of sCr ≥0.3 mg/dL above the baseline value
Full response	Return of sCR to a value within 0.3 mg/dL of the baseline value

TABLE 47.2	Diagnostic Criteria for the Hepatorenal Syndrome (HRS)

Diagnosis of cirrhosis and ascites
Diagnosis of AKI
No response after 2 consecutive days of diuretic withdrawal and plasma volume
  expansion with albumin 1 g/kg body weight
Absence of shock
No current or recent use of nephrotoxic drugs
No macroscopic signs of parenchymal kidney injury, defined as:
  Absence of proteinuria (>500 mg/day)
  Absence of microhematuria (>50 RBCs per high-power field)
  Normal findings on renal ultrasonography

Treatment of HRS begins with intravascular volume expansion. Albumin (25%
is a particularly effective volume expander, and support for its role is provided by the
success of albumin in conjunction with vasoactive agents in improving HRS compared to vasoactive agents and saline. The coadministration with vasoactive agents
such as octreotide (100 to 200 mcg SC q8h) and midodrine (7.5 to 12.5 mg q8h) o
terlipressin (a vasoconstrictor not currently approved in the United States) has been
studied for the treatment of HRS in clinical trials of varying quality. Liver transplantation remains the most effective approach for the treatment of HRS.

ENCEPHALOPATHY

Early symptoms of hepatic encephalopathy are often subtle and can include changes
in mood and insomnia that only later progress to agitation and coma. The development of encephalopathy of any severity should prompt a search for precipitants that
commonly include infection, gastrointestinal hemorrhage, or medication exposure.
The mediators of hepatic encephalopathy are unknown. Serum ammonia is a biomarker of hepatic encephalopathy, but may not correlate well with the severity of the
encephalopathy.

Treatment options include cathartics (lactulose 30 cc PO q2–8h or lactulose
retention enemas) or nonabsorbable, oral antibiotics (neomycin 500 mg PO q6h o
rifaximin 550 mg bid). In a randomized, double-blind placebo-controlled study in
which 90% of patients were receiving lactulose, the addition of rifaximin significantly
reduced the risk of recurrent episodes of hepatic encephalopathy.

VARICEAL HEMORRHAGE

Variceal hemorrhage has an annual incidence rate of 20% in cirrhosis, and each episode carries a 20% to 40% mortality rate. There is no typical presentation of variceal
bleeding, and it should be suspected in those with known chronic liver disease and
gastrointestinal hemorrhage. The initial steps in the management of acute variceal
bleeding involve treatment of shock and protection of the airway (Table 47.3). Volume resuscitation in the form of packed red blood cells should be privileged to other
blood products. Octreotide (50 mcg IV bolus followed by 50 mcg/hr IV infusion)
should be started. Diagnostic paracentesis should be performed, and prophylactic

TABLE 47.3 Guidelines for the Management of Variceal Hemorrhage

Resuscitate hypovolemic shock

Assessment of airway and intubation if airway protection necessary

Octreotide 50 mcg IV bolus followed by 50 mcg/hr IV infusion

Blood and urine culture; diagnostic paracentesis

Prophylactic parenteral antibiotics

Upper endoscopy

TIPS, BRTO, or Blakemore tube for variceal bleeding refractory to endoscopic management

parenteral antibiotics should be given; the latter intervention is associated with decreased risk of rebleeding.

Upper endoscopy should be performed promptly as both band ligation and sclerotherapy can result in effective hemostasis for esophageal varices. TIPS is an option for esophageal variceal bleeding that is refractory to endoscopy or for bleeding gastric varices. Early TIPS placement (within 24 to 48 hours following hospitalization for variceal hemorrhage) in Child class B and C cirrhosis has also been advocated as a strategy that prolongs survival based on randomized trials.

Balloon-occluded retrograde transvenous obliteration (BRTO) is another potential therapy that may be particularly helpful in the management of bleeding gastric or ectopic varices. Balloon tamponade devices (Blakemore tube) can also be inserted temporary in cases where either TIPS or endoscopy is delayed or unsuccessful. Nonselective beta blockers (e.g., propranolol, nadolol, or carvedilol) are effective at reducing the risk of initial and recurrent variceal bleeding; however, they should be introduced only after acute bleeding is controlled and the patient is hemodynamically stable.

There are conflicting data on the safety of beta blockers in patients with decompensated cirrhosis. Until their role is clarified by further clinical studies, a reasoned approach would be to continue the medication except for those with manifestations of extreme vasodilation such as those with refractory ascites, AKI, hypotension (systolic blood pressure <90 mm Hg), or hyponatremia (serum sodium <130 mg/dL).

TRANSJUGULAR INTRAHEPATIC PORTOSYSTEMIC SHUNT (TIPS)

TIPS is a channel created between the hepatic vein and the intrahepatic portion of the portal vein. It is placed to reduce portal pressure in patients with complications related to portal hypertension, most commonly variceal hemorrhage or refractory ascites. Contraindications to TIPS placement can include pulmonary hypertension, right heart failure, severe encephalopathy, polycystic liver disease, or tumor within the path of the TIPS.

ACUTE ON CHRONIC LIVER FAILURE

An acute deterioration of liver function in patients with cirrhosis that results in the failure of one or more organs has been used to describe the category of acute on chronic liver failure (ACLF). This is distinct from both acute liver failure and

decompensated liver disease. Not surprisingly, the development of ACLF has b
associated with alcohol consumption within 3 months and bacterial infections. I
many as 45% of cases, the cause is unknown. The mortality risk increases with
increase in organ failure; for example, in the setting of the failure of three or m
organs, the 28-day transplant-free mortality risk was 78%.

SUGGESTED READINGS

Angeli P, Gines P, Wong F, et al. Diagnosis and management of acute kidney injury in pati
with cirrhosis: revised consensus recommendations of the international club of asc
J Hepatol. 2015;62(4):968–974.
   *Revised definitions and diagnostic criteria for acute kidney injury by the International As
   Club (IAC).*
DellaVolpe JD, Garavaglia JM, Huang DT. Management of complications of end-stage l
disease in the intensive care unit. *J Intensive Care Med.* 2016;31(2):94–103.
   *A useful and readable summary of common complications encountered in the ICU care of pat
   with end-stage liver disease.*
Jalan R, Fernandez J, Wiest R, et al. Bacterial infections in cirrhosis: a position statement ba
on the EASL special conference 2013. *J Hepatol.* 2014;60(6):1310–1324.
Moreau R, Arroyo V. Acute-on-chronic liver failure: a new clinical entity. *Clin Gastroen
Hepatol.* 2015;13(5):836–841.
   *A summary of current research on acute on chronic liver failure, including definitions,
   factors, and outcomes.*
Nadim MK., Durand F, Kellum JA, et al. Management of the critically ill patient with cirrho
a multidisciplinary perspective. *J Hepatol.* 2016;64(3):717–735.
   Review of the multidisciplinary management of critically ill patients with cirrhosis.
Tandon P, Delisle A, Topal JE, et al. High prevalence of antibiotic-resistant bacterial in
tions among patients with cirrhosis at a US liver center. *Clin Gastroenterol Hepatol.* 20
10(11):1291–1298.
   *Analysis on the frequency of multidrug resistant infections in hospitalized patients w
   cirrhosis.*

48

Upper Gastrointestinal Bleeding

Jason G. Bill and C. Prakash Gyawali

Acute upper gastrointestinal bleeding (UGIB) is a common medical emergency that frequently results in emergency department evaluations and intensive care unit admissions. The annual incidence of acute UGIB is estimated to range between 80 and 90 cases per 100,000 population, carrying a mortality rate of 6% to 12%. In the last decade, the incidence of nonvariceal gastrointestinal hemorrhage has declined in all populations, possibly because of lower *Helicobacter pylori* incidence and widespread use of proton pump inhibitors (PPIs). Common causes of acute UGIB are listed in Table 48.1.

One of the first assessments in any patient with acute gastrointestinal bleeding is determining the severity of the bleeding episode (Algorithm 48.1). Bleeding is considered massive with loss of one-fifth to one-fourth of the circulating volume if a previously normotensive or hypertensive patient develops resting hypotension. In the absence of resting hypotension, evidence of postural or orthostatic hypotension (drop in systolic blood pressure of 15 mm Hg or increase in heart rate of 20 beats per minute) indicates loss of 10% to 20% of the circulating volume. Bleeding is considered minor if neither of these conditions is met, indicating loss of <10% of circulating volume. In all instances, two large-bore intravenous (IV) lines or a central line must be urgently placed, and normal saline or lactated Ringer's solution administered intravenously.

TABLE 48.1	Etiology of Upper Gastrointestinal Bleeding

Peptic ulcer disease (accounts for ~50%)
  Gastric ulcers
  Duodenal ulcers
  Gastric erosions and gastritis
Esophageal and/or gastric varices (accounts for 10%–20%)
Stress ulcers
Mallory–Weiss tear
Esophagitis and esophageal ulcers
Vascular abnormalities (angiodysplasia, Dieulafoy lesion, telangiectasia)
Portal hypertensive gastropathy
Neoplasms, benign and malignant
Hemobilia (bleeding into bile ducts)
Hemosuccus (bleeding into pancreatic ducts)
Aortoenteric fistula

ALGORITHM 48.1 — Initial Management of Acute Gastrointestinal (GI) Bleeding

Resuscitation

- Establish two large-bore IVs or central line
- Obtain blood for blood typing, CBC, CMP, INR, PTT
- Infuse isotonic saline, Ringer's lactate, or 5% hetastarch
- Blood transfusion: O negative if extremely urgent
- Oxygen by nasal canula

Factors propagating bleeding

- Discontinue anticoagulants (warfarin, heparin), thrombolytic agents
- Discontinue antiplatelet agents if possible (aspirin, clopidogrel)
- Discontinue antithrombotic agents[a] if possible
- Correct prolonged PT/INR with FFP infusions and/or vitamin K injection
- Correct prolonged PTT with protamine infusion if necessary

Level of bleeding[b]

- Hematemesis, coffee ground emesis indicate upper GI bleeding
- Melena usually indicates upper GI bleeding but can originate more distally
- Maroon stool, red blood in the stool typically indicate lower GI bleeding
- Any bleeding in the presence of hemodynamic compromise can be upper GI in origin

Etiology of bleeding[b]

- Presence of cirrhosis may indicate variceal bleeding
- Hypotension or shock preceding bleeding may indicate ischemic colitis
- Recent polypectomy may indicate postpolypectomy bleeding
- Prior aortic graft surgery may indicate aortoenteric fistula
- Prior radiation therapy may indicate radiation enteritis or proctopathy
- Prior emesis may indicate Mallory–Weiss tear

ABBREVIATIONS
CBC: complete blood count
CMP: complete metabolic panel
INR: international normalized ratio
PTT: partial thromboplastin time
PT: prothrombin time
FFP: fresh-frozen plasma

[a]Antithrombotic agents can also propagate bleeding, and include glycoprotein IIb/IIIa receptor antagonists (abciximab [ReoPro], eptifibatide [Integrilin], tirofiban [Aggrastat]) and direct thrombin inhibitors (argatroban, bivalirudin).
[b]These will dictate the nature of further investigation.

id repletion of circulating volume is crucial when blood loss approaches massive, transfusion of packed red blood cells needs to be arranged, requiring a blood w for blood count, metabolic profile, coagulation parameters, blood type, and ss-matching. When type-specific blood is not immediately available, O negative od may need to be transfused, using rapid infusing devices if necessary. Blood sfusions are performed with target hemoglobin ≥7 g/dL; higher hemoglobin values r ultimately be necessary in patients with clinical evidence of intravascular volume letion or comorbidities such as coronary artery disease. In stable patients without morbidities, transfusion is only required if hemoglobin is <7 g/dL. Oxygen is ninistered by nasal cannula to improve oxygen-carrying capacity of the blood, and l signs and urine output are constantly monitored.

Factors propagating bleeding must be rapidly assessed during this initial evaluation. Patients receiving heparin infusion, thrombolytic therapy, or newer antiombotic agents (Algorithm 48.1) need to be assessed to determine if it is safe to porarily discontinue these medications. Oral anticoagulants are held, and the coagulation reversed with vitamin K and/or fresh-frozen plasma, if possible. As use of novel oral anticoagulants increases, reversal agents are under development. e only currently available reversal agent is idarucizumab (Praxbind), which has n approved for patients with life-threatening hemorrhage while taking dabigatran daxa). Otherwise, prothrombin complex concentrates (PCC) may be considered patients with severe or life-threatening bleeding. Hemodialysis can be used to uce the blood concentration of dabigatran, but not rivaroxaban and apixaban, ich are more tightly plasma protien bound.

Once the patient is stabilized hemodynamically, further evaluation can resume gorithm 48.1). A history of hematemesis or coffee-ground emesis establishes the diagis of UGIB. Melena (passage of dark, tarry, sticky, and foul-smelling stool) typically icates a proximal gut source for blood loss, but melena can develop from bleeding s as far distal as the proximal or even middle colon. Nevertheless, upper endoscopy he first investigation to be done in the presence of melena. Up to 10% to 11% of ients presenting with hematochezia and altered hemodynamic parameters are found lave an upper gastrointestinal source for their bleeding. Therefore, in the presence of nificant hemodynamic compromise, upper gastrointestinal tract evaluation is indied even if the bleeding presentation resembles lower gastrointestinal bleeding.

Aspiration of bloody gastric contents through a nasogastric tube establishes the gnosis of UGIB and can be useful in identifying patients with high-risk lesions o may benefit from emergent endoscopy. On the other hand, dark blood or coffee unds that clear quickly on nasogastric tube lavage may indicate that active bleeding ceased, and elective endoscopy within 24 hours may be adequate (Table 48.2). The ence of a bloody aspirate does not exclude active upper gastrointestinal bleeding, d bleeding can be present despite a negative aspirate in approximately 15% of cases. rly indicators for the need for intensive care unit admission include massive bleeding, nodynamic compromise, variceal bleeding, bleeding onset while hospitalized for an related illness, and the presence of factors that predict a poor outcome (Table 48.3). moccult testing of nasogastric aspirates has very little value in the assessment of acute GIB. If the nasogastric aspirate is clear, or clears quickly with a tap water lavage, the sogastric tube can be removed; with bloody aspirates that do not clear, the nasogastric be may provide an assessment of the acuity and ongoing nature of bleeding.

Acute UGIB consists of two broad categories: acute variceal UGIB and acute nvariceal UGIB (Algorithm 48.2). These categories require differing investigative

TABLE 48.2	Triage of Patients With Acute Upper Gastrointestinal Bleeding

Admission to Intensive Care Unit

Hypotension at presentation

Moderate-to-severe bleeding onset while admitted for an unrelated illness

Ongoing hemodynamic instability despite resuscitation

Absence of adequate hematocrit increase despite blood transfusion

Low initial blood count (hematocrit <25% with cardiopulmonary disease or stroke <20% otherwise)

Bright or dark red NG tube aspirate, especially if it does not clear with lavage

Prolonged coagulation parameters (prothrombin time >1.2 times the control value)

Myocardial infarction, stroke, or other systemic complications of rapid blood loss

Any unstable comorbid disease, including altered mental status

Variceal bleeding

Evidence of active oozing, spurting, or visible vessel on endoscopy

Admission to Regular Hospital Floor

Stable hemodynamic parameters after initial resuscitation

Mild hematocrit drop (<5% from baseline and/or baseline hematocrit >30%)

Stable coagulation parameters

Coffee grounds on NG tube aspirate that clears with lavage

No systemic complications from blood loss

No bleeding source found on upper endoscopy

Nonvariceal bleeding source without active bleeding; bleeding lesion with a clean base or pigmented base

Emergent or Urgent Upper Endoscopy

Suspected or known variceal bleeding

Hemodynamic instability despite resuscitation

Bright red or dark red NG aspirate, especially if it does not clear with lavage

Absence of appropriate hematocrit increase despite blood transfusion

NG, nasogastric.

TABLE 48.3	Factors of Predicting Poor Outcome After Acute Upper Gastrointestinal Bleeding

Age >65 yrs

Comorbid medical illnesses (liver disease, COPD, renal failure, coronary artery disease, malignancy)

Variceal bleeding

Systolic blood pressure <100 mm Hg at presentation

Large peptic ulcers >3 cm

Active bleeding (spurting blood vessel) at endoscopy

Multiple units of blood transfusion

Onset of acute bleeding when hospitalized for unrelated illness

Need for emergency surgery for bleeding control

COPD, chronic obstructive pulmonary disease.

nd therapeutic approaches, and are associated with different short- and long-term
morbidity and mortality. For instance, variceal UGIB is associated with a higher rate
f rebleeding (30% to 40% vs. 15% to 20% for nonvariceal bleeding), and a signifi-
antly higher mortality (20% to 30% vs. 6% to 9%, respectively). Acute nonvariceal
UGIB that develops in patients hospitalized for an unrelated illness is associated with
orse morbidity and mortality (estimated at 35%) compared with patients admitted
hrough emergency departments for acute bleeding.

The initial management of acute variceal UGIB includes IV infusion of octreotide,
while IV PPI administration is considered routine in nonvariceal UGIB. Early clinical
valuation of acute UGIB should therefore include an assessment to determine which
ategory the patient falls into, with the understanding that such an assessment may
ot always be accurate or even possible.

The initial mode of therapy for acute UGIB is pharmacologic (Algorithm 48.2).
Octreotide, a somatostatin analog, lowers splanchnic and portal venous pressure in
he short term, with slowing or cessation of variceal UGIB. Early administration of
ctreotide is encouraged (25 to 50 mcg bolus, followed by 50 to 100 mcg/hr infu-
ion) when acute variceal UGIB is suspected. Intravenous antibiotics with coverage of
nteric pathogens are administered for 7 to 10 days in patients with variceal bleeding
o prevent infectious complications, particularly spontaneous bacterial peritonitis.
n all other instances, PPIs are administered to suppress gastric acid (Table 48.4) as
lot formation and stabilization are facilitated in an alkaline environment. Intrave-
ous administration is recommended for the first 72 hours in patients with ongoing
leeding. Intravenous bolus administration (omeprazole, 40 mg every 12 hours IV)
as been shown to be equivalent to continuous infusion; however, IV bolus followed

TABLE 48.4	Doses of Antisecretory Medication	
Medication	Oral Therapy (mg)	Parenteral Therapy (mg)
Cimetidine[a]	300 qid 400 bid 800 qhs	300 q6h
Ranitidine[a]	150 bid 300 qhs	50 q8h
Famotidine[a]	20 bid 40 qhs	20 q12h
Nizatidine[a]	150 bid 300 qhs	
Omeprazole	20 qd	
Esomeprazole	40 qd	20–40 q24h
Lansoprazole	15–30 qd	30 q12–24h
Pantoprazole	20 qd	40 q12–24h or 80 IV, then 8 mg/hr infusion

Dosage adjustment required in renal insufficiency.
qid, four times daily; bid, two times daily; qhs, at bedtime; qd, daily.

ALGORITHM 48.2 Management of Acute Upper Gastrointestinal (GI) Bleeding

- Hematemesis: emesis of blood or coffee grounds
- Blood or coffee grounds in NG tube aspirate
- Melena
- Maroon or red blood in stool with hemodynamic compromise

Variceal bleeding
Clinical indicators
- History of varices/variceal bleeding
- History of liver disease/cirrhosis
- Spider angiomata
- Caput medusa
- Ascites
- Splenomegaly
- Hepatic encephalopathy
- Pancytopenia, low albumin

Nonvariceal bleeding
Clinical indicators
- Absence of liver disease
- History of peptic ulcers
- History of *Helicobacter pylori*
- History of retching/vomiting
- NSAID/aspirin use
- Chronic renal disease
- Valvular heart disease
- History of hereditary hemorrhagic telangiectasia

Initial resuscitation
- Consider elective intubation for airway protection
- Tamponade (Sengstaken–Blakemore tube) if endoscopic therapy is delayed or not immediately available

Blood pressure tends to run low in cirrhotic patients, caution against over hydration and fluid overload

Initial resuscitation

Pharmacologic therapy
Octreotide bolus and infusion
Vasopressin infusion is an alternative, but side effects may be limiting; rarely used
IV antibiotics to prevent SBP

Pharmacologic therapy
Intravenous PPI bolus or infusion OR
High-dose oral PPI bid if oral intake tolerated

Endoscopic therapy
- Variceal band ligation
- Variceal sclerotherapy
- Glue injection for gastric varices
Can be repeated if bleeding recurs

Endoscopic therapy
Therapy based on presence of stigmata of recent bleeding

Angiography
- Placement of TIPS if endoscopic therapy fails
- Early TIPS for gastric varices from portal hypertension

Angiography
If endoscopy fails or if bleeding is too fast for adequate endoscopic localization and therapy

Surgery
- Splenectomy for gastric varices from splenic vein thrombosis
- Surgical shunts for portal hypertension

Surgery
- As an alternative to angiography if endoscopy fails
- Neoplasms, both benign and malignant
- Isolated vascular abnormalities, e.g., Dieulafoy lesion
- Aortoenteric fistula; emergent surgery

ABBREVIATIONS

NG:	nasogastric
IV:	intravenous
SBP:	spontaneous bacterial peritonitis
TIPS:	transjugular intrahepatic portosystemic shunt
NSAIDs:	nonsteroidal anti-inflammatory drugs
PPI:	proton pump inhibitor

sion (pantoprazole 80 mg then 8 mg/hr or equivalent) has been advocated for d ongoing bleeding. Intravenous PPI therapy significantly decreases identification igh-risk stigmata of bleeding on endoscopy, and has decreased the need for endo-ic therapy. In patients who do not undergo endoscopy, double-dose PPI (ome-zole, 40 mg or equivalent) administered two times daily has been demonstrated to ice the likelihood of rebleeding or the need for surgery in acute peptic ulcer bleed-Stable patients without active ongoing bleeding can tolerate oral PPI adminis-ion, and double-dose two times daily may be beneficial at least until endoscopy erformed; some centers administer this higher dose for 5 days. PPI therapy is used in the prophylaxis of erosive upper gut disease in predisposed patients on rin, nonsteroidal anti-inflammatory drugs (NSAIDs), especially when there are factors for peptic ulcer disease. While the use of PPI with clopidogrel may result ecreased clopidogrel effect in vitro, large randomized placebo-controlled studies gest that the interaction does not appear to translate into worse vascular outcomes.

A crucial adjunct to pharmacologic therapy is endoscopy (Algorithm 48.2), both definitive diagnosis of the bleeding lesion and for administration of endoscopic rapy to lower the risks for rebleeding, surgery, and other morbidities or mortality. ning of endoscopy depends on the degree of bleeding, whether bleeding is ongo-, and the patient's overall condition (Table 48.2). Urgent endoscopy is generally icated in any patient with significant or ongoing bleeding. Hemodynamic param-'s should be in the process of being normalized when endoscopy is performed. nscious sedation can be administered when hemodynamic stability is achieved the patient is no longer hypotensive. Rapid bleeding or the presence of blood clots within the upper gastrointestinal tract may preclude complete examination. ministration of a prokinetic agent such as metoclopramide (5 to 10 mg IV) or thromycin (250 mg IV) is recommended to induce gastric-emptying and to allow aner endoscopic field, thus reducing the need for repeat endoscopy. Lavage using re-bore, double-lumen orogastric tubes can be performed to clear the stomach of od and clots. Positioning the patient so that the intraluminal blood pool is away m the area of interest during endoscopy can be useful. In some instances, especially arge volumes of luminal blood or massive intraluminal clots are encountered, loscopy may need to be repeated at a later time, or angiography used for bleeding alization. Therapy administered during endoscopy can include variceal band liga-n, sclerotherapy, glue injection for variceal UGIB, epinephrine injection, thermal tery, bipolar or monopolar electrocautery, and hemoclip deployment.

Short- and long-term outcomes of therapy depend on the etiology of the bleed. bleeding rates are typically high in variceal bleeding, to the order of 30% to 40%. nselective beta-blocker therapy is initiated if the patient can tolerate. Repeat var-al band ligation or sclerotherapy can be considered when bleeding recurs. When ess to definitive therapy is not immediately available, placement of a Sengstaken–kemore or similar tube can tamponade varices and temporarily stabilize the ient (Table 48.5). Rebleeding refractory to endoscopic therapy is managed by the cement of a transjugular intrahepatic portosystemic shunt (TIPS). Gastric varices ated to portal hypertension are likewise managed with TIPS or balloon-occluded rograde transvenous occlusion (BRTO) earlier in the course, and those resulting m splenic vein thrombosis may require splenectomy for successful management.

In nonvariceal bleeds, rebleeding rates approximate 15% to 20% when stratified the presence or absence of stigmata of recent hemorrhage in the case of peptic ulcer eding (Table 48.6). Rebleeding from peptic ulcers can be treated endoscopically,

TABLE 48.5	Balloon Tamponade for Variceal Bleeding

Indications

Temporary control of variceal bleeding (gastric, esophageal or both)

Access to endoscopic or radiologic therapy not immediately available, to stabilize patient for transport

Efficacy is thought to be better when combined with pharmacologic therapy (Algorithm 48.2)

Equipment

Sengstaken-Blakemore tube (three lumen), Minnesota tube (four lumen), Linton-Nachlas tube (gastric balloon alone) or similar tube

Nasogastric tube when three-lumen tube or gastric balloon alone is used

Soft restraints

Traction mechanism (typically a football helmet, weights, or orthopedic traction system)

Manometer

Tube clamps, surgical scissors

Topical anesthetic, tube connectors, syringes

Technique

Patient needs to be intubated and sedated, with soft restraints in place

Test balloons, check intraluminal pressures at full inflation using manometer

Gastric lavage till clear through nasogastric tube, which is then removed

Introduce lubricated tube through mouth

When gastric juice or blood is aspirated through gastric lumen, check tube position radiographically

With manometer attached to measuring port, fill gastric lumen with air in 100-mL increments to recommended volume for particular tube (typically 450–500 mL)

If rapid pressure increase noted on manometer, tube may have been inflated in esophagus; deflate immediately, advance tube, reinflate

Clamp air inlet for gastric balloon, pull back, secure to traction device

If esophageal balloon inflation is desired, inflate esophageal balloon to 30–45 mm Hg pressure as measured by manometer on measuring port

Further traction can be applied if bright red blood continues to be aspirated through gastric port

With three-lumen tubes, place nasogastric tube so the tip is 3–4 cm above esophageal balloon, and connect to intermittent suction

Deflate balloons for 5 min every 5–6 hrs to reduce risk of pressure necrosis

Keep balloons inflated for up to 24 hrs as needed

Efficacy is around 80% when correctly placed

Complications

Complications occur in 15%–30%; mortality rate is around 6%

Major complications include asphyxia, airway occlusion, esophageal rupture, esophageal and gastric pressure necrosis

Aspiration pneumonia, epistaxis, pharyngeal erosions are other complications

TABLE 48.6	Outcome After Endoscopic Therapy of Peptic Ulcers	
Endoscopic Finding	Risk for Rebleeding (%) (After Treatment)	Mortality (%) (After Treatment)
Clean ulcer base	<5	2
Flat pigmented spot	10 (<1)	3 (<1)
Adherent clot	22 (5)	7 (<3)
Visible vessel	43 (15)	11 (<5)
Active bleeding	55 (20)	11 (<5)

Modified from Laine L, Petersen WL. Bleeding peptic ulcer. *N Engl J Med.* 1994;331:717–727.

reserving angiographic measures (such as embolization) or surgery for repeated endoscopic failures. Eradication of *H. pylori* accelerates healing of peptic ulcers (Algorithm 48.3, Table 48.7). When aspirin or NSAIDs are the etiologic factors, discontinuation, substitution of a less toxic NSAID or a cyclo-oxygenase-2 inhibitor, continuous acid suppression with a PPI, or addition of a mucosal protective agent such as misoprostol may reduce the risk for recurrence of bleeding. Bleeding from

TABLE 48.7	Regimens for *Helicobacter pylori* Eradication	
Medications	Dose	Comments[a]
Clarithromycin	500 mg bid	First line
Amoxicillin	1 g bid	
PPI[b]	bid	
Pepto-Bismol	524 mg qid	First line in penicillin-allergic patients
Metronidazole	250 mg qid	Salvage regimen if three-drug regimen fails
Tetracycline	500 mg qid	
PPI[b] or H2RA[c]	bid	
Clarithromycin	500 mg bid	Alternate regimen, if four-drug therapy is not tolerated
Metronidazole	500 mg bid	
PPI[b]	bid	
Levofloxacin	250 mg bid	Alternate salvage regimen
Amoxicillin	1 g bid	
PPI[b]	bid	
Rifabutin	300 mg qd	Alternate salvage regimen
Amoxicillin	1 g bid	
PPI[b]	bid	

[a] Duration of therapy: 10–14 days. When using salvage regimens after initial treatment failure, choose drugs that have not been used before.

[b] Standard doses for PPI: omeprazole, 20 mg; lansoprazole, 30 mg; pantoprazole, 40 mg, rabeprazole 20 mg, all twice daily. Esomeprazole is used as a single 40 mg dose once daily.

[c] Standard doses for H2RA: ranitidine, 150 mg; famotidine, 20 mg; nizatidine, 150 mg; cimetidine, 400 mg; all twice daily.

bid, twice daily; PPI, proton pump inhibitor; qid, four times daily; H2RA, H$_2$-receptor antagonists.

ALGORITHM 48.3   Management of Peptic Ulcers

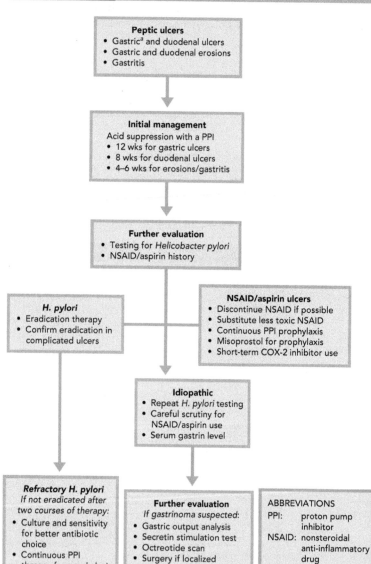

Peptic ulcers
- Gastric[a] and duodenal ulcers
- Gastric and duodenal erosions
- Gastritis

Initial management
Acid suppression with a PPI
- 12 wks for gastric ulcers
- 8 wks for duodenal ulcers
- 4–6 wks for erosions/gastritis

Further evaluation
- Testing for *Helicobacter pylori*
- NSAID/aspirin history

H. pylori
- Eradication therapy
- Confirm eradication in complicated ulcers

NSAID/aspirin ulcers
- Discontinue NSAID if possible
- Substitute less toxic NSAID
- Continuous PPI prophylaxis
- Misoprostol for prophylaxis
- Short-term COX-2 inhibitor use

Idiopathic
- Repeat *H. pylori* testing
- Careful scrutiny for NSAID/aspirin use
- Serum gastrin level

Refractory H. pylori
If not eradicated after two courses of therapy:
- Culture and sensitivity for better antibiotic choice
- Continuous PPI therapy for prophylaxis

Further evaluation
If gastrinoma suspected:
- Gastric output analysis
- Secretin stimulation test
- Octreotide scan
- Surgery if localized
- Long-term PPI if refractory

ABBREVIATIONS
PPI: proton pump inhibitor
NSAID: nonsteroidal anti-inflammatory drug
COX-2: cyclo-oxygenase-2

[a]Evaluation with endoscopy or barium contrast study is repeated at 3 months in all patients with gastric ulcers to confirm healing. If the ulcer is not completely healed, multiple biopsies are taken to exclude other nonpeptic causes, including malignancy.

plastic lesions responds poorly to endoscopic or angiographic hemostasis, and
ery is frequently required. Isolated vascular lesions such as Dieulafoy lesion can be
cessfully treated endoscopically, angiographically, or surgically with low likelihood
recurrence. On the other hand, angiodysplasia or telangiectasia can redevelop after
oscopic ablation, or may be present elsewhere in the luminal gut, and blood loss
uently recurs.

GGESTED READINGS

t DL, Cryer BL, Contant CF, et al. Clopidogrel with or without omeprazole in coronary
  artery disease. *N Engl J Med*. 2010;363:1909–1917.

ung FK, Lau JY. Management of massive peptic ulcer bleeding. *Gastroenterol Clin N Am.*
  2009;38:231–243.

cia-Tsao G, Sanyal AJ, Grace ND, et al. Prevention and management of gastroesophageal
  varices and variceal hemorrhage in cirrhosis. *Hepatology.* 2007;46(3):922–938.

ang JH, Fisher DA, Ben-Menachem T, et al. The role of endoscopy in the management of
  acute non-variceal upper GI bleeding. *Gastrointest Endosc.* 2012;75(6):1132–1138.

ang JH, Shergill AK, Acosta RD, et al. Gastrointest Endosc. 2014;80(2):221–227.

e L, Jensen D. Management of patients with ulcer bleeding: ACG practice guidelines. *Am J
  Gastroenterol.* 2012;107:345–360.

e L, Peterson WL. Bleeding peptic ulcer. *N Engl J Med.* 1994;331:717–727.

za FL, Chan FK, Quigley EM, et al. Guidelines for prevention of NSAID-related ulcer complications. *Am J Gastroenterol.* 2009;104:728–738.

ntiadis GI, McIntyre L, Sharma VK, et al. Proton pump inhibitor treatment for acute peptic
  ulcer bleeding. *Cochrane Database Syst Rev.* 2004;3:CD002094.

ack C, Reilly P, Eikelboom J, et al. Idarucizumab for dabigatran reversal. *N Engl J Med.* 2015;
  373:511–520.

anueva C, Colomo A, Bosch A, et al. Transfusion strategies for acute upper gastrointestinal
  bleeding. *N Engl J Med.* 2013;368:12–21.

49 Lower Gastrointestinal Bleeding

Pierre Blais and C. Prakash Gyawali

Acute lower gastrointestinal bleeding (LGIB) was traditionally defined as re[] onset bleeding originating distal to the ligament of Trietz. Advances in endosc[] and radiologic diagnostic modalities, however, have given rise to the introductio[] small bowel bleeding defined as blood loss between the ampulla of Vater and the[] ocecal valve. LGIB, then, is a term restricted to bleeding distal to the ileocecal v[] The new definitions reflect an improved ability to accurately and promptly loc[] bleeding sites, but they also serve as useful clinical tools to stratify management b[] on the type of bleed.

Incidence of acute LGIB in the literature ranges anywhere from 20 to[] out of 100,000 in the population, making it one-fifth as frequent as acute u[] gastrointestinal bleed (UGIB). Nevertheless, the increase in clinical indicati[] for use of antiplatelet and anticoagulation therapies, compounded with ref[] guidelines for prophylaxis of peptic ulcers and nonsteroidal anti-inflammat[] drug (NSAID)-induced enteropathies, likely has pushed the total burden of dis[] toward a more even distribution between upper and lower sources. In contras[] UGIB, acute LGIB is associated with an overall lower rate of hemodynamic c[] promise, fewer transfusions, and lower 1-year mortality (4.2%). Typically, a[] LGIB is self-limiting, but bleeding can be severe, and recurrence rates are hig[] than that for UGIB (46% at 5 years). Similar to acute UGIB, patients who dev[] acute LGIB while hospitalized for any other indication have a worse outcome, v[] estimated mortality of 23% during admission. In recent years, advances in en[] scopic and radiologic therapies for actively bleeding patients (such as hemoclip[] and superselective embolization of the bleeding vessel) have reduced the need[] emergent surgery.

Presentation can range from scant bright red blood around formed stool or[] toilet tissue to massive uncontrolled bloody bowel movements with hemodyna[] collapse and shock. The color of bloody stool has been demonstrated to be a go[] predictor of the location of the bleeding source in patients without hemodyna[] compromise. Patients pointing to a bright red or a dark red color on a color card[] the highest positive predictive value for acute LGIB in one study, higher than ph[] cian reports of the same color data. Conversely, patients pointing to a black color[] a color card effectively ruled themselves out of a colonic or anorectal bleed.

Bloody diarrhea is sometimes interpreted as acute LGIB by patients, and a go[] clinical history usually distinguishes between the two. If the presentation is blo[] diarrhea rather than acute LGIB, stool culture, including culture for *Escherichia*[] O157:H7, and stool *Clostridium difficile* toxin are ordered. Parasitic infestati[]

TABLE 49.1	Causes of Acute Lower Gastrointestinal Bleeding

Colonic Sources

Diverticulosis

Angiodysplasia

Neoplasia: includes large polyps and cancers

Post polypectomy bleeding

Colitis: includes inflammatory and infectious causes

Ischemia

Anorectal causes: hemorrhoids, anal fissure

Radiation proctopathy and colopathy

Aortoenteric fistula (rare)

Dieulafoy lesion (rare)

Rectal varices (rare)

Small Bowel Sources

Angiodysplasia

Neoplasia: includes cancers, stromal tumors, lymphoma

Enteritis: includes inflammatory and infectious causes

Radiation enteritis and enteropathy

Meckel diverticulum

Aortoenteric fistula (rare)

such as amebiasis may need to be considered and ameba serology ordered, when relevant. In immunosuppressed patients, cytomegalovirus colitis can present with bloody diarrhea. Bleeding presentations of inflammatory bowel disease (Crohn's disease, ulcerative colitis) are more often bloody diarrhea than acute LGIB. The upper gastrointestinal tract can also be the source for bright or dark red blood in the stool if bleeding is brisk and massive. Small bowel bleeding may resemble UGIB or LGIB in its clinical presentation, but because the small intestine is the least accessible portion of the bowel, initial work-up proceeds with an assessment for upper and lower sources first (Table 49.1). The small bowel is then investigated if an alternate source is not identified elsewhere in the luminal gut. Therefore, the spectrum of acute LGIB is broad.

Initial resuscitation and early management of acute LGIB do not vary from that of acute UGIB (see Algorithm 48.1, Chapter 48). In addition to adequate intravenous (IV) access (two 18-gauge or larger IV, central line, or introducer catheter—in the case of massive hemorrhage and shock), volume expansion with normal saline, lactated Ringer's solution, or blood products may be appropriate depending on severity of bleeding and acuity of presentation. Anticoagulants, antiplatelet agents, and medications that affect the coagulation cascade are discontinued if possible. When clotting parameters are significantly abnormal, infusions of fresh-frozen plasma, injections of vitamin K, and protamine are administered as indicated.

Several clinical and laboratory features at presentation help identify patients at risk for higher short-term morbidity or mortality. These include recurrent bleeding, hemodynamic compromise, syncope, aspirin or anticoagulant use, more than two comorbid medical conditions, and continued bleeding 4 hours after initial presentation. A prolonged prothrombin time (PT/INR) >1.2 times the control value and altered mental status have been identified as additional predictors of poor outcome.

TABLE 49.2 Triage of Patients With Acute Lower Gastrointestinal Bleeding

Admission to Intensive Care Unit
Hypotension (systolic blood pressure <115 mm Hg) at presentation
Moderate-to-severe bleeding onset while admitted for an unrelated illness
Ongoing hemodynamic instability despite resuscitation
Absence of adequate hematocrit increase despite blood transfusion
Low initial blood count (hematocrit <25% with cardiopulmonary disease or stroke,
  <20% otherwise)
Prolonged coagulation parameters (prothrombin time 1.2 times ≥ the control value)
Myocardial infarction, stroke, or other systemic complications of rapid blood loss
Any unstable comorbid disease, including altered mental status
Ongoing significant bleeding 4 hours after presentation
Evidence of active oozing, spurting, or visible vessel on endoscopy
Requirement of angiography for localization or control of bleeding

Admission to Regular Hospital Floor
Stable hemodynamic parameters after initial resuscitation
Mild hematocrit drop <5% from baseline and/or baseline hematocrit >30%)
Stable coagulation parameters
No systemic complications from blood loss
Absence of ongoing bleeding 4 hours after presentation

Emergent *Upper* Endoscopy in Patients with Bloody Stool
Bright red or dark red blood in stool with hemodynamic compromise
Bloody NG aspirate
Suspicion of aortoenteric fistula (distal duodenum needs to be evaluated)

NG, nasogastric.

These characteristics are useful in making triage decisions, especially in identifying patients who could benefit from admission to an intensive care unit and patients who need urgent investigational procedures (Table 49.2).

An important decision point in the initial triage of patients with hematochezia is to rule out a brisk UGIB, since as many as 10% of hemodynamically unstable patients with bright red blood per rectum may have a bleeding source within the reach of an upper endoscope. These patients should be evaluated with the initial intent to exclude an upper source, as upper endoscopy is easier to perform than colonoscopy in the setting of an acute bleed. A nasogastric tube can be placed to assess for a bloody aspirate. However, only a bilious, nonbloody aspirate can reliably exclude UGIB. Regardless of the aspirate appearance, if suspicion remains high, an upper endoscopic examination is indicated. Patients with acute unstable bleeding in the setting of past aortic graft repair need an emergent upper endoscopy for evaluation of the distal duodenum, the most common location for an aortoenteric fistula.

Further evaluation of the patient depends on several factors: the severity and acuity of bleeding, hemodynamic state of the patient, coagulation parameters, and investigative facilities available at the institution. In patients with minimal bleeding with historical features suggesting a distal source (red blood coating outside of formed

l, pain with defecation, tenesmus, passage of fresh clots), inspection of the peri-
area, anal canal, rectum, and sometimes the distal colon is often a useful initial
. This can be achieved with anoscopy and/or flexible sigmoidoscopy. However,
oidoscopy rarely replaces full colonoscopy after bowel preparation, as a concur-
more proximal bleeding source cannot be excluded with this approach alone.

In cases of rapid bleeding, hemodynamic instability, significantly impaired coag-
ion parameters, comorbid illnesses, or inability to tolerate a bowel preparation,
gged red blood cell (RBC) scan helps triage actively bleeding patients to more
sive procedures such as mesenteric angiography and angiotherapy. In the research
ng, bleeding rates as low as 0.1 to 0.5 mL/min are picked up by tagged RBC
s, but in the clinical setting, only 45% of tagged RBC scans in patients with acute
atochezia will demonstrate extravasation. Rapidly positive scans have the highest
racy and predict the best likelihood of identification of the bleeding site at subse-
nt angiography. Delayed positive scans have a much lower sensitivity in accurately
lizing the bleeding source, as intestinal peristalsis may impact the reading. The
continues to be used as a screening tool prior to more invasive testing, although
e suggest that the test unnecessarily delays more definitive studies and reduces
nces of early bleeding localization. For example, studies suggest a 22% to 42%
of false localization of bleeding sites in patients subsequently taken to surgery.

In patients with intact renal function and bleeds faster than 0.5 mL/min, mul-
tector computed tomography angiography (CT angiography) may represent a
er and more convenient means to localize bleeding. Arterial-phase images may
n demonstrate vascular abnormalities such as angiodysplasia. It is less sensitive
n the tagged RBC scan at detecting bleeds, but when the results are positive, it
more rapidly and accurately localize the segment of bleeding bowel. Another new
ging modality that can be considered in refractory situations and in obscure gas-
ntestinal bleeding is magnetic resonance enterography (MRE). Overall, both CT
iography and MRE have not been systematically studied as diagnostic modalities
acute LGIB.

For patients with positive imaging findings for a bleeding source or for those
unstable to receive the aforementioned localizing studies, selective angiography
resents the final option in acute LGIB prior to surgery. If a rapidly bleeding site
dentified on angiography, vasopressin can be infused after selective catheterization
the bleeding vessel. This may induce vasoconstriction and cessation of bleeding.
ernatively, embolization of the bleeding vessel can be attempted. Complications
angiography can be dye-related (renal failure), procedure-related (hematoma for-
tion, retroperitoneal bleeding, intestinal ischemia), or as a result of vasopressin
usion (arrhythmias, myocardial infarction).

All patients presenting with acute hematochezia eventually need a full colo-
scopy for diagnosis of the bleeding source and biopsy of suspicious lesions. For
tain bleeding sources, therapeutic measures including epinephrine injection, ther-
l therapy, and mechanical therapy with hemoclips can be attempted (Table 49.3).
ll, it remains uncertain if urgent colonoscopy has any clinical benefit for patients.
hough diagnostic rates for sources of bleeding are higher in patients undergoing
onoscopy within 24 hours of presentation (45% to 90%), intervention is not indied for many of the etiologies of bleeding (Algorithm 49.1). To this end, two recent
domized clinical trials comparing urgent versus eventual colonoscopy for patients
h LGIB showed no change in mortality, hospital length of stay, rebleeding rates, or
es of receiving surgery. Ultimately, early colonoscopy is preferable to maximize the

TABLE 49.3	Management of Vascular Lesions[a]

Initial Management

Endoscopic ablation when possible, using thermal cautery, argon plasma coagulation or laser:

  Lesions accessible with conventional endoscopy

  Double-balloon enteroscopy in specialized cases

  Numerous lesions may not be amenable to endoscopic therapy

Iron repletion

  Oral iron therapy, ferrous sulfate 325 mg tid or equivalent

  Intravenous or parenteral iron repletion when oral iron is not tolerated or inadequate

Intermittent blood transfusions

Surgery: rare, only for isolated, discrete, limited vascular lesions such as hamartoma or Dieulafoy lesion

Refractory Situations

Continue above measures

Consider adding medications with anecdotal and limited evidence in decreasing blood loss:

  Epsilon-amino caproic acid

  Combination estrogen-progesterone hormone therapy

  Danazol

  Octreotide by subcutaneous injection

[a]Vascular lesions include angiodysplasia, telangiectasia, hamartoma, arteriovenous malformation, nevus, Dieulafoy lesion.

tid, three times daily.

diagnostic yield of the procedure, but the patient's overall clinical picture will dictate the timing of colonscopy.

When blood is seen throughout the colon as well as within the terminal ileum or if a potential colonic source is not evident despite a careful and adequate examination, the bleeding source could reside in the small bowel. Capsule endoscopy is the recommended test to begin with in situations where a small bowel source of bleeding is suspected following negative upper and lower endoscopy (Table 49.3). The drawbacks of capsule endoscopy include the fact that real-time reading is not possible, accurate localization of findings is almost impossible, and no therapeutics can be administered. Actively bleeding sources identified in the small bowel have required surgery in the past, either for surgical resection or for endoscopic therapy during intraoperative enteroscopy. More recently, newer endoscopic techniques such as double-balloon enteroscopy have been developed that allow reach of almost the entire small bowel for endoscopic therapy, but these may be associated with a higher degree of morbidity and complications compared with routine endoscopic procedures. These studies can be considered in refractory situations or in obscure gastrointestinal bleeding.

Diverticulosis and angiodysplasia account for >50% of colonic bleeding sources. Diverticular bleeding is arterial bleeding, and therefore presents with clinically significant painless episodes of bright red blood in the stool. Bleeding spontaneously

ALGORITHM 49.1 Investigation of Acute Lower Gastrointestinal Bleeding

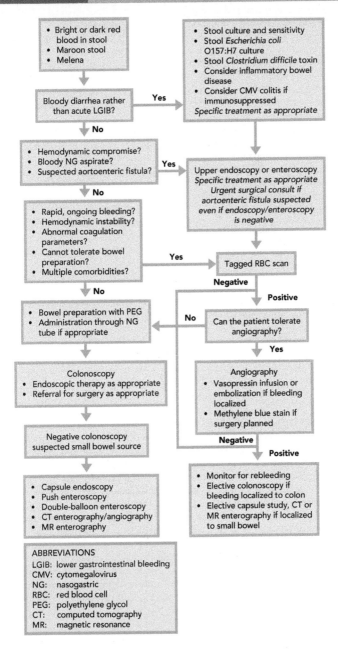

- Bright or dark red blood in stool
- Maroon stool
- Melena

- Stool culture and sensitivity
- Stool *Escherichia coli* O157:H7 culture
- Stool *Clostridium difficile* toxin
- Consider inflammatory bowel disease
- Consider CMV colitis if immunosuppressed
Specific treatment as appropriate

Bloody diarrhea rather than acute LGIB? — **Yes** →

↓ **No**

- Hemodynamic compromise?
- Bloody NG aspirate?
- Suspected aortoenteric fistula?

— **Yes** →

Upper endoscopy or enteroscopy
Specific treatment as appropriate
Urgent surgical consult if aortoenteric fistula suspected even if endoscopy/enteroscopy is negative

↓ **No**

- Rapid, ongoing bleeding?
- Hemodynamic instability?
- Abnormal coagulation parameters?
- Cannot tolerate bowel preparation?
- Multiple comorbidities?

— **Yes** →

Tagged RBC scan

Negative ↓   **Positive** →

↓ **No**

- Bowel preparation with PEG
- Administration through NG tube if appropriate

← **No** — Can the patient tolerate angiography?

↓   ↓ **Yes**

Colonoscopy
- Endoscopic therapy as appropriate
- Referral for surgery as appropriate

Angiography
- Vasopressin infusion or embolization if bleeding localized
- Methylene blue stain if surgery planned

↓

Negative colonoscopy suspected small bowel source

Negative ↓

↓

Positive ↓

- Capsule endoscopy
- Push enteroscopy
- Double-balloon enteroscopy
- CT enterography/angiography
- MR enterography

- Monitor for rebleeding
- Elective colonoscopy if bleeding localized to colon
- Elective capsule study, CT or MR enterography if localized to small bowel

ABBREVIATIONS
LGIB: lower gastrointestinal bleeding
CMV: cytomegalovirus
NG: nasogastric
RBC: red blood cell
PEG: polyethylene glycol
CT: computed tomography
MR: magnetic resonance

TABLE 49.4	Suspected Small Bowel Bleeding[a]

Approach

    If bleeding is rapid and severe with hemodynamic compromise, consider immediate selective angiography and embolization of bleeding site

    If bleeding is rapid but patient can be stabilized, perform tagged RBC scan or CT angiography

    If bleeding is not rapid and patient is stable, or initial radiographic studies show no active bleeding, perform upper and lower endoscopy and consider second-look upper endoscopy in cases of recurrent melena

    If small bowel bleeding is suspected at presentation, consider push enteroscopy as the initial choice for upper endoscopy

After nondiagnostic upper and lower endoscopy, perform video capsule endoscopy

Consider CT or MR enterography in cases of suspected bowel obstruction or negative capsule endoscopy to look for luminal or mural small bowel lesions

If capsule endoscopy or radiographic studies confirm small bowel bleeding, perform single-balloon or double-balloon enteroscopy to treat lesions

Consider retrograde balloon enteroscopy in instances of ileal bleeding

Consider intraoperative enteroscopy:

    Healthy individuals with significant bleeding recurrences and a potential small bowel source

    For small bowel bleeding after ineffective repeated attempts at endoscopic treatment

    For localization of a likely small bowel source, for surgical resection

Provocative measures (administration of heparin, thrombolytic agents, or vasodilators) are very rarely used, and should not be recommended except in very refractory situations, in patients without comorbidities, under very close observation by experienced personnel

[a]Small bowel bleeding, formerly obscure gastrointestinal bleeding, consists of persistent or recurrent bleeding, with no bleeding source evident on conventional upper and lower endoscopy. RBC, red blood cell; CT, computed tomography; MR, magnetic resonance.

ceases in >80% of patients, but one-quarter may develop recurrent bleeding. Multiple recurrences of diverticular bleeding are an indication for resection of the offending segment of colon. Bleeding from angiodysplasia can be slow and more persistent and may be associated with iron deficiency anemia. Endoscopic ablation of bleeding lesions may decrease the rate of bleeding, but patients typically require iron repletion and supplementation. In refractory situations, medications with anecdotal or limited evidence can be considered, but these approaches can be associated with serious adverse effects including thrombotic complications (Table 49.3). Hemorrhoids account for 5% to 10% of episodes of acute LGIB, and are the most common cause of bright red blood in the stool or toilet tissue in the ambulatory patient. Other causes are less common, and include neoplasia, colitis, Meckel diverticulum, and radiation proctopathy. Angiodysplasias are the most common small bowel cause of acute LGIB. Other small bowel causes include stromal tumors, lymphoma, adenocarcinoma, inflammatory disorders including Crohn's disease, and ulcers/erosions from NSAID use (Table 49.1).

BLE 49.5	Levels of Diagnostic Certainty in Interpreting Test for Acute Lower Gastrointestinal Bleeding

finitive Evidence of a Bleeding Source

ve oozing or bleeding visualized at colonoscopy or angiography

mata of recent bleeding (adherent clot, nonbleeding visible vessel) identified on lonoscopy

itive tagged RBC scan associated with either of above

cumstantial Evidence of a Bleeding Source

gle potential bleeding source on colonoscopy with fresh blood in the same gment

gle potential bleeding source on colonoscopy or angiography in the same area a positive tagged RBC scan

ght or dark red blood on objective stool testing, single potential source (without idoscopic stigmata) on colonoscopy, negative upper endoscopy, and capsule idoscopy

ght or dark red blood, maroon stool, or melena on objective stool testing, single tential source (without endoscopic stigmata) on capsule endoscopy, negative pper endoscopy, and colonoscopy

uivocal Evidence of a Bleeding Source

ematochezia" unconfirmed by objective testing, potential sources (without endo-opic stigmata) on colonoscopy or capsule endoscopy

, red blood cell.

One of the dilemmas in patients with acute LGIB is making a clinical determi-on as to whether the lesion identified on diagnostic testing is indeed the source the patient's bleeding episode. This is particularly important as active bleeding or mata of recent bleeding are not always identified on potential bleeding lesions. At es, more than one potential bleeding lesion may be identified. Criteria have been gested to assess the level of diagnostic certainty in interpreting diagnostic tests cute LGIB, which may help determine the nature of definitive management or ow-up needed, especially when surgery is recommended based on the results of gnostic tests (Table 49.5).

JGGESTED READINGS

i T, Nagata N, Niikura R, et al. Recurrence and mortality among patients hospitalized for acute lower gastrointestinal bleeding. *Clin Gastroenterol Hepatol.* 2015;13:488–494.

n FK. Lower gastrointestinal bleeding: what have we learned from the past 3 decades? *Clin Gastroenterol Hepatol.* 2015;13(3):495–497.

rie GM, Kiat H, Wheat JM. Scintigraphic evaluation of acute lower gastrointestinal hemor-rhage: current status and future directions. *J Clin Gastroenterol.* 2011;45:92–99.

son LB, Fidler JL, Cave DR, et al. ACG clinical guideline: diagnosis and management of small bowel bleeding. *Am J Gastroenterol.* 2015;110(9):1265–87; quiz 1288.

en BT, Rockey DC, Portwood G, et al. Urgent colonoscopy for evaluation and management of acute lower gastrointestinal hemorrhage: a randomized controlled trial. *Am J Gastroen-terol.* 2005;100(11):2395.

Lanas A, Garcia-Rodriguez LA, Polo-Tomas M, et al. Time trends and impact of upper and gastrointestinal bleeding and perforation in clinical practice. *Am J Gastroenterol.* 104:1633–1641.

Lanas A, Perez-Aisa MA, Feu F, et al. A nationwide study of mortality associated with ho admission due to severe gastrointestinal events and those associated with nonsteroidal inflammatory drug use. *Am J Gastroenterol.* 2005;100(8):1685.

Laine L, Shah A. Randomized trial of urgent vs. elective colonoscopy in patients hospit with lower GI bleeding. *Am J Gastroenterol.* 2010;105(12):2636–2641; quiz 2642.

Navaneethan U, Njei B, Venkatesh PG, et al. Timing of colonoscopy and outcomes in pa with lower GI bleeding: a nationwide population-based study. *Gastrointest Endosc.* : 79(2):297–306.e12.

Strate LL, Naumann CR. The role of colonoscopy and radiological procedures in the ma ment of acute lower intestinal bleeding. *Clin Gastroenterol Hepatol.* 2010;8:333–343

Zink SI, Ohki SK, Stein B, et al. Noninvasive evaluation of active lower gastrointestinal blee comparison between contrast-enhanced MDCT and 99m Tc-labeled RBC scintigr *AJR Am J Roentgenol.* 2008;191(4):1107–1114.

Zuccaro G. Epidemiology of lower gastrointestinal bleeding. *Best Pract Res Clin Gastroenterol.* : 22(2):225–232.

Zuckerman GR, Trellis DR, Sherman TM, et al. An objective measure of stool color for d entiating upper from lower gastrointestinal bleeding. *Dig Dis Sci.* 1995;40(8):1614–1

50

Acute Pancreatitis

Gabriel D. Lang and Daniel K. Mullady

BACKGROUND

Acute pancreatitis is the most common reason for gastrointestinal inpatient admission in the United States and is associated with significant morbidity, mortality, and cost. The incidence of acute pancreatitis is rising, and mortality rates of 5% to 20% have been reported. There are a variety of causes of acute pancreatitis, but gallstones and alcohol account for nearly 70% (Table 50.1).

Acute pancreatitis is inflammation of the pancreas associated with varying degrees of autodigestion, edema, necrosis, and hemorrhage of pancreatic tissue. Acute pancreatitis can be associated with a systemic inflammatory response that can impair the function of other organs and evolve to persistent organ failure. The clinical course varies from mild, self-limited episodes to severe pancreatitis with associated multiorgan dysfunction, local complications such as infected peripancreatic fluid collections, or extra-pancreatic complications such as venous thrombosis. Up to 20% of patients presenting with pancreatitis have a severe course often requiring critical care. The mortality rate of severe pancreatitis with infectious complications is 10% to 20% and can increase to over 50% in the presence of persistent organ failure.

EVALUATION

The diagnosis of acute pancreatitis should be suspected in patients with acute onset of severe epigastric pain with tenderness to palpation. The diagnosis of acute pancreatitis

TABLE 50.1	Causes of Acute Pancreatitis	
Common	Uncommon	Rare
Gallstones	Pancreas divisum	Malignancy
Alcohol	Autoimmune pancreatitis	Hereditary
	Hypertriglyceridemia	Vascular (e.g., ischemia)
	Medications	Abdominal trauma
	Iatrogenic (post-ERCP)	Toxins (e.g., scorpion bite)
	Sphincter of Oddi dysfunction	Hypercalcemia
	Idiopathic	Infection (e.g., mumps, coxsackie)

ERCP, endoscopic retrograde cholangiopanreatography.

TABLE 50.2	Indications for Monitoring in Intensive Care Setting

- Patients with severe acute pancreatitis
- Patients with acute pancreatitis and one or more of the following:
  - Pulse <40 or >150 beats per minute
  - Systolic arterial pressure <80 or mean arterial pressure <60 mm Hg or diastolic arterial pressure >120 mm Hg
  - Respiratory rate >35 breaths per minute
  - Serum sodium <110 or >170 mg/dL
  - Serum Potassium <2 or >7 mg/dL
  - PaO2 <50 mm Hg
  - pH <7.1 or >7.7
  - Serum glucose >800 mg/dL
  - Serum calcium >15 mg/dL
  - Anuria
  - Coma

requires two of the following three criteria: (1) acute onset severe epigastric pa which may radiate to the back, (2) elevation in serum amylase or lipase three tin the upper limit of normal, and (3) characteristic findings of pancreatic inflammati on imaging. Indications for monitored or intensive care are described in Table 50.

The evaluation of a patient with suspected acute pancreatitis should begin w a careful history with attention to symptom onset, alcohol use, gallstone disease, pr pancreatitis, review of medications, and family history of pancreatitis. The princi symptom on history is abdominal pain, typically in the epigastric region, which c radiate to the back. It typically presents acutely and can be associated with naus and vomiting. On physical examination, palpation demonstrates severe abdomin tenderness and guarding. Inactive bowel sounds may be indicative of ileus. In sev cases, signs of the systemic inflammatory response syndrome (SIRS) with fever, tach cardia, and tachypnea may be present. Additional findings suggesting severe disea include diminished breath sounds, hypoxia, and altered mental status. Cullen's si (periumbilical ecchymosis) and Grey Turner's sign (flank ecchymosis) are rare fin ings and indicate hemorrhagic pancreatitis in the setting of pancreatic necrosis.

Early in the course of pancreatitis, digestive enzymes leak out of pancreatic a nar cells and enter the systemic circulation. Serum lipase levels rise earlier and rema elevated longer than serum amylase. Serum lipase levels elevated to three times t upper level of normal are a more sensitive marker than serum amylase for the dia nosis of acute pancreatitis (82% to 100% vs. 67% to 83%). It should be noted th enzyme levels may be normal in 5% of patients at the time of hospital admission.

Additional laboratory investigations required at the onset of suspected acu pancreatitis to aid in risk stratification include liver function tests, complete blo count (CBC), blood urea nitrogen (BUN), calcium, and creatinine. Elevations liver enzymes (particularly transaminases) with or without associated hyperbilir binemia suggest the presence of bile duct stones or compression of the common b duct by edema.

Imaging studies may be needed when there is doubt in the diagnosis or f documentation of the severity of illness. It is important to note that in patients wi acteristic abdominal pain and elevation in serum amylase/lipase, imaging is not ssary to establish the diagnosis of acute pancreatitis. An abdominal ultrasound ld be performed to assess for cholelithiasis or choledocholithiasis, especially in s of suspected gallstone pancreatitis. Early detection of gallstones helps dictate ner management either by endoscopic retrograde cholangiopancreatography CP) or cholecystectomy.

Cross-sectional imaging is not a mandatory part of the initial evaluation but can performed if there is concern for complications of acute pancreatitis. Contrast-inced computed tomography (CECT) is the best modality for evaluating pancre-inflammation, necrosis, and peripancreatic fluid collections. The most common ings on imaging in uncomplicated interstitial pancreatitis are enlargement of all or of the pancreas with blurring of the margins and inflammatory changes. CECT e at the initial presentation may underestimate disease severity since it can take up 2 hours for necrosis to develop. Therefore, CECT should be delayed unless there concern for other complications or if the diagnosis is in doubt.

For recurrent acute pancreatitis (two or more episodes), a detailed work-up is ranted, including immunoglobulin G4 (IgG4) levels to check for autoimmune creatitis, triglycerides, and serum calcium levels. Medications should be thor-nly reviewed as iatrogenic causes account for 2% of pancreatitis. An endoscopic asound can be performed to evaluate for pancreatic cancer in patients who do have an identified etiology. Further workup may also include a genetic workup, uation for pancreas divisum, and an infectious workup. Empiric cholecystec-y should be considered in patients with no identifiable cause for recurrent acute creatitis, even if liver function tests and gallbladder imaging are normal. No r etiology of pancreatitis will be found in 10% to 20% of patients (idiopathic creatitis).

EDICTION OF SEVERITY

ly prediction of severity in acute pancreatitis is important in identifying patients increased risk for morbidity and mortality. This can be challenging, as there is no le, reliable way to predict severity. Current severity indices are based on clinical radiographic parameters. An important clinical factor in the determination of ase severity is persistent organ failure for more than 48 hours.

Various grading and scoring systems have been developed to risk-stratify acute creatitis patients. Historically, the Ranson criteria and Glasgow scoring systems e been used, but these are cumbersome and can take 48 hours to complete. More ntly, the APACHE II (Acute Physiology and Chronic Health Examination II) has n used to predict severity in acute pancreatitis, but it is not pancreatitis-specific. ents with an APACHE II score >8 usually have severe disease. A new prognostic ring system, the bedside index for severity in acute pancreatitis (BISAP), has n proposed as a simple method for early identification of patients at risk for in-pital mortality and is as accurate as other scoring systems (Table 50.3). One point ssigned for each of the following signs within 24 hours of presentation: BUN l >25 mg/dL, impaired mental status, presence of SIRS, age >60, and pleural sion on imaging studies. A BISAP score ≥3 is associated with an increased risk complications.

Other single factors on admission that are associated with a severe course lude hemoconcentration (hematocrit >44%), obesity, C-reactive protein (CRP)

TABLE 50.3	BISAP Score for Predicting Severity and Complications in Acute Pancreatitis

- BUN >25
- Impaired mental status
- Systemic inflammatory response
- Age >60
- Pleural effusion

Calculate within 24 hours; increased risk for complications in patients with score of 3 or more.

>150 mg/dL, albumin <2.5 mg/dL, calcium <8.5 mg/dL, BUN >20, and e hyperglycemia (Table 50.4). Other markers of immune activation such as interle (IL)-6, IL-8, IL-10, and tumor necrosis factor (TNF) have also been associated v acute pancreatitis, although are not routinely checked in clinical practice. Var studies have found the BUN to be a good predictor of mortality in acute pancrea A BUN >20 is associated with an increased risk of death, as is any increase in B at 24 hours post admission.

The CT severity index (CTSI) is a scoring system based on a contrast-enhar CT grading system (A-E) and percentage of pancreatic necrosis (Table 50.5). Pan atic necrosis appears as a sharply demarcated region that does not enhance after in venous contrast. A score >6 indicates severe disease and a poorer prognosis. There a variety of local complications that can be diagnosed on cross-sectional imagin severe acute pancreatitis. Early findings include pancreatic necrosis and acute f collections, which are almost always sterile. Other complications that can occu various stages include peripancreatic artery pseudoaneurysm (e.g., gastroduode hepatic, and splenic arteries) and venous thrombosis (e.g., portal, superior mes teric, and splenic veins). Pancreatic necrosis can be sterile (Fig. 50.1A) or infe (Fig. 50.1B). Infected necrosis is a delayed complication, generally occurring n than 2 weeks after symptom onset; however, early cases of infected necrosis h been reported. Persistent fevers, leukocytosis, and hemodynamic instability associ with gas within the necrotic area are clinical indicators of infected necrosis. Pati with gas-containing pancreatic necrosis who are hemodynamically stable likely h developed a pancreaticoenteric fistula. The diagnosis can be confirmed with nee aspiration of the necrotic area, but the decision to proceed with invasive treatm is based on the patient's overall stability. Stable patients, even with infected necro can be managed conservatively without drainage.

TABLE 50.4	Other Single Factors on Admission Associated With Severe Acute

- Hematocrit >44%
- Obesity
- C-reactive protein (CRP) >150 mg/dL
- Albumin <2.5 mg/dL
- Calcium <8.5 mg/dL
- Early hyperglycemia

TABLE 50.5	Computed Tomography (CT) Grading of Acute Pancreatitis: CT Severity Index[a]	
Grade[b]	Findings	Score
A	Normal pancreas: normal size, sharply defined, smooth contour, homogeneous enhancement, retroperitoneal peripancreatic fat without enhancement	0
B	Focal or diffuse enlargement of the pancreas; contour may show irregularity, enhancement may be inhomogeneous, but there is on peripancreatic inflammation	1
C	Peripancreatic inflammation with intrinsic pancreatic abnormalities	2
D	Intrapancreatic or extrapancreatic fluid collections	3
E	Two or more large collections of gas in the pancreas or retroperitoneum	4

Necrosis Score Based on Contrast-Enhanced CT	
Necrosis (%)	Score
0	0
<33	2
33–50	4
≥50	6

[a] CT severity index equals unenhanced CT score plus necrosis score: maximum = 10, ≥6 = severe disease.
[b] Grading based on findings on unenhanced CT.

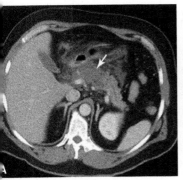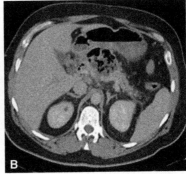

Figure 50.1. A: Necrotizing pancreatitis. Area of decreased attenuation in the pancreatic head and neck (arrow) represents necrosis in a patient with severe ethanol induced pancreatitis. The body and tail are viable. **B:** Imaging in the same patient several weeks after presentation with gas within the fluid collection indicating infected necrosis.

TABLE 50.6	Revised Atlanta Classification of Acute Pancreatitis Definitions of Severity

Mild
- No organ failure
- No local or systemic complications

Moderately Severe
- Organ failure that resolves within 48 hrs (transient)
- Local or systemic complications without persistent organ failure

Severe
- Persistent organ failure (>48 hrs): single organ or multiple organ failure

The revised Atlanta Classification (2012) recognized three levels of severity acute pancreatitis: mild, moderately severe, and severe (Table 50.6). In mild pancreatitis, there are no local/systemic complications or organ failure. These patients typically recover with supportive care within a week without complication. Patients with moderately severe acute pancreatitis have transient organ failure that resolve within 48 hours or a local complication such as a pancreatic fluid collection without persistent organ failure. Severe acute pancreatitis is defined by >48 hours of persistent organ failure. Persistent organ failure has been found to be associated with a 33% risk of mortality.

MANAGEMENT

This section will address the treatment strategies in severe acute pancreatitis, including intravenous fluids (IVF), pain control, nutritional support, the role of ERCP, use antibiotics, and management of peripancreatic fluid collections (Table 50.7).

Hypovolemia is thought to be the principal etiology of pancreatic hypoperfusion and inflammation in acute pancreatitis. Thus, rapid restoration of intravascular volume is the first and most effective therapy. Fluid resuscitation maintains intravascular

TABLE 50.7	Management of Severe Acute Pancreatitis in the Intensive Care Unit

- Supportive care: aggressive IVF, pain control
- Early ERCP (<48–72 hours) in patients with suspected concurrent cholangitis or biliary obstruction
- Early enteral nutrition via nasojejunal tube
- No role for antibiotics in infection prophylaxis
- Reserve drainage[a] for:
  - Acute fluid collections with abdominal compartment syndrome
  - Suspected infected necrosis in an unstable patient (usually occurs 2–3 wks into illness)

[a]Current evidence supports "step-up" approach to peripancreatic fluid collections and infected necrosis (endoscopic or percutaneous drainage initially followed by surgery if necessary).

me in the setting of massive capillary leak associated with the inflammatory
onse to acute pancreatitis. Fluid resuscitation prevents local ischemia and the
lopment of pancreatic necrosis, SIRS, and multiorgan failure. Recommendations
rding fluid rate, type, and duration vary and should be individualized, although
t studies have shown that early hydration within the first 24 hours decreases mor-
y and mortality. In general, all patients with suspicion for acute pancreatitis should
eated aggressively, as if they have severe disease, until proven otherwise. At the very
, a patient presenting with acute pancreatitis should be started on IVF at 250 to
mL/hr in order to maintain urine output of at least 0.5 mL/kg/hr. In patients with
s of severe volume depletion, maximal fluid resuscitation of 500 to 1,000 mL/hr
ild be initiated and can be decreased once evidence of hypoperfusion subsides.
American College of Gastroenterology guidelines recommend goal-directed fluid
scitation with 250 to 500 mL/hr of isotonic crystalloid for the first 12 to 24 hours
t frequent re-evaluation every 6 hours, with a therapeutic goal of decreasing the
N level from the admission value. In one randomized study, the use of lactated
ers (LR) had a more substantial effect on decreasing SIRS and CRP levels than
nal saline. Care should be taken to avoid using LR on patients with hypercalcemia,
is solution contains calcium. Although routine use of invasive intravascular moni-
ig is not routinely recommended, it may be useful in severe disease.

With the cardinal symptom of acute pancreatitis being severe epigastric abdom-
pain, intravenous opiate pain medication should be administered, and it may be
essary to administer pain medications via a patient-controlled anesthesia (PCA)
ip. Uncontrolled pain can contribute to hemodynamic instability. Nausea and vom-
g associated with pancreatitis usually respond well to parenteral antiemetics. Patients
i mild pancreatitis should begin to eat as soon as they feel able and typically
rate a solid, low fat diet within 1 week of admission. In patients with severe pan-
titis, enteral nutrition is preferred over total parenteral nutrition. Enteral nutri-
i preserves the intestinal mucosa and thereby potentially reduces the incidence of
terial translocation from the gut and subsequent infectious complications. Enteral
rition is associated with reduced central line infections, sepsis, need for surgical
rvention, length of hospital stay, and cost when compared to total parenteral
rition. There is no consensus on the preferred route of enteral nutrition, for exam-
oral versus gastric versus post-pyloric feeding. A recently published, randomized
trolled trial demonstrated that early nasoenteric tube feeding was no different
n an oral diet started at 72 hours in reducing the rates of infection or death in
ients with acute pancreatitis at high risk of complications.

In cases of gallstone pancreatitis, antibiotics should be initiated and biliary
ompression via ERCP should be performed early (within the first 72 hours) if
ending cholangitis is suspected. In some cases in which patients are too unstable for
ation or in which ERCP is unavailable, a percutaneous transhepatic cholangiogram
C) with catheter placement can be performed. Early ERCP does little to affect the
rse of pancreatitis, but reduces morbidity associated with concurrent cholangitis. If
atient with acute pancreatitis has abnormal liver enzymes and an intact gallbladder,
lecystectomy should be performed during the same hospital stay or within 30 days
lischarge to decrease the risk of recurrent acute pancreatitis. An ERCP with biliary
incterotomy should be performed in patients who are not surgical candidates.

In general, routine use of prophylactic antibiotics is not recommended in severe
icreatitis. Antibiotics are recommended if there is a concern for concurrent cholan-
s or for other documented infections. Early in the course of disease, patients with

TABLE 50.8	Pancreatic Fluid Collections

Acute Peripancreatic Fluid Collection
Associated with interstitial, edematous pancreatitis and no necrosis
Occur within first 4 weeks
No wall or encapsulation

Pancreatic Pseudocyst
Well circumscribed with well-defined wall
No non-liquid component
Maturation requires >4 weeks after onset of acute pancreatitis

Acute Necrotic Collection
Occurs in setting of acute necrotizing pancreatitis
Heterogeneous and non-liquid components
No definable wall

Walled-off Necrosis
Heterogeneous with non-liquid components
Encapsulated
Maturation requires 4 weeks after onset of acute necrotizing pancreatitis

severe pancreatitis can be febrile and have leukocytosis from inflammation associ
with pancreatitis, and antibiotics are not warranted for these signs alone. Antibi
should not be given routinely in necrotizing pancreatitis, since infected necrosis
late complication, generally occurring at least 2 weeks after symptom onset. C
all, antibiotics may decrease infectious complications but have not been show
decrease mortality. Treatment with antibiotics is appropriate for documented pos
blood cultures and/or a fine needle aspiration of pancreatic necrosis reveals infect
The preferred antibiotics for pancreatic necrosis are carbapenems, quinolones
metronidazole because these antibiotics penetrate the necrotic pancreas. Probic
have no role in the management of severe pancreatitis.

Local complications of acute pancreatitis include peripancreatic fluid collec
pancreatic pseudocyst, necrotic fluid collections, and walled off necrosis (Table 5
Acute fluid collections (enzyme-rich pancreatic fluid and tissue debris in and aro
the pancreas) occur in up to 40% of patients with severe pancreatitis. They represe
serous or exudative reaction to pancreatic injury and inflammation. There is little rol
draining acute fluid collections unless abdominal compartment syndrome, severe ga
outlet obstruction, or early infection is suspected. The majority of acute fluid collec
resolve spontaneously. These fluid collections lack definable walls and as such are
amenable to endoscopic intervention and require percutaneous drainage when indica

Fluid collections that persist gradually encapsulate over 4 to 6 weeks and incl
a spectrum of collections ranging from pseudocysts that are mostly fluid (no necr
to walled-off pancreatic necrosis (WOPN) that contains varying amounts of necr
debris. Drainage should be performed in those patients with sterile necrosis
become symptomatic (e.g., pain, gastric outlet obstruction) or in those with infe
necrosis who do not respond to antibiotics.

Treatment of infected necrosis is based on the patient's clinical course,
infected necrosis should be suspected in patients with pancreatic necrosis who l

nical deterioration. Unstable patients with infected necrosis or abdominal compart-
ent syndrome usually require drainage. Traditionally, this has been accomplished
th exploratory laparotomy, debridement, and drain placement, but is associated
th high morbidity and mortality. There is now compelling evidence that endo-
opic or percutaneous drainage results in lower morbidity and mortality than open
rgery; therefore, there has been a move toward delayed intervention and minimally
vasive approaches, including direct endoscopic pancreatic necrosectomy and per-
taneous drainage.

UMMARY

ute pancreatitis is a frequently encountered medical condition requiring hospital
mission and is associated with high rates or morbidity and mortality. Numerous
oring systems have been used to predict disease severity and direct medical treat-
ents. Early diagnosis and aggressive medical management with intravenous fluids,
in control, and early feeding are paramount to improve patient outcomes.

UGGESTED READINGS

-Omran M, Albalawi ZH, Tashkandi MF, et al. Enteral versus parenteral nutrition for acute
    pancreatitis. *Cochrane Database Syst Rev.* 2010;20;(1):CD002837.

kker J, Van Brunschot S, Van Santvoort J, et al. Early versus on-demand nasoenteric tube
    feeding in acute pancreatitis. *NEJM.* 2014;371:1983–1993.

nks PA, Bollen TL, Dervenis C, et al. Classification of acute pancreatitis—2012: revisions
    of the Atlanta classification and definitions by international consensus. *Gut.* 2013;62:
    102–111.

nks PA, Freeman ML. Practice guidelines in acute pancreatitis. *Am J Gastro.* 2006;101:2379–2400.

reer SE, Burchard KW. Acute pancreatitis and critical illness: a pancreatic tale of hypoperfusion
    and inflammation. *Chest.* 2009;136:1413–1419.

ohnson CD, Besselink MG, Carter R. Acute pancreatitis. *BMJ.* 2014;12:349–357.

andol SJ, Saluja AK, Imrie CW, et al. Acute pancreatitis: bench to bedside. *Gastroenterology.*
    2007;132:1127–1151.

apachristou GI, Muddana V, Yadav D, et al. Comparison of BISAP, Ranson's, APACHE-II, and
    CTSI scores in predicting organ failure, complications, and mortality in acute pancreatitis.
    Am J Gastroenterol. 2010;105(2):435–441; quiz 442.

ezzilli R, Zerbi A, DiCarlo V, et al. Practical guidelines for acute pancreatitis. *Pancreatology.*
    2010;10:523–535.

enner S, Baillie J, DeWitt J, et al. Management of acute pancreatitis. *Am J Gastroenterol.*
    2013;108:1400–1415.

an Santvoort HC, Besselink MG, Bakker OJ, et al. A step-up approach or open necrosectomy
    for necrotizing pancreatitis. *NEJM.* 2010;362:1491–1502.

51

Status Epilepticus

Rajat Dhar

DEFINITION OF STATUS EPILEPTICUS

Status epilepticus (SE) is formally defined as any seizure lasting longer than 30 minu[es] or repetitive seizures without return to baseline level of consciousness. As m[ost] seizures stop without treatment within 2 to 3 minutes, any seizure lasting ov[er] 5 minutes is unlikely to stop spontaneously and requires treatment. There is a[lso] greater risk of neuronal injury if seizures persist beyond 30 minutes, so aggress[ive,] prompt intervention (especially for convulsive seizures) is paramount. SE is classifi[ed] by seizure type (generalized vs. either simple or complex partial) and by manifes[ta-] tions (e.g., tonic–clonic, focal motor, nonconvulsive). SE occurs in over 100,000 p[er]sons each year in the United States. Mortality is between 5% and 30% for SE, vary[ing] with type and duration, but outcome is largely determined by etiology (Table 51.[1]). Causes of SE can be divided into acute processes, either in the central nervous syste[m] or systemically, or chronic disorders such as pre-existing epilepsy or an old stro[ke] or brain tumor. It is imperative to evaluate and manage the underlying etiology [in] parallel with attempts to control seizures.

INITIAL MANAGEMENT OF STATUS EPILEPTICUS

The first priorities are stabilization of the airway, breathing, and circulation. Not [all] patients with incipient SE require intubation, but all require close attention to paten[cy] of the airway. The head should be positioned to avoid obstruction and an artificial a[ir]way may be placed. Placing an oral airway may be challenging in a patient with tee[th] clenched, but a nasal airway can usually be inserted. Oxygen can be applied via nas[al] cannula or face mask. Many patients with SE will maintain oxygen saturation wi[th] these basic measures and continue to ventilate. It is common for patients with seizur[es] to develop an acute lactic acidosis that resolves as SE is controlled. Hypertension [is] more common than hypotension in the early stages of SE, while hemodynamic su[p]port and invasive monitoring are often required later as treatment intensifies.

Benzodiazepines are usually the first-line agents to stop persistent seizur[es] (Algorithm 51.1). Lorazepam can be given in 2 to 4 mg aliquots repeated every [2] to 3 minutes to a maximum of 0.1 mg/kg intravenously. If intravenous (IV) acce[ss] is not immediately available, then rectal diazepam gel (Diastat: 0.2 mg/kg in adul[ts,] usually 10 to 20 mg) can be used. Midazolam can also be squirted into the mouth [or] delivered intranasally (5 to 10 mg, with rapid absorption by both routes). Such ra[p]idly acting agents will be effective in 50% or more of SE cases treated early. Howev[er,]

BLE 51.1	Causes of Status Epilepticus

⁀ses	Evaluation
⁀te symptomatic CNS lesion ⁀ncephalitis/meningitis ⁀erebrovascular (ischemic stroke, ICH, SAH, CVST) ⁀raumatic brain injury ⁀lobal hypoxic–ischemic brain injury (post-cardiac arrest) ⁀ypertensive encephalopathy/PRES	Brain imaging (head CT, MRI) Lumbar puncture
⁀onic CNS lesion ⁀xisting stroke ⁀rain tumor (primary or metastatic, paraneoplastic), vascular malformation	Brain imaging (head CT, MRI)
⁀ic/metabolic derangement: ⁀rug intoxication or overdose (TCA, amphetamine) ⁀rug withdrawal (alcohol, benzodiazepines) ⁀atrogenic: medications (beta-lactams, theophylline, others) ⁀ypoglycemia ± hyperglycemia ⁀lectrolytes (hyponatremia, hypocalcemia) ⁀ebrile seizures (in young children)	Drug screen and drug history, EKG Glucose level Electrolytes
⁀lepsy ⁀oncompliance with AEDs ⁀ecent change in dose or AED ⁀sychogenic seizures ("pseudo-status")	Medication history Serum AED levels

, antiepileptic drugs; ICH, intracerebral hemorrhage; SAH, subarachnoid hemorrhage; CVST,
⁀bral venous sinus thrombosis; TCA, tricyclic antidepressant; PRES, posterior reversible
⁀ephalopathy syndrome.

duration of anticonvulsant action of these agents is relatively short (longest for
⁀zepam), so a longer-acting antiepileptic drug (AED) should be given concur-
⁀ly or immediately after benzodiazepines in cases of SE. **Phenytoin** is the most
⁀monly used maintenance AED, as it is available IV and has rapid onset of action
⁀hout significant respiratory or neurologic depression. A dose of 18 to 20 mg/kg
⁀uld be given at a maximum rate of 50 mg/min. Rapid infusions of phenytoin can
⁀se bradycardia, arrhythmias, hypotension, and even cardiac arrest. It can also cause
⁀ple glove syndrome and infusion site reactions. Therefore, acute IV administration
⁀osphenytoin may be preferred if central access is not available. Fosphenytoin is a
⁀-drug that is dose in "phenytoin equivalents" or PE and can be given at a rate of
⁀ mg PE per minute through a peripheral IV without potential for such serious
⁀usion problems. If seizures are still not controlled after initial phenytoin load,
⁀n an additional 5 to 10 mg/kg can be given. A phenytoin level should be drawn
⁀our after loading is complete and further IV or enteral doses given as necessary
⁀maintain total blood levels of 15 to 25 µg/mL. Several other IV AEDs are now
⁀ilable and can be used in lieu or in conjunction with phenytoin if seizures are not
⁀trolled (see Algorithm 51.1). These include the newer agents, Levetiracetam and
⁀osamide, which can be given rapidly without major hemodynamic effects, and

ALGORITHM 51.1 Initial Management of Status Epilepticus

- Assess and protect airway
- Monitor vital signs (including oxygen saturation, BP, EKG)
- Check bedside glucose level
- Obtain IV access
- Send labs (CBC, electrolytes, calcium, renal/hepatic function, toxicology, AED levels, ABG)

↓

Initial anticonvulsant treatment
- Consider giving thiamine (100 mg IV) with glucose (50 mL of D50)
- Lorazepam 4 mg IV, repeat 2–4 mg IV to a maximum of 0.1 mg/kg; AND
- Phenytoin/fosphenytoin IV load of 18–20 mg/kg; maximum rate of 50 mg/min (phenytoin) or 150 mg/min (fosphenytoin)

Convulsive seizures stop
- Check phenytoin level 1–2 hours post load
- Perform additional diagnostic studies to evaluate cause of SE (head CT, lumbar puncture)
- Consider stat EEG if not waking up to exclude ongoing (nonconvulsive) seizures

Seizures continue
- Additional 5–10 mg/kg of phenytoin
- Consider other 2nd-line agents including:
- Valproate 20–40 mg/kg IV bolus over 10 minutes
- Levetiracetam 2g IV bolus
- Lacosamide 100–200 mg IV bolus
- Phenobarbital 5 mg/kg IV to max of 20 mg/kg given q15min

ABBREVIATIONS

BP:	blood pressure
EKG:	electrocardiogram
CBC:	complete blood cell count
AED:	antiepileptic drugs
ABG:	arienal blood gas
SE:	status epilepticus
CT:	computed tomography
EEG:	electroencephalogram

the older broad-acting AED, Valproic acid (which should not be used in conjunction with phenytoin as significant drug–drug interactions exist).

REFRACTORY STATUS EPILEPTICUS

A subset of patients presenting with SE (~20% to 30%) will fail to respond to both benzodiazepines and phenytoin (or another second-line agent, such as IV valproate or phenobarbital). By this time, seizures will have usually persisted for 60 minutes, if not longer. This subgroup is designated to have *refractory status epilepticus* (RSE), which carries a significantly higher mortality and worse functional outcome. Most will require continuous infusions of anesthetic anticonvulsants to control RSE (although an additional nonanesthetic agent can be given for focal RSE without significantly impaired level of consciousness prior to initiating aggressive anesthetic agents). Patients receiving deep sedation to control RSE need to be admitted to the intensive care unit and usually require both ventilatory support and electroencephalogram (EEG) monitoring (Algorithm 51.2). If intubation is required, use of paralytics should ideally be avoided or restricted to short-acting agents so as not to mask ongoing convulsive movements. SE that begins with convulsions (e.g., generalized tonic–clonic seizures) often evolves into a state of dissociation between ongoing electrical seizure activity and lack of obvious motor expression; such nonconvulsive RSE requires EEG to diagnose and monitor its treatment. Subtle motor manifestations may be observed, including facial myoclonus, tonic eye deviation, or nystagmus. Continuous EEG with video monitoring is preferable to correlate electrographic changes with states of arousal, clinical manifestations, and stimulation.

Choice of anesthetic agent to control RSE is not guided by rigorous comparative evidence. It should be based on a consideration of patient factors, including hemodynamic stability, seizure severity and duration, and goal of treatment (i.e., seizure cessation vs. burst suppression), as well as local (physician and institutional) experience. The major choices are compared in Table 51.2. There is a definite risk of "propofol-related infusion syndrome (PRIS)" with the high cumulative doses of propofol often required to control RSE; this manifests as a variable combination of metabolic acidosis, hyperkalemia, rhabdomyolysis, renal failure, bradycardia, and arrhythmias (including cardiac arrest). Even in the absence of PRIS, hypotension can be considerable with propofol. For this reason, midazolam is a reasonable first-line option for RSE if EEG seizure cessation is the target. Propofol or pentobarbital may be used as second-line agents if midazolam either fails to control seizures or there are breakthrough or recurrent seizures during maintenance or weaning of the infusion. These two agents are better able to induce a burst suppression pattern on EEG. While burst suppression has been associated with worse outcome (than seizure control alone) in some series with RSE, it may be reasonable to target this more aggressive goal in more resistant/recurrent cases. Volatile anesthetics have been used in limited series and require specialized equipment and monitoring. Their major advantages are short half-life and ability to rapidly induce burst suppression.

Once the EEG treatment goal has been achieved (i.e., seizure cessation and/or burst suppression), it may be advisable to maintain infusion rates and EEG targets for 24 hours before gradually weaning. Avoidance of all epileptic activity on EEG (e.g., periodic discharges) may not be necessary unless these are clearly associated with persistent alterations in mental status or build/evolve enough to resemble incipient seizures. Many patients requiring deep sedation will develop hypotension requiring fluid

ALGORITHM 51.2 Treatment of Refractory Status Epilepticus

Persistent seizure activity (clinically or on EEG) despite two+ anticonvulsants

General management
- Intubate for airway protection
- Continuous EEG monitoring
- Close hemodynamic monitoring
- Fluids and vasopressors as needed
- Continue maintenance AEDs (e.g., phenytoin, levetiracetam) at high therapeutic levels
- Treat underlying cause of seizures
- Consider neurology consultation

Seizure control
- Initiate infusion to control clinical and electrographic seizures (see Table 51.2), e.g., midazolam
- Can give loading bolus of same agent (e.g., at time of intubation) to rapidly control seizures
- Titrate infusion to maintain seizure control

Seizures not controlled
- Still having seizures despite increasing infusion rate (i.e., treatment failure), breakthrough seizures after initial control, or recurrent seizures on trying to wean infusion

Seizures controlled
- Continue infusion for 24 hours at rate that achieved target
- Monitor closely for complications of treatment (infections, hemodynamic instability, ileus)
- After 24 hours try to gradually wean infusion off and watch for recurrent seizures

Burst suppression
- Consider alternate agent (e.g., propofol, pentobarbital) with goal of inducing burst suppression
- Consider therapeutic hypothermia
- Add additional enteral AEDs (e.g., topiramate, lacosamide)

Refractory status epilepticus controlled
- Continue EEG for 12–24 hours off all infusions
- Continue other AEDs

ABBREVIATIONS

EEG: electroencephalogram
AED: antiepileptic drugs

BLE 51.2	**Anesthetic Infusions for Refractory Status Epilepticus**			
	Midazolam	Propofol	Pentobarbital	Volatile Anesthetics
hanism	Benzodiazepine (GABA)	Unclear (GABA modulation)	Barbiturate (GABA)	Polysynaptic GABA
ding se[a]	0.2 mg/kg	1–2 mg/kg	5 mg/kg	N/A
ting usion	0.05 mg/kg/hr	1–2 mg/kg/hr (15–30 mcg/kg/min)	1 mg/kg/hr	N/A
sion nge	0.05–0.8 mg/kg/hr	1–15 mg/kg/hr (15–250 mcg/kg/min)	0.5–10 mg/kg/hr	0.8%–2.0%
-life	1–2 hrs[b]	<1 hr[b]	15–40 hrs	<1 hr
erse fects	Hypotension Tachyphylaxis	Hypotension "Infusion syndrome" Lipemia	Hypotension Bradycardia Poikilothermia Pulmonary infections	Hypotension Ileus

repeat loading dose boluses till seizures controlled.
accumulate with prolonged infusions.

scitation and vasopressor support. Respiratory drive will be severely inhibited or lished, and all patients require mechanical ventilation with meticulous attention l to prevention of ventilator-associated pneumonia and other nosocomial infec- s. If background levels of AEDs are not maintained, then seizures will recur n anesthetic agents are weaned off. Phenytoin, levetiracetam, lacosamide, val- ate, topiramate, and/or other agents should be continued and titrated in patients n RSE during and after use of anesthetic infusions. Phenytoin levels should be nitored frequently, if possible, with a therapeutic target in the high therapeutic ge. Induced hypothermia offers another treatment option in resistant cases (e.g., are of midazolam) and may avoid the use of long-lasting barbiturates or the risks of pofol. This has only been shown effective in a small series where temperature was ered to between 31°C and 35°C and titrated to EEG response. The major advan- is rapid offset of metabolic suppression once temperature is normalized (in com- ison to pentobarbital that persists for days after infusion is stopped). **Ketamine**, NMDA-receptor antagonist, has also shown anecdotal promise in controlling RSE has the advantages of working independent of gamma-aminobutyric acid (GABA) ptors, which are downregulated after prolonged seizures, and also not worsening nodynamic instability. It can be loaded at 1.5 mg/kg IV (repeated every 3 to 5 min- s till seizures stop to max 4.5 mg/kg) and then infused at 1.2 mg/kg/hr (range 0.3 7.5 mg/kg/hr). Other options for super RSE include induction of a ketogenic state h specialized feeding or the application of electroconvulsive therapy (ECT). Young ients with RSE (even those requiring a month or more of sedative therapies) may make gratifying recoveries if ICU complications are avoided and the underlying rce of seizures is reversible (e.g., encephalitis) and treated successfully. This may involve immunotherapies, such as steroids, intravenous immunoglobulin (IVIG plasmapheresis in some cases. Neurosurgical resection of an epileptic lesion may aid in seizure control.

SE in comatose survivors of cardiac arrest (i.e., *post-anoxic* SE) is usuall ominous sign of diffuse cerebral damage. Especially when accompanied by myoc jerking, the presence of SE is one of the most consistent predictors of death/ne covery after cardiac arrest. The one exception is when SE occurs in conjunction a preserved brainstem examination and EEG shows evidence of reactivity. Post-ar myoclonus and SE may be transiently controlled by agents such as valproate, clc epam, or levetiracetam, but SE is usually refractory and aggressive measures sh be withheld pending discussion of prognosis with the family.

SUGGESTED READINGS

Abou Khaled KJ, Hirsch LJ. Advances in the management of seizures and status epileptic critically ill patients. *Crit Care Clin.* 2007;22:637–659.

Brophy GM, Bell R, Claassen J, et al. Guidelines for the management of status epilep *Neurocrit Care* 2012;17:3–23.

Chen JW, Wasterlain CG. Status epilepticus: pathophysiology and management in adults. *L Neurol* 2006;5:246–256.

Corry JJ, Dhar R, Murphy T, et al. Hypothermia for refractory status epilepticus. *Neurocrit* 2008;9:189–197.

Grover EH, Nazzal Y, Hirsch LJ. Treatment of convulsive status epilepticus. *Curr Treat Op Neurol* 2016;18:11.

Lowenstein D. The management of refractory status epilepticus. An update. *Epilpesia.* 2 47(Suppl. 1):35–40.

Shorvon S, Ferlisi M. The treatment of super-refractory status epilepticus: a critical revie available therapies and a clinical treatment protocol. *Brain.* 2011;134:2802–2818.

52

Acute Ischemic Stroke

Tobias B. Kulik and Salah G. Keyrouz

roke is the fifth leading cause of death in the United States and a major cause of disility. Approximately 85% of all strokes are ischemic, with the remainder being hemrhagic. Although most ischemic strokes can be managed on a regular hospital floor, me warrant admission to intensive care unit (ICU). Patients who have undergone rombolysis or endovascular recanalization are usually admitted to a specialized stroke ICU for tight blood pressure control and monitoring for hemorrhagic complications. urge hemispheric, cerebellar, or brainstem strokes require frequent neurologic moniring in a critical care setting given the potential need for osmotic therapy or surgical ecompression to treat cerebral edema. In addition, decreased alertness and weak bulbar uscle tone may lead to respiratory compromise necessitating airway management and echanical ventilation. Finally, the underlying stroke etiology could pose management allenges that need to be dealt within an ICU, like arrhythmias, myocardial infarction, idocarditis with valvular dysfunction, and hypertensive emergencies to name a few.

RESENTATION

stroke occurs when there is sudden inadequate perfusion of a brain region causing euronal death and irreversible damage. Clinical presentation varies considerably id depends on the region of the brain that is affected. It may be as subtle as minor insory loss or as impressive as the complete loss of motor function and speech npairment. Thalamic and brainstem infarctions may cause alteration of mental sta-is that may be difficult to distinguish from metabolic or infectious encephalopathy. linical diagnosis is usually possible when acute deficits match the pattern of a typical roke syndrome. A suspicion for stroke should always lead the clinician to perform ead computed tomography (CT) or magnetic resonance imaging (MRI) to exclude itracranial hemorrhage and evaluate the presence of other structural lesions, such ; neoplasia or abscess ("stroke mimics"). Other pathologies that may mimic stroke iclude postictal neurologic deficits (typically paralysis), complicated migraine, met-bolic derangements (hypo-/hyperglycemia), and psychosomatic disorders.

MANAGEMENT

General critical care management is similar to that of other ICU patients: maintenance nd restoration of normal acid–base physiology, oxygenation, euvolemia, and glycemic ontrol. However, there are other considerations that are inherent to ischemic stroke ictims. Fever has been shown to worsen outcome in stroke, and effective temperature

control likely mitigates this effect. The practice of permissive hypercapnia should
minimized if at all possible; the rise in CO_2 dilates intracranial vessels, especially a
rioles, and leads to a rise in intracranial pressure, which could be detrimental in th
with cerebral edema complicating large strokes. Aspirin (or another antiplatelet age
should be given to ischemic stroke patients as soon as feasible or 24 hours after receiv
thrombolytics. The combination of aspirin and dipyridamole appears equally effecti
Conversely, combining clopidogrel and aspirin increases the odds of intra- and extrac
nial hemorrhagic complications. Therefore, dual antiplatelet therapy in the immedi
poststroke period should be avoided in the absence of a strong cardiac indication.

Heparin is no longer recommended for the treatment of acute ischemic stro
There are rare occasions where it might be considered, for example, a left ventricular
a carotid thrombus. Anticoagulation for atrial fibrillation reduces the chance of fut
stroke and is therefore indicated in instances of stroke or transient ischemic attac
Generally, therapeutic anticoagulation is not started in the acute stroke period given
concern for hemorrhagic conversion of an infarct. Depending on the size of the infarc
brain tissue, most experts recommend starting anticoagulation between 7 and 14 d
post stroke. Mechanical and pharmacologic prophylaxis of venous thromboemboli
should be initiated as soon as feasible. Enoxaparin is superior to unfractionated hepa
in preventing deep venous thrombosis but not pulmonary embolism. Seizure prophi
laxis is not indicated in ischemic stroke, and some agents, in fact, have been shown
worsen outcome (i.e., phenytoin, valproic acid). However, suspicion for seizure shou
be evaluated with routine or extended electroencephalography and treated if appropria

For ischemic strokes <4.5 hours old, intravenous thrombolysis with tissue pl
minogen activator (tPA) is the intervention of choice in selected patients. Howeve
critically ill patients with multiple failing organs are seldom candidates for int
venous thrombolysis. This is often due to thrombocytopenia, coagulopathy, act
bleeding, or failure to establish time of last-known-normal, among other reaso
With the advent of new embolectomy devices ("stentrievers"), such patients cou
benefit from more aggressive interventions to potentially restore blood flow to at-r
brain regions. Embolectomy using the Solitaire® and Trevo® devices are associat
with better odds of recanalization and a lower risk of symptomatic hemorrhage wh
compared to earlier generation devices (Table 52.1).

Stroke often causes reactive hypertension which helps to perfuse the ischemic pe
umbra. High blood pressure should be tolerated up to 220/120 mm Hg unless the
is evidence of ongoing end-organ damage (i.e., acute myocardial infarction, dissecti
aneurysms, heart failure, renal failure) or if tPA was administered; for the first 24 hou
after thrombolysis, systolic and diastolic blood pressure are kept under 180 and 105 m
Hg, respectively to avoid hemorrhagic complications. Labetalol, nicardipine, or hydra
zine can be used. Nitrates are avoided because of their potential for venous dilatation a
subsequent intracranial pressure elevation. Inducing hypertension to salvage ischem
penumbra is a debated therapeutic approach and should only be utilized when a clo
relationship between clinical deterioration and relatively low blood pressure is observe

Determining the cause of stroke is necessary to guide therapy for seconda
prevention. Telemetry, echocardiography, brain MRI, carotid Doppler study, and
form of intracranial vascular imaging may be used. Proper use and interpretation
these diagnostic tests should be done by or with the consultation of a stroke speciali
given the increasing complexity of stroke management. General methods of the pa
such as universal anticoagulation and carotid endarterectomy, have changed to mo
complex algorithms and will likely evolve even further.

BLE 52.1   Indications and Contraindications for Thrombolysis

ications

te onset of focal neurologic symptoms in a defined vascular territory, consistent
h ischemic stroke

rly defined onset of stroke less than 3 or 4.5 hrs (extended window) prior to
anned start of treatment (if patient awakens with symptoms, onset is defined as
st seen normal")

18 or older

evidence of intracranial hemorrhage, nonvascular lesions (e.g., brain tumor,
scess), or signs of advanced cerebral infarction such as sulcal edema, hemi-
heric swelling, or large areas of low attenuation consistent with acute stroke
CT.

traindications

set of stroke greater than 3 or 4.5 hrs (extended window) prior to planned start
treatment

idly improving symptoms or mild symptoms (relative)

ICA stroke, an obtunded or comatose state may be a relative contraindication

zure at onset of stroke symptoms or within 3 hrs prior to tPA administration

ical presentation suggestive of subarachnoid hemorrhage regardless of CT result

pertension, SBP >185 mm Hg or DBP >110 mm Hg

or ischemic stroke within 1 mo or major ischemic stroke/head trauma within
mo

tory of intracerebral or subarachnoid hemorrhage if recurrence risk is substantial

treated cerebral aneurysm, arteriovenous malformation, or brain tumor

strointestinal or genitourinary hemorrhage within the last 21 days

erial puncture at a noncompressible site within 7 days or lumbar puncture within
days

jor surgery or major trauma within the last 14 days

ical presentation suggestive of acute myocardial infarction or post-MI
ericarditis

tient taking oral anticoagulants (warfarin, dabigatran [Pradaxa®], rivaroxaban
arelto®], apixaban [Eliquis®])

tient receiving heparin within 48 hrs or LMWH within 24 hrs

ceived tPA less than 7 days previously

own hemorrhagic diathesis or unsupported coagulation factor deficiency

ucose <50 or >400 mg/dL

telet count <100,000/mm^3

R >1.7 or elevated aPTT

sitive pregnancy test

lditional Contraindications for 4.5-hr Window

mbination of previous stroke *and* diabetes

ed for intravenous drip to obtain SBP <185 or DBP <110

---

tissue plasminogen activator; CT, computed tomography; MCA, middle cerebral artery; SBP,
olic blood pressure; DBP, diastolic blood pressure; MI, myocardial infarction; INR, international
malized ratio; aPTT, activated partial thromboplastin time; LMWH, low–molecular-weight heparin.

ALGORITHM 52.1 — Management of Malignant Cerebral Edema Due to Stroke

Stage 1: Initial intensive care and monitoring
- Monitoring of vitals and mental status at least every 2 hours
- Keep head of bed at 30 degrees elevation
- Avoid jugular compression by keeping head midline
- Maintain normothermia and euglycemia
- Avoid hypotonic solutions
- Permissive hypertension, treat only SBP >220 mm Hg or DBP >120 mm Hg
- Intubation for airway protection (GCS <9 or bulbar weakness).

Stage 2: Osmotic therapy for intracranial hypertension
- Avoid hypercarbia (ascertain adequate minute ventilation, treat fever)
- Give intravenous boluses of mannitol (see Chapter 60)
- Consider hypertonic saline if mannitol is unsuccessful or contraindicated.

Stage 3: Surgery for cerebral edema—consult neurosurgeon for possible decompressive hemicraniectomy
- Allow surgical evaluation *before* offering to family
- Continue osmotic therapy and medical management

Stage 4: Experimental techniques (induced hypothermia)

ABBREVIATIONS
SBP: systolic blood pressure
DBP: diastolic blood pressure
GCS: Glasgow Coma Scale

CEREBRAL EDEMA

A large acute ischemic stroke is typically complicated by cytotoxic edema. Edema, escially in young patients without age-related cerebral atrophy, may have dire consequen essitating close monitoring and requiring aggressive interventions. Some strokes may se compression of the cerebral ventricular system and lead to obstructive hydro-halus requiring a ventriculostomy. Edema will create pressure differentials between bral compartments created by dural folds leading to herniation syndromes. Cere-lar infarction is notorious for compressing the fourth ventricle and brainstem and sing hydrocephalus and catastrophic herniation. Edema typically peaks within 3 to ays, but in severe cases, rapid deterioration can occur within the first 48 hours with a rtality rate that approaches 80% to 90%. Risk factors for early deterioration include ing age, large infarcts, and use of thrombolytics. Simple measures such as keeping the d elevated at >30 degrees, avoiding hypotonic solutions which lead to hyponatremia worsening cerebral edema, and careful monitoring may be sufficient. In cases with re severe edema, osmotic therapy (mannitol or hypertonic saline), external ventricular inage, or decompressive craniectomy and duraplasty may be necessary.

As with all major interventions, the physician must establish a clear under-nding of the patient's and family's wishes regarding the degree of interventions ired for treating malignant cerebral edema. Chapter 60 offers further details on : of osmotic therapy. Algorithm 52.1 demonstrates a step-wise approach to man- : patients with stroke complicated by cerebral edema, beginning with intubation airway protection, osmotic therapy, considering decompressive craniectomy, and illy, the use of experimental interventions such as hypothermia.

Several trials have confirmed the mortality benefit of hemicraniectomy in large mispheric strokes, when performed within 48 hours from the ictus. Functional out-ne, however, was not significantly improved. Patients who would have died without gical intervention ended up with severe disability in long-term nursing facilities, ly dependent on others for care. Hence, it is important to have a discussion with : next-of-kin regarding patient's expectations before offering this surgical option.

While initially only patients age 60 and younger were thought to benefit from : procedure, it is now believed that older individuals could undergo decompressive niectomy, reaping similar benefits.

JGGESTED READINGS

ams HP Jr, del Zoppo G, Alberts MJ, et al. Guidelines for the early management adults with ischemic stroke: a guideline from the American Heart Association/American Stroke Associa-tion Stroke Council, Clinical Cardiology Council, Cardiovascular Radiology and Intervention Council, and the Atherosclerotic Peripheral Vascular Disease and Quality of Care Outcomes in Research Interdisciplinary Working Groups: the American Academy of Neurology affirms the value of this guideline as an educational tool for neurologists. *Stroke.* 2007;38:1655–1711.
An evidence-based review and most up-to-date guidelines for the management of patients with acute ischemic stroke.

drews PJ. Critical care management of acute ischemic stroke. *Curr Opin Crit Care.* 2004;10: 110–115.
A retrospective and prospective review on the management of acute stroke in the critical care setting.

l Zoppo GJ, Saver JL, Jauch EC, et al. Expansion of the time window for treatment of acute ischemic stroke with intravenous tissue plasminogen activator: a science advisory from the American Heart Association/American Stroke Association. *Stroke.* 2009;40:2945–2948.
Update on new time window for tPA.

pta R, Connolly ES, Mayer S, et al. Hemicraniectomy for massive middle cerebral artery territory infarction: a systematic review. *Stroke.* 2004;35:539–543.
An excellent review of factors to account for when deciding whether to proceed with decompres-sive hemicraniectomy for hemispheric malignant infarction.

53 Aneurysmal Subarachnoid Hemorrhage

Rajat Dhar

Subarachnoid hemorrhage (SAH) is an acute cerebrovascular disorder that encom passes various sources of usually diffuse bleeding into the subarachnoid space (co taining cerebrospinal fluid [CSF]) that surrounds the brain and spinal cord. The me common etiology of SAH is rupture of an intracranial aneurysm, although oth etiologies may be responsible (Table 53.1); 10% to 20% remain cryptogenic af angiographic evaluation: many of these have a *perimesencephalic* pattern of bleedi (i.e., localized around the brainstem without extension into the lateral Sylvi fissures, ventricles, or brain parenchyma). This form of SAH is more benign a likely has a venous origin. Although SAH comprises only 10% of all cerebrovascu events, it affects a younger population, and carries a significant mortality (20% 30% within 30 days) as well as persistent neurologic disability (due to the init bleed and effects of delayed ischemia). Risk factors for aneurysmal rupture inclu hypertension, cigarette smoking, heavy alcohol use, polycystic kidney disease, anc history of aneurysms/SAH in first-degree relatives. Patients with SAH should idea be managed in centers with expertise in both neurocritical care and endovascula surgical management of intracranial aneurysms (Algorithm 53.1).

DIAGNOSIS AND INITIAL MANAGEMENT

Patients with SAH usually present with sudden severe headache that reaches max mum intensity within seconds (i.e., thunderclap headache). This may be associat with syncope or persistent alteration in level of consciousness. Meningismus develo often over hours. The diagnosis is confirmed by noncontrast computed tomograph (CT) of the head that has almost perfect (99%) sensitivity if performed with 24 hours of symptom onset. Those presenting in a delayed fashion (i.e., headache f >24 hours) or with negative CT despite clinical suspicion should undergo lumb puncture to evaluate for red blood cells and *xanthochromia* (the yellow discoloratic of centrifuged CSF seen with blood breakdown). It is critical to fully evaluate a patient with a sudden or new headache for SAH as delay or misdiagnosis places the at risk for aneurysmal rebleeding, with a mortality approaching 50%. Those wi confirmed SAH but negative initial angiogram should undergo repeat angiograph (or CT angiography) in 1 to 3 weeks to exclude a missed aneurysm (especially if t bleeding is diffuse and not just localized in a perimesencephalic pattern).

Acute hydrocephalus from obstruction to CSF flow is seen in half patien and may lead to impaired mental status, requiring urgent ventriculostomy. On the patient has been diagnosed and stabilized, cerebral angiography should b

ALGORITHM 53.1 Initial Evaluation and Management of Patients with Subarachnoid Hemorrhage

Patient has subarachnoid hemorrhage
- Presents with sudden onset of the worst headache of his or her life ± LOC
- Noncontrast head CT shows hyperdensity (blood) in the basal cisterns, Sylvian fissure and sulci of the brain; blood may also be present in the ventricles
- Lumbar puncture shows xanthochromia in a patient with negative head CT

↓

- Admission to intensive care unit, preferably specialized neuro-ICU
- Bed rest, airway protection, maintain MAP <110 mm Hg and consider antifibrinolytic agent to prevent rebleeding, frequent neurological examinations, EKG
- Institute anticonvulsant prophylaxis, laxatives, pain, and anxiety control
- Order **cerebral angiography**
- Place EVD if signs of hydrocephalus (drowsiness, large ventricles on head CT)

↓

Aneurysm or other vascular malformation found → **No** →
- Consider digital subtraction angiography if initially used CTA or MRA
- Consider other cause (trauma, PMSAH)
- Repeat angiography in 1–3 weeks

Yes
↓

Treat aneurysm/vascular malformation to prevent rebleeding
- Consult neurosurgery and neurointerventionalist to determine optimal treatment plan (clipping vs. coiling of aneurysms, embolization vs. resection of AVM)
- Treatment of aneurysms within 24 hours is strongly recommended
- Evacuation of hematoma if focal deficits complicated by herniation or increased ICP

↓

Aneurysm "protected" (clipped or coiled successfully)

↓

Initial preventative measures for vasospasm
- Maintain euvolemia
- Permissive hypertension (hold antihypertensives)
- Nimodipine 60 mg orally or enterally every 4 hours

Monitor closely for common complications
- Frequent neurologic examination
- Monitoring of ICP if appropriate
- Frequent monitoring of vitals, heart rhythm, electrolytes
- Place Foley catheter to monitor input and output closely
- See Algorithm 53.2

ABBREVIATIONS	
LOC:	loss of consciousness
CT:	computed tomography
ICU:	intensive care unit
MAP:	mean arterial pressure
EKG:	electrocardiography
EVD:	external ventricular drain
CTA:	CT angiography
MRA:	magnetic resonance angiography
PMSAH:	perimesencephalic SAH
AVM:	arteriovenous malformation
ICP:	intracranial pressure.

TABLE 53.1	Cause of Subarachnoid Hemorrhage
Etiology	Clues/Comments
Intracranial aneurysm	Most common cause of spontaneous SAH, usually presents with "thunderclap headache", diffuse hemorrhage on imag
Arteriovenous malformation	Often associated with intra-parenchymal bleeding
Trauma	Blood usually more focal, located around cerebral convexit and associated with parenchymal contusions
Perimesencephalic	Angiogram negative, blood confined to cisterns around brains
Arterial dissection	Only if dissection extends intracranially
Coagulopathy	May be focal (with minor trauma) or diffuse, angiogram nega
Venous thrombosis	Often associated with edema and parenchymal hemorrhage
Pituitary apoplexy	Sudden headache with visual complaints and ophthalmopl
Reversible cerebral vasoconstriction syndrome	Focal SAH, often at convexity Angiogram reveals diffuse segmental vasoconstriction Associated with certain medications, post-partum state, dr abuse

performed to evaluate for an aneurysm or other vascular lesion. Conventional eter angiography remains the gold standard but CT angiography may be used a initial screening test (but may miss small aneurysms). The clinical severity of is graded using either the Hunt and Hess or World Federation of Neurosur Societies' scales (Table 53.2); survival is inversely proportional to grade, with g V patients who do not improve with initial stabilization (sometimes with ven ulostomy to drain CSF if hydrocephalus is present) invariably doing poorly. amount of blood on admission CT scan is also graded using the modified Fi scale (Table 53.3); higher grade patients are at greater risk for vasospasm, del ischemic deficits, and strokes.

TABLE 53.2	Clinical Grading Scales
Grade	Criteria
Hunt and Hess Grading System	
1	Asymptomatic or mild headache
2	Moderate to severe headache, nuchal rigidity, or cranial nerve palsy
3	Confusion, lethargy, and/or mild focal neurologic deficit
4	Stupor and/or hemiparesis
5	Comatose, posturing
World Federation of Neurosurgical Societies' Scale	
I	GCS 15, no motor deficit
II	GCS 13–14, no motor deficit
III	GCS 13–14 or motor deficit
IV	GCS 7–12
V	GCS 3–6

ABLE 53.3	CT Grading Scale for Risk of Vasospasm		
mount of SAH in Basal Cisterns		IVH	Modified Fisher Grade
iffuse or localized, thick		Present	4
iffuse or localized, thick		Absent	3
iffuse or localized only thin SAH		Present	2
nly thin SAH		Absent	1
o SAH		Present	2
o SAH		Absent	0

H is considered thick if it completely fills at least one cistern or fissure. IVH (intraventricular morrhage) is considered present if there is blood in both lateral ventricles.

The risk of **rebleeding** is as high as 20% in the first 24 to 48 hours after SAH d is the most common cause of early death (along with ventricular arrhythmias). rly treatment of the ruptured aneurysm is critical to prevent rebleeding, and may be complished by surgical clipping (with craniotomy) or endovascular approach with iling. The patient's age, clinical condition, and anatomy/location of the aneurysm ll inform the preferred treatment, made in discussion between the neurosurgeon d endovascular specialist. Prior to definitive aneurysmal treatment, blood pres-re should be controlled to prevent further bleeding; mean arterial pressure (MAP) ould be kept below 110 mm Hg and/or systolic blood pressure below 140 mm Hg. ort-acting antihypertensives (e.g., labetalol, nicardipine), analgesics, and sedatives e preferred. Blood pressure can be liberalized after successful securing of the aneu-sm. Administration of antifibrinolytic agents such as tranexamic acid (1g IV q 4 to hours, prior to aneurysm treatment) has been shown to reduce the risk of rebleeding.

Aneurysmal rupture triggers a molecular cascade culminating in release of cate-iolamines and cytokines. This sympathetic hyperactivity may induce cardiopulmo-iry dysfunction. EKG changes are common and troponin levels are elevated (usually 5 to 10 mcg/L) in 20% to 30%. Ten percent of patients (especially those with severe AH and elevated cardiac enzymes) will have **stunned myocardium** with wall-motion inormalities or globally depressed systolic function on echocardiography. Coronary igiography is not necessary in most and is invariably unrevealing (i.e., no obstructive sion). This form of "stress-induced cardiomyopathy" is reversible and usually resolves ithin 1 to 2 weeks; some patients will require inotropic support in the acute period. ilmonary edema and hypoxemia is seen in 10% to 20% and may have both cardio-nic as well as neurogenic origins.

OMPLICATIONS OF SAH

eizures most often occur early after SAH (either at ictus or prior to hospitalization 5% to 10%). However, there is an approximately 5% risk of seizures in-hospital id, despite lack of evidence for their benefit, many provide anticonvulsant prophy-xis for patients after SAH. This can either be given for just the immediate periop-rative period (e.g., 3-day course) or continued till hospital discharge in high-risk atients (e.g., with parenchymal hematoma) or those having seizures after admission. evetiracetam at a dose of 1000 mg twice daily is one commonly used regimen. Those

remaining or becoming poorly responsive after SAH should undergo EEG monit
ing to exclude subclinical seizures.

Hyponatremia occurs in 30%, most often 4 to 10 days after admission. It m
be due to syndrome of inappropriate antidiuretic hormone secretion (SIADH, euvo
mic) and/or cerebral salt wasting (CSW, hypovolemic). Distinguishing between t
two is important (but often challenging) as therapeutic strategies are different; ave
excess water intake with SIADH versus replace volume with isotonic or hypertor
saline solutions in CSW. Total fluid restriction should never be utilized for hyp
natremia after SAH (even with SIADH) as hypovolemia has been shown to eleva
the risk of cerebral infarction. As SIADH and CSW often overlap, it is advisable
assess volume status, and unless hypovolemia can be confidently excluded, then sali
replacement (either with normal or hypertonic saline infusions) is the safer approac
This can be accompanied by oral fluid restriction of 1 to 1.5 L/day. All patients wi
SAH should have daily measurements of serum sodium as well as close monitori
of fluid balance. They should not receive hypotonic fluids and diuretics should
restricted as hypovolemia promotes cerebral ischemia. Central **fever** is also commo
seen and may be part of a systemic inflammatory response (SIRS) making true infe
tion difficult to differentiate and diagnose in these patients.

CEREBRAL VASOSPASM AND DELAYED CEREBRAL ISCHEMIA

Cerebral infarction as a result of delayed ischemia is the major source of seconda
disability after SAH. Arterial narrowing (i.e., vasospasm) is seen on angiography in
majority of SAH patients between 4 and 21 days after bleeding (peaking around d
7 to 10) and is more likely in those with greater thickness of SAH and intraventricul
hemorrhage (estimated by the modified Fisher scale, Table 53.3). Some patients wi
vasospasm will remain asymptomatic, but others will develop neurological defic
related to reductions in cerebral blood flow (CBF) below ischemic thresholds. Th
reduction in CBF and oxygen delivery may be worsened by hypovolemia, hypote
sion, and anemia. For this reason, patients with SAH should be kept euvolemic I
adjustment of intravenous fluids and normotensive (avoiding BP-lowering medic
tions). The optimal hemoglobin and role of transfusion are less clear. All patier
should receive nimodipine, a calcium channel antagonist that has demonstrated ef
cacy in improving neurological outcome (at a dose of 60 mg every 4 hours enteral
continued for 21 days). The dose may be halved and given q 2h if blood pressu
drops after each dose. Some centers employ Transcranial Doppler (TCD) to screen f
vasospasm, as an increase in velocities in the basal cerebral vessels suggests a decrea
in their caliber. Prophylactic hypervolemia or hypertensive therapy is not effective
either improving cerebral perfusion or preventing deficits from vasospasm.

Any alteration in neurological status (new or worsening of neurological defici
or persistent alteration in mentation) after SAH requires prompt evaluation for isc
emia (Algorithm 53.2). Confounders should be excluded, usually with head CT
rule out hydrocephalus, new bleeding, or cerebral edema. Metabolic derangemen
including hyponatremia, fever, hypoxemia or hypercapnia, and seizures can also cau
neurological worsening and should be excluded. If ischemia remains suspected, the
hemodynamic augmentation to raise cerebral perfusion should be initiated. So-calle
"Triple H" therapy (hypervolemia, hypertension, hemodilution) is instituted with
fluid bolus and vasopressors titrated to raise MAP 10% to 15% above the patien

ALGORITHM 53.2 Management of Complications After Subarachnoid Hemorrhage

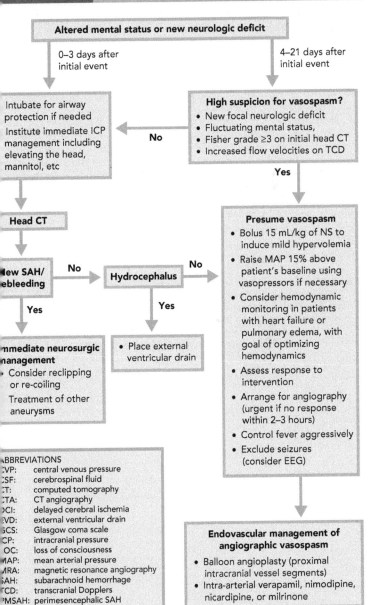

Altered mental status or new neurologic deficit

0–3 days after initial event

4–21 days after initial event

High suspicion for vasospasm?
- New focal neurologic deficit
- Fluctuating mental status,
- Fisher grade ≥3 on initial head CT
- Increased flow velocities on TCD

No

Intubate for airway protection if needed

Institute immediate ICP management including elevating the head, mannitol, etc

Yes

Head CT

New SAH/rebleeding

No → Hydrocephalus **No** →

Yes

Immediate neurosurgic management
- Consider reclipping or re-coiling
- Treatment of other aneurysms

Yes

- Place external ventricular drain

Presume vasospasm
- Bolus 15 mL/kg of NS to induce mild hypervolemia
- Raise MAP 15% above patient's baseline using vasopressors if necessary
- Consider hemodynamic monitoring in patients with heart failure or pulmonary edema, with goal of optimizing hemodynamics
- Assess response to intervention
- Arrange for angiography (urgent if no response within 2–3 hours)
- Control fever aggressively
- Exclude seizures (consider EEG)

ABBREVIATIONS

CVP: central venous pressure
CSF: cerebrospinal fluid
CT: computed tomography
CTA: CT angiography
DCI: delayed cerebral ischemia
EVD: external ventricular drain
GCS: Glasgow coma scale
ICP: intracranial pressure
LOC: loss of consciousness
MAP: mean arterial pressure
MRA: magnetic resonance angiography
SAH: subarachnoid hemorrhage
TCD: transcranial Dopplers
PMSAH: perimesencephalic SAH

Endovascular management of angiographic vasospasm
- Balloon angioplasty (proximal intracranial vessel segments)
- Intra-arterial verapamil, nimodipine, nicardipine, or milrinone

baseline. Hemodilution is generally avoided unless polycythemia is present. In c
of cardiac failure, inotropic support may be helpful in reversing neurological defi
Noninvasive cardiac monitoring may be helpful to optimizing hemodynamics (
diac index, stroke volume, and pulse pressure variability). Patients with suspe
ischemia should undergo angiography to evaluate for vasospasm (further confirn
the clinical diagnosis). While CT angiography (sometimes with CT perfusion)
be used to screen for vasospasm and hypoperfusion, angiography allows endovasc
therapies to be administered, including intra-arterial injections of vasodilators (
verapamil, nimodipine, nicardipine, milrinone) and balloon angioplasty of access
proximal arterial segments. While vasodilators usually only offer transient relie
arterial narrowing, angioplasty more durably reverses vasospasm.

Hemodynamic augmentation should be titrated to clinical effect (i.e., reve
of new/worsening deficits) rather than a specific blood pressure target. High d
of vasopressors may be required for induced hypertension. Close observation
complications from this therapy (e.g., pulmonary edema, arrhythmias, cardiac inj
worsening cerebral edema or hemorrhagic transformation of an established infa
hypertensive encephalopathy) is mandatory. Once clinical response is achieved,
goal MAP should be maintained for at least 48 to 72 hours before cautious
gradual weaning of MAP and vasopressors is attempted. Improvement on a rep
angiogram may be helpful in guiding when to wean therapy in more complex ca

SUGGESTED READINGS

Connoly ES Jr, Rabinstein AA, Carhuapoma JR, et al. Guidelines for the management of a
rysmal subarachnoid hemorrhage. *Stroke*. 2012;43:1711–1737.
Diringer MN, Bleck TP, Hemphill CJ, et al. Critical care management of patients follov
aneurysmal subarachnoid hemorrhage: recommendations from the neurocritical
society's multidisciplinary consensus conference. *Neurocrit Care*. 2011;15:211–240.
Keyrouz SG, Diringer MN. Clinical review: prevention and therapy of vasospasm in subarachn
hemorrhage. *Crit Care*. 2007;11:220. Available online at http://ccforum.com/cont
11/4/220
Suarez J, Tarr RW, Selman WR. Aneurysmal subarachnoid hemorrhage. *N Engl J Med*. 2006;:
387–396.

54 Intracerebral Hemorrhage

Tobias B. Kulik and Salah G. Keyrouz

racerebral hemorrhage (ICH) is a focal collection of blood within the brain paren-
yma with potential extension into adjacent brain compartments (ventricles, sub-
chnoid, or subdural space). The overall incidence of ICH is estimated at 24.6 cases
r 100,000 person-years. It is the second most common stroke subtype accounting
10% to 15% of all strokes with a higher proportion in the African-American and
ian population. The case fatality rate reaches 40% at 1 month and 54% at 1 year.
ly 12% to 39% of patients achieve long-term functional independence.

ICH is a heterogeneous group of conditions and can be divided into primary
d secondary ICH (Table 54.1). The two most common causes of ICH are hyper-
sion and cerebral amyloid angiopathy. Chronic arterial hypertension leads to a
sculopathy (lipohyalinosis) involving the lenticulostriate arteries arising from the
ddle cerebral artery, the small thalamic arteries branching off the posterior com-
nicating and posterior cerebral arteries, as well as pontine perforators originating
m the basilar artery. Therefore, hypertensive hemorrhages are usually found in the
ep gray matter (basal ganglia and thalamus), pons, or cerebellum (Fig. 54.1). Cere-
al amyloid angiopathy results from deposition of amyloid-β peptide in the walls of
all- to medium-sized leptomeningeal and cortical vessels. It typically affects older
dividuals, and leads to cortical-subcortical (lobar) hemorrhages. Anticoagulation
ses the risk and severity of ICH and rebleeding in any of these settings.

LINICAL PRESENTATION

ne presenting symptoms of ICH are nonspecific and include the tetrad of headache,
ered level of consciousness, nausea, vomiting, and focal neurologic symptoms
cording to the anatomic distribution of the hematoma. Symptom onset can be
sidious or abrupt depending on the underlying etiology. Headaches are seen in
) to 30% of patients. Nausea and vomiting are frequently observed in posterior
ssa ICH due to vestibular dysfunction or hemorrhage into the fourth ventricle.
onetheless, it can also herald increased intracranial pressure (ICP) in supratentorial
emorrhages. The majority of patients present with depressed level of consciousness.
izures, focal in two third and generalized tonic-clonic in one third, are associated
ith cortical involvement. Progressive clinical deterioration is common and patients
ould initially be cared for in an intensive care setting. Early hematoma growth,
en in the absence of a coagulopathy, is mostly observed within 3 to 4 hours but
n be seen up to 20 hours after hemorrhage onset. Hematoma expansion has been
sociated with clinical deterioration and affects approximately one third of patients.

TABLE 54.1	Etiologies of Intracranial Hemorrhage	
Primary ICH	Clues to the Etiology	Imaging Findings
Hypertension	History of and stigmata of hypertension	Typical locations: Basal ganglia (55%), thalamus (26%), cerebral hemispheres (11%), pons (8%), cerebellum (7%)
Cerebral amyloid angiopathy	Older age, history of cognitive impairment, prior TIA or prior ICH	Superficial, lobar distribution; lobulated appearance, rupture into subarachnoid or subdural spaces, secondary IVH; more frequent in temporal and occipital regions; less common in cerebellum; spares deep hemispheric structures and brainstem; "microbleeds" on MRI (gradient echo, T2* weighted sequences)
Sympathomimetic drug use, for example • Cocaine • Methamphetamine • Pseudoephedrine	Younger age, history of use of said drugs	More frequent subcortical pattern and IVH
Coagulopathy	History of anticoagulant use	Lobulated, fluid—fluid levels within hematoma
Secondary ICH		
Vascular malformations • Arteriovenous malformations • Cavernous malformations • Saccular aneurysm • Mycotic aneurysm Dural arteriovenous fistula	Younger patients (<45 years), normotensive, family history, prior seizure or hemorrhage in same brain region	CT-A or DSA with typical findings
Moyamoya	African-American, Asian, sickle cell disease. Might also result in cerebral infarcts, IVH, or SAH	Puff of smoke on DSA
Hemorrhagic conversion of ischemic stroke	Prior ischemic stroke; the latter and the deficits it caused could have gone unnoticed, until the hemorrhagic conversion.	Petechial hemorrhages, patchy, scattered throughout the infarcted tissue. An outline of the infarct is often easy to delineate on CT.

BLE 54.1	Etiologies of Intracranial Hemorrhage (*Continued*)	
:ondary ICH	Clues to the Etiology	Imaging Findings
:ebral sinus venous rombosis	Eclampsia, pregnancy	Noncontrast CT with hyperdensity of sinus, CT venogram, or MR venogram with filling defect in cerebral sinus
:ebral vasculitis	Young individual, history of headache	Nonspecific findings. Infarcts and white matter disease in multiple brain regions.
nor	Known primary tumor, prior hemorrhage in same territory	Significant edema surrounding acute hemorrhage, contrast enhancement contiguous to acute hematoma.

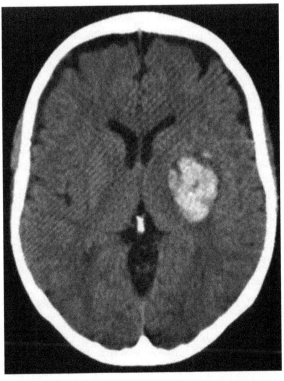

ıre 54.1. Hypertensive ICH. Acute left putaminal intracerebral hemorrhage; axial, noncontrasted head CT.

ICH causes damage to brain parenchyma through several mechanisms. expanding hematoma dissects neuronal pathways and brain tissue. Blood and its radation products are highly toxic and can contribute to seizures, electrolyte dera ments, fever, and autonomic changes. A recently ruptured vessel is also pro rebleeding. Finally, elevated ICP due to the hematoma and subsequent edema damage other areas of the brain and result in herniation.

DIAGNOSIS

Patients with suspected intracranial hemorrhage should receive an expedited ne logical assessment and workup. A brief medical history should be obtained, foc on a prior history of anticoagulant use, illicit drug use, recent head trauma, a history of prior hemorrhage or stroke. Noncontrast head CT is the most rapid readily available tool to establish the diagnosis of ICH. Within the first week, has a high sensitivity (89%) and specificity (100%) for acute ICH. It allows fo anatomic localization of the hematoma and possible extension into the ventri system and the estimation of hematoma volume. A "spot sign" may be visua with the addition of contrast. It represents active contrast extravasation into hematoma and has been associated with hematoma expansion in 60% of patien CT-angiogram performed with contrast during the acute phase has an overall sens ity of 97% and specificity of 98.9% for causal vascular abnormalities, compared digital subtraction angiography (DSA) as a gold standard (Algorithm 54.1).

MANAGEMENT

Any patient with suspected ICH constitutes a neurological emergency and due significant risk for early deterioration and cardiorespiratory compromise shoul medically stabilized in an expedited fashion before diagnostic imaging is initiate

Airway

The initial management includes a brief assessment of the patient's ability to pr their own airway. In a setting of impaired arousal with concomitant risk of aspirat hypoxemia, and hypercarbia, rapid sequence intubation should be undertaken ventilator support initiated. Given concerns for transient elevations of intracr pressure during laryngoscopy and associated worsening of mass effect, induc agents should be chosen that minimize side effect. Pretreatment with lidoc (1.5 mg/kg) 2 to 3 minutes prior to intubation is felt to mitigate the rise in intr nial pressure. Etomidate is thought to have the least impact on blood pressure ar a preferred induction agent baring any contraindications.

Blood Pressure Management

Extreme increases in blood pressure in the immediate period after ICH are thou to raise the risk of early neurologic deterioration and contribute to hemat expansion. However, sound scientific evidence proving reduced hematoma volu with aggressive blood pressure management is lacking. The results of the Inten Blood Pressure Reduction in Acute Cerebral Hemorrhage Trial 2 (INTERAC demonstrated that patients randomized to early intensive lowering of blood p sure to a target SBP less than 140 mm Hg (compared to an SBP of 180 mm had no difference in death or major disability at 90 days, but significantly be

ALGORITHM 54.1 Approach to the Patient With Suspected ICH

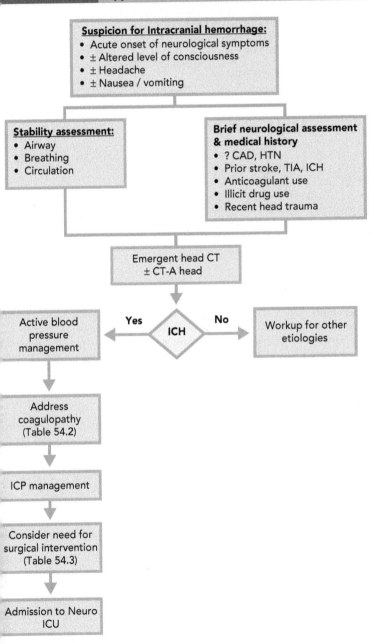

Suspicion for Intracranial hemorrhage:
- Acute onset of neurological symptoms
- ± Altered level of consciousness
- ± Headache
- ± Nausea / vomiting

Stability assessment:
- Airway
- Breathing
- Circulation

Brief neurological assessment & medical history
- ? CAD, HTN
- Prior stroke, TIA, ICH
- Anticoagulant use
- Illicit drug use
- Recent head trauma

Emergent head CT
± CT-A head

ICH

Yes → Active blood pressure management

No → Workup for other etiologies

Active blood pressure management →
Address coagulopathy (Table 54.2) →
ICP management →
Consider need for surgical intervention (Table 54.3) →
Admission to Neuro ICU

TABLE 54.2 Stabilizing Coagulation Status After Intracerebral Hemorrha

- Discontinue all antiplatelet and anticoagulant medications.
- Reverse anticoagulation or correct coagulopathy:
  - Vitamin K 10 mg IV or enterally daily for 3 days
  - Fresh-frozen plasma 15–20 mL/kg
  - Prothrombin complex concentrate (PCC) for urgent surgical procedure or with risk for volume overload):
    - INR 2–3.9: 25 units/kg (max 2,500 units)
    - INR 4–6: 35 units/kg (max 3,500 units)
    - INR >6: 50 units/kg (max 5,000 units)
  - Platelet and coagulation factor replacement as needed for thrombocytopenia and coagulation factor deficiency, respectively
- LMWH (last dose < 8 hr ago): Protamine 1 mg/100 anti-Xa units (max 50 mg)
- Pradaxa: Idarucizumab (Praxbind) 5 g once
- Apixaban and Rivaroxaban:
  - Consider activated charcoal if last dose less than 3 hr
  - Consider PCC 50 units/kg (max. 5,000 units)
- Follow coagulation panel frequently, keep corrected for 24–48 hr

IV, intravenous.

modified 90-day Rankin scores. It appears safe to acutely lower blood pressure a target SBP of 140 mm Hg or MAP <110 mm Hg to prevent ongoing damage other organs (heart or kidneys) and maximize patient outcomes as no adverse eff on perihematomal cerebral blood flow has been demonstrated. Common dru used are short-acting and titrated rapidly, for example intravenous beta-block or calcium channel blockers. Nitrates are avoided because of the risk of cereb vasodilatation with worsening edema. Addressing pain may also help to contr elevated BP.

Coagulopathy

All anticoagulants and antiplatelet agents should be stopped immediately. Existi guidelines emphasize the rapid correction of coagulopathy in patients with intrac nial hemorrhage (Table 54.2). Options for correction of warfarin-induced coagulo athy include fresh frozen plasma (FFP), prothrombin complex concentrates (PCC) recombinant activated factor VIIa (rFVIIa). If available, PCC are generally preferr over FFP. They can be administered more rapidly, correct the coagulopathy fast and require less volume of infusion. rFVIIa is not recommended as a sole agent f warfarin reversal as it may normalize the international normalized ratio (INR) b not completely correct the coagulopathy. Patients using warfarin should in additi receive vitamin K. Optimal reversal of coagulopathy associated with newer oral an coagulants remains unclear. PCC can be given for Rivaroxaban (Xarelto), Apixab (Eliquis), or Edoxaban (Savaysa), however, they are more likely to partially reverse t coagulopathy. More recently, a monoclonal antibody (Idarucizumab, Praxbind) h become available for the rapid and reliable reversal of Dabigatran (Pradaxa). Despi lack of scientific evidence, some transfuse platelets in patients with prior use of clop dogrel (Plavix) or aspirin presenting with ICH.

BLE 54.3	Indications for Neurosurgical Intervention After Intracerebral Hemorrhage

osterior fossa or temporal lobe hemorrhage >3 cm
CH causing hydrocephalus or brainstem compression
ydrocephalus or IVH requiring EVD
Complicated cases requiring ICP monitoring

intracerebral hemorrhage; EVD, external ventricular drain; IVH, intraventricular hemorrhage; intracranial pressure.

triculostomy and ICP Management

drocephalus complicates up to 50% of ICH cases, and is associated with younger lower Glasgow Coma Scale score, deep hemorrhages, intubation, and mortality. In ents with decreased level of consciousness (Glasgow Coma Scale score ≤8), clinical ence of cerebral herniation, or those with significant intraventicular hemorrhage H) or hydrocephalus, monitoring of intracranial pressure with a ventricular or paren- mal catheter should be considered. ICP greater than 20 mm Hg was seen in 70% atients in one retrospective study and was most common in young patients with atentorial hemorrhage. Increased ICP can be treated with hyperosmolar therapy, for nple mannitol or hypertonic saline, cerebrospinal fluid diversion via ventriculostomy, ition, or therapeutic hypothermia (see ICP treatment Algorithm 60.1 in Chapter 60).

zures

e primary neuronal damage and blood degradation products increase seizure risk r ICH. Seizures occur in 5% to 15% of these patients, usually in the first few days ospitalization. Prophylactic anticonvulsant therapy is not indicated in ICH. In ents with depressed mental status out of proportion to the degree of brain injury, tinuous electroencephalography should be considered. Patients with clinical ures and those with mental status changes and electrographic seizures should be ted with anticonvulsant drugs.

urosurgical Intervention

patients with cerebellar hemorrhage who are deteriorating neurologically or who e brainstem compression and/or hydrocephalus from ventricular obstruction, surgical oval of the hemorrhage is recommended as soon as possible (Table 54.3). In most er cases of ICH, the utility of surgical evacuation remains controversial. For patients h supratentorial lobar hemorrhage >30 mL and within 1 cm of the surface, evacuation tandard craniotomy may be considered, although strong evidence is lacking (Fig. 54.2).

ver

er after ICH is common and should be treated aggressively given an independent ciation with poor outcome. Sustained temperature elevations greater than 38.5°C uld be treated with acetaminophen, chilled saline infusions, and cooling blankets. ncurrently, a thorough search for a potential source of infection should be started. the case of medically refractory fever, consideration should be paid to initiate face, or endovascular cooling with heat exchange catheters. Fever of central origin diagnosis of exclusions but can be seen more frequently with intraventricular ension of hemorrhage and hemorrhages in the pons.

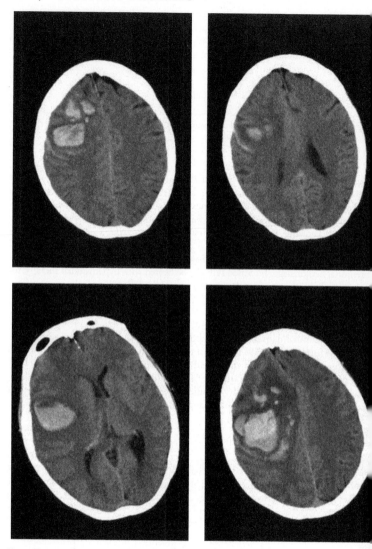

Figure 54.2. CAA-related intracranial hemorrhage. Lobar hemorrhage due to cerebral amyloid angiopathy. panel: admission noncontrasted, axial head CT; Bottom panel: axial, noncontrasted head CT 4.5 hours lat

General Care

Patients with ICH, like all critically ill patients, are at risk for a myriad of comp cations including myocardial infarctions, heart failure with pulmonary edema, d vein thrombosis (DVT), aspiration pneumonia, urinary tract infections, press ulcers, and orthopedic complications (contractures etc.). Sequential compress

ices in addition to elastic stockings should be used on admission, and subcuta-
ous low–molecular-weight heparin or unfractionated heparin for DVT prophy-
is can be started after 48 hours if there is no evidence of hematoma expansion.
ontaneous lobar ICH in particular carries a relatively high risk of recurrence, thus
idance of long-term anticoagulation for nonvalvular atrial fibrillation in these
ients is recommended. In the presence of a clear indication for anticoagulation
., mechanical heart valve) or antiplatelet therapy (i.e., coronary artery stents), it is
sonable to restart anticoagulation in nonlobar ICH in 2 to 4 weeks and antiplatelet
rapy in all ICH, 1 to 2 weeks after documentation of cessation of bleeding.

ROGNOSIS

spite recent advances in the care of ischemic strokes with subsequent improved
tcomes, ICH remains one of the acute neurological disorders with the worst prog-
sis; case fatality rates reach 40% at 1 month and 54% at 1 year, and only 12% to
% of patients achieve long-term functional independence. Glasgow Coma Score,
matoma volume, intraventricular extension, infratentorial origin, and advanced
e form the basis of the ICH score, a frequently used, validated grading scale for
k stratification of patients upon presentation (Table 54.4). Hematoma volume in

ABLE 54.4	ICH Score
H Score Component	Points
CS score	
3–4	2
5–12	1
13–15	0
H volume, cm^3	
>30	1
<30	0
traventricular hemorrhage	
Yes	1
No	0
fratentorial origin	
Yes	1
No	0
ge, years	
>80	1
<80	0
otal ICH score (0–6):	30-day mortality:
0	• 0%
1	• 13%
2	• 26%
3	• 72%
4	• 97%
5	• 100%

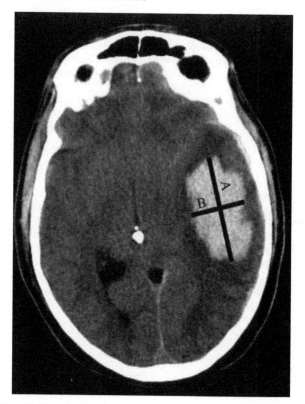

Figure 54.3. ABC/2 formula for calculation of hematoma volume. Estimation of hematoma volume usi the ABC/2 method (A, maximum diameter of hematoma on the reference axial slice with the largest area hematoma; B, maximum hematoma diameter perpendicular to A; and C (not depicted), the number of sli in the vertical plane with visible hematoma multiplied by slice thickness (typically 0.5 cm); the hemato volume in milliliters is (A*B*C*0.5 cm)/2.

milliliters is reliably approximated using the ABC/2 method (Fig. 54.3): A represen the largest hematoma diameter on axial head CT, B the largest diameter perpendi ular to A, and C the approximate number of CT slices with hemorrhage multipli by slice thickness (usually 0.5 cm). The total is divided by 2.

SUGGESTED READINGS

Anderson CS, Heeley E, Huang Y, et al. Rapid blood-pressure lowering in patients with acu intracerebral hemorrhage. *N Engl J Med.* 2013;368:2355–2365.

Hemphill JC 3rd, Bonovich DC, Besmertis L, et al. The ICH score: a simple, reliable, gradi scale for intracerebral hemorrhage. *Stroke.* 2001;23(4):891–897.

Hemphill JC 3rd, Greenberg SM, Anderson CS, et al.; Guidelines for the management of spo taneous intracerebral hemorrhage: a guideline for healthcare professionals from the Ame can Heart Association/American Stroke Association. *Stroke.* 2015;46;2032–2060.

55 Coma

Baback Arshi

...na is a persistent state of unresponsiveness. Key findings include closed eyes and ...xive responses to external stimuli. Coma typically arises from injury to bilat-...cerebral hemispheres, bilateral thalami, or brainstem injury at the level of the ...nding reticular activating system. Conditions that mimic coma include brain ...h and hypersomnia. In contrast, unresponsive states with open eyes include ...istent vegetative state, minimally conscious state, locked-in syndrome, abulia, ...akinetic mutism. Differentiating between coma and these other diagnoses has ...nostic implications as well as management differences. Confounders when eval-...ng the comatose patient include eyelid apraxia (eyelid opening impairment) and ...sedation.

...CALIZATION OF COMA

...na occurs as a result of injury to bilateral cerebral hemispheres, diencephalon ...ateral thalamus), or ascending reticular activating system (midbrain and pons). ...ry may occur as a result of structural lesions, toxic ingestion, metabolic encepha-...thies, or infectious diseases (Table 55.1).

...proach to Coma

...mination of the comatose patient is crucial for diagnosis and prognosis. Coma ...mination should begin with observation of the patient in their undisturbed state ...le taking note of any interactions with the environment. Initial examination should ...ays focus on level of consciousness. If the patient is not awake at baseline, begin ...ssment of level of consciousness initially with verbal cues and subsequently with ...ile stimulus. If there is no response to verbal cues and tactile stimuli, then assess ...onse to noxious stimuli (sternal rub, supraorbital pressure, nail bed pressure). If ...patient does not respond during the examination and the eyes remain closed, ...patient is in a coma.

Further examination should focus on brainstem reflexes and motor responses. ...mination of the brainstem reflexes cues the examiner to focal injury at the level of ...midbrain, pons, or medulla. Examination should consist of testing the pupillary ...t reflex (assesses CN II, III), oculocephalic reflex (CN III, VI, and VIII), corneal ...ex (CN V, VII), and cough and gag reflex (CN IX and X). Motor response should ...aimed at assessing voluntary versus involuntary motor activity. In the comatose ...ient motor examination can be assessed with noxious stimulus. Fold the arms ...the patient's lap and administer a noxious stimulus. Differing responses include

TABLE 55.1	Causes of Coma

Drugs/Toxins

Opiates, alcohol, sedatives, amphetamines, barbiturates, tranquilizers, bromide salicylates, acetaminophen, lithium, anticholinergics, lead, methanol, ethylene glycol, carbon monoxide, arsenic

Metabolic

Anoxia or hypoxia, hypercapnia, hypotension, hypoglycemia, hyperglycemia, diabetic ketoacidosis, hypernatremia, hyponatremia, hypercalcemia, hypocalcem hypermagnesemia, hypothermia, hyperthermia, Wernicke's encephalopathy, hepatic failure, uremia, adrenal insufficiency, myxedema

Infectious/Inflammatory

Bacterial, viral, or fungal meningitis/meningoencephalitis, acute disseminated encephalomyelitis, sepsis, malaria, Waterhouse–Friderichsen syndrome

Structural brain lesions

Subarachnoid hemorrhage, intraparenchymal hemorrhage, ischemic strokes, global cerebral hypoperfusion, cerebral venous sinus thrombosis, traumatic bra injury, hydrocephalus, basilar occlusion, central pontine myelinolysis, large her spheric masses, pituitary apoplexy, cerebral abscess, or multifocal infection

Other

Nonconvulsive status epilepticus, catatonia, hypertensive encephalopathy, heat stroke, psychogenic coma

localization, withdrawal, flexor posturing, and extensor posturing. Care shoul taken to note laterality. These findings will allow calculation of the Glasgow c scale or FOUR score (Tables 55.2 and 55.3). When possible, the examiner may assess tone, muscle bulk, and reflexes in the coma patient to aid with localizatio

Diagnostic Studies in Coma

Initial screening of the coma patient should be geared towards examination diagnostics. During assessment in the emergency room, workup should include (glucose, sodium, calcium), drug screen, and imaging. Noncontrast head CT she be first line for imaging for all newly found coma patients. Advanced imaging s as MRI or angiography can be completed after the patient is stabilized. If labora data and imaging are negative, electroencephalography can be considered to eval for nonconvulsive seizures or lumbar puncture to evaluate for infectious or infl matory causes of coma.

Stabilization of the Coma Patient

Stabilization of the coma patient should occur in tandem with diagnostics. W care should be taken to maintain ABCs, the patient with GCS <8 may not necessa require endotracheal intubation. Airway protection refers to maintenance of a pa passage of air from the mouth and nose to the lungs. Many comatose patients are to maintain gas exchange without requiring invasive endotracheal intubation. W deciding whether to intubate the comatose patient, consider other factors prio intubation including bulbar function, cough, and secretions. Other efforts to prevent intubation include bronchial hygiene such as elevation of the head of

TABLE 55.2	Glasgow Coma Scale (GCS)

Test eye opening

Spontaneous	4
With voice only	3
With pain only	2
None at all	1

Test verbal response

Coherent speech	5
Confused intelligible speech	4
Inappropriate words	3
Incomprehensible sounds	2
No verbal output	1

Test motor response

Follows commands	6
Localizes pain stimuli[a]	5
Withdraws to pain stimuli	4
Decorticate posturing	3
Decerebrate posturing	2
No movements at all	1

Localizing pain stimuli refers to gaze deviation, head turning, or hand movements toward the stimulus.

TABLE 55.3	Full Outline of UnResponsiveness (FOUR) Score

Eye response

Eyelid open or opened, tracking, or blinking to command	4
Eyelids open but not tracking	3
Eyelids closed but open to loud voice	2
Eyelids closed but open to pain	1
Eyelids remain closed with pain	0

Motor response

Thumbs-up fist or peace sign	4
Localizing to pain	3
Flexion response to pain	2
Extension response to pain	1
No response to pain or generalized myoclonus status	0

Brainstem reflexes

Pupil and corneal reflexes present	4
One pupil wide and fixed	3
Pupil or corneal reflexes are absent	2
Pupils and corneal reflexes absent	1
Absent pupil, corneal, and cough reflex	0

Respiration

Not intubated, regular breathing pattern	4
Not intubated, Cheyne–Stokes breathing pattern	3
Not intubated, irregular breathing	2
Breathes above ventilator rate	1
Breathes at ventilator rate or apnea	0

ALGORITHM 55.1 Prognosis of Coma Following Anoxic Brain Injury

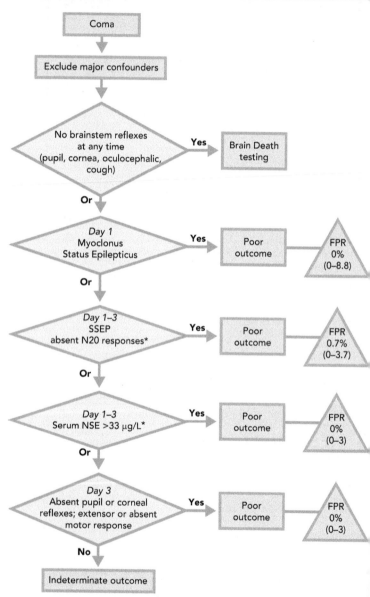

Adapted from Wijdicks (2006). FPR refers to false positives at each clinical day with associated 95% CI in parentheses. Major confounders include use of sedatives, neuromuscular blockers, or hypothermia.

strategic suctioning, and cough assist, which can be used in the coma patient
duce cough, clear secretions, and prevent atelectasis. When intubating the coma
ent, pharmacologic assistance including sedation and analgesia are indicated. Do
assume that the patient cannot sense pain because they are not awake. Use anal-
and sedation, in particular when paralyzing this group of patients.

In addition to basic life-saving treatments, the coma patient often requires other
agement strategies. If history is unobtainable, C-spine precautions should be
n. In particular, with signs of other traumatic injuries such as bruising or frac-
s, C-spine protection with a C-collar should be performed. A nasogastric tube
be necessary both for aspirating gastric contents in the coma patient and for
entation. Exclude and treat hypoglycemia and opiate overdose. Physicians or
ses should perform neurologic examinations frequently. Hourly neurologic checks
be indicated in the acute setting.

OGNOSIS

gnosis of the coma patient depends upon the etiology of coma. Infectious, toxic,
metabolic causes of coma can be reversible and may carry a favorable progno-
Conversely coma from hypoxia depends on the associated neurologic findings
orithm 55.1). In contrast, brain death carries a uniformly fatal prognosis, and
e have been no cases of brain death reversal reported in the literature. Persistent
tative states typically occur after anoxic brain injury. Persistent vegetative state
nes a state of wakefulness without awareness. Minimally conscious state represents
ss severe form of persistent vegetative states where patients may be aware of the
ronment or themselves but with significantly impaired interaction with their
ronment. Prognosis for minimally conscious state is better than for persistent
tative state but overall prognosis for both is poor.

GGESTED READINGS

DE, Caronna JJ, Singer BH, et al. Predicting outcome from hypoxic-ischemic coma.
JAMA. 1985;253:1420–1426.
*Early observational study evaluating prognosis in postanoxic coma including an algorithm for
predicting outcomes based on exam findings.*

er JB, Saper CB, Schiff ND, et al. *Plum and Posner's Diagnosis of Stupor and Coma.* 4th ed.
Oxford: Oxford University Press; 2007.
Comprehensive textbook about coma.

dicks EF, Hijdra A, Young GB, et al. Practice parameter: prediction of outcome in comatose survivors after cardiopulmonary resuscitation (an evidence-based review): report of
the Quality Standards Subcommittee of the American Academy of Neurology. *Neurology.*
2006;67:203–210.
*Concise review about the current approach to postanoxic coma and an algorithm for predicting
outcomes with current diagnostics.*

56 Declaration of Brain Death

Rajat Dhar

THE CONCEPT OF BRAIN DEATH

Death may be legally determined based on the complete absence of either all car
respiratory or cerebral activity. The latter (i.e., brain death) emerged as an import
distinct concept with the advent of intensive care and artificial ventilation in
1950s and was first formally delineated in the 1960s. Brain death is defined in
United States as the irreversible cessation of all brain functions, including the br
stem. The specific laws and policies governing determination of death by neurolog
criteria vary among countries, states, and different medical institutions, albeit ba
on this overarching concept. The person is declared dead at the time that final de
mination of brain death has been made. Although declaration does not require c
sent of the family or surrogate decision-makers, it is always preferable to explain
concept and process explicitly at all stages of testing. Physicians should be sensi
to both religious and ethnic perspectives of the family while allowing them time
process an often sudden catastrophic loss.

DIAGNOSING BRAIN DEATH

In essence, brain death comprises irreversible coma of a known etiology accompan
by absence of all brainstem reflexes and respiratory drive. It may result from a var
of severe brain injuries, most commonly cerebral trauma, hemorrhage (subarachnc
subdural, or intracerebral), and hypoxic-ischemic injury after cardiac arrest or d
overdose. Cerebral edema with raised intracranial pressure resulting from large br
tumors, meningitis/encephalitis, hydrocephalus, or fulminant liver failure may a
progress to brain death. The particular etiology for coma should be known in ea
patient (from history or with adjunctive brain imaging) and brain death sho
never be diagnosed without a clear cause capable of inducing the observed degree
cerebral dysfunction. Any confounders must be carefully excluded, chief among th
hypothermia and drug intoxication. Overdose of a variety of medications (includ
barbiturates, tricyclic antidepressants, baclofen, and lidocaine) can mimic a bra
dead state with coma and absent brainstem reflexes. The metabolic milieu must a
be normalized as much as possible to avoid confounding from systemic disturbar
including hypoglycemia, hypotension, severe electrolyte imbalances, or acid–base c
orders that could result in cerebral dysfunction. Any deep sedation or neuromuscu
blockade must have been allowed to wear off before testing (the latter can be tes
by train-of-four stimulation). Patients in a locked-in state from lesions in the vent

ts may appear unresponsive, are unable to move to stimulation, and lack some
instem function, but on closer testing are able to respond (with vertical eye move-
nts or blinking) and have reactive electroencephalography (EEG); a somewhat
ilar picture may be seen with high cervical spine injuries. Severe Guillain–Barré
drome may induce a complete deafferented state where the patient cannot move
respond, and can even lose brainstem and respiratory functions. Careful history,
mination, and sometimes ancillary testing will exclude such confounding cases.

Once confounders have been excluded, homeostasis normalized (temperature,
ctrolytes, acid–base), and shock resuscitated, then the process of brain death test-
can begin (Algorithm 56.1). One must remember to document the temperature
d blood pressure at the time of each examination. First, an unresponsive comatose
te without motor response should be verified. Central painful stimulation (e.g.,
raorbital ridge, temporomandibular joint) should neither elicit eye opening nor
rposeful or reflexive movements (i.e., posturing of the upper extremities). There
uld be no spontaneous movements in the cranial nerve territory and no signs of
zure activity. All brainstem reflexes must then be tested on both sides to verify
nplete cessation of all brainstem function. This includes absence of midbrain func-
n by lack of pupillary constriction to bright light; pupils should be mid-position
dilated. Pontine function is assessed with corneal reflex and cold water caloric
ting of vestibular-ocular reactivity. Medullary failure is documented with lack of
ugh reflex to deep suctioning. This whole sequence of testing should be repeated
ween 1 and 24 hours after the first examination if the underlying process is still
olving. Short intervals may be appropriate in catastrophic conditions where devas-
ing injury is clearly seen on imaging and condition has been unchanged prior to
ting (new recommendations suggest one exam may be adequate in such a case).
longer duration is recommended in children and in the postcardiac arrest patient
ere imaging is usually normal and the early exam can fluctuate. Testing should also
deferred till 12 to 24 hours after rewarming from induced-hypothermia if utilized
such patients. At some institutions, only certain (qualified) personnel can perform
her all or parts of the brain death testing. In complicated cases, regardless, it is
visable to have assistance from a neurologist or neurosurgeon in the determination
death by neurologic criteria.

Clinical confirmation of complete cerebral death requires absence of spontaneous
piratory efforts despite adequate stimuli of hypercapnia and acidemia, as assessed by
e **apnea test**; the time of death is set when the patient fails to breath and a blood gas
monstrates adequate acidemia (usually pH <7.28 to 7.30) and hypercapnia ($PaCO_2$
ove 60 mm Hg and/or a rise of 20 mm Hg from baseline). Prior to performing the
nea test, the patient should receive preoxygenation for at least 10 minutes on 100%
O_2 (to minimize the risk of desaturation during testing). A baseline arterial blood
s (ABG) should be reviewed and ventilator settings adjusted to obtain a $PaCO_2$ in
e normal range (ideally 40 to 45 mm Hg) with a pH as close to normal as possible.
oper apnea testing may be impossible in significant CO_2 retainers or those who are
arkedly acidotic from metabolic derangements; ancillary testing (see later) should
en be performed in lieu. Occasionally, ventilator self-cycling may falsely suggest
e persistence of patient respiratory effort; changing from flow-triggered breaths to
essure-triggered (or a higher threshold) usually abolishes this artifact.

For apnea testing, the patient is disconnected from the ventilator and a suction
theter (with thumb-hole taped closed) attached to oxygen at a flow rate of 2 to
L/min is placed through the endotracheal tube down to the level of the carina.

ALGORITHM 56.1 Approach to Determination of Death by Neurologic Criteria

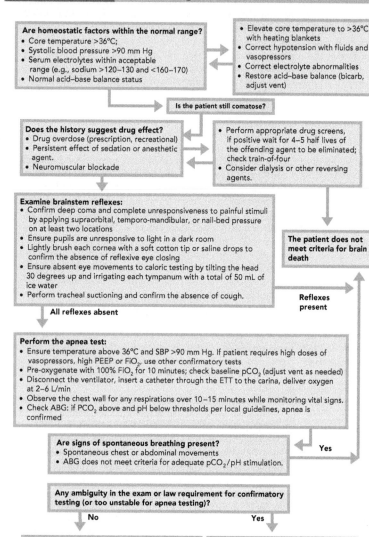

Are homeostatic factors within the normal range?
- Core temperature >36°C;
- Systolic blood pressure >90 mm Hg
- Serum electrolytes within acceptable range (e.g., sodium >120–130 and <160–170)
- Normal acid–base balance status

- Elevate core temperature to >36°C with heating blankets
- Correct hypotension with fluids and vasopressors
- Correct electrolyte abnormalities
- Restore acid–base balance (bicarb, adjust vent)

Is the patient still comatose?

Does the history suggest drug effect?
- Drug overdose (prescription, recreational)
- Persistent effect of sedation or anesthetic agent.
- Neuromuscular blockade

- Perform appropriate drug screens, if positive wait for 4–5 half lives of the offending agent to be eliminated; check train-of-four
- Consider dialysis or other reversing agents.

Examine brainstem reflexes:
- Confirm deep coma and complete unresponsiveness to painful stimuli by applying supraorbital, temporo-mandibular, or nail-bed pressure on at least two locations
- Ensure pupils are unresponsive to light in a dark room
- Lightly brush each cornea with a soft cotton tip or saline drops to confirm the absence of reflexive eye closing
- Ensure absent eye movements to caloric testing by tilting the head 30 degrees up and irrigating each tympanum with a total of 50 mL of ice water
- Perform tracheal suctioning and confirm the absence of cough.

The patient does not meet criteria for brain death

Reflexes present

All reflexes absent

Perform the apnea test:
- Ensure temperature above 36°C and SBP >90 mm Hg. If patient requires high doses of vasopressors, high PEEP or FiO₂, use other confirmatory tests
- Pre-oxygenate with 100% FiO₂ for 10 minutes; check baseline pCO₂ (adjust vent as needed)
- Disconnect the ventilator, insert a catheter through the ETT to the carina, deliver oxygen at 2–6 L/min
- Observe the chest wall for any respirations over 10–15 minutes while monitoring vital signs.
- Check ABG: if PCO₂ above and pH below thresholds per local guidelines, apnea is confirmed

Are signs of spontaneous breathing present?
- Spontaneous chest or abdominal movements
- ABG does not meet criteria for adequate pCO₂/pH stimulation.

Yes

Any ambiguity in the exam or law requirement for confirmatory testing (or too unstable for apnea testing)?

No   Yes

- Patient meets clinical criteria for brain death
- Notify organ procurement agency immediately.

Perform confirmatory testing
- Use method required by law or hospital

ABBREVIATIONS

pCO₂: partial pressure of arterial carbon dioxide
ETT: endotracheal tube
PEEP: positive end-expiratory pressure
SBP: systolic blood pressure

chest should be exposed and the patient observed for visible respiratory efforts a duration of 10 to 15 minutes (to allow adequate CO_2 retention to occur). A d gas must be obtained prior to placing the patient back on the ventilator. Many ents will become hemodynamically unstable as acidemia develops, so one must repared to titrate up any vasopressors. An arterial line can be very helpful to monitor blood pressure and draw ABGs during apnea testing. If desaturation rs then increase the flow of oxygen to 6 L/min; should the patient not tolerate ter testing (due to refractory hypotension or desaturation), then they should laced back on the ventilator and an ABG should be obtained at that time, because meets criteria for hypercapnia and acidemia and no respiratory efforts were seen, apnea test is still positive. Care should be taken not to occlude the endotracheal by the oxygen catheter (preventing air from releasing) or infusing too high a of oxygen as these may lead to air trapping and lung hyperinflation, with risk neumothorax. If acute decompensation occurs during apnea testing, look for utaneous air and consider urgent evaluation for pneumothorax. Patients who hemodynamically unstable, requiring high doses of vasopressors at baseline or e with hypoxemic respiratory failure (requiring high FiO_2 and/or positive end-ratory pressure) may not tolerate apnea testing, and rather than risk instability even cardiac arrest during the procedure; such patients may benefit from substi-1g a confirmatory test for apnea testing as discussed below.

Certain reflexive and spontaneous movements may be seen in a significant pro-ion of those declared dead by cerebral criteria. These are likely generated by spinal or generators and do not invalidate an otherwise complete and clear diagnosis of n death. Common movements include triple flexion of the lower limb (at the ankle, e, and hip), either spontaneously or in response to stimulation, and extension-nation of the arms (which can mimic decerebrate posturing). Deep tendon and ominal reflexes are often preserved. Fine jerking of the finger or toe may be erved in some cases, and rarely more complex movements are seen. The **Lazarus** , with abdominal flexion, adduction and flexion of the arms, can be extremely ling to both family and healthcare personnel present; it may also raise questions ut the correctness of the diagnosis of death. It is commonly triggered by neck ion but has also been seen with hypoxic stimulation of cervical neurons during ea testing or with hypotension. When brain perfusion scans are performed on ents with such movements, they invariably have confirmed lack of cerebral func-. Reassuring those witnessing the events is the most important part of managing se phenomena.

NFIRMATORY TESTING

dults and children above the age of 1 year, if the above sequence of clinical tests luding positive apnea test) confirms absence of all brain function, then death can ronounced without any ancillary tests. In cases where the above testing cannot be pleted, due to patient instability (for apnea testing) or impediment to full brain-n testing (e.g., eye swollen shut or missing), or in rare cases where family dissent historical ambiguity necessitates it, ancillary tests can be performed to confirm state of total brain failure (Table 56.1). Such testing must never supersede clin-examination; for example, if someone manifests respiratory effort during apnea ing, it is inappropriate to then perform a confirmatory test to negate that finding.

TABLE 56.1	Confirmatory Tests Used to Declare Brain Death		
Method	Finding	Pros	Cons
Nuclear scintigraphy	Absence of uptake (empty light bulb)	Safe Bedside	None—preferre[d] test (reliable, high specificity[)]
Cerebral angiography	No filling of intra-cranial arteries (high pressure injection)	Reliable Not affected by sedation or temperature	Requires transportation Contrast injectio[n]
EEG	Isoelectric Lack of reactivity to stimuli	Safe Bedside	Prone to artifact[s] Only test cortica[l] function Affected by sedation and hypothermia
TCD	Absence of diastolic or reverberating flow with high pulsatility index—2 studies, bilateral anterior + posterior	Safe Bedside	Requires bone windows and skilled technici[an] Absence of sign[al] not equate wit[h] brain death

EEG, electroencephalography; TCD, transcranial Doppler ultrasonography.

The most common method of confirming brain death is by demonstrati[ng] lack of effective intracranial perfusion. This can be achieved by nuclear scintigra[phy] or cerebral angiography. CT angiography and transcranial Doppler (TCD) are b[eing] tested as simpler alternatives to conventional angiography. While these are not [con]founded by sedation or metabolic disturbances, they do require stable blood pres[sure.] Alternatively, isoelectric and nonreactive EEG is often used as an ancillary test [but] may be confounded by artifacts and sedation, so is not suitable in all situations.

CARE OF THE POTENTIAL BRAIN DEAD ORGAN DONO[R]

The dead-donor rule states that the diagnosis of (brain) death is an absolute prere[qui]site for organ and tissue donation. Donation should not be discussed with the fa[mily] prior to determination of death to avoid the appearance of a conflict of interest. [The] United States and other countries, however, require physicians to contact local o[rgan] procurement agencies as soon as a patient is deemed to be a potential organ d[onor] (i.e., any patient with severe brain injury who has lost significant brainstem functi[on] even before the final confirmation of brain death. The role of the intensivist [thus] extends to stabilizing the potentially brain-dead patient to allow safe diagnostic, [and] confirmatory testing while avoiding further organ injury should the person bec[ome] an organ donor.

Important metabolic and hemodynamic derangements are commonly see[n as] a result of herniation with brain death. Sympathetic failure can trigger a stat[e]

urogenic shock with hypotension (although a transient state of hypertension and
:hycardia may occur as the patient progresses to brain death, with abrupt cate-
olamine release). Vasopressors are often required to maintain systemic perfusion
ıd only short-acting antihypertensive agents should be administered in cases of
pertension). Neurogenic pulmonary edema can occur, usually with rapid herni-
on, while cardiac injury from catecholamine excess can contribute to pulmonary
ngestion/edema. Diabetes insipidus occurs frequently and loss of excess free
ater can precipitate hypovolemia and exacerbate hypotension. If large volumes
300 mL/hr) of dilute urine output are seen (in the absence of recent mannitol
ses), especially with rising serum sodium, vasopressin agonists should be given to
op water loss. Desmopressin can be administered as a bolus of 1 to 4 μg IV or SQ
th a half-life of ~12 hours. Alternately, vasopressin 2 to 5 U can be given IV or SQ
d a vasopressin infusion is started, both to maintain blood pressure (infusion of
04 U/min or less) and prevent polyuria.

UGGESTED READINGS

otloff RM, Blosser S, Fulda GJ, et al. Management of the potential organ donor in the ICU:
    Society of Critical Care Medicine/American College of Chest Physicians/Association of
    Organ Procurement Organizations Consensus Statement. *Crit Care Med.* 2015;43:1291–
    1325.
actice parameters for determining brain death in adults (summary statement). The Quality
    Standards Subcommittee of the American Academy of Neurology. *Neurology.* 1995;45:
    1012–1014.
ijdicks EF. The diagnosis of brain death. *N Engl J Med.* 2001;344:1215–1221.
ood KE, Becker BN, McCartney JG, et al. Care of the potential organ donor. *N Engl J Med.*
    2004;351:2730–2739.

57

Sedation and Delirium in the Intensive Care Unit

Theresa Human

SEDATION

Significant advances have been made in our understanding of how to provide physical and psychological comfort for patients in the ICU. Important concepts to consider include ensuring reliable assessment tools are being used to evaluate pain, agitation and delirium and establishing goals for each. Of the available sedation assessment scales, the Riker Sedation–Agitation Scale (SAS) (Table 57.1) and Richmond Agitation Sedation Scale (RASS) (Table 57.2) are the most valid and reliable. Preventative strategies and protocol-driven dosing algorithms for pharmacologic interventions are key to keeping the patients calm, comfortable, and cooperative in their care while minimizing the doses of medications and avoiding oversedation.

Maintaining patient comfort, frequent reorientation, and optimization of the environment to maintain normal sleep–wake patterns are key interventions to reduce anxiety and agitation. Prompt identification and treatment of possible underlying causes of agitation, such as pain, hypoxemia, hypoglycemia, hypotension, fever, and alcohol or drug withdrawal, are important. Evidence from multiple randomized, controlled trials supports the use of the lowest possible level of sedation and dose of sedative for most ICU patients. Studies that compare the level of sedation demonstrate that deeper sedation is independently associated with longer duration of mechanical ventilation, longer length of ICU stay, and reduced survival. Similarly, scheduled daily interruptions of sedative infusions have also shown to contribute to using lower doses of benzodiazepine sedatives, reduce the duration of mechanical ventilation

TABLE 57.1	Riker Sedation–Agitation Scale (SAS)
7	Pulling at tube(s) or catheter(s), climbing over bed rails, striking at staff, thrashing
6	Requires restraints and frequent verbal cues, biting endotracheal tube
5	Anxious or physically agitated, calmed by verbal instructions
4	Calm, easily arousable, follows commands
3	Difficult to arouse but awakens to verbal stimuli or gentle touch; follows simple commands but drifts off again
2	Arouses to physical stimuli but does not communicate or follow commands, moves spontaneously
1	Minimal or no response to noxious stimuli, does not follow commands

BLE 57.2	Richmond Agitation–Sedation Scale (RASS)

Combative, violent, danger to staff
Pulls or removes tube(s) or catheter(s); aggressive
Frequent nonpurposeful movement, fights ventilator
Anxious, apprehensive but not aggressive
Alert and calm
Awakens to voice (eye opening/contact) >10 s
Light sedation, briefly awakens to voice (eye opening/contact) <10 s
Moderate sedation, movement or eye opening. No eye contact
Deep sedation, no response to voice, but movement or eye opening to
  physical stimulation
Unarousable, no response to voice or physical stimulation

reduce ICU length of stay. These results need to be interpreted within the pop-
ions studied and may not apply to all ICU patients; for example, patients with
acranial hypertension, severe respiratory failure, concurrent treatment with neu-
uscular blockers, and severe burns require deeper levels of sedation.

Despite the plethora of trials comparing sedative regimens, no sedative drug is
rly superior. Common agents used in the ICU include benzodiazepines, propofol,
dexmedetomidine (Table 57.3). Since the goal should be to minimize the depth
duration of sedation, short-acting agents without an active metabolite would be
ferred. In studies that compared propofol to benzodiazepines, propofol did not
uce overall mortality, but did show a reduction in the ICU length of stay. Dex-
letomidine may also have advantages over benzodiazepines, as it does not cause
iratory depression and provides some analgesia properties. When compared to
izepam and midazolam, dexmedetomidine resulted in less delirium and reduced
chanical ventilator days, but did not reduce hospital or ICU length of stay. When
pofol and dexmedetomidine were compared, no difference in time at target seda-
1 level, duration of mechanical ventilation, or ICU length of stay was noted. A
ta-analysis comparing clinical outcomes in patients sedated with a benzodiaze-
e regimen to those sedated with nonbenzodiazepine regimens, suggested a slightly
ger length of stay and longer mechanical ventilation times in patients receiving
enzodiazepine-based regimen. In general, a nonbenzodiazepine-based regimen is
ommended; however, the choice of sedative agent used should be driven by the
cific indication and sedation goal, the clinical pharmacology of the medication
luding onset and offset, medication side effect profile, and the patient's specific
hophysiology including organ function and concomitant illnesses.

LIRIUM

lirium is recognized as a frequent and serious event that may occur in critically
patients. Cognition is the most metabolically demanding process in the human
anism and is easily disturbed by systemic or neurologic pathology, medications,
he routine of ICU care. Estimates for the incidence of delirium in the ICU range
m 16% to 89%, although the diagnosis is often overlooked unless active bedside
eening is implemented. Delirium remains a clinical diagnosis, as there are no diag-
tic imaging or laboratory tests available to detect delirium. Delirium is associated

TABLE 57.3 Sedation Medications in ICU

Drug	Dose	Time to Arousal	Clinical Pearls
Midazolam (Versed)	Bolus: 1–5 mg IVP Infusion 1–10 mg/hr	Bolus: 1–2 hrs	• Reversed with Flumazenil • Active metabolite may accumulate in renal dysfunction • Arousal time prolonged with continuous infusion due to active metabolite • Can be given IV/IM/nasal/infusion • Hepatic metabolism and is a cytochrome P450 substrate • Intubation required when administering infusion
Lorazepam (Ativan)	Bolus 1–4 mg IVP Infusion 1–10 mg/hr	Bolus: 2–6 hrs	• Reversed with Flumazenil • Can be given IV/PO/PT/infusion • Intubation required when administering infusion • Propylene glycol toxicity may occur with high-dose infusion (symptoms include hypotension, bradycardia, lactic acidosis, hyperosmolality, and seizures)

Propofol (Diprivan)	20–100 mcg/kg/min	10–15 min	• Caution propofol-related infusion syndrome (PRIS)
			<u>Characteristics of PRIS</u>
			  • Metabolic acidosis
			  • Cardiac dysfunction
			  • Hyperlipidemia
			  • Hyperkalemia
			  • Rhabdomyolysis
			  • Hypertriglyceridemia
			  • Renal failure
			<u>Risk factors for development of PRIS</u>
			  • Increased doses (>80 mcg/kg/min)
			  • Prolonged infusion (>48 hrs)
			  • Low BMI
			  • Younger age
			  • Concurrent vasopressors use
			• Dose-limiting ADR: hypotension
			• In a 10% lipid emulsion and provides 1.1 kcal/mL
			• May cause hypertriglyceridemia

Dexmedetomidine (Precedex)	0.1–1.5 mg/kg/hr	6–10 min	• Does not cause respiratory depression • Does not achieve deep levels of sedation • Avoid bolus due to hypotension • Dose-limiting ADR: hypotension, bradycardia

		Time to	
ABLE 57.3	**Sedation Medications in ICU (Continued)**		
rug	Dose	Arousal	Clinical Pearls
etamine	2 mg/kg IV bolus 0.5–3 mg/kg/hr infusion	5–10 min	• Does not inhibit pharyngeal or laryngeal protective reflexes—No respiratory depression • May be beneficial for wheezing secondary to bronchospasm • May cause hypertension, tachycardia, hypersalivation • Patients may experience reemergence hallucinations, which may be treated with low-dose benzodiazepines

intravenous; IM, intramuscular; PT, per tube; BMI, body mass index; ADR, adverse drug reaction.

th higher rates of mortality, increased ICU and hospital length of stay, increase cost care, and a risk of permanent cognitive disability.

Delirium is defined as an *acute* change in global cognitive function affecting ention, arousal, orientation, or perception. The course is usually fluctuating and mptoms often worsen at night. Knowing a patient's baseline cognitive ability is ential, as delirium must be distinguished from dementia (a chronic problem of paired cognition) and neurologic emergencies (cerebral herniation) producing acutely decreased level of alertness. Risk factors for delirium can be found in ble 57.4. There are three types of delirium: hypoactive, hyperactive, and mixed. tients with hyperactive delirium may be loud, agitated, and/or combative, eliciting a high degree of attention from staff. They often require medical and physical straints. Although hypoactive delirium is more common, particularly among the lerly, it tends to be overlooked and underdiagnosed. These patients may be quiet sleepy yet profoundly confused and disoriented. Mixed delirium occurs when tients fluctuate between hyperactive and hypoactive delirium and is the most common type of delirium. Monitoring for all types of delirium should be routine in all Us; regardless of the type of delirium, the etiology is often the same. Patients with poactive delirium are least likely to survive, but those who do survive may have tter long-term function than those with agitated or mixed delirium.

Routine bedside monitoring of all ICU patients for delirium is recommended. he confusion assessment method for the ICU (CAM-ICU) (Algorithm 57.1) and e intensive care delirium screening checklist (ICDSC) (Fig. 57.1) are the most valid

ABLE 57.4	**Risk Factors for Delirium in the ICU**

re-existing dementia or cognitive impairment
istory of alcohol or drug abuse
istory of hypertension
igh severity of illness on admission
edative-induced and multifactorial coma
ge (data is variable)

ALGORITHM 57.1 Confusion Assessment Method for the ICU (CAM-ICU) Flowsheet

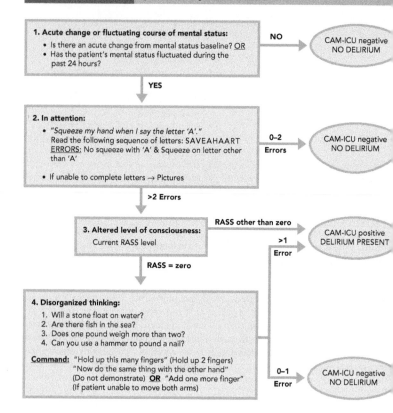

and reliable delirium monitoring tools within the ICU. Both tools demonstrate re‐
able psychometric properties and are designed to detect delirium in both intubate
and nonintubated patients. Furthermore, both scales demonstrate high interra
reliability among practicing ICU nurses and physicians. The CAM-ICU reports a
assessment at a single time point, whereas the ICDSC reports observations in sym
toms over a period of time. Neither scale quantifies the severity of the delirium b
rather report only if it is present or not. Furthermore, neither scale distinguish
hyperactive from hypoactive delirium; therefore, it is recommended to use in co
junction with an endorsed sedation assessment. Because delirium is a fluctuatin
change in the patient's mental status, patients should be screened more than one tim
per day (usually once per shift).

The workup of altered mental status in the ICU begins with knowledge
their baseline cognitive function, including known dementia and level of fun
tional independence. The timeline of the delirium is essential to distinguish th
cause from a primary neurologic insult to the sequelae of medications, abnorm

...ore your patient over the entire shift. Components don't all need to be present at the same time.

...mponents #1 to #4 require a focused bedside patient assessment. This cannot be completed when the patient is ...eply sedated or comatose (i.e., SAS = 1 or 2; RASS = –4 or –5).

...mponents #5 to #8 are based on observations throughout the entire shift. Information from the prior 24 hours (i.e., ...om prior 1–2 nursing shifts) should be obtained for components #7 and #8.

...tered level of consciousness				
...o sedation/coma over entire shift [SAS = 1, 2; RASS = –4, –5]	= Not assessable			
...ation [SAS = 5, 6, or 7; RASS = 1–4] at any point	= 1 point	No	0	1 Yes
...mal wakefulness [SAS = 4; RASS = 0] over the entire shift	= 0 points			
	= 1 point (if no recent sedatives)			
...t sedation [SAS = 3; RASS = –1, –2, –3]	= 0 points (if recent sedatives)			
...attention				
...culty following instructions or conversation; easily distracted by external stimuli. ...not reliably squeeze hands to spoken letter "A": S A V E A H A A R T		No	0	1 Yes
...isorientation				
...ddition to name, place, and date, does the patient recognize ICU caregivers? ...s patient know what kind of place they are in? (List examples such as dentist's office, ...ome, work, hospital.)		No	0	1 Yes
...allucination, delusion, or psychosis				
...the patient if they are having hallucinations or delusions (e.g., trying to catch an ...bject that is not there). ...they afraid of the people or things around them?		No	0	1 Yes
...sychomotor agitation or retardation				
...HER: Hyperactivity requiring the use of sedative drugs or restraints to control ...otentially dangerous behaviour (e.g., pulling IV lines out or hitting staff). ...Hypoactive or clinically noticeable psychomotor slowing or retardation.		No	0	1 Yes
...nappropriate speech or mood				
...ent displays inappropriate emotion, disorganized or incoherent speech, sexual or ...ppropriate interactions, or is apathetic or overly demanding.		No	0	1 Yes
...leep–wake cycle disturbance				
...HER: Frequent awakening/<4 hours sleep at night. ...Sleeping during much of the day.		No	0	1 Yes
...ymptom fluctuation				
...ctuation of any of the above symptoms over a 24-hour period.		No	0	1 Yes
TOTAL SHIFT SCORE (Min 0 – Max 8)				

...re **57.1.** Intensive care delirium screening checklist (ICDSC).

...p patterns, and metabolic disturbances. It is important to see delirium as both ...indication of an evolving pathology and a problem in itself that needs to be ...ated; giving a sedative without consideration of etiology may lead to masking a ...eloping issue.

...The list of diagnoses that contribute to delirium is broad (Table 57.5). A careful ...rologic examination, medication review, and basic laboratory studies will address ...st causes. Medications are among the most common causes of delirium in the ...U. In addition to newly added medications, recently discontinued medicines with

TABLE 57.5	Etiologies that Cause Delirium
Vascular	Stroke, hemorrhage, reversible posterior leukoencephalopathy, vasospasm, migraine
Toxins	Alcohol, illicit drugs, occupational exposures
Seizures	Aura, ictal state, nonconvulsive status epilepticus, postictal state
Other organs	Hepatic, uremia, cardiac disease, lung disease
Electrolytes	Hypoglycemia, hyponatremia, hypocalcemia, hypomagnesemia
Neoplastic	Primary tumor, metastases, carcinomatous meningitis, paraneoplastic syndromes
Infection	Urinary tract infection, pneumonia, meningitis/encephalitis, sepsis
Trauma	Direct trauma, edema, diffuse axonal injury, postconcussive syndrome
Autoimmune	Neuropsychiatric lupus, Hashimoto's encephalopathy, CNS vascul limbic encephalitis
Endocrine	Hypo/hyperthyroidism, hypopituitary state, hyper/hypoparathyroidi
Nutritional	Vitamin B_{12} deficiency, Wernicke's encephalopathy (thiamine deficiency), Marchiafava–Bignami disease
Medication withdrawal	Appetite suppressants, cough/cold remedies, alcohol (even witho delirium tremens), selective serotonin reuptake inhibitors, nicotin baclofen
Medications	Anticholinergic agents, sedatives, antipsychotics, antiemetics, ant spasmodics, tricyclic antidepressants, muscle relaxants, digoxin anticonvulsants, corticosteroids, lithium, benzodiazepine, opioid barbiturate

CNS, central nervous system.

a withdrawal potential, new drug interactions, or a change in the metabolism previously well-tolerated medications should be considered. It is important to the development of new-onset liver and/or renal dysfunction, as these may medication levels and their effect; elderly patients may become delirious even "therapeutic" levels.

If the cause of delirium is not found, neurologic consultation should be sidered. Serious conditions can exhibit subtle findings or even a nonfocal exam tion. For instance, strokes in the nondominant hemisphere can cause deliriur the absence of hemiparesis, or fluent aphasia may be mistaken for delirium. Pat experiencing nonconvulsive status epilepticus may have no symptoms except d ium. Lumbar puncture, electroencephalography, brain imaging, and more spe laboratory studies are usually warranted in these cases.

Prevention of Delirium

Studies suggest that early mobilization in ICU patients may reduce the incide and duration of delirium, shorten ICU and hospital length of stay (LOS), and lo hospital cost. There are currently no high-quality trials to indicate prophyla pharmacologic agents are effective in preventing delirium in high-risk patients, therefore, generally are not recommended.

Treatment of Delirium

A methodical and thorough approach will help identify the cause of delirium in most cases and should guide treatment. A useful technique that combats the contribution of routine ICU care to the development of delirium is to have family members bring familiar objects (glasses, hearing aids, clocks, calendars, photographs of friends, and family) to the bedside, and regular reorientation of the patient by a familiar person. Placing patients in rooms with natural light helps restore normal sleep–wake cycles, and if possible, efforts should be made to limit stimulation at night. Next, one should consider pharmacologic etiologies, such as drug interactions and withdrawal syndromes, and efforts made to eliminate potential inciting medications (Tables 57.5 and 57.6). Neurologic and neurosurgical causes should also be sought and treated appropriately. Finally, one should address and correct any metabolic derangement or dysfunction.

If delirium persists despite treating possible causes or if treating of the underlying etiologie(s) is not feasible, one can consider treating symptoms pharmacologically. The goal should not be to make the patients unconscious, but to treat them to the point that they are not a danger to themselves or staff members. Although hypoactive delirium is more common, we do not recommend trying to improve level of consciousness in the acute setting with activating medications.

Atypical antipsychotics may reduce the duration of delirium in adult ICU patients. In a small single-center, double-blind, placebo-controlled study comparing quetiapine 50 mg twice daily to placebo, where quetiapine could be increased based on the number of breakthrough haloperidol doses administered in 24 hours, patients that received quetiapine had a shorter duration of delirium. Patients treated with antipsychotics need to be carefully monitored for fever or rigidity (indicating neuroleptic malignant syndrome), extrapyramidal symptoms (tremors, stereotypic movements,

TABLE 57.6	Environmental Contributors that Cause Delirium
Cause	Treatment
Disorientation	Frequent reorientation
Sleep cycle change	Provide stimulating activity, keep out of bed during day, no interruptions at night
Sensory deficits	Put on glasses, hearing aids, dentures
Poor communication	Communication devices
Catheters, restraints	Remove catheters, tubes, and restraints as early as possible
Dehydration	Assess for dehydration and hydrate
Malnutrition	Feed with parenteral nutrition if needed
Pain	Assess for and treat pain
Immobility	Remove restraints early, range-of-motion exercises, keep out of bed
Urinary retention	Place a bladder catheter or start scheduled catheterizations
Constipation	Disimpact if needed, start bowel routine
Fever	Antipyretics, scheduled if necessary
Infection	Search for and treat underlying infection
Hypoxemia, hypercarbia	Check arterial blood gases, ventilate or oxygenate as needed

dystonia), and QT interval prolongation, which can lead to fatal arrhythmias. patients should have a baseline and daily electrocardiogram.

Dexmedetomidine is the drug of choice in patients with delirium that requ continuous intravenous infusions of a sedative agent. Two randomized controlled als comparing dexmedetomidine to benzodiazepines for sedation showed an appr imate 20% reduction in delirium in the dexmedetomidine group. It is not cl whether dexmedetomidine reduced the incidence of delirium or if benzodiazepi increased the risk for delirium in this population. Currently, no additional data ex to recommend other sedation agents to treat delirium.

CONCLUSION

Our ability to effectively diagnosis, treat, and manage pain, agitation, and deliri in the ICU is key to reduce cost and improve ICU outcomes. A multidisciplina protocolized approach can significantly assist clinician's in identifying the diagno direct choice of treatment goals, and assist in mitigating oversedation with sedati algorithms. Central to these principles is that pain should always be addres simultaneously.

SUGGESTED READINGS

Barr J, Fraser GL, Puntillo K, et al; American College of Critical Care Medicine. Clinical pr tice guidelines for the management of pain, agitation, and delirium in adult patients in intensive care unit. *Crit Care Med.* 2013;41(1):263–306.

O'Mahony R, Murthy L, Akunne A, et al; Guideline Development Group. Synopsis of National Institute for Health and Clinical Excellence guideline for prevention of deliriu *Ann Intern Med.* 2011;154(11):746–751.

Reston JT, Schoelles KM. In-facility delirium prevention programs as a patient safety strategy systematic review. *Ann Intern Med.* 2013;158(5 Pt 2):375–380.

Roberts DJ, Haroon B, Hall RI. Sedation for critically ill or injured adults in the intensive ca unit: a shifting paradigm. *Drugs.* 2012;72(14):1881–1916.

58

Acute Spinal Cord Disorders

Terrance T. Kummer

te spinal cord injury (SCI) or myelopathy, may be traumatic or nontraumatic le 58.1). Traumatic SCI affects approximately 12,000 individuals annually in the ted States. Causes include motor vehicle collisions, recreational accidents, sports ries, and work-related injuries. Nontraumatic causes of myelopathy include emic, hemorrhagic, infectious, inflammatory, and neoplastic. SCI may lead to astating life-long disability with major health, psychological, and financial impact, :cially if one considers that injuries most commonly occur in the fourth decade of when victims are in their most productive years. Despite extensive public educa- campaigns, licensing requirements, occupational and sports safety measures, SCI tinues to increase in prevalence.

Certain types of myelopathy can be reversed if addressed in a timely fash- . Prompt recognition of clinical symptoms is imperative. The usual clinical sentation involves a triad of motor impairment (may be asymmetric), sensory , and sphincter dysfunction (i.e., urinary retention or incontinence of stool /or urine) with preservation of cerebral function (unless there is concomitant umatic brain injury). Pain at the corresponding level of the spine is not always sent. A group of well-described syndromes help localize the level of the injury ble 58.2). Algorithm 58.1 presents a detailed initial approach to this medical ergency. In addition to surgical care and medical interventions for improving rologic outcome, ICU management may be necessary due to the systemic plications of SCI.

ABLE 58.1	Causes of Spinal Cord Injury

Traumatic and degenerative (compression fractures, disc herniation)
Vascular (infarcts, epidural hematoma, arteriovenous malformations)
Infections (abscesses, myelitis, empyema, tuberculosis)
Inflammatory/demyelinating (transverse myelitis, acute disseminating encephalo-myelitis, multiple sclerosis)
Neoplastic (tumors and metastases, postradiation)
Other (vitamin B_{12} deficiency, syringomyelia, amyotrophic lateral sclerosis, spinal canal stenosis, spondylosis)—usually more chronic course

TABLE 58.2	Spinal Cord Syndromes

- Complete transection—loss of bilateral motor and sensory function below level
- Hemisection (Brown–Sequard)—loss of ipsilateral motor and proprioception/vibration; contralateral loss of pain and temperature
- Central cord—impairment of hands and arms more than legs
- Anterior cord—loss of all modalities except proprioception/vibration
- Posterior cord—preservation of motor and pain/temperature, loss of proprioception/vibration
- Cauda equina—extremely painful, asymmetric, lower motor neuron findings, la[?] urinary retention
- Conus medullaris—less painful, symmetric, mixed upper and lower motor neuro[?] findings, early urinary retention

TRAUMATIC SPINAL CORD INJURY

Cervical cord injury is the most common type of traumatic SCI. Traumatic b[?] injury is found in up to a half of these patients; just as many may have injurie[?] other organs. Almost 50% of victims of cord trauma will present with "spinal sho[?] a condition characterized by flaccid areflexic paralysis and lack of sensation in[?] modalities. This usually improves in the first few days post injury. Spine stab[?] is assessed with multiple-view plain films, CT, and often MRI (to evaluate for l[?] mentous injury) to direct surgical intervention or guide stabilization with a cerv[?] collar. The appropriate type of spinal imaging is dictated by the mechanism of trau[?] and suspicion for spinal injury. Surgical decompression, when required, is usu[?] emergent. The surgical plan and the stability of the spine are important factors[?] intensivists to consider, as limitations of mobility ("log roll precautions") and n[?] extension are important for airway management. Immobilization, performed to li[?] secondary cord damage due to improper positioning of the unstable spine, is[?] without its own risks, such as increasing intracranial hypertension, airway comp[?] mise, diminished chest wall mobility, pressure sores, and pain.

Neuroprotection

There are no proven neuroprotective agents for SCI. In the past, high-dose me[?] ylprednisolone infusion was common. A critical review of prior studies, howe[?] does not support this tradition, and the practice has fallen out of fashion as mult[?] societies have stated there is insufficient evidence to recommend its use. There[?] however evidence that methylprednisolone results in increased mortality in moder[?] to severe traumatic brain injury, which often coexists in traumatic SCI. A num[?] of additional experimental therapies are under investigation, but none are pro[?] effective or are in use clinically.

Cardiovascular Management

Many patients with cervical or upper thoracic cord injury may develop neuroge[?] shock (note the difference between spinal shock, described above, and neuroge[?] shock) because of the interruption of the spinal sympathetic chain. Decreased sy[?] pathetic innervation to the heart and blood vessels results in cardiovascular depress[?] with bradycardia, hypotension, and low systemic vascular resistance. Hemodyna[?]

ALGORITHM 58.1 **Initial Approach to a Patient with Suspected Spinal Cord Injury (SCI)/Acute Myelopathy**

Suspect SCI or myelopathy:
- New onset of weakness (both legs or all four extremities)
- Sensory deficits
- Intact cerebral function
- Sphincter dysfunction (check rectal tone and catheterize the bladder)

↓

Initial stabilization:
- Immobilize patient with cervical or thoracic cord lesions
- Address airway, breathing, and circulation

↓

Obtain imaging:
- CT of spine if suspect bony abnormalities (fractures)
- MRI of spine if soft tissue or cord may be involved (hematoma, abscess, neoplasms)

Trauma:
- Neurosurgery consult

Epidural hematoma:
- Neurosurgery consult
- Immediately reverse anticoagulation with FFP and vitamin K

Epidural abscess:
- Neurosurgery consult
- Broad spectrum antibiotics
- Look for source (blood cultures, echocardiogram, CT)

Tumor or metastases:
- Neurosurgery consult
- Dexamethasone 10 mg IV, followed by 4 mg IV q 6 hours
- Look for primary tumor

Demyelinating lesions:
- Neurology consult
- MP 1 g IV daily for 5 days

Spinal cord infarct:
- Neurology consult
- Consider anticoagulation (if known embolic source)
- Consider maintaining mean arterial pressure >70–80 mm Hg
- Consider lumbar drain

ABBREVIATIONS

CT: computed tomography
MRI: magnetic resonance imaging
MP: methylprednisolone
FFP: freshfrozen plasma
IV: intravenous

monitoring is advisable and treatment with fluids and vasopressors to preserve organ perfusion is essential. Vasopressors with chronotropic/inotropic features (norepinephrine, dopamine) are preferred to augment cardiac function as well as to increase vascular tone. The optimal blood pressure goal is unclear; experimental data show that hypotension further worsens SCI due to hypoperfusion. Limited evidence suggests there may be a benefit to augmentation of blood pressure, though this is not proven. As a result, the practice of maintaining mean arterial pressure at supraphysiologic levels (>85 mm Hg) for several days post injury is inconsistently implemented. Atropine should be kept at bedside for severe bradycardia. Transcutaneous pacing may be needed in rare refractory cases.

Airway and Breathing

The most common indication for endotracheal intubation after SCI is for high cervical injuries that impair diaphragmatic function. Injuries above the level of C5 almost universally require mechanical ventilation. Injuries at C3 or above often result in respiratory arrest. Endotracheal intubation is recommended for those cord trauma victims who have associated traumatic brain injury with Glasgow Coma Scale <8 or signs of elevated intracranial pressure. Any airway compromise due to focal edema, fractures, and/or hemorrhages of the neck may also require intubation. Only physicians with advanced airway skills should attempt intubation with an unstable spine. Fiberoptic intubation is often required as the cervical spine often cannot be manipulated. Measures should be taken to avoid hypotension during intubation. Succinylcholine is contraindicated in cases in which SCI occurred >24 hours ago. Neurosurgeons should be at bedside to help with spine immobilization if the cervical collar or halo must be removed.

Close respiratory monitoring in a critical care setting is generally necessary as SCI victims encounter multiple pulmonary complications (neurogenic pulmonary edema, pneumonia, atelectasis, pleural effusions, pulmonary embolism) and are prone to respiratory failure even days after the initial injury. Patients who require extensive operative courses with or without prone positioning may have massive fluid shifts in the first few postoperative days and are at risk for rapid pulmonary edema. This is particularly dangerous in combination with limited neck mobility. Keep in mind that with lesions below C5, while diaphragmatic function is generally preserved, intercostal muscles may be compromised leading to diminished lung volumes, poor cough, aspiration, and hypoventilation.

Thromboembolism Prevention

The majority of patients with SCI eventually develop deep venous thromboses, with the highest risk in the first 3 months after the injury. Prophylactic IVC filter placement, however, is not indicated. Surveillance Doppler venous studies are an option. Pneumatic compression devices and elastic stockings should be applied as soon as possible. Pharmacologic prophylaxis (low–molecular-weight heparin or adjusted dose unfractionated heparin) should be started as soon as possible after trauma or surgery, generally within 2 days of surgery, when the risk of bleeding is lower. Therapeutic anticoagulation should generally be withheld in the immediate postoperative period. Placement of an IVC filter in these cases may be required if a DVT develops.

Gastrointestinal Management

Acute gastroparesis may require gastric suctioning and administration of prokinetic agents to avoid aspiration. Ileus and constipation commonly complicate the course

atients with SCI. A bowel regimen (e.g., scheduled laxatives, suppositories every
r day) should be instituted early to prevent fecal impaction. H$_2$-antagonists or
on pump inhibitors are indicated in these patients for prophylaxis of stress ulcer
gastrointestinal bleeding.

n

s population is highly prone to pressure ulcers. Frequent alteration of position to
w pressure relief and meticulous care of wounds is necessary. Low–air-loss sus-
sion beds and automatically rotating beds may diminish the incidence of pressure
rs and facilitate healing of existing ulcers.

er Issues

sticity and contractures become a major problem within weeks post injury. Early
sical and occupational therapy should be initiated. Baclofen, diazepam, and
trolene are potentially useful agents for spasticity. Pulmonary, urinary tract, and
aneous infections are common. Universal precautions for ventilator-associated pneu-
aia should be instituted. Urinary retention is seen commonly and may require self-
.eterization or indwelling catheters. Pain and depression are common and should be
ressed promptly. A pain management specialist is often helpful, and psychological
port systems are essential.

NTRAUMATIC MYELOPATHY

st patients with nontraumatic SCI do not require ICU admission, unless the
er cord is involved, in which case, it is important to identify those at risk for respi-
ry failure or hemodynamic instability and supply the supportive care described
ve. Treatment for nontraumatic myelopathy is tailored to the condition, and may
olve surgical and/or medical interventions. Further discussion of nontraumatic
elopathys is outside the scope of this text.

GGESTED READINGS

sortium for Spinal Cord Medicine. Early acute management in adults with spinal cord
    injury: a clinical practice guideline for health care professionals. *J Spinal Cord Med.*
    2008;31(4):403–479.
    Guidelines form the Consortium for Spinal Cord Medicine.
ens RD, Bhardwaj A, Kirsch JR, et al. Critical care and perioperative management in trau-
    matic spinal cord injury. *J Neurosurg Anesthesiol.* 2003;15(3):215–229.
    *An excellent evidence-based review on multifaceted approach to patients with traumatic spinal
        cord injury.*

59

Neuromuscular Disorders in the Critically Ill

Rajat Dhar

The neuromuscular system encompasses the connections between the motor rons in the spinal anterior horn and the effector muscles that allow us to move breathe. Disorders of this system usually lead to generalized weakness and ma best divided into community-acquired (those with onset prior to hospital admiss and hospital-acquired (those developing in patients admitted to the hospital/inter care unit [ICU] for a separate illness). They are further classified based on neurol localization (Table 59.1). Occasionally, a disorder with onset prior to admission not be recognized until a patient is admitted for another related problem (e.g., ration pneumonia) or develop as a secondary feature of a multisystem disorder vasculitis, porphyria).

NEUROMUSCULAR RESPIRATORY FAILURE

Respiratory muscles may be affected in almost any of the acute neuromuscular orders, but most commonly are prominently involved in Guillain–Barré syndr (GBS), myasthenia gravis (MG), and amyotrophic lateral sclerosis (ALS). In some patients with ALS present with isolated or predominant respiratory invo ment without much extremity weakness, making the diagnosis challenging. Bu dysfunction with dysphagia and dysphonia often accompanies respiratory invo ment in all these disorders. Weakness of the respiratory system (i.e., diaphragm well as intercostal muscles of the chest wall) leads to impaired ventilation and red cough and clearance of secretions. Accessory muscles, including the sternocleido toid and scalenes, may compensate in part, but hypercapnic respiratory failure result from progressive weakness. Hypoxemia may develop due to atelectasis airway plugging from retained secretions. However, it is critical not to solely rel arterial blood gas or pulse oximetry evidence of hypercapnia or hypoxemia as mar of neuromuscular respiratory failure (NMRF) as these signs occur late in the cou when decompensation is imminent. There are a number of clinical markers that be detected much earlier, and should be tracked closely in patients with acute qua paresis and suggestion of respiratory involvement (Table 59.2). Observing the pa breathe (especially when lying flat), speak, lift their head, and cough can pro important information. Shallow supine breathing, weak voice, inability to main neck posture, and poor cough, all provide early clues to development of NMRF.

Objective ancillary testing can confirm the suspicion and be followed ser during the course to monitor progression. These tests involve bedside spirometr measure negative inspiratory force (NIF) and forced vital capacity (FVC). NIF is

TABLE 59.1	Causes of Neuromuscular Respiratory Failure by Localization	
Localization of Disorder	Onset Prior to ICU Admission	ICU-Acquired Weakness
Muscle	Inflammatory myopathies Acid maltase deficiency Mitochondrial myopathies Myotonic dystrophy Periodic paralysis	Critical illness myopathy Acute necrotizing myopathy Rhabdomyolysis (incl. drugs) Electrolytes ($\downarrow PO_4$, $\downarrow K$)
Neuromuscular junction	Myasthenia gravis Lambert–Eaton syndrome Botulism, Tick paralysis Organophosphate toxicity	Prolonged neuromuscular blockade Hypermagnesemia
Peripheral nerve/root	Guillain–Barré syndrome Multifocal motor neuropathy Porphyria, Vasculitis, CMT Heavy metals and toxins HIV, Diphtheria, Lyme disease Paraproteinemia, Paraneoplastic	Critical illness polyneuropathy Phrenic nerve injury
Anterior horn cell	Amyotrophic lateral sclerosis Poliomyelitis (including West Nile and Enterovirus infections)	
Central (spinal cord/ brain)	Acute myelopathy (ischemic, compressive, inflammatory) Brainstem infarction	Spinal cord ischemia (e.g., post-operative), epidural abscess Central pontinemyelinolysis

CMT, Charcot–Marie–Tooth (inherited neuropathy).

maximal inspiratory pressure generated after forceful exhalation, as measured with a mouthpiece attached to a pressure gauge; it is normally −50 to −70 cm H_2O. Values decreasing below −30 suggest significant weakness. FVC measures the amount of air exhaled and normally exceeds 3 to 4 L. Values below 30 mL/kg require close monitoring. A consistent downward trend or values below 20 mL/kg may signal impending respiratory failure and warrant evaluation for preemptive mechanical ventilation. Spirometry can be performed at regular intervals (one to four times per day) in patients with progressive weakness, but not too frequently as to induce fatigue. Facial weakness may prevent the patient forming a tight seal around the mouthpiece, making results artifactually low; a facemask pressed tightly against the lips may overcome this limitation. The trend and overall clinical evaluation should guide decision making rather than any single isolated FVC or NIF value.

Intubation of patients with NMRF should be performed prior to acute decompensation and ideally before hypercapnia, significant atelectasis, or aspiration has developed (Algorithm 59.1). Neuromuscular blocking agents (NMBs) should be avoided, if possible; succinylcholine can precipitate lethal hyperkalemia in patients with denervation, and non-depolarizing NMBs can cause prolonged paralysis in MG. A trial of noninvasive ventilation may be considered in select patients with NMRF as long as mental status and airway reflexes are preserved. Some patients with neuromuscular

TABLE 59.2	Signs of Impending Neuromuscular Respiratory Failure
Sign	Red Flag
Clinical	
Progressive weakness	Quadriplegia, inability to lift head off bed
Bulbar involvement	Dysphagia, weak voice, bifacial weakness
Weak cough	Trouble expelling secretions, "wet" voice
Respiratory complaints	
Dyspnea	Complains of respiratory fatigue
Tachypnea	Unable to speak in full sentences, count to 20
Orthopnea	Nocturnal desaturations, prefers to sit up
Accessory muscle use	Using neck and abdominal muscles
Abdominal paradox	Inward motion of abdomen with inspiration
Signs of distress	
Tachycardia	Restless
Diaphoresis	Staccato speech
Monitoring	
Vital capacity testing (bedside)	VC <15–20 mL/kg, falling, drop by 30%
Arterial oxygen saturation	Desaturation (late sign)
Arterial blood gas: $PaCO_2$	Hypercapnia = hypoventilation (late sign)
Chest radiographs	Atelectasis, Pneumonia

failure may not have diaphragmatic weakness requiring ventilatory support (i.e. normal FVC and NIF) but severe enough bulbar weakness to cause an inability to manage secretions and therefore, necessitate intubation for airway protection. Such patients will not benefit from BiPAP but also not require much ventilator support once intubated. The use of BiPAP in GBS may be unsuccessful partially for this reason (i.e., failure of airway protection) but also because these patients usually progress rapidly beyond the support that noninvasive positive pressure ventilation (NIPPV) is able to provide. Overventilation (to fully normalize PCO_2) should be avoided in those with chronic CO_2 retention otherwise alkalemia will develop, impairing subsequent weaning. Decisions about tracheostomy should be deferred in GBS and MG patients till after immunomodulatory treatment with plasmapheresis or intravenous immunoglobulin (IVIG) is completed, as rapid improvement can be seen in some cases. Decisions on tracheostomy and weaning can also be facilitated by daily measurements of FVC and NIF on the ventilator. When FVC rises above 7 to 10 mL/kg and NIF becomes less than −20 cm H_2O, the patient may be ready for weaning and possibly avoid tracheostomy. It is advisable to wait for 24 hours of spontaneous breathing (with an ABG to exclude CO_2 retention) in patients recovering from NMRF prior to extubation, as delayed fatigue can occur.

GUILLAIN–BARRÉ SYNDROME

GBS is an acute inflammatory demyelinating polyneuropathy (AIDP) that is the most common cause of flaccid paralysis worldwide. It is a monophasic autoimmune process often triggered by an upper respiratory or gastrointestinal infection

ALGORITHM 59.1 Managing Neuromuscular Respiratory Failure

Identify patient at risk for neuromuscular respiratory failure
(Table 59.2)

Close respiratory monitoring
- Spirometry (NIF, FVC) q6–12 hr
- Oxygen saturation
- Assess if patient is able to lift head off bed, count to 20
- Monitor adequacy of cough and secretion clearance
- ABG if respiratory symptoms or concern about hypoventilation
- CXR if desaturation or fever

Aggressive pulmonary toilet
- Incentive spirometry (q1h)
- Mobilization to prevent atelectasis
- Suctioning as required
- Glycopyrrolate if copious thin secretions
- Minimize sedative use
- Swallowing evaluation for dysphagia
- Prevent aspiration by using post-pyloric feeding and/or motility agents

Signs of impending NMRF
- FVC <15 mL/kg or drop by 30%
- NIF below −30 cm H$_2$O
- Inability to clear secretions
- Desaturation
- Hypercapnia

Endotracheal intubation
- Avoid succinylcholine/NMBs
- Mechanical ventilation (setting based on degree of weakness)
- Follow NIF/FVC daily on vent
- Wean when weakness improving with daily SBT as FVC >7 mL/kg
- Delay tracheostomy 1–2 weeks

Treat underlying disorder if possible
- EMG/NCS for diagnosis if required
- Plasmapharesis or IVIG for GBS or MG
- Corticosteroids for inflammatory myopathy, CIDP, or MG (low-dose)
- Antibiotics for pneumonia/infections

ABBREVIATIONS
NIF:	negative inspiratory force
FVC:	forced vital capacity
ABG:	arterial blood gas
CXR:	chest x-ray
NMBs:	neuromuscular blocking drugs
SBT:	spontaneous breathing trial
EMG/NCS:	electromyography and nerve conduction studies
IVIG:	intravenous immunoglobulin
GBS:	Guillain-Barré syndrome
MG:	myasthenia gravis
CIDP:	chronic inflammatory demyelinating polyneuropathy

Clinical hallmarks include symmetric proximal and distal muscle weakness in legs and arms associated with areflexia and frequent bulbar, facial, and respirat muscle involvement. *Dysautonomia* is seen in over half the patients with GBS may manifest as wide fluctuations in blood pressure, tachycardia and/or bradyca (sometimes leading to cardiac arrest), and gastrointestinal symptoms, including ile Caution should be exercised in treating blood pressure due to potential lability, atropine should be kept at the bedside as suctioning may induce bradycardia. S sory complaints and back pain are common in GBS, although patients with ac para- or quadriparesis and sensory dysfunction (especially a "sensory level") sho be evaluated for spinal cord compression or other causes of myelopathy. Find elevated protein levels in CSF without pleocytosis supports the diagnosis of G Nerve conduction studies (NCS) and electromyography (EMG) may be obtained assist with diagnosis and prognosis, but may be relatively normal if performed e in the course. The incidence of NMRF requiring intubation is 30%, and alm half of these patients require tracheostomy for prolonged ventilation. Treatmen with IVIG (total dose 2 g/kg over 2 to 5 days) or plasmapheresis, and although r complete recovery is the rule, it may be delayed in severe cases. ICU stay is most p longed in those with complete quadriplegia and axonal changes (e.g., reduced mc amplitudes) on EMG/NCS.

MYASTHENIA GRAVIS

MG is an autoimmune disease where antibodies are directed against the acetylcho receptor (Ach-R) at the neuromuscular junction. This impairment of neuromuscu synaptic transmission leads to fatigable weakness with predominant ocular (ptc restriction of ocular movements with diplopia) and bulbar involvement. NM occurs with diaphragmatic involvement and is the hallmark of *myasthenic crisis*, wh occurs in 20% of patients with MG. There is often an identifiable precipitant suck intercurrent infection, surgery (including thymectomy), or medications (commo antibiotics, see Table 59.3). Worsening of MG is seen in a subset of patients sho after initiating corticosteroid therapy (especially at doses above 20 mg/day) a may precipitate crisis. The diagnosis of MG is primarily clinical, confirmed either presence of Ach-R antibodies in the serum or by the finding of "decrement" of mc amplitudes on repetitive nerve stimulation. Treatment of MG consists of cholines ase inhibitors (pyridostigmine) and immunosuppression (including corticosteroi Crises are usually treated with IVIG or plasmapheresis (as in GBS). Recovery

TABLE 59.3	Medications That Can Aggravate Weakness in Myasthenia Gravis
Antibiotics	Aminoglycosides, ciprofloxacin, clindamycin, erythromy cin, azithromycin, tetracyclines, polymixin B, colistin
Antiarrhythmics	Quinidine, procainamide, lidocaine, beta-blockers, calciu channel blockers
Hormones	Corticosteroids
Neuromuscular blockers	Succinylcholine, vecuronium, pancuronium, etc.
Other	Lithium, phenytoin, quinine, statins

usually more rapid than in GBS, and most patients do not require prolonged ventilation or tracheostomy.

In patients on high doses of pyridostigmine, there may be concern that increasing weakness is a sign of cholinergic toxicity and not worsening MG. Cholinergic crisis will be associated with excessive salivation, muscle cramping, diarrhea, and fasciculations, peaking shortly after drug dosing. This is a rare toxidrome in MG but can be excluded by discontinuing the medication and reevaluating symptoms. Pyridostigmine can exacerbate pulmonary secretions and is usually held during periods of respiratory failure. Imaging of the chest may be obtained when a new patient with MG is stabilized to evaluate for thymoma. However, thymectomy should be delayed till after crisis has resolved to avoid exacerbation postoperatively.

ICU-ACQUIRED WEAKNESS

Patients who are critically ill often develop neuromuscular weakness that not only prolongs duration of mechanical ventilation, but may also contribute to residual disability in survivors. There has been considerable confusion and overlap in terminology and classification of such disorders. Dysfunction commonly occurs at both the level of the peripheral nerve and muscle (even in the same patient) and can be hard to distinguish clinically or even with EMG/NCS. The term "ICU-acquired weakness" may be preferable to label the clinical syndrome in the absence of electrodiagnostic or pathologic testing. The diagnosis is often suspected in the setting of failure to wean after recovery from critical illness (most often sepsis and ARDS). Testing muscle groups in the upper and lower extremities when a patient awakens from sedation and encephalopathy can assess weakness; it may be suspected even in uncooperative patients when painful stimulation elicits a grimace but limited limb movement.

Critical illness polyneuropathy (CIP) reflects noninflammatory axonal nerve damage as a result of sepsis; it may be best viewed as another end-organ failure resulting from cytokine-mediated systemic inflammatory response with nerve edema and tissue hypoxia. It may be exacerbated by hyperglycemia, and attempts at intensive glucose control have yielded reductions in CIP. Myopathy has been related to corticosteroid and NMB exposure and was first described in a patient with status asthmaticus. Creatine kinase (CK) levels may be elevated early in the course but are often normal by the time weakness is recognized. The pathologic hallmark is selective loss of the thick (myosin) muscle filaments. It is difficult to clinically distinguish CIP from myopathy, because sensory loss, which is absent in myopathy, is difficult to test in ICU patients and the pattern of weakness (both proximal and distal muscles) is similar in both conditions. NCS will also show reduced motor amplitudes in both states. Evaluation of motor units with EMG may help (as neuropathic and myopathic changes in unit morphology are different) but weak encephalopathic ICU patients rarely cooperate adequately to allow recruitment of motor units. Muscle biopsy will show the hallmark of "myosin loss myopathy" but is not mandatory in most cases of ICU-acquired weakness. Once a clinical diagnosis has been made, supportive care and avoiding additional precipitants are required for both subtypes. Muscle and nerve biopsy may be useful if the patient does not improve or there is suspicion of an underlying systemic disorder (e.g., inflammatory myopathy with elevated CK, nerve vasculitis). Restricting use of neuromuscular blockers (or monitoring level of paralysis, if used), daily sedative holidays, early mobilization of ICU patients, and intensive insulin therapy may minimize the risk of these disorders; however, they must be weighed against their potential risks, and individualized based on each patient's clinical condition.

SUGGESTED READINGS

Chalela JA. Pearls and pitfalls in the intensive care management of Guillain-Barré syndrome. *Semin Neurol.* 2001;21:399–405.

Dhar R, Stitt L, Hahn AF. The morbidity and outcome of patients with Guillain-Barré syndrome admitted to the intensive care unit. *J Neurol Sci.* 2008;264:121–128.

Gorson K. Approach to neuromuscular disorders in the intensive care unit. *Neurocrit Care.* 2005;3:195–212.

Lawn ND, Fletcher DD, Henderson RD, et al. Anticipating mechanical ventilation in Guillain-Barré syndrome. *Arch Neurol.* 2001;58:893–898.

Schweickert WD, Hall J. ICU-acquired weakness. *Chest.* 2007;131:1541–1549.

60 Traumatic Brain Injury and Elevated Intracranial Pressure

Terrance T. Kummer

Severe head trauma is a leading cause of morbidity and mortality worldwide, especially among young adults. About 2.5 million people in the United States are treated in the hospital for a traumatic brain injury (TBI) each year; the most common causes are falls, motor vehicle accidents, and assaults. Mortality rates in severe TBI have decreased from 50% to 25% over the last 25 years, emphasizing the impact of improvements in medical and surgical management. This improvement is particularly related to the prevention of secondary brain injury, which occurs hours to days after the initial trauma.

INITIAL STABILIZATION AND MANAGEMENT

Initial management focuses on airway, breathing, and circulation. The Glasgow Coma Scale (GCS) is widely used for classification and prognosis (Table 60.1).

TABLE 60.1	Glasgow Coma Scale
Best eye opening	
Spontaneous	4
With voice only	3
With pain only	2
None at all	1
Best verbal response	
Coherent speech	5
Confused intelligible speech	4
Inappropriate words	3
Incomprehensible sounds	2
No verbal output	1
Best motor response	
Follows commands	6
Localizes pain stimuli[a]	5
Withdraws to pain stimuli	4
Decorticate posturing	3
Decerebrate posturing	2
No movements at all	1

Localizing pain stimuli refers to gaze deviation, head turning or hand movements towards the stimulus.

The GCS consists of an assessment of eye opening/level of consciousness, m and verbal responses. According to this scale, head injuries are classified as or concussive (GCS, 13.15 to 15), moderate (GCS, 9 to 12), and severe (C 3 to 8). Those patients with GCS ≤8 usually require endotracheal intubation mechanical ventilation. Fluid resuscitation, blood transfusion, and/or vasopre to maintain adequate perfusion are initiated in cases of ongoing bleeding hypotension. Because approximately 15% of patients with TBI have an assoc spinal cord injury, an effort should be made to stabilize and immobilize the s (see Chapter 58). Once initial stabilization has been achieved, a noncontrast computed tomography (CT) and films of the spine to assess the magnitude type of injury should be obtained. The range of head injuries includes simple lacerations, skull fractures, cerebral contusions, intracranial hemorrhage (epid subdural, intraparenchymal, and subarachnoid hemorrhages), and diffuse ax injury. Emergent neurosurgical consultation is indicated in penetrating wou skull fractures, intracranial hematoma, or cerebral hemorrhages, as these may re immediate operative management. Further management of head injury is base prevention, recognition, and aggressive treatment of secondary injury to the b These include hypoxia, hypotension, hypoperfusion, elevated intracranial pre (ICP), and seizures or status epilepticus.

ICU MANAGEMENT OF PATIENTS WITH SEVERE TBI

Once stabilized, patients with severe TBI should be monitored in an intensive unit with ICP and cerebral perfusion pressure (CPP) monitoring. ICP monitori indicated in all cases of severe TBI (GCS ≤8) with an abnormal CT scan (Table 6 ICP can be measured using either a ventricular catheter (which has the advan of allowing CSF drainage) or a parenchymal fiberoptic probe. Routine ventric catheter exchange and prophylactic antibiotic use for ventricular catheter placer are not recommended. CPP is the difference between mean arterial pressure (M and ICP. MAP is most accurately measured by direct arterial cannulation (e.g., ra femoral).

ICP CONTROL

Elevated ICP (>20 mm Hg) after head injury is associated with unfavorable comes. In approximately half of those who die after severe TBI, increased ICP

TABLE 60.2	Indications for ICP and CPP Monitoring
Patients with GCS ≤8 and an abnormal CT scan (i.e., hematoma, contusion, swellir herniation, or compressed basal cisterns)	
Patients with a normal CT scan and at least two of the following on admission:	
Age >40	
Unilateral or bilateral motor posturing	
Systolic BP <90 mm Hg	

ICP, intracranial pressure; CPP, cerebral perfusion pressure; GCS, Glasgow Coma Scale; CT, cc puted tomography; BP, blood pressure.

herniation is the primary cause of death. In all patients who have ICP monitors, universal measures should be instituted, including elevating the head of bed to 30 degrees, keeping the chin midline to avoid jugular compression, maintaining normocarbia, normothermia, and euvolemia, and avoiding hyponatremia. For refractory ICPs (>20 mm Hg for >5 minutes), sedation, osmotherapy, hyperventilation, hypothermia, and surgical decompression should be considered (Algorithm 60.1). Hyperventilation is not recommended for management of elevated ICP because it results in intracranial vasoconstriction, therefore worsening cerebral perfusion; it is reserved only as a brief temporizing measure for acute symptoms of herniation while more definitive interventions are arranged.

CPP THRESHOLD

Maintenance of CPP at 60 to 70 mm Hg is generally necessary following severe TBI to maintain adequate cerebral blood flow; any reduction below these levels increases risk for cerebral ischemia. CPP may drop because of a decrease in MAP, an increase in ICP, or by a combination of these mechanisms. Maintenance of CPP is achieved by maintaining euvolemia, avoiding hypotension, controlling elevated ICP, and in refractory cases, using vasopressors to augment MAP (Table 60.3).

SEIZURE PROPHYLAXIS

Up to 25% of TBI patients will experience a posttraumatic seizure within 7 days of injury, thus seizure prevention with anticonvulsants is indicated for 7 days after TBI. Prophylaxis should not extend beyond 1 week as it does not affect the development of late posttraumatic seizures.

VENOUS THROMBOEMBOLISM PREVENTION

Sequential compression devices should be used from admission, and subcutaneous low–molecular-weight heparin or unfractionated heparin for DVT prophylaxis can be started 48 hours after documented cessation of bleeding.

NUTRITIONAL SUPPORT

Metabolic expenditures are higher in patients with severe TBI, therefore, caloric intake should be adjusted to provide approximately 140% of expected requirements. At least 15% of calories should be supplied as protein. Early feeding (within 48 to

TABLE 60.3	CPP Management
Keep MAP above 80 mm Hg until CPP can be measured	
Use normal saline boluses and vasopressors if needed to avoid hypotension	
Once ICP monitor is inserted, CPP goal 60–70 mm Hg (CPP = MAP – ICP)	
Control ICP, see Algorithm 60.1	
Use vasopressors to augment MAP and CPP in refractory cases	

MAP, mean arterial pressure; CPP, cerebral perfusion pressure; ICP, intracranial pressure.

ALGORITHM 60.1 Management of Elevated Intracranial Pressure

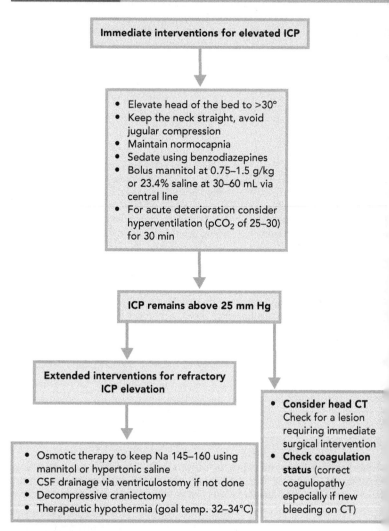

Immediate interventions for elevated ICP

- Elevate head of the bed to >30°
- Keep the neck straight, avoid jugular compression
- Maintain normocapnia
- Sedate using benzodiazepines
- Bolus mannitol at 0.75–1.5 g/kg or 23.4% saline at 30–60 mL via central line
- For acute deterioration consider hyperventilation (pCO$_2$ of 25–30) for 30 min

ICP remains above 25 mm Hg

Extended interventions for refractory ICP elevation

- Osmotic therapy to keep Na 145–160 using mannitol or hypertonic saline
- CSF drainage via ventriculostomy if not done
- Decompressive craniectomy
- Therapeutic hypothermia (goal temp. 32–34°C)

- **Consider head CT** Check for a lesion requiring immediate surgical intervention
- **Check coagulation status** (correct coagulopathy especially if new bleeding on CT)

ABBREVIATIONS
CSF: cerebrospinal fluid
CT: computed tomography
ICP: intracranial pressure
PCO$_2$: partial pressure of carbon dioxide

ours of insult) is important, resulting in a trend toward fewer infectious compli-
ns and lower mortality.

GGESTED READING

n Trauma Foundation; American Association of Neurological Surgeons; Congress of
    Neurological Surgeons. Guidelines for the management of severe traumatic brain injury.
    J Neurotrauma. 2007;24(suppl 1):S1–S106.
    For most up-todate version of the Brain Trauma Foundation guidelines, visit www.braintrauma.
        org

61 Neurologic Approach t Central Nervous Syste Infections

Baback Arshi and Salah G. Keyrouz

Central nervous system (CNS) infections can progress rapidly from onset to threatening in a matter of hours; therefore, any suspicion should prompt ra evaluation and treatment. The classic triad of headache, fever, and meningis may only be seen in half of patients with bacterial meningitis and only some have focal neurologic deficits and peripheral leukocytosis. The index of suspicio even higher in immunocompromised patients, as any one of these symptoms r be the sole manifestation of infection. In addition to the devastation caused by infection, complications like abscess formation, hydrocephalus, cerebral infarcts, seizures may supervene. In addition, neurosurgical procedures, indwelling hardw and penetrating skull injuries may further complicate the treatment of meningiti

GENERAL MEASURES

Blood cultures and a coagulation profile should be promptly obtained. Those who immunocompromised, have depressed level of consciousness, papilledema, or fe neurologic deficits should undergo brain imaging prior to lumbar puncture (LP) to the risk of herniation from a mass lesion (see Table 61.1). Correction of any co ulopathy should be done prior to LP in order to prevent the development of a spi epidural hematoma. Opening pressure should always be measured and the stand lab profile sent as shown in Table 61.2. Treatment with antimicrobials should be delayed by LP. Although antimicrobials may reduce the yield of CSF culture started prior to LP, a a gram stain may still provide positive results. Treatment sho be appropriate for age and other risk factors and should remain broad until offending organism is identified (see Algorithm 61.1). Current data suggest impro neurologic outcomes with early initiation of dexamethasone when given before

TABLE 61.1	Contraindications to Lumbar Puncture
Absolute	Relative
Space-occupying lesion in the posterior fossa	International normalized ratio above 1.
Presence of midline shift	Platelet count below 50,000/mcL
Effacement of basal cisterns or fourth ventricle	
Skin infection in the area of puncture	
Lumbar epidural abscess or empyema	

	Bacterial	Viral	Fungal
TABLE 61.2	**Cerebrospinal Fluid (CSF) Findings Suggestive of Infection**		
CSF Parameter	Bacterial Meningitis	Viral Meningitis	Fungal Meningitis
Opening pressure (cm H₂O)	>18	9–18	>18
White cell count	100–10,000	5–1,000	5–1,000
Percent neutrophils	>80	<20	<20
Protein	100–500	<100	>100
Glucose	<40	>40	<40
Gram stain (% positive)	60–90	0	0
Culture (% positive)	70–85	50	25–50

during the first dose of antibiotics, particularly with *Streptococcus pneumoniae* meningitis. It is useful to save CSF for future studies; once results of cell count, protein, and glucose are available, they could suggest an infection caused by a likely class of organisms and therefore extra agglutination or PCR testing might be warranted. Table 61.2 lists the various cerebrospinal fluid (CSF) patterns according to cause.

MENINGITIS

In general, meningitides are the most common type of CNS infection, with mortality reaching 60% in bacterial meningitis; delay in diagnosis and timely treatment can be catastrophic.

Bacterial Meningitis

An accurate history may elucidate the source and allow a more narrow differential diagnosis. Bacterial meningitis can commonly be preceded by a pneumonia, otitis media, mastoiditis, or acute sinusitis. Common organisms in the adult population include *S. pneumoniae*, *Neisseria meningitides*, *Haemophilus influenzae*, and *Staphylococcus aureus*. In the elderly, chronic alcoholic, or immunocompromised patient *Listeria monocytogenes* should be considered. Those with neurosurgical hardware or penetrating skull injuries should also be covered for aerobic gram-negative bacilli and methicillin-resistant *Staphylococcus*. The Infectious Disease Society of America (IDSA) recommended initial empiric regimen of antibiotics include ceftriaxone (or meropenem) and vancomycin. If *Listeria* is suspected, ampicillin should be added to the initial regimen of antibiotics. Patients should be monitored closely for complications including septic shock, cerebral edema, hydrocephalus, cerebral venous sinus thrombosis, seizures, disseminated intravascular coagulation, hearing loss, and syndrome of inappropriate antidiuretic hormone secretion. Often neurologic consultation is valuable not merely for help in diagnosis and treatment, but also for identification of associated neurologic complications.

Aseptic Meningitis

Aseptic meningitis refers to inflammation of the meninges without an isolated bacterium in the CSF. Etiologies range from infectious to noninfectious. Infectious

ALGORITHM 61.1 Approach to Treatment of Suspected Infection of the Central Nervous System

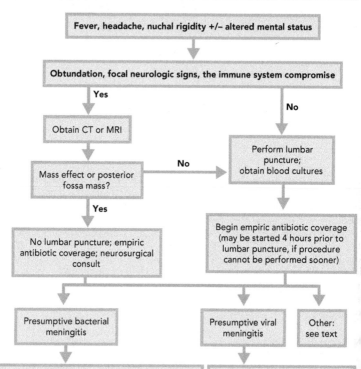

Fever, headache, nuchal rigidity +/− altered mental status

↓

Obtundation, focal neurologic signs, the immune system compromise

Yes ↓   **No** →

Obtain CT or MRI

↓

Mass effect or posterior fossa mass?   **No** → Perform lumbar puncture; obtain blood cultures

Yes ↓

No lumbar puncture; empiric antibiotic coverage; neurosurgical consult

Begin empiric antibiotic coverage (may be started 4 hours prior to lumbar puncture, if procedure cannot be performed sooner)

↓

Presumptive bacterial meningitis   Presumptive viral meningitis   Other: see text

- Vancomycin 20 mg/kg q8 and ceftriaxone 2 g q12 hours IV;
- Add ampicillin 2 g q4 hours IV for *Listeria* coverage in elderly, alcohol abusers, immunocompromised;
- Dexamethasone 10 mg IV q6 hours for 4 days for *Streptococcus*;
- Finish full course antibiotics even if no organism recovered;
- Monitor for hydrocephalus, seizures, DIC, SIADH, venous sinus thrombosis.

- Continue IV acyclovir 10 mg/kg q8 hours for 21 days if PCR is positive;
- Stop acyclovir if HSV or VZV PCR results are negative;
- Monitor for seizure.

ABBREVIATIONS

CT:	computed tomography
MRI:	magnetic resonance imaging
IV:	intravenous
DIC:	disseminated intravascular coagulation
SIADH:	syndrome of inappropriate antidiuretic hormone secretion
PCR:	polymerase chain reaction
HSV:	herpes simplex virus
VZV:	varicella-zoster virus

TABLE 61.3	Noninfectious Causes of Meningitis

- Medications and toxins
  Nonsteroidal anti-inflammatory medications (ibuprofen, ketorolac)
  Chemotherapy agents (especially intrathecal preparations)
  Antibiotics (metronidazole, trimethoprim-sulfamethoxazole, isoniazid)
  Vaccinations
  Intravenous immunoglobulin G
  Intravenous contrast
- Neoplastic (leptomeningeal metastases)
- Autoimmune or inflammatory disorders
  Systemic lupus erythematosus
  Sjögren's syndrome
  Primary central nervous system angiitis
  Behçet's disease

eptic meningitis could occur in the setting of syphilis, Lyme disease, Rocky Moun-
in spotted fever, HIV, and West Nile virus. The incidence of viral meningitides is
gher than that of bacterial meningitides. While the presentation is similar to that
bacterial meningitis including headache, fever, meningismus, and photophobia,
tients usually have a less toxic appearance, and sensorium is less likely to be altered.
ost cases of aseptic meningitis are self-limited and carry a favorable outcome. If
icrobiologic tests yield negative results, and there is no clinical improvement with
tibiotics, consider noninfectious causes of meningitis (Table 61.3). CSF cytology
th flow cytometry should be requested if malignancy is suspected (leptomeningeal
rcinomatosis).

NCEPHALITIS

cephalitis is an infection/inflammation of brain parenchyma. Cerebral dysfunc-
n is the key trait that differentiates encephalitis from meningitis. This can be
aracterized by altered mental status, motor or sensory deficits, and personality
anges. In common practice, many patients will exhibit signs of parenchymal and
eningeal inflammation, and should more appropriately be diagnosed as having a
eningoencephalitis.

rpes Simplex Virus Encephalitis

SV encephalitis is known for its high morbidity and mortality, but also its respon-
eness to timely institution of antiviral therapy. Common presentation includes
er and altered mental status. Other presenting signs may include focal neurologic
dings such as hemiparesis, aphasia, ataxia, or focal seizures. CSF is usually hem-
hagic with a moderate lymphocytic pleocytosis and elevated protein. Patients
pected of having HSV encephalitis should be started on acyclovir until HSV PCR
onfirmed negative. EEG performed in the setting of HSV encephalitis can show
al slowing or epileptiform activity, typically over the temporal lobes. Hemorrhagic
ons on head CT or brain MRI may be present in the subacute or chronic phase
he disease or if treatment is not initiated promptly. Prompt diagnosis and timely
atment of this infection is of paramount importance given its significant morbidity

and mortality; acyclovir should be given intravenously for the entire duration treatment. Mortality approaches 70% in untreated cases.

Arthropod-Borne Encephalitis

This class of viral encephalitides is typically spread via mosquito or tick. They inclue St. Louis encephalitis, California encephalitis, Japanese B encephalitis, Eastern ar Western equine encephalitis, and West Nile encephalitis. Treatment of these infetions is generally supportive.

BRAIN ABSCESS

Brain abscess, subdural empyema, and epidural abscess represent a subset of less fiquently seen CNS infections. Patients typically present with focal neurologic deficial Brain abscess arises from one of three sources: direct spread (such as from an infect sinus), hematogenous spread from another source (e.g., pneumonia, endocarditi or penetrating trauma. Similarly, subdural and epidural abscesses develop from dirispread or after surgical manipulation. The presentation of a brain abscess typical involves headache lateralizing to the side of the abscess, accompanied by focal neurolog signs. Evidence of elevated intracranial pressure (papilledema, vomiting, or depres level of consciousness) may also be present. Diagnosis relies primarily on neuroiming with a contrast agent. The typical abscess appears as a ring-enhancing lesion w surrounding edema. Abscesses resulting from hematogenous spread (septic emboli c to endocarditis) may present as multiple lesions. In case of endocarditis patients shoundergo cerebral vascular imaging to evaluate for mycotic aneurysms and imaging the neuraxis to evaluate for metastatic sites of abscess (e.g., spinal epidural or subdur Subdural empyema and epidural abscess are classified as neurosurgical emergencies. should not be performed when signs of elevated intracranial pressure are present.

The workup for the source should include blood and urine cultures, ecl cardiography, and possibly further body imaging. Toxoplasma titers are checked immunocompromised patients. Antimicrobial coverage for brain abscesses va with the presumptive source of infection. Empiric treatment should include van mycin, metronidazole, and a third-generation cephalosporin (ceftriaxone or ceft dime). Immunocompromised patients (including neutropenic and recent transpl patients) should also receive amphotericin B for additional fungal coverage.

Neurosurgical patients are at risk in the months or even years after a proced Most brain abscesses are bacterial and often polymicrobial, although fungal intions are also possible, especially in the immunocompromised patient. Common obes include *Streptococcus* species (including *viridans* in endocarditis), *Staphyloco* species (especially after surgical procedures), *Pseudomonas* species, and *Enteroba* species (otitis media). Anaerobic abscesses (*Bacteroides* and *Actinomyces* species) arise from oral sources (dental carries) and abdominal or pelvic infections. Neu penic patients and transplant recipients have a particular predilection for *Asperg* abscesses. Toxoplasmosis is the most common intracranial infection in patients acquired immune deficiency syndrome (AIDS).

INFECTIONS RELATED TO NEUROSURGERY

Infections following neurosurgery include meningitis, encephalitis, ventricul abscess, and hardware infection. These typically occur within weeks of surg although vulnerability to infections remains for years. Ventriculoperitoneal shunt infections may present with symptoms of hydrocephalus (increasing headaches, vomiting, lethargy) and abdominal distention; otherwise, symptoms are similar to other types of CNS infections. Shunts are assessed with imaging to determine their functional status and tapped to sample CSF and identify the organism. Infected hardware should be removed if possible. The most common organisms causing post-neurosurgical infection include *Staphylococcus* species and gram-negative organisms.

TROPICAL CNS INFECTIONS

Tuberculous meningitis, West Nile encephalomyelitis, and neurocysticercosis comprise a group of tropical diseases that have become increasingly common in the United States. Tuberculous meningitis carries a high mortality and presentation includes altered mental status, lethargy, cranial neuropathies, and hemiparesis. West Nile encephalomyelitis, typically encountered in warm-climate months, is spread by mosquitos and causes fever, encephalitis, meningitis, and a polio-like illness presenting with flaccid paralysis. Neurocysticercosis, the world's leading cause of adult-onset seizure, is transmitted by consumption of undercooked pork that contains *Taenia solium* larvae.

IMMUNOCOMPROMISED PATIENTS

These include patients with AIDS, solid-organ or bone marrow transplantation recipients, and those receiving chemotherapy or immunosuppression for autoimmune conditions. The most common infections include toxoplasmosis, cryptococcal meningitis, fungal abscess (*Aspergillus*), and progressive multifocal leukoencephalopathy (JC virus). Special CSF testing includes polymerase chain reaction testing for *Toxoplasma*, JC virus, Epstein–Barr virus, and cytomegalovirus, as well as *Cryptococcus* and *Histoplasma* antigen testing. The Venereal Disease Research Laboratory test should also be requested, given the higher incidence of neurosyphilis in AIDS patients. An infectious diseases consult is strongly recommended if CNS infection is suspected in an immunocompromised patient.

SUGGESTED READINGS

Pruitt AA. Infections of the nervous system. *Neurol Clin.* 1998;16:419–447.
> *An excellent review of comprehensive approach to infections of the central nervous system with special attention to the immunocompromised patients.*

Tunkel AR, Hartman BJ, Kaplan SL, et al. Practice guidelines for the management of bacterial meningitis. *Clin Infect Dis.* 2004;39(9):1267–1284.
> *Current recommendations for the diagnosis and management of bacterial meningitis representing data published through May 2004.*

Ziai WC, Lewin JJ 3rd. Advances in the management of central nervous system infections in the ICU. *Crit Care Clin.* 2006;22(4):661–694.
> *Most recent review of management of various acute central nervous system infections in the critical care setting.*

Hunt JR, Marra CM. Cerebrospinal fluid testing for the diagnosis of central nervous system infection. *Neurol Clin.* 1999;17(4):675–689.
> *A detailed review of various methods of testing cerebrospinal fluid for suspected infection of the central nervous system.*

62

Thrombocytopenia in the Intensive Care Unit

Warren Isakow

Thrombocytopenia is a very common occurrence in the intensive care unit (ICU), occurring in as many as 60% of patients, either before ICU admission or during the course of the ICU stay. The normal platelet count ranges between 150,000 and 450,000/mcL. In the ICU, it is important to recognize that the absolute platelet count is important, but trends in the platelet count, specifically a decline by more than 50% may be evidence of a serious clinical problem such as heparin-induced thrombocytopenia (HIT), which requires urgent attention. A systematic approach to the diagnosis allows for the common causes to be detected early and enables rational use of platelet transfusions (Algorithm 62.1). Platelet survival in the circulation is approximately 7 to 10 days, and one-third of the platelets are sequestered in the spleen under normal circumstances.

Recognition of thrombocytopenia normally occurs after a complete blood count is drawn, but it is important to remember that mucocutaneous bleeding is a classic sign of thrombocytopenia. Bleeding from thrombocytopenia normally occurs only once the platelet count is <50,000/mcL in postsurgical patients; spontaneous bleeding can occur with counts <5,000/mcL. The diagnostic approach starts with a thorough history and physical examination, followed by examination of the peripheral smear. A pathophysiologic approach to thrombocytopenia enables all common causes to be rapidly screened for and facilitates recognition of potential causes (Table 62.1). Careful attention should be paid to prescription and over-the-counter drugs (Table 62.2).

The common causes of thrombocytopenia in an ICU setting are as follows:

- Drug-induced (heparin, H_2-receptor blockers, GP2b3a inhibitors, antibiotics, and alcohol)
- Sepsis
- Massive bleeding
- Thrombocytopenia with microangiopathic hemolytic anemia (thrombocytopenic thrombotic purpura [TTP], hemolytic uremic syndrome [HUS], and disseminated intravascular coagulation [DIC]).

Clinical recognition of the cause is vital as the therapies differ considerably depending on the etiology. For example, a patient with thrombocytopenia secondary to bleeding should be treated with platelets, compared with a patient with TTP/HUS, in whom platelet transfusion is generally contraindicated and treatment entails use of plasmapheresis. A few common conditions will be discussed and readers are encouraged to refer to the suggested reading for further details.

ALGORITHM 62.1 Diagnostic Algorithm for Thrombocytopenia

Thrombocytopenia

ABBREVIATIONS
ETOH: alcohol
TTP: thrombocytopenic thrombotic purpura

History and physical examination
- Drugs
- Current bleeding
- Neurological symptoms and signs
- Recent viral illness
- Gastrointestinal bleeding
- Family history
- Travel history (malaria)
- Tick exposure
- ETOH use
- Splenomegaly
- Lymphadenopathy
- Petechiae
- Fundal hemorrhage

Peripheral smear
- Pseudothrombocytopenia (artifact)
- Schistocytes (TTP)
- Spherocytes (hemolysis)
- Left shift, bands (sepsis)
- Blasts (leukemia)
- Large platelets (peripheral destruction)
- Macrocytosis (liver disease, ETOH)

Review of complete blood count
- Concomitant cytopenias

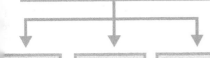

Decreased platelet production

Increased platelet destruction

Increased platelet sequestration

TABLE 62.1	Pathophysiologic Classification of Thrombocytopenia	
Decreased Production	**Increased Destruction**	**Increased Sequestration**
Aplastic anemia	Immunologic	Hypersplenism from any cause:
Hematologic malignancies	ITP	Cirrhosis
Lymphoma	Heparin-induced (HIT)	Portal hypertension
Leukemia	Drug-induced (see Table 62.2)	Congestive heart failure
Myelodysplasia	HIV	Hematologic malignancies
Metastatic malignancy	Autoimmune disease	Lipid storage disorders
Nutritional (vitamin B_{12} and folate)	Infectious	
Drugs (see Table 62.2)	Posttransfusion purpura	
Chemotherapy and radiation	Antiphospholipid antibody syndrome	
Alcohol	Nonimmunologic	
Viral infections	DIC	
HIV	HUS/TTP	
Mumps	HELLP syndrome	
Parvovirus	Preeclampsia/eclampsia	
Varicella	Malignant HTN	
Rubella	Sepsis	
Epstein–Barr	Cardiac valves	
Hepatitis C	Burns	
	Massive bleeding	

HIV, human immunodeficiency virus; ITP, immune thrombocytopenic purpura; HIT, heparin-induc[ed] thrombocytopenia; DIC, disseminated intravascular coagulation; HUS, hemolytic uremic syndrom[e]; TTP, thrombotic thrombocytopenic purpura; HELLP, hemolysis, elevated liver enzyme levels and a[nd] low platelet count; HTN, hypertension.

IMMUNE THROMBOCYTOPENIC PURPURA

Immune thrombocytopenic purpura (ITP) is a condition caused by autoantibod[ies] directed against the platelets surface glycoproteins. Binding of the antibodies resu[lts] in accelerated platelet removal by the spleen. *Evans syndrome* refers to ITP togeth[er] with autoimmune hemolytic anemia. The diagnosis of ITP is made by exclusio[n]; checking for antiplatelet antibodies has no role in the diagnosis. Treatment consi[sts] of corticosteroids, intravenous immunoglobulin, anti-RhD antibodies, rituxima[b], danazol, cyclophosphamide, azathioprine, or splenectomy.

HEPARIN-INDUCED THROMBOCYTOPENIA

Type 1 Heparin-Induced Thrombocytopenia

Platelet counts often decline modestly in the first few days after starting thera[py] with a heparin product. This is a spontaneously resolving, reversible decline with[in]

TABLE 62.2	Common Drugs Associated with Thrombocytopenia	
Decreased Production	**Immune-Mediated Destruction**	**Unknown Mechanism**
Chemotherapeutic agents	Abciximab (all GP2b3a inhibitors)	Fluconazole
Busulfan	Amphotericin B	Ganciclovir
Cyclophosphamide	Aspirin	Nitrofurantoin
Cytosine arabinoside	Carbamazepine	Rifampin
Daunorubicin	Chloroquine	Valganciclovir
Methotrexate	Cimetidine	
6-Mercaptopurine	Clopidogrel	
Vinca alkaloids	Digoxin	
Estrogens	Eptifibatide	
Ethanol	Heparin	
Linezolid	Meropenem	
Thiazide diuretics	Phenytoin	
	Piperacillin	
	Quinine	
	Ranitidine	
	Trimethoprim/sulfamethoxazole	
	Valproic acid	
	Vancomycin	

platelet nadir above 100,000/mcL. This condition is not normally associated with complications.

Type 2 Heparin-Induced Thrombocytopenia

This is a much more serious disorder that occurs when patients develop antibodies against the heparin-platelet factor-4 complex. It can be induced by exposure to unfractionated or low–molecular-weight heparins. Important clues to the diagnosis include a >50% decline in the platelet count 5 to 10 days after being exposed to heparin for the first time. A more rapid decline in platelet counts can occur with prior heparin exposures. The platelet count is often well below 100,000/mcL without clinical evidence of bleeding. In addition, patients may develop erythema or necrosis at heparin injection sites and systemic symptoms like fever, wheezing, and tachycardia from heparin boluses. The major clinical problem with continued heparin exposure is not bleeding but devastating thrombotic complications in up to 50% of patients. These thromboses can be venous or arterial and can result in life-threatening complications such as limb ischemia, deep venous thrombosis, pulmonary embolism, myocardial infarction, cerebral sinus thrombosis, stroke as well as mesenteric and renal infarction. When this diagnosis is suspected, all sources of heparin products should be immediately stopped, a serologic test (ELISA) for heparin-dependent antibodies should be requested, and the patient should be started on a direct thrombin inhibitor. The current ELISA for heparin-platelet factor-4 antibodies is highly sensitive but has low specificity. A more specific functional assay which measures platelet degranulation and serotonin release in response to heparin-platelet factor-4 complexes is available to confirm the diagnosis, however therapy with a direct thrombin inhibitor should not be delayed if there is significant clinical concern for HIT. Currently available direct thrombin inhibitors include lepirudin (renally metabolized), argatroban (hepatically metabolized), and bivalirudin (FDA approved for use in patients with HIT or suspected HIT undergoing percutaneous coronary interventions). Appropriate dosing of the thrombin inhibitors is critical to avoid bleeding complications and should be discussed with an ICU pharmacist, taking into account the patient's renal and hepatic function. An additional option is fondaparinux, a synthetic selective factor Xa inhibitor, the dosing of which is weight based and dependent on renal function. Platelets should not be given to patients with HIT unless there is life-threatening bleeding. Once the platelet count has demonstrated recovery to greater than 100,000/mcL, warfarin therapy should be initiated and the direct thrombin inhibitor should be continued until therapeutic anticoagulation with warfarin has been achieved.

SEPSIS-INDUCED THROMBOCYTOPENIA

Sepsis-induced thrombocytopenia is usually multifactorial and caused by marrow suppression, increased platelet destruction, drugs used to treat the septic patient and associated DIC. Treatment is supportive and possible offending drugs should be stopped. Specific infections tend to cause thrombocytopenia, and physicians should be aware of the common culprits, according to their geographic location. In Missouri, ehrlichiosis needs to be considered and travelers from endemic areas should be screened for malaria. DIC is recognized by the combination of microvascular thrombosis and bleeding, thrombocytopenia, coagulopathy, and low fibrinogen levels. Treatment for this complication is supportive with therapy directed at the underlying cause and occasional use of platelets, fresh-frozen plasma, and cryoprecipitate for the actively bleeding patient.

THROMBOTIC THROMBOCYTOPENIC PURPURA

The diagnostic pentad of TTP is:

* Microangiopathic hemolytic anemia
* Thrombocytopenia
* Renal failure
* Fever
* Altered mental status

However, all five criteria are met in <40% of patients. The major differential diagnosis is DIC. Both TTP and DIC are associated with thrombocytopenia, microangiopathic hemolytic anemia, and schistocytes. In DIC, there is often an associated coagulopathy with prolonged PT, aPTT, and thrombin time which should all be normal in TTP. In addition, fibrinogen levels in DIC are low and fibrin degradation product (FDP) levels are high which should not be seen in TTP. The degree of thrombocytopenia is often more severe in TTP compared to DIC and the associated elevation in LDH levels is also more profound.

Management of patients with TTP is challenging. Importantly, platelet transfusions in these patients are contraindicated in the absence of life-threatening bleeding as they can precipitate vasoocclusive crises of vital organs, such as the brain and

1yocardium. This disorder is caused by an acquired deficiency of ADAMTS13, which normally cleaves von Willebrand factor multimers. Absence of ADAMTS13 activity results in large circulating multimers of von Willebrand factor, which cause latelets to adhere to the endothelium with resultant thrombosis, thrombocytopenia, nd shearing of red cells as they pass the thrombi, which causes a microangiopathic emolytic anemia. The syndrome is most commonly precipitated by infections (*Escherichia coli* O157:H7 enteritis, human immunodeficiency virus) or drugs (ticlopidine, yclosporine, tacrolimus, and clopidogrel). Treatment consists of plasma exchange or esh-frozen plasma/intravenous immunoglobulin if plasma exchange is not immediately available. The assay for ADAMTS13 plays no role in diagnosis in the acute tting.

LATELET TRANSFUSIONS

he indications for transfusing platelets depend on the cause of the thrombocytopenia and the presence of bleeding. As previously noted, transfusions should be avoided TTP and HIT unless the patient is experiencing life-threatening bleeding. For her causes, platelets should be transfused prophylactically when the platelet count <10,000/mcL to prevent spontaneous intracranial bleeding. For major surgery, e counts should be >100,000/mcL; for minor procedures, the counts should be 50,000/mcL.

UGGESTED READINGS

ca S, Haji-Michael P, de Mendonca A, et al. Time course of platelet counts in critically ill patients. *Crit Care Med.* 2002;30(4):753–756.

> *This prospective, observational multicenter cohort study identified late thrombocytopenia (day 14) as being predictive of death and related changes in platelet count over time to patient outcome.*

epally GM, Ortel TL. Clinical practice. Heparin-induced thrombocytopenia. *N Engl J Med.* 2006;355(8):809–817.

> *An excellent recent review of the incidence, diagnostic algorithm, and therapies available.*

1es DB, Bussel JB. How I treat idiopathic thrombocytopenic purpura. *Blood.* 2005;106(7): 2244–2251.

> *A thorough review of the topic for clinicians.*

orge JN. Clinical practice. Thrombotic thrombocytopenic purpura. *N Engl J Med.* 2006; 354(18):1927–1935.

> *An excellent review of the topic for clinicians.*

einacher A. Clinical Practice. Heparin-induced thrombocytopenia. *N Engl J Med.* 2015; 373(3):252–261.

> *An excellent case based review article which covers risk factors, diagnosis, and treatment of HIT.*

GK, Juhl D, Warkentin TE, et al. Evaluation of pretest clinical score (4T's) for the diagnosis of heparin-induced thrombocytopenia in two clinical settings. *J Thromb Haemost.* 2006;4(4):759–765.

> *A prospective study evaluating the diagnostic utility of a clinical scoring system for HIT based on using the 4 T's: Severity of the thrombocytopenia, timing of the thrombocytopenia, presence of thrombosis, and evaluating other causes of thrombocytopenia.*

e TW, Wheeler AP. Coagulopathy in critically ill patients: part 1: platelet disorders. *Chest.* 2009;136(6):1622–1630.

> *An excellent clinically focused 2 part review of the common coagulopathies and platelet disorders encountered in the ICU.*

Salter BS, Weiner MM, Trinh MA, et al. Heparin-induced thrombocytopenia: a comprehensi clinical review. *J Am Coll Cardiol.* 2016;67(21):2519–2532.

Comprehensive review of the topic including scoring systems and a nice section on the dr used to treat HIT.

Sekhon SS, Roy V. Thrombocytopenia in adults: a practical approach to evaluation and manag ment. *South Med J.* 2006;99(5):491–498.

A concise review for clinicians with relevant suggestions for daily clinical practice.

Strauss R, Wehler M, Mehler, K, et al. Thrombocytopenia in patients in the medical intensi care unit: bleeding prevalence, transfusion requirements, and outcome. *Crit Care M* 2002;30(8):1765–1771.

Prospective observational study in a university hospital, found that 44% of patients develop ICU-acquired thrombocytopenia. These patients had higher mortality, more bleed and greater transfusion requirements.

Vanderschueren S, De Weerdt A, Malbrain M, et al. Thrombocytopenia and prognosis in inte sive care. *Crit Care Med.* 2000;28(6):1871–1876.

Prospective observational cohort study which identified thrombocytopenia as a readily availa risk marker for mortality, independent of severity of disease indices.

Vincent JL, Yagushi A, Pradier O. Platelet function in sepsis. *Crit Care Med.* 2002;30(5 sup S313–S317.

A review of the multifactorial etiology of thrombocytopenia in septic patients and the role of plate in modulating sepsis.

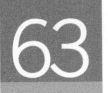

63

Acute Management of the Bleeding Patient/ Coagulopathy

Zaher K. Otrock and Ronald Jackups, Jr.

Bleeding in the intensive care unit (ICU) is common and associated with several known etiologies. Initial evaluation of the patient by history and physical examination will usually lead to a cause of bleeding. A patient bleeding from a single site will most likely have a structural defect (e.g., site of trauma, gastrointestinal bleed), whereas a patient bleeding from multiple mucosal surfaces or from puncture sites most likely has a derangement in the coagulation or fibrinolytic systems of hemostasis (e.g., disseminated intravascular coagulation [DIC], factor deficiency). No history of bleeding suggests an acquired reason for bleeding, whereas a lifelong history of bleeding suggests a genetic or congenital etiology. Determining the cause of bleeding in the patient is paramount to rapid management and control of the bleeding.

Hemostasis is a tightly regulated process that involves complex interactions between circulating proteins, blood cells, and vascular endothelial cells. This process can be divided into two phases: primary and secondary hemostasis. *Primary hemostasis* refers to a process that requires interactions between intact platelets, endothelial cells, and von Willebrand factor (vWF), which leads to the formation of a platelet plug. Abnormal primary hemostasis typically results in bleeding from mucosal surfaces (e.g., epistaxis, gastrointestinal bleeding, vaginal bleeding, or hematuria) and skin (petechiae or prolonged bleeding at venipuncture sites). *Secondary hemostasis* refers to the formation of the fibrin clot and is achieved through the activation of coagulation proteins. Any significant deficiency in coagulation proteins or interference with their activations, and hence the formation of the fibrin clot, will lead to excessive bleeding. Abnormal secondary hemostasis may be clinically manifested by spontaneous bleeding from deep tissue sites (e.g., intraperitoneal bleeding, hemarthroses, and intramuscular hematomas). This chapter focuses on the identification and the management of bleeding that is primarily due to abnormalities in secondary hemostasis. Thrombocytopenia-related bleeding is addressed in a Chapter 62. Structural bleeding, such as gastrointestinal bleeding, is addressed in Chapters 48 and 49.

COAGULATION

Coagulation and subsequent fibrin formation have been historically represented as occurring by two distinct pathways (Fig. 63.1). The extrinsic or tissue factor (TF) pathway is classically triggered by tissue injury and release of TF into circulation, which then activates factor VII. The intrinsic pathway or contact activation pathway classically occurs in response to blood contact with an artificial or negatively charged surface. Each pathway is depicted as the sequential activation of coagulation factors

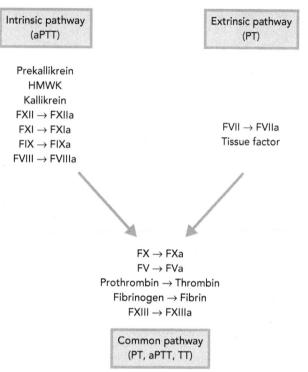

Figure 63.1. Classical Model of Hemostasis. The classical coagulation cascade is depicted as two distinct pathways converging on a common pathway. Although the pathways are not distinct *in vivo*, the distinct pathways can be measured *in vitro*. Disorders of the intrinsic pathway are measured by the activated partial thromboplastin time (aPTT), and disorders of the extrinsic pathway are measured by the prothrombin time (PT). HMWK, high–molecular-weight kininogen; FV/VII/VIII/IX/X/XI/XII, factors V/VII/VIII/IX/X/XI/XII.

in the presence of calcium and phospholipids and converges onto a common pathway to form thrombin. Thrombin, in turn, cleaves fibrinogen to form fibrin, and thus clot is formed. These pathways do not act independently *in vivo*, but this concept useful in laboratory diagnosis and treatment of coagulopathies; defects in the extrinsic pathway are measured by the prothrombin time (PT) and defects in the intrinsic pathway by the activated partial thromboplastin time (aPTT).

More recently, a cell-based model of thrombin generation has been proposed show the *in vivo* interaction between the classical pathways. This model proposes that the TF pathway initiates activation, whereas the contact activation pathway amplifies the activation.

Screening Tests for Coagulation

Initial testing to determine the cause of bleeding should include a PT, aPTT, and platelet count. If these fail to elucidate the cause of bleeding, further testing for platelet function and deficiencies in the fibrinolytic pathway may be necessary. Table 63 lists the interpretation of the most common patterns of coagulation screening tests

TABLE 63.1	Rapid Interpretations of Abnormal Prothrombin Time and/or Activated Partial Thromboplastin Time in a Bleeding Patient	
PT Result	aPTT Result	Possible Interpretation and Associating Conditions/Coagulopathy
Normal	Normal	Platelet dysfunction, thrombocytopenia, factor XIII deficiency, α2-antiplasmin deficiency, plasminogen activator inhibitor-1 deficiency
Prolonged	Normal	Liver diseases (early), warfarin therapy factor VII deficiency/defect
Normal	Prolonged	Heparin therapy, hemophilia A/B/C, factor XII deficiency, a lupus anticoagulant[a]
Prolonged	Prolonged	Liver disease (end stage), vitamin K deficiency, oral anti-coagulants, disseminated intravascular coagulopathy, isolated fibrinogen, factor II, V, or X deficiency/defect

Although factor XII deficiency and lupus anticoagulant may cause an isolated prolonged aPTT, they are not associated with bleeding.

Further Tests to Assess Acute Bleeding

Thrombin Time (TT): It measures the conversion of fibrinogen to fibrin. Prolonged results occur when

- heparin or a direct thrombin inhibitor is in the test system;
- fibrinogen is decreased or abnormal;
- therapeutic fibrinolysis or fibrinogen degradation products (FDPs) are present; and
- liver disease is severe.

Mixing Studies: These studies are conducted to determine the cause of a prolonged aPTT or PT.

These tests are performed to distinguish between factor deficiencies and inhibitors of coagulation. A 50:50 mix of patient's plasma and pooled normal plasma is tested immediately and after 1 hour incubation at 37°C. Figure 63.2 depicts the interpretation of mixing studies.

Platelet Function Test (e.g., **PFA-100**): In the presence of a normal platelet count and a hemoglobin level of at least 10 g/dL, PFA-100 is useful in detecting platelet dysfunction, including inherited defects and acquired defects due to aspirin therapy. Further laboratory testing such as platelet aggregation tests may be needed to characterize the platelet defect, but will not alter the initial therapy.

Viscoelastic Tests of Coagulation: Rotational thromboelastometry (ROTEM) and thromboelastography (TEG) are two systems that allow near real-time hemostasis evaluation within 10 to 30 minutes from blood draw. Both devices measure changes in the physical properties of the clot by monitoring the movement of a suspended in activated blood. As the clot begins to form, its physical properties, including elasticity and shear modulus, are displayed on the tracing, giving physicians information on global hemostatic properties during complicated surgical procedures and trauma. Both coagulation pathways (intrinsic or extrinsic) can be simulated depending on the choice of the activator.

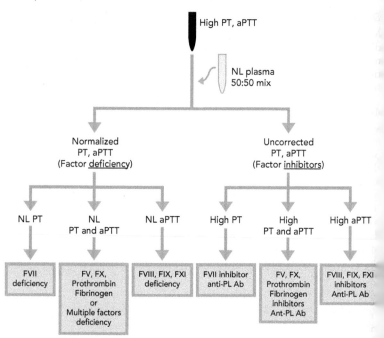

Figure 63.2. Mixing Analysis of Elevated Prothrombin Time (PT) and Activated Partial Thromboplastin Time (aPTT) in a Bleeding Patient. Patient's plasma is mixed with normal pooled plasma at 1:1 rat followed by subsequent retesting of PT and aPTT. Normalization of PT or aPTT suggests a factor deficien However, if mixing study does not correct the prolongation, this favors the presence of factor-specific nonspecific inhibitors. NL, normal; FV/VII/VIII/IX/X/XI, factors V/VII/VIII/IX/X/XI; anti-PL Ab, ar phospholipid antibody.

COMMON ACQUIRED DISORDERS OF COAGULATION IN THE CRITICAL CARE SETTING

Vitamin K Deficiency and Warfarin Therapy

Causes

- Inadequate oral vitamin K intake
- Antibiotics
- Generalized fat malabsorption
- Warfarin therapy

Pathophysiology

Vitamin K is a cofactor for γ-glutamyl carboxylation, which is required for the fu tion of factors II, VII, IX, and X, protein C, and protein S. Therefore, patients w vitamin K deficiency often present with prolonged PT and elevated internatio normalized ratio (INR). Major sources of vitamin K are green leafy vegetables, and colonic flora. With daily intake of 100 to 200 μg of vitamin K, a healthy ad has 1 week reserve of vitamin K.

Diagnosis

Measuring vitamin K–independent coagulation factors (e.g., factor V) is useful to distinguish vitamin K deficiency from liver disease. Vitamin K levels are not routinely measured. Ultimately, the diagnosis is made by a shortening of the PT in response to treatment with vitamin K. Failure to correct the PT after vitamin K administration suggests an alternative cause of PT prolongation.

Management

Vitamin K therapy may be given through intravenous (IV), subcutaneous (SC), or enteral routes. In a critically ill bleeding patient, the enteral route should generally be avoided because of high likelihood of gut dysfunction, whereas the SC route should be avoided in patients with perfusion defects or edema. There is a risk of anaphylaxis with IV administration of vitamin K; therefore, this route should be restricted to those situations where the SC or enteral routes are not feasible and the risk of anaphylaxis is considered justified. Unfortunately, in the critically ill patient, this is the most reliable route. A dose of 1 to 2 mg should be given either daily until the PT has corrected or for 3 days. Patients with milder forms of vitamin K deficiency may be treated with oral vitamin K of 5 to 20 mg, depending on the severity of the deficiency. The effect of vitamin K supplementation should be observed within 24 hours. In the setting of life-threatening bleeding (e.g., intracranial bleeding), fresh-frozen plasma (FFP) should be given at the initial dose of 10 to 15 mL/kg with concurrent slow administration of 10 mg of IV vitamin K. If 4-factor prothrombin complex concentrates (PCCs) (see next paragraph) are available, they may be used instead of FFP for rapid correction; the dose is based on the patient's weight and INR.

PCCs are also used for reversal of warfarin. PCCs contain coagulation factors II, IX, and X, with variable amounts of factor VII, protein C, protein S, antithrombin III, and heparin. The available concentrates are 3- and 4-factor PCC, with 4-PCC containing higher concentrations of factor VII. PCCs are advantageous over FFP in that they offer faster normalization of INR, smaller infusion volume, and no need for ABO blood-type matching. Both are relatively safe, with 4-PCC being superior to 3-PCC in correcting INR.

Liver Disease

Causes

Shock liver due to hypoperfusion
Acute hepatitis
Chronic liver disease
Acute liver injury

Pathophysiology

The liver is the major organ that produces coagulation factors (except vWF and factor VIII) and fibrinolytic proteins. It is also important in clearing activated factors and inhibitors of coagulation. Insults to the liver are associated with bleeding abnormalities caused by factor deficiencies and accumulation of activated factors and inhibitors of coagulation, which may interfere with platelet function. In addition, hypersplenism is often associated with liver cirrhosis and portal hypertension and may cause thrombocytopenia.

Diagnosis

PT and aPTT are often prolonged, and fibrinogen may be low. In the absence additional coagulation factor inhibitors, the abnormal clotting time may be correc *in vitro* by the 50:50 mixing study. Measuring factor V and factor VII levels may b differentiate liver disease from vitamin K deficiency. Both factors are deficient in l disease, whereas only factor VII is deficient in vitamin K deficiency.

Management

FFP, cryoprecipitate (rich source of fibrinogen), and platelets should be used in setting of active bleeding. In general, a platelet count of 50,000/μL, a fibrino level of >60 mg/dL, and PT less than two times normal control should be adequ to achieve hemostasis. The initial dose of FFP should be 10 to 15 mL/kg (~4 6 units). For thrombocytopenic patients, one unit of single donor platelets (or f units of random platelet concentrates) should be given with a posttransfusion plat count dictating further dosing. Cryoprecipitate is usually given in pools of up to units, which generally contain 1500–2000 mg of fibrinogen in 150 mL. In rare ca where bleeding is not controlled after adequate resuscitation with blood produ recombinant factor VIIa (RFVIIa) might be considered. RFVIIa has been associa with clinically significant thrombosis and should be used with caution. There is well-defined study for the dosing in off-label use of RFVIIa; however, 20 to 90 μg should provide adequate hemostatic control. In the absence of active bleeding, p phylactic FFP, cryoprecipitate, or platelet transfusion has not been shown to red bleeding risk or improve outcome.

Disseminated Intravascular Coagulation

Cause

There are many causes of DIC (Table 63.2). Common conditions associated w DIC include tissue damage, neoplasia, infection, or obstetric emergencies.

Pathophysiology

DIC is a consumptive coagulopathy with rapid and enhanced systemic activation normal coagulation. Through consumption of coagulation and fibrinolytic fact and their inhibitors, an imbalance in this tightly regulated process occurs. Excess

TABLE 63.2	Underlying Conditions Commonly Associated with Disseminated Intravascular Coagulation
Sepsis	Pregnancy complications (abruptio placentae, septic
Trauma/crush injury	abortion, amniotic fluid embolus, HELLP syndrome,
CNS injury	eclampsia, and severe preeclampsia)
Heat stroke	Uterine atony
Burns	Fat emboli
Venomous snake bites	Tumor lysis syndrome
	Acute hemolytic transfusion reaction
	Liver disease

CNS, central nervous system; HELLP, hemolysis, elevated liver enzyme levels, and a low platelet count.

brin clots are formed in small and mid-size blood vessels causing thrombotic occlu-
ions and ultimately end-organ damage. Coagulation factors are quickly exhausted
ithout adequate physiologic compensation, and bleeding occurs.

Diagnosis

DIC is characterized by prolonged PT/aPTT/TT, thrombocytopenia, and microan-
iopathic hemolytic anemia. The level of fibrinogen may be normal due to pathologic
ompensation in the early disease stage; however, significant hypofibrinogenemia is
ound in severe DIC. D-dimer will be markedly elevated and is useful to distinguish
DIC from other coagulopathies with thrombocytopenia.

Management

he primary goal of management is to treat the underlying disease causing DIC.
ometimes this is all it takes to stop the process. However, in most cases, this is
ot easily or rapidly accomplished, and the patient will need further support.
esuscitation to maintain adequate perfusion is necessary, as acidosis will only
acerbate the coagulopathy. The role of FFP, cryoprecipitate, and platelets is
nclear. In a bleeding patient, platelet transfusions (usually as a single-donor
atelet or 4 to 6 platelet concentrates) are generally given to keep the platelet
ount above 50,000/μL and cryoprecipitate (usually in pools of 10 units) to keep
e fibrinogen above 60 mg/dL. The role of antithrombin III concentrates and
parin is controversial in most cases of DIC. Heparin has been useful in cases
subacute DIC associated with acute promyelocytic leukemia, abdominal aortic
eurysm, and purpura fulminans.

Uremic Bleeding

Causes

eeding in patients with uremia is multifactorial, including intrinsic platelet dys-
nction and abnormal platelet–vessel wall interactions. In addition, anemia contrib-
es to increased bleeding, because platelets flow more centrally in the vessel, making
ess likely that they would interact with the injured vessel wall.

Pathophysiology

cumulation of toxin (e.g., guanidinosuccinic acid) in plasma inhibits normal
atelet activation and aggregation. Increased levels of nitric oxide and prostacyclin
found in patients with uremia compared to nonuremic individuals, and these
gatively impact platelet adhesion to endothelium and platelet–platelet interactions.
fects in platelet function have been attributed to the environment in which the
atelets exist, as incubation of platelets from a uremic patient in normal plasma cor-
ts the dysfunction, whereas placement of platelets from a nonuremic individual in
emic plasma reproduces the defect.

Diagnosis

ients with uremia usually present with mucosal bleeding, such as gingival bleed-
, epistaxis, and hematuria. Less commonly, central nervous system and severe
rointestinal bleeding may occur. In addition to laboratory changes associated
h decreased renal function, patients may present with a decrease in hemoglobin
mild thrombocytopenia. The most common laboratory abnormality, although

not routinely performed, is decreased platelet aggregation in response to exogenous agents. PT and aPTT are usually normal.

Management

Hemodialysis or peritoneal dialysis is the most effective method to improve platelet function in patients with uremia. Red blood cell transfusions to correct anemia have been shown to decrease bleeding in the acute situation. Desmopressin (DDAVP) at a dose of 0.3 μg/kg IV or SC every 24 hours (or 10 units of cryoprecipitate when DDAVP has been ineffective or contraindicated) may temporarily control the bleeding. Platelet transfusions will not be effective in the setting of uremia. Once uremia is corrected, the patient's endogenous platelets should be functional.

Bleeding Due to Direct Oral Anticoagulants

Causes

Since 2010, direct oral anticoagulants (DOACs) have emerged as alternatives to warfarin to treat deep vein thrombosis (DVT) and pulmonary embolism (PE) and to prevent thrombosis in certain conditions (e.g., atrial fibrillation). However, they also present new challenges due to bleeding risk.

Pathophysiology

Direct thrombin inhibitors (e.g., dabigatran, argatroban, bivalirodin) bind to and inhibit the action of thrombin in cleaving fibrinogen. Factor Xa inhibitors (e.g., rivaroxaban, apixaban, edoxaban) bind to and inhibit the action of factor Xa in cleaving prothrombin. These drugs are taken once or twice a day and do not require routine therapeutic drug monitoring, unlike warfarin. Patients are anticoagulated within a few hours of taking the first dose and will return to their hemostasis baseline within 1 to 2 days of discontinuing the drug, assuming adequate renal function.

Diagnosis

A thorough history from the bleeding patient should include recent use of any anticoagulant medication. While there are currently no FDA-approved tests to measure DOAC activity, existing tests are sufficiently sensitive to detect the presence of DOACs. A normal thrombin time effectively rules out a direct thrombin inhibitor. A negative anti-factor Xa inhibitor assay, usually used for dosing of heparin or low-molecular-weight heparin, effectively rules out a factor Xa inhibitor. PT and/or aPTT are generally prolonged, but the degree of prolongation does not necessarily correlate with drug concentrations or bleeding risk.

Management

Reversal of DOACs with FFP, or even PCCs, is likely to be inadequate; in most cases, bleeding will need to be managed expectantly while the drug is cleared naturally. Dabigatran can potentially be removed by hemodialysis. A new specific reversal agent for dabigatran called idarucizumab may be used if available. There is currently no specific reversal agent for factor Xa inhibitors, but trials of potential agents (e.g., andexanet alfa) are in progress.

COMMON CONGENITAL DISORDERS OF COAGULATION

Hemophilia A and B

Cause

Hemophilia is a genetic deficiency in a specific coagulation factor that is associated with increased bleeding risk. Most individuals inherit the gene causing the deficiency, but up to 30% of deficiencies are caused by a spontaneous mutation. *Hemophilia A* (factor VIII deficiency), the most common type, is an X-linked genetic disorder that affects 1 in 5,000 male births and up to 80% of all hemophiliac individuals. The severity of hemophilia is categorized into mild, moderate, and severe forms correlating with the degree of factor VIII deficiency (6% to 30%, 2% to 5%, and <1%, respectively). *Hemophilia B* (factor IX deficiency) is also an X-linked genetic disorder and has an incidence of 1 in 25,000 male births worldwide, which contributes to 20% to 25% of the hemophilia cases. In contrast to factor VIII, which has a half-life of 8 to 12 hours, factor IX has longer half-life (24 to 25 hours) and wider tissue distribution. *Hemophilia C* (factor XI deficiency) is an autosomal genetic disorder that tends to have a milder course than hemophilia A or B, and will not be discussed here.

Pathophysiology

In general, factor VIII and factor IX levels of ≥30% are sufficient for normal coagulation. With decreasing amounts of these factors, *in vivo* hemostasis is impaired. Primary hemostasis and platelet function are normal.

Diagnosis

Individuals with hemophilia will have an isolated prolongation of the aPTT. Those with severe hemophilia present with a lifelong history of spontaneous bleeding, which may include hemarthroses. Up to 30% of patients will present without a family history of bleeding. Individuals with moderate hemophilia will usually have an excessive bleeding history if trauma or surgery has occurred. Individuals with mild hemophilia might present with a prolongation of the aPTT without a history of excessive bleeding. The final diagnosis is made with the finding of decreased factor VIII or IX levels in patient's plasma.

Management

Treatment depends on the severity of the hemophilia and severity of bleeding.

Hemophilia A: DDAVP may be used to increase factor VIII activities by three-to fivefold in patients with mild and moderate forms of hemophilia A and should be tried in cases of mild bleeding. The typical dose, given intravenously or subcutaneously, is 0.3 µg/kg. The expected rise in factor VIII should occur within 5 to 8 hours. Patients with severe hemophilia and any bleeding will require factor concentrates or factor replacement. Factor VIII concentrates are either viral-inactivated plasma-derived or recombinant products. Both are effective, and an individual choice is usually made on the basis of availability. Factor VIII concentrate is dosed by the patient's weight. A unit of factor VIII concentrate should increase the plasma activity of factor VIII by 2% per kg of body weight. The goal of replacement therapy in patients with minor bleeding is a factor VIII activity of 25% to 30%; with moderate to severe bleeding, it is 50%; and with surgical or life-threatening bleeding, it is 75% to 100%. Factor VIII concentrate has a half-life of 8 hours, and activities should be monitored during treatment. Dosing is usually repeated every 8 to 12 hours, depending on the measured plasma activities of factor VIII. Treatment should be continued until the bleeding is stabilized. In the surgical patient, factor replacement is typically continued for 10 to 12 days after the procedure.

Some patients with hemophilia A will develop inhibitors to factor VIII, which will prevent the concentrates from working. In these patients, RFVIIa at a dose of 90 to 120 µg/kg every 2 hours may be given until hemostasis is achieved. These patients may consume an enormous amount of concentrates and should be managed by an experienced hematologist.

Hemophilia B: Plasma-derived and recombinant factor IX products are available for replacement therapy. Each unit of factor IX concentrate should raise the plasma factor IX activity by 1% per kg of body weight. Factor IX half-life is 24 hours and therefore dosing should occur at 18- to 24-hour intervals. The subsequent doses are usually half the initial dose, but monitoring of plasma activities will help to adjust the dose as necessary. The target plasma activities of factor IX are similar to those noted earlier for factor VIII. Bleeding patients with inhibitors to factor IX should be treated with RFVIIa, as noted earlier for patients with inhibitors to factor VIII.

von Willebrand Disease

Causes

von Willebrand disease (vWD) is a genetic disease caused by a deficiency or qualitative defect in vWF. It is the most common inherited bleeding disorder, and is most often inherited in an autosomal dominant manner; therefore, men and women are equally affected.

Pathophysiology

vWF is a carrier molecule for factor VIII, and normal levels are needed to maintain adequate levels of factor VIII in circulation. In addition, vWF is necessary for platelet adhesion to the vessel wall at sites of injury and thus is essential for normal platelet function. There are several types of vWD, ranging from mild to severe quantitative disorders and several types with qualitative defects.

Diagnosis

Patients with vWD present with mucocutaneus bleeding (e.g., bleeding from gums, menorrhagia in women) and easy bruising. vWF antigen, vWF activity (by immuno assay or ristocetin cofactor [RCo] activity), and factor VIII activity are measured to determine the type of vWD. Types I (mild) and III (severe) are quantitative defects of vWF, whereas type II (subdivided into several different defects) is a qualitative defect. von Willebrand multimer studies may be necessary to determine the type of vWD.

Management

DDAVP, which promotes the release of vWF, has been shown to be beneficial in raising the vWF in type 1 and certain type 2 vWD patients. It should not be used in individuals diagnosed with type IIB vWD or type III. If individuals are refractory to DDAVP or are severely deficient in vWF (type III vWD), vWF/FVIII concentrate should be given. The initial dose in severe bleeding or surgery is 40 to 60 RCo units/kg ollowed by 20 to 40 RCo units/kg every 12 to 24 hours to keep vWF activities at 0% to 100% for 7 to 14 days. For milder bleeding and surgery, an initial dose of 30 o 60 RCo units/kg should be given, followed by 20 to 40 RCo units/kg every 12 to 8 hours to keep the vWF above 30% for 3 to 5 days. Antifibrinolytic agents (e.g., minocaproic acid, tranexamic acid) may be helpful adjuvant treatments to achieve emostasis in patients bleeding from mucosal surfaces.

UGGESTED READINGS

loffman M. A cell-based model of coagulation and the role of factor VIIa. *Blood Rev.* 2003; 17:51–55.
  A succinct review highlighting the importance of the cellular control of hemostasis in vivo.

evi M, Hugo TC. Disseminated intravascular coagulation. *N Engl J Med.* 1999;341:586–592.
  Review of diagnosis and management of DIC.

evi M, Levy JH, Andersen HF, et al. Safety of recombinant activated factor VII in randomized clinical trials. *N Engl J Med.* 2010;363:1791–1800.
  Analysis of thrombotic events in 35 randomized trials of off label use of recombinant FVIIa.

lacLaren R, Wilson SJ, Campbell A, et al. Evaluation and survey of intravenous vitamin K1 for treatment of coagulopathy in critically ill patients. *Pharmacotherapy.* 2001;21:175–182.
  Observational study and survey of vitamin K usage in ICU patients.

annucci PM. Treatment of von Willebrand's disease. *N Engl J Med.* 2004;351:683–694.
  Review of laboratory diagnosis and treatment of VWD.

annucci PM, Tuddenham EG. The hemophilias–from royal genes to gene therapy. *N Engl J Med.* 2001;344:1773–1779.
  Review of history, biology and treatment of hemophilias, including discussion on plasma-derived and recombinant products.

arks PW. Coagulation disorders in the ICU. *Clin Chest Med.* 2009;30:123–129.
  Review of mechanisms, laboratory abnormalities and management of coagulation disorder in ICU patients.

oris M, Remuzzi G. Uremic bleeding: closing the circle after 30 years of controversies. *Blood.* 1999;94:2569–2574.
  Review of mechanism of bleeding in uremia.

shal M. Thromboelastography/Thromboelastometry. Chapter 154. In: Shaz BH, Hillyer CD, Roshal M, Abrams CS, eds. Transfusion Medicine and Hemostasis: Clinical and Laboratory Aspects London, Waltham, San Diego: Elsevier; 2013.
  Review of ROTEM/TEG.

avitz RT. Critical management decisions in patients with acute liver failure. *Chest.* 2008; 134:1092–1102.
  Review of etiology, treatment and management of complications of acute liver failure.

ils SA, Holder MC, Premraj S, et al. Comparative effectiveness of 3- versus 4-factor prothrombin complex concentrate for emergent warfarin reversal. *Thromb Res.* 2015;136:595–598.
  Comparative study between the effectiveness of 3- and 4-PCC for emergent warfarin reversal.

64 Transfusion Practices

Vladimir N. Despotovic and Morey A. Blinder

Anemia is a common problem in the intensive care unit (ICU) setting. In the critically ill patient, oxygen delivery and oxygen consumption may be impaired by factors such as decreased cardiac output, decreased red cell mass, decreased circulating blood volume from red blood cell (RBC) loss, and altered acid–base status. Causes of anemia in this setting are varied and include overt blood loss from bleeding, frequent blood draws or hemolysis, a functional decrease in usable iron, and decreased erythropoietin production.

Anemia is traditionally treated with infusions of RBCs to increase oxygen-carrying capacity and tissue delivery of oxygen. Various studies have estimated that more than 40% of all ICU patients receive blood transfusions and that more than two-thirds of these transfusions were not for acute blood loss.

In most critically ill patients the transfusion trigger of hemoglobin (Hb) <7 g/dL is recommended. This is based on the recent multicenter randomized trials and systematic reviews showing decreased complications and decreased mortality when compared to the higher transfusion triggers of 9 to 10. Transfusion Requirements in Critical Care (TRICC) trial was the original large multicenter RCT that showed decreased hospital mortality with the hemoglobin goal of 7 to 9 g/dL as opposed 10 to 12 g/dL. Transfusion thresholds in septic shock (TRISS) trial showed that septic shock a restrictive transfusion strategy that maintained Hb ≥7 g/dL had similar mortality at 90 days to the Hb ≥9 g/dL with 50% fewer units of blood transfused. In the setting of an acute upper GI bleed Hb ≥7 g/dL had a higher probability survival compared to the hemoglobin target of ≥9 g/dL at 6 weeks and fewer over complications. Notably massive gastrointestinal bleeds and hemodynamically unstable patients were excluded from the trial and 51% of the patients in the restrictive transfusion trigger group never received any blood. In the setting of a massive bleed the transfusion practices and blood product ratios should be guided by the clinical situation and the clinician experience. Under circumstances of coronary artery disease and acute coronary syndromes (ACSs), more trials are needed to clarify the beneficial transfusion goals. In ACS, a trend toward increased survival has been demonstrated with transfusions for hemoglobin levels 8 to 10 g/dL. Recent pilot trial looking patients with ACS undergoing cardiac catheterization found death at 30 days to less frequent in the liberal transfusion goal group for Hb <10 g/dL as compared to more restrictive goal for Hb <8 g/dL. Nevertheless, transfusion practices must take into account systemic organ dysfunction that may affect oxygen delivery, anticipated blood losses, and overall patient morbidity, resulting in patient and situation-specific use of RBCs and other blood products.

In massive transfusions, various protocols have been institutionally developed, and the data comes from the severe trauma patients. The initial transfusions are based on the bleeding and the hemodynamic instability. Serial monitoring of hemoglobin level, platelets, PT/INR, PTT, fibrinogen and if available viscoelastic testing should be performed. In the initial resuscitation in a severe trauma setting, FFP:Plt:RBC ratio of 1:1:1 appears to be well supported. In the nontraumatic setting there is insufficient data available, and the ratios from 1:1:1 to 2:1:4 are used. Following and correcting the acid–base status, hypocalcemia and hypothermia should be a part of the protocol. Antifibrinolytic therapies, factor concentrates, and recombinant factor VII use should also be considered.

In patient populations who refuse blood transfusions on cultural, religious, or personal belief basis, their wishes should be honored. The most well-known religious group that commonly declines blood transfusions are Jehovah's Witnesses. Confirmation of the patient's understanding of short- and long-term risks and the benefits should be obtained. For a bleeding, anemic patient in the ICU setting aggressively controlling the bleeding source, minimizing phlebotomy, administration of erythropoiesis stimulating agents and IV iron are most commonly used. Careful review of medications should be performed, and if possible, medications that could increase the bleeding diathesis should be discontinued and antifibrinolytic or if acceptable recombinant factor therapy should be considered.

DOSING AND ADMINISTRATION

Each unit of packed RBCs is approximately 300 mL and is generally given during 2 to 3 hours. One unit of packed RBCs is expected to increase hemoglobin by approximately 1 g/dL and raise the hematocrit by approximately 3% in a healthy individual without ongoing blood loss or destruction. Prior to transfusions, the patients' blood should be tested for ABO status, but type O-negative RBCs can be given in emergency situations.

TYPES OF RBC PRODUCTS

Table 64.1 presents some of the various blood products and their indications. Included in this section is further discussion of common products.

Whole Blood

Whole blood is currently used in autologous donation situations (prior to surgery, and so forth). Whole blood contains all normal constituents of human plasma, including RBCs, platelets, and plasma proteins.

Packed RBCs

Packed RBCs contain approximately 200 mL of RBCs resuspended in a preservative solution. Each bag has a hematocrit of approximately 55% to 60% and approximately 200 to 250 mg of iron.

Gamma-Irradiated

External-beam radiation is applied to the unit of blood to produce gamma-irradiated blood. This allows for destruction of donor T lymphocytes for prevention of

TABLE 64.1	Blood Products	
Product	Indications	Comments
Packed red blood cells	• Increase oxygen-carrying capacity in patients with anemia • Can be used to increase blood volume in acute loss	• Transfusions to keep Hgb ≥7 g/dL in ICU setting • Data support higher levels in ACS, from Hb >8 g/dL to Hb >10 g/dL (see text)
Platelets	• Thrombocytopenia with high risk of bleeding • *Not* indicated in presence of increased destruction without bleeding	• Prophylactic transfusion only if platelet count <10,000/μL • Maintain platelet count ≥50,000/μL with active bleeding or in anticipation of an invasive procedure • Thresholds for procedures vary by institution
Fresh-frozen plasma	• Bleeding in setting of factor deficiency or coagulopathy • Warfarin reversal • Severe DIC	• Dosage ranges from 5–15 mL/kg, but generally start with 2 units and recheck PT/PTT
Cryoprecipitate	• Fibrinogen deficiency	• Contains fibrinogen as well as vWF, factors VIII, XIII, and fibronectin
Humate-P	• vWD types 2B, 2N, 3	• A specific vWF-containing factor VIII concentrate
Factors VIII and IX concentrates	• Hemophilia A and B treatment, respectively	• Virally inactivated • Recombinant technologies have eliminated infectious risks
Recombinant Factor VIIa	• Bleeding complications in acquired hemophilia A and B • Factor VII deficiency	• Recombinant • Used for surgery and acute bleeding in hemophilia

Hgb, hemoglobin; ICU, intensive care unit; ACS, acute coronary syndrome; DIC, disseminated intravascular coagulation; PT/PTT, prothrombin time/partial thromboplastin time; vWF, von Willebrand factor; vWD, von Willebrand disease.

graft-versus-host disease in stem cell transplant patients and severely immunocom promised patients.

Cytomegalovirus Antibody-Negative

Cytomegalovirus (CMV) antibody-negative blood is used in patients who are know to be CMV-negative and at high risk for complications if infected with CMV (e.g transplant patients and pregnant patients). Leukocyte reduction is also a relative

ffective method for reducing risk of CMV infection. Leukocyte reduction is per-
ormed most often at the time of product collection.

Washed RBCs

The donor cells are processed with normal saline to remove as much of the donor
serum as possible. This is most commonly used in patients who are immunoglobulin
(IgA)-deficient and at a high risk for anaphylaxis during transfusions, as well as in
paroxysmal nocturnal hemoglobinuria patients to deplete complement.

RISK OF TRANSFUSIONS

Transfusion of blood products carries risks. These risks can be divided on the basis
of whether the complication is short term (related to each unit that is transfused) or
long term (proportional to the total number of units that a patient receives over his
or her lifetime).

Short-Term Transfusion Risks

Acute Hemolytic Reactions

The most serious and immediately life-threatening complication of transfusions is an
acute hemolytic reaction. This is due to antibodies, usually immunoglobulin M, in
the recipient's serum against major antigens present on the donor RBCs, and occurs
with an estimated frequency of 1 in 250,000 to 1 in 1,000,000. This is initially manifested acutely as fever, dyspnea, tachycardia, back pain, hypotension, chills, and chest
pain, within the first several minutes of the transfusion. If an acute hemolytic reaction
is suspected, *the infusion should be stopped immediately,* and the blood bank notified.
Algorithm 64.1 outlines management strategies for acute hemolytic reactions.

Delayed Hemolytic Reactions

Delayed hemolytic reactions usually occur more than 24 to 48 hours, and up to 7
to 10 days, after a transfusion. Delayed reactions result from antibodies in the recipient's serum that are directed toward minor antigens on the donor's RBCs, which
are produced by an anamnestic response. This usually manifests as an asymptomatic
but sudden decrease in hemoglobin concentration, with laboratory evidence of
hemolysis, including a positive direct Coombs test and increased indirect bilirubin
concentration.

Nonhemolytic Febrile Reactions

Nonhemolytic febrile reactions occur in approximately 1% of transfusions and are
the result of antibodies in the recipient's serum against white blood cells in the donor's
product. This manifests acutely as an increase in body temperature and is more common in patients who have been previously alloimmunized by numerous transfusions.
This reaction is treated with antipyretic medications.

Allergic Reactions

Allergic reactions occur because of transfused allergens in the donor's product, with
symptoms such as urticaria and bronchospasm; they occur in approximately 1 in 100
transfusions. This condition is treated with antihistamine medications. However, a
potentially severe form may be encountered in IgA-deficient individuals who can

ALGORITHM 64.1 **Management of Acute Hemolytic Reaction**

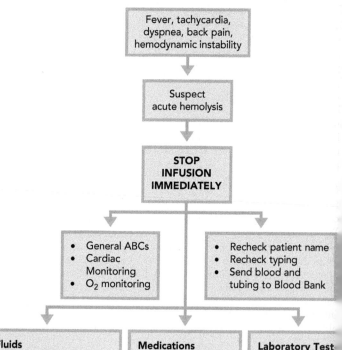

Fever, tachycardia, dyspnea, back pain, hemodynamic instability

↓

Suspect acute hemolysis

↓

STOP INFUSION IMMEDIATELY

- General ABCs
- Cardiac Monitoring
- O$_2$ monitoring

- Recheck patient name
- Recheck typing
- Send blood and tubing to Blood Bank

IV Fluids
- D5W with 3 amps NaHCO$_3$ at 250 mL/hr
- Keep UOP >30–50 mL/hr

Medications
- Hydrocortisone 100 mg IV
- Diphenhydramine 50 mg IV
- Acetaminophen 650 mg PO
- Epinephrine 0.3 mL of 1:1000 SC

Laboratory Test
- CBC
- Coombs test
- Urine free hemoglobin
- Haptoglobin
- PT/PTT
- Fibrinogen
- Bilirubin
- LDH

ABBREVIATIONS

IV:	intravenous
D5W:	5% dextrose in water
UOP:	PO, orally
SC:	subcutaneously
CBC:	complete blood count
PT/PTT:	prothrombin time/partial thromboplastin time
LDH:	lactate dehydrogenase

have anaphylactic reactions to serum from non–IgA-deficient donors. This is best prevented with washed RBCs, but can be treated with high-dose corticosteroids, airway protection, and antihistamines.

Transfusion-Related Acute Lung Injury

Transfusion-related acute lung injury (TRALI) occurs by an incompletely understood mechanism, but an immune antibody-mediated process has been established in a majority of cases. A nonimmune mechanism has been postulated as well. Data from animal models and recent clinical studies suggest that both processes occur and that TRALI may be the end result of diffuse neutrophil activation and capillary leak by these mechanisms. TRALI presents with diffuse capillary damage in the pulmonary vasculature with rapid-onset dyspnea, hypoxia, fever, and bilateral pulmonary infiltrates resembling acute respiratory distress syndrome, in the absence of volume overload or heart failure. Treatment is supportive as most cases are self-limiting, but patients may require mechanical ventilation.

Bacterial Infection

Blood units can be contaminated with bacterial agents, including cold-growing organisms such as *Yersinia enterocolitica*, as well as various gram-negative organisms. With chronic infections like syphilis, currently routine testing for Treponema pallidum is performed. Incidence of bacterial infection has dramatically decreased since the introduction of disposable plastic blood bags.

Long-Term Transfusion Risks

Viral Infections

Infectious complications of blood transfusions are located in Table 64.2. All blood products are currently screened for hepatitis B, hepatitis C, human immunodeficiency virus 1 and 2, and human T-lymphotropic virus I and II. In the United States, West Nile virus and Zika virus testing have recently been added to the screening process. Other infectious risks include viruses that are not universally screened for, such as CMV and parvovirus B19, and the prion-transmitted Creutzfeldt–Jacob disease.

TABLE 64.2	Transfusion-Associated Infections		
Virus	**Risk Factor (per million)**	**Estimated Frequency (per unit)**	**No. of Deaths (per million units)**
Hepatitis A	1	1/1,000,000	0
Hepatitis B	7–32	1/30,000–1/250,000	0–0.14
Hepatitis C	4–36	1/30,000–1/150,000	0.5–17
HIV	0.4–5	1/200,000–1/2,000,000	0.5–5
HTLV I and II	0.5–4	1/250,000–1/2,000,000	0
Parvovirus B19	100	1/10,000	0

HIV, human immunodeficiency virus; HTLV, human T-lymphotropic virus.
Adapted from Goodnough LT, Brecher ME, Kanter MH, et al. Transfusion medicine. First of two parts–blood transfusion. *N Engl J Med.* 1999;6:438–441. With permission.

Other Infections

Chronic protozoan infections like Chagas disease and babesiosis can occasionally be transmitted through transfusion, and are minimized through selective screening processes.

Iron Overload

Although not typically an issue in the ICU setting, secondary iron overload syndromes occur in proportion to the number of blood products a patient receives. Patients at highest risk include those with multiple transfusions over long periods of time (e.g., sickle-cell disease, thalassemias, myelodysplastic syndromes). Each milliliter of packed RBCs contains approximately 1 mg of iron. Patients who are repeatedly transfused in the absence of blood loss are at risk of overwhelming the body's ability to use iron with resultant deposition into tissues such as the myocardium, bone marrow, and liver.

SUGGESTED READINGS

Carson JL, Brooks MM, Abbott JD, et al. Liberal versus restrictive transfusion thresholds fo patients with symptomatic coronary artery disease. *Am Heart J.* 2013;165(6):964–971.

Drews RE. Critical issues in hematology: anemia, thrombocytopenia, coagulopathy, and blood product transfusions in critically ill patients. *Clin Chest Med.* 2003;24:607–622.
  A systematic review of diagnosis, evaluation, and treatment of blood and bleeding disorder commonly encountered in the critical care setting.

Garfinkle M, Lawler PR, Filion KB, et al. Red blood cell transfusion and mortality amon patients hospitalized for acute coronary syndromes: a systematic review. *Int J Cardio* 2013;164(2):151–157.

Goodnough LT, Brecher ME, Kanter MH, et al. Transfusion medicine. First of two parts-bloo transfusion. *N Engl J Med.* 1999;6:438–441.
  A review article on principles of basic transfusion medicine, including complications an indications for transfusion.

Herbert PC, Wells G, Blajchman MA, et al. A multicenter, randomized, controlled clinical tri of transfusion requirement in critical care. *N Engl J Med.* 1999;6:409–417.
  A randomized trial of 838 ICU patients to receive transfusions for hemoglobin levels of less tha 10 g/dL, or 7 g/dL. Overall 30-day mortality was similar in the two groups, but the was significantly less in-hospital mortality in patients transfused for hemoglobin levels le than 7 g/dL (22.2% vs. 28.1%, p 0.05), demonstrating that a "restrictive" transfusio strategy is well tolerated and potentially superior to liberal transfusion strategies.

Holcomb JB, Pati S. Optimal trauma resuscitation with plasma as the primary resuscitative flui the surgeon's perspective. *Hematology Am Soc Hematol Educ Program.* 2013;2013(1):656 659.

Holcomb JB, Tilley BC, Baraniuk S, et al. Transfusion of plasma, platelets, and red blood cel in a 1: 1: 1 vs a 1: 1: 2 ratio and mortality in patients with severe trauma: the PROPP randomized clinical trial. *JAMA.* 2015;313(5):471–482.

Holst LB, Haase N, Wetterslev J, et al. Lower versus higher hemoglobin threshold for transf sion in septic shock. *N Engl J Med.* 2014;371(15):1381–1391.

McLellan SA, McClelland DB, Walsh TS. Anaemia and red blood cell transfusion in the cri cally ill patient. *Blood Rev.* 2003;17:195–208.
  A review of anemia and transfusion strategies in critically ill patients.

Pajoumand M, Erstad BL, Camamo JM. Use of Epoetin Alfa in critically ill patients. *Ann Ph macother.* 2004;38:641–648.
  A review of the use of Epoetin Alfa for reduction of red blood cell transfusions in critically patients with anemia.

riulzi DJ. Transfusion-related acute lung injury: an update. *Hematology Am Soc Hematol Educ Program.* 2006;497–501.

Review of current research and proposed mechanisms of TRALI.

Jy GL. Transfusion medicine. In: Lin TL, ed. *Hematology and Oncology Subspecialty Consult.* Baltimore, MD: Lippincott, Williams & Wilkins; 2004:73–79.

Book chapter focusing on basic transfusion medicine and practical information about blood products and proper use.

illanueva C, Colomo A, Bosch A, et al. Transfusion strategies for acute upper gastrointestinal bleeding. *N Engl J Med.* 2013;368(1):11–21.

incent JL, Baron JF, Reinhart K, et al. Anemia and blood transfusion in critically ill patients. *JAMA.* 2002;12:1499–1507.

*A prospective observational study of patients in European ICUs evaluating the prevalence of anemia and transfusion use in this setting.*AQ1: Permission needed

65

Hypercoagulable States

Vladimir N. Despotovic and Morey A. Blinder

Hypercoagulable states are a heterogeneous group of inherited or acquired disorders that predispose individuals to the inappropriate formation of a clot in the venous or arterial circulation. The inappropriate formations of thrombi occur in the presence of Virchow's triad of hypercoagulability, stasis, and endothelial damage. Embolization of these clots can occur, resulting in pulmonary embolism (PE) in the case of venous embolic disease, or emboli to vital organs in the setting of arterial thrombosis.

Various manifestations of hypercoagulability are demonstrated in the intensive care unit (ICU) setting. Patients are at an increased risk of venous thromboembolic disease because of their prolonged immobilization, procedures, and intravascular devices that they are exposed to, and their underlying disease states. Patients in the ICU setting may have transient risk factors for thromboembolic disease, or may in addition have underlying predisposing genetic or acquired conditions that increase their risk. Notably previous thromboembolic events are a prominent risk factor for future thromboembolism, particularly if they occurred without surgical or clear precipitating factors. The common causes of hypercoagulability are listed in Table 65.1.

DEEP VENOUS THROMBOSIS AND PULMONARY EMBOLISM

Deep venous thrombosis (DVT) and PE are very common in the ICU and are likely underdiagnosed. Some observational studies have demonstrated a 20% to 40% incidence of DVT in the ICU setting.

Diagnosis of DVT and PE in the ICU can be challenging (Algorithms 65.1 and 65.2). Various studies have demonstrated that 10% to 100% of DVTs diagnosed ultrasound in this setting were not found on physical examination. Furthermore, patients in the ICU setting have a number of factors confounding the diagnosis, including their numerous comorbid conditions, inability to communicate symptoms, numerous procedures and medications, and inability to undergo various diagnostic tests. Table 65.2 lists the diagnostic modalities for DVT and PE.

Treatment of DVT and PE should commence when clinically suspected if contraindications exist. As previously mentioned, diagnosis can be difficult in the ICU setting, but delay in treatment can lead to increased morbidity and mortality. Clinically suspected DVT or PE should be treated with weight-based unfractionated heparin or in a more stable patient with low–molecular-weight heparin. Our preference in critically ill patients is unfractionated heparin or in the setting of suspected heparin-induced thrombocytopenia (HIT), bivalirudin, or argatroban.

TABLE 65.1	Causes of Hypercoagulability	
Acquired Causes		**Inherited Causes**
Trauma/surgery		Factor V Leiden mutation
Malignancy		Prothrombin G20210A mutation
Immobilization		Protein C deficiency
Nephrotic syndrome		Protein S deficiency
Obesity		Antithrombin deficiency
Pregnancy		Increased factor VIII activity
Oral contraceptive use		Dysfibrinogenemia
Congestive heart failure		
Myeloproliferative disorders		
Antiphospholipid antibodies		
Lupus anticoagulant		
Anticardiolipin antibodies		
Heparin-induced thrombocytopenia (HIT)		
Paroxysmal nocturnal hemoglobinuria (PNH)		

since both agents are shorter acting, can be stopped for bleeding or procedures and can be adjusted for renal dysfunction. In addition to the oral vitamin K antagonist, warfarin, recently multiple new direct oral anticoagulants (DOACs) that function as direct thrombin inhibitors (dabigatran) or direct factor Xa inhibitors (rivaroxaban, apixaban, and edoxaban) have been introduced. Due to their long half-life and renally affected pharmacokinetics, these agents should have limited use in the ICU

TABLE 65.2	Diagnostic Tests for Deep Venous Thrombosis (DVT) and Pulmonary Embolism (PE) in the Intensive Care Unit Setting	
Test	**Indication for Testing**	**Key Points**
Venous duplex ultrasound	Suspected DVT in extremities	• Good sensitivity and specificity for proximal DVT
Spiral computed tomography	Suspected PE	• Good sensitivity for large PEs • Contrast bolus predisposes to nephrotoxicity
Ventilation–perfusion scanning	Suspected PE	• Good sensitivity for PEs • Difficult to interpret in setting of recent pneumonia or other infiltrative process
Computed tomography angiography/venography	Suspected DVT or PE	• Not widely available • Large bolus of contrast used

Adapted from Cook D, Douketis J, Crowther MA, et al. The diagnosis of deep venous thrombosis and pulmonary embolism in medical-surgical intensive care unit patients. *J Crit Care.* 2005;20(4):314–319, with permission.

ALGORITHM 65.1 Algorithm for Diagnosis of Deep Venous Thrombosis (DVT)

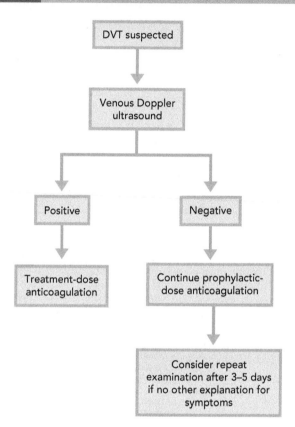

DVT suspected

↓

Venous Doppler ultrasound

Positive

↓

Treatment-dose anticoagulation

Negative

↓

Continue prophylactic-dose anticoagulation

↓

Consider repeat examination after 3–5 days if no other explanation for symptoms

ABBREVIATIONS
DVT: deep venous thrombosis
PE: pulmonary embolism
SC: subcutaneously
HIT: heparin-induced thrombocytopenia
IV: intravenous

ALGORITHM 65.2 Algorithm for Diagnosis of Pulmonary Embolism (PE)

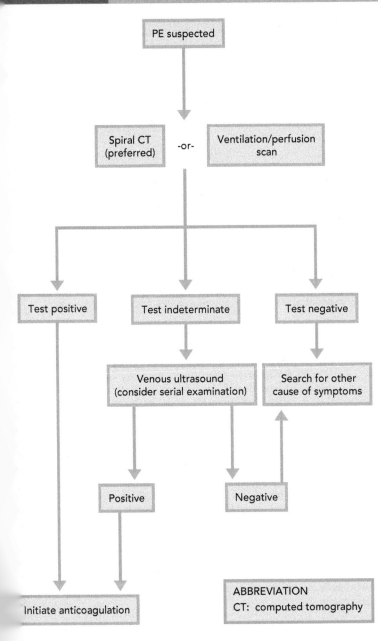

ABBREVIATION
CT: computed tomography

TABLE 65.3	Weight-Based Unfractionated Heparin Dosing
Initial Dose	
Bolus 60–80 U/kg	
Infusion 14–18 U/kg/hr	
Adjustment: aPTT[a]	
<40	2.000 units IV bolus and increase infusion rate by 2 U/kg/hr
40–44	Increase infusion rate by 1 U/kg/hr
45–70	No change
71–80	Decrease infusion by 1 U/kg/hr
81–90	Hold infusion for 30 min, decrease infusion rate by 2 U/kg/hr
>90	Hold infusion for 1 hr, decrease infusion rate by 3 U/kg/hr

aPTT, activated partial thromboplastin time; IV, intravenous.
[a]aPTT should be drawn 6 hrs after any adjustment to dose.

setting. Dosing guidelines for unfractionated heparin and some alternatives are list in Tables 65.3 and 65.4.

DVT prophylaxis decreases the incidence of PE and venous thromboemboli in the ICU patient. In general, all patients in the ICU should receive pharmacolo and/or mechanical DVT prophylaxis if no contraindication exists.

ARTERIAL THROMBOEMBOLISM

Acute arterial thrombosis can be secondary to embolization of material (e.g., fr the atria in atrial fibrillation or from a proximal source secondary to a damag artery), or an in situ formation of clot. Symptoms are generally related to the te tory served by the artery that has thrombosed, and generally is noted as a pain pale, and cool extremity, or an acute neurologic deficit in the case of a stro However, in the ICU setting, these symptoms may be masked by the patie comorbidities.

Clues from the physical examination can yield evidence as to the source of thrombosis. Multiple sites of ischemia are typical of an embolic phenomenon (h ever can also be seen in the setting of vasculitis), whereas isolated ischemia is m typical of in situ thrombosis. Further evaluation of suspected arterial thrombosis be performed with Doppler signal assessment and compression ultrasound, altho computed tomographic angiography (CTA) can be more anatomically revealing helpful.

Treatment of suspected arterial thrombosis should be instituted immedia as delay in treatment can result in irreversible damage due to tissue ischemia. A coagulation should be initiated as outlined in Tables 65.3 and 65.4, and surgic percutaneous interventionalist consultation should be sought for possible opera management.

TABLE 65.4	Alternative Anticoagulants			
Drug	Mechanism of Action	Use	Prophylaxis Dosing	Therapeutic Dosing
Enoxaparin	Inactivation of factor Xa	Prophylaxis and treatment of DVT/PE	40 mg SC q24h	1 mg/kg SC q12h or 1.5 mg/kg SC q24h
Dalteparin	Inactivation of factor Xa	Prophylaxis and treatment of DVT/PE	5000 units SC q24h	100 U/kg SC q12h or 200 U/kg SC q24h
Fondaparinux	Inactivation of factor Xa	Prophylaxis and treatment of DVT/PE, HIT	2.5 mg SC q24h	7.5 mg SC q24h or 10 mg SC q24h if >100 kg
Argatroban	Direct thrombin inhibitor	Treatment of thrombosis in HIT		2 µg/kg/min IV
Bivalirudin	Direct thrombin inhibitor	Treatment of thrombosis most commonly in the setting of HIT	None	Adjusted by CrCl 0.15 mg/kg/hr (see reference below)

DVT, deep venous thrombosis; PE, pulmonary embolism; SC, subcutaneous; HIT, heparin-induced thrombocytopenia; IV, intravenous.

HYPERCOAGULABILITY EVALUATION

Patients in the ICU have many transient risk factors for the development of thromboembolic disease. Because of this, most instances of thromboembolism do not warrant workup for an underlying hypercoagulable state. The optimal time for laboratory evaluation of hypercoagulable states is unclear, but is often undertaken approximately weeks to 6 months after the event. Laboratory evaluation in the immediate days to weeks following a thrombosis can yield false results because of the increase in acute-phase reactants associated with acute clot formation, which can result in false-positive tests for hypercoagulable states. However, in the setting of recurrent or atypical thrombosis, such as cerebral vein or visceral vein thrombosis, and nonembolic arterial thrombosis, further evaluation is warranted. Minimal workup should include evaluation for HIT, lupus anticoagulant, anticardiolipin antibody, and fasting plasma homocysteine level. In cases marked by recurrent thrombosis or cerebral or visceral vein thrombosis, further workup should include a prothrombin G20210A mutation analysis, paroxysmal nocturnal hemoglobinuria (PNH) testing, as well as a factor V Leiden mutation analysis. Hematology consultation should be obtained for further evaluation and long-term treatment planning.

CONDITIONS ASSOCIATED WITH DECREASED PLATELETS AND HYPERCOAGULABILITY

There are occasional conditions that present with thrombocytopenia as well as hyper-coagulability. HIT is a serious condition manifested by the formation of antibodies to platelets in response to heparin administration. This condition can cause thrombosis in the setting of severe thrombocytopenia, and is discussed in detail in Chapter 62.

Thrombotic thrombocytopenia purpura is another condition associated with hypercoagulability and thrombocytopenia. This serious condition is the result of a deficiency of or inhibitor to the von Willebrand factor cleaving protease, ADAMTS 13. It is manifested by thrombocytopenia, microangiopathic changes on peripheral blood smear (schistocytes), fever, mental status changes, and varying degrees of renal insufficiency. Treatment is emergent and requires immediate hematology consultation and plasma exchange. This condition is discussed further in the Chapter 61.

Disseminated intravascular coagulation can also present with thrombocytopenia and coagulopathy in the setting of hypercoagulability. Underlying conditions such as sepsis, ischemia, acidosis, and multiorgan failure can induce a consumptive coagulopathy, resulting in the formation of diffuse thrombi as well as diffuse hemorrhage.

SUGGESTED READINGS

Burnett AE, Mahan CE, Vazguez SR, et al. Guidance for the practical management of the direct oral anticoagulants (DOACs) in VTE treatment. *J Thromb Thrombolysis.* 2016;41(1):206–232.

Cook D, Douketis J, Crowther MA, et al. The diagnosis of deep venous thrombosis and pulmonary embolism in medical--surgical intensive care unit patients. *J Crit Care.* 2005 20(4):314–319.
  Review of current data investigating diagnostic modalities for DVT and PE with focus on patients in the critical care setting.

Geerts WH. Prevention of venous thromboembolism in high-risk patients. Hematology Am Soc Hematol Educ Program. 2006:462–466.
  Review of prophylactic modalities for DVT in patients in various clinical circumstances.

Kiser TH, Burch JC, Klem PM, et al. Safety, efficacy, and dosing requirements of bivalirudin in patients with heparin-induced thrombocytopenia. *Pharmacotherapy.* 2008;28(9):1115–1124.

Levine JS, Branch DW, Rauch J. The antiphospholipid syndrome. *N Engl J Med.* 2002;346(10) 752–763.
  A review of the pathogenesis, diagnosis, and treatment strategies of the Antiphospholipid Antibody Syndrome.

Nachman RL, Silverstein R. Hypercoagulable states. *Ann Intern Med.* 1993;119(8):819–827.
  A review of the major pathophysiologic mechanisms underlying inherited and secondary hypercoagulable states and review of the frequency, natural history, diagnosis, and management of the disorders.

Nakashima MO, Rogers HJ. Hypercoagulable states: an algorithmic approach to laboratory testing and update on monitoring of direct oral anticoagulants. *Blood Res.* 2014;49(2):85–9.

eles S, Pillot, G. Thrombotic disease. In: Pillot G, Chantler M, Magiera H, et al., eds. Hematology and Oncology Subspecialty Consult. Baltimore, MD: Lippincott, Williams & Wilkins; 2004:25–32.

Edited book chapter describing hypercoagulable disease states, with focus on diagnosis and treatment strategies.

osenberg RD, Aird WC. Vascular-Bed–specific hemostasis and hypercoagulable states. *N Engl J Med.* 1999;340(20):1555–1564.

A review of the pathophysiologic mechanisms underlying coagulation disorders on a cellular level, describing the interaction of coagulation factors with vascular-bed–specific cellular signaling pathways.

abatabai A. Disorders of hemostasis. In: Ahya SN, Flood K, Parajothi S, eds. Washington Manual of Medical Therapeutics. 30th ed. Baltimore, MD: Lippincott, Williams & Wilkins; 2001:394–412.

Edited book chapter describing differential diagnosis, diagnostic strategies, and treatment modalities for hypercoagulable states, as well as bleeding disorders.

66 Critical Care Rheumatology

Dany Thekkemuriyil and Vladimir N. Despotovic

ICU admissions due to rheumatologic conditions are not very common. When the occur they are often complex with multisystem involvement. Rapid diagnosis of th condition and initiation of treatment can minimize morbidity and mortality of th patient population in the intensive care unit. In addition to the appropriate initi: diagnostic workup and initiation of treatment, early consultation with the Rheuma tology service and other affected organ system–specific consultants can optimize th management and follow-up of these often complicated patients.

GENERAL RULES

1. Most common cause for ICU admission for patients with rheumatologic illne is infection. The second most common cause is the autoimmune disease exace bation or complication.
2. Most common rheumatologic conditions in the ICU are rheumatoid arthrit systemic lupus erythematosus (SLE), and systemic sclerosis.
3. Most likely cause of fever in patients with a rheumatologic diagnosis is infectio
4. All serologic testing must be interpreted in context of the patient's clinical conditic
5. Inflammatory markers like ESR and CRP are acute phase reactants and are no specific in the critical care setting.
6. Caution should be exercised in the intubation of patients with rheumatoid arth tis (RA) particularly seropositive, erosive RA. Anterior atlantoaxial subluxation C1 on C2 may occur and compress the anterior spinal cord. Hyperextension the neck during intubation could result in quadriplegia. If no previous C-spi imaging is available inline stabilization of the spine should be done. Alternative fiberoptically guided endotracheal intubation can be performed.
7. Cricoarytenoid joint disease may cause difficulty with intubation in an I patient. It may present with hoarseness, inspiratory stridor, dyspnea, or wheezi
8. In SLE with heart failure symptoms consider myocarditis, valvular vege tions (Libman-Sacks), tamponade, premature atherosclerosis, or pulmon hypertension.
9. Suspect mesenteric ischemia or vasculitis for unexplainable abdominal pain SLE.
10. Cognitive impairment or coma without focal neurologic signs is extremely ra related to CNS vasculitis.
11. Septic arthritis is a medical emergency and if suspicion is high pursue the arth centesis promptly.

Steroid dosing:

- To treat RA flares dose equivalent of 20 mg of prednisone daily is usually adequate
- For acute management of gout if having contraindication for NSAIDs/Colchicine use prednisone 40 to 60 mg with quick taper over 7 to 10 days. Another option is 40 mg for 5 days without a taper.
- Mild SLE or vasculitis flare will usually respond to 40-mg prednisone equivalent with a 2-week taper.
- Moderate SLE or vasculitis flare will require high doses of steroids of 1 mg/kg/day (up to 60 to 80 mg/day) with a taper over 2 to 4 weeks usually with the adjustment of the chronic underlying immunosuppressive therapy.
- Severe life-threatening SLE or vasculitis, high doses of intravenous glucocorticoids are preferred (methylprednisolone 500 mg to 1 g IV daily for 3 to 5 days) followed by oral or parenteral therapy with the equivalent of 1 mg/kg of prednisone per day.
- In severe life-threatening illness with strong suspicion for autoimmune etiology do not delay therapeutic intervention. Once infection has been reasonably excluded, empiric glucocorticoids can be initiated and rheumatology or other appropriate service can be consulted.
- Patients who have been chronically on corticosteroids (even if none currently) will require stress dose steroids (hydrocortisone 50 mg IV Q 6 hours or equivalent) during critical illness or surgical procedures to avoid shock and acute adrenal insufficiency.

PULMONARY RENAL SYNDROME (PRS) AND DIFFUSE ALVEOLAR HEMORRHAGE (DAH)

PRS is a combination of DAH and rapidly progressive glomerulonephritis (RPGN) (Table 66.1).

When to suspect: Worsening diffuse pulmonary infiltrates, falling hemoglobin, often with low-grade fevers, in the setting of hematuria, RBC casts, and worsening renal failure.

Clinical Findings: Hemoptysis (absent in 30% of DAH), purpuric rash, active urinary sediment (RBC casts most specific, often not present), renal impairment, fall in hemoglobin levels, arthralgias/arthritis, mononeuritis multiplex, pericarditis/myocarditis/pleuritis, sinusitis, cerebral ischemia.

Investigation: Complete blood count with Hb and platelets, basic coagulation tests, hemolysis labs including a blood smear, BUN and Cr levels, urinalysis, spun urine sediment assessment, serologies including ANA, ANCA and anti-GBM, also consider RF/anti-CCP, myositis panel. Chest radiograph/chest CT scan. Flexible bronchoscopy with bronchoalveolar lavage with increasingly bloody returns on subsequent passes through a wedged bronchoscope. Biopsy is usually not necessary. Percutaneous renal biopsies with histopathology and immunohistochemistry can finalize the diagnosis.

Management: Treat the underlying condition, maintain adequate oxygenation, provide ventilatory support, correct the coagulopathy, provide adequate PEEP, if autoimmune condition suspected and no active infection consider high-dose steroids (pulse dose 1000 mg for 3 days followed by 1 mg/kg methylprednisolone equivalent) as well as possible plasmapheresis, IVIG, or specific immunosuppression

TABLE 66.1 Causes for Pulmonary Renal Syndrome and DAH	
ANCA-Associated Vasculitis	**Isolated DAH**
Granulomatosis with polyangiitis (GPA) (Wegener's granulomatosis)	Idiopathic pulmonary hemosiderosis
Microscopic polyangiitis (MPA)	Isolated pulmonary capillaritis
Eosinophilic granulomatosis with polyangiitis (EGPA) (Churg–Strauss syndrome)	**Other Causes**
Other Autoimmune Etiologies	
Anti-GBM disease (Goodpasture's syndrome)	Coagulopathies including DIC and iatrogeni
Antiphospholipid antibody syndrome (APS)	Thrombocytopenia including ITP
Systemic lupus erythematosus (SLE)	Thrombotic microangiopathy (TMA) includir TTP and HUS
Systemic sclerosis (SSc)	Hematopoietic cell transplantation
Idiopathic inflammatory myopathies (IIM)	Infections (particularly in the setting of coagulopathy)
Henoch–Schönlein purpura (HSP)	Drugs
Cryoglobulinemia	ARDS (particularly in the setting of coagulopathy)
Behcet's syndrome	Mitral stenosis
IgA nephropathy	Pulmonary infarct
Rheumatoid arthritis	Acute interstitial pneumonia (AIP)
Pauci-immune glomerulonephritis	Radiation pneumonitis
Mixed connective tissue disease	Infective endocarditis

depending on the condition and the diagnosis. ECMO assessment if available the appropriate candidates with difficulty oxygenating should be considered, a the presence of bleeding and potential need for anticoagulation should not considered absolute contraindications.

VASCULITIS (Fig. 66.1)

Large Vessel Vasculitis

Giant Cell Arteritis (GCA)

Most common systemic vasculitis with the lifetime risk of 1% in women and I percent in men (Table 66.2).

> **Clinical Features of ANCA Vasculitis** (Table 66.3, Fig. 66.2)
> **Additional considerations in ANCA-associated vasculitis:**

- The RAVE trial showed similar outcomes between cyclophosphamide and rit imab in nonintubated patients with serum creatinine less than 4. Lower-qua data support use of rituximab without the above exclusions.
- MAINRITSAN trial and its long-term follow-up study showed rituximab superi ity to azathioprine in maintenance of remission and improved long-term surviva

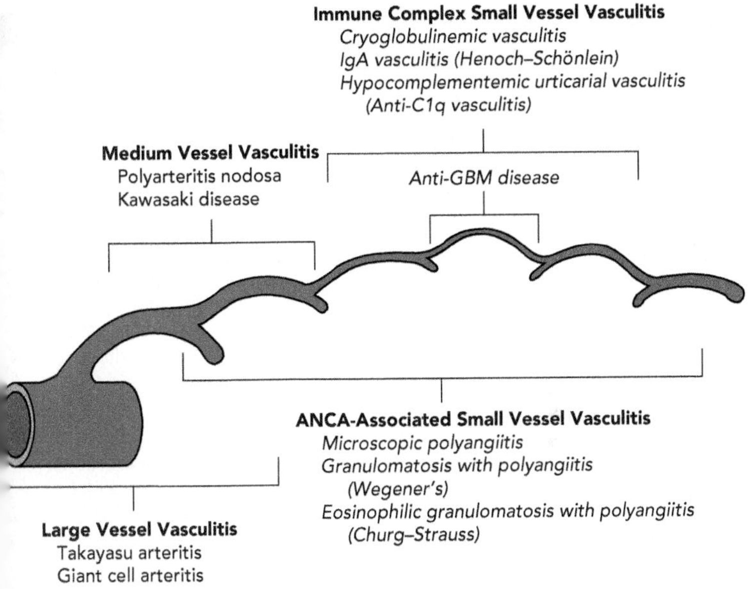

Immune Complex Small Vessel Vasculitis
Cryoglobulinemic vasculitis
IgA vasculitis (Henoch–Schönlein)
Hypocomplementemic urticarial vasculitis
(Anti-C1q vasculitis)

Medium Vessel Vasculitis
Polyarteritis nodosa
Kawasaki disease

Anti-GBM disease

ANCA-Associated Small Vessel Vasculitis
Microscopic polyangiitis
Granulomatosis with polyangiitis
(Wegener's)
Eosinophilic granulomatosis with polyangiitis
(Churg–Strauss)

Large Vessel Vasculitis
Takayasu arteritis
Giant cell arteritis

Figure 66.1. Predominant types of vessels affected by major categories of systemic vasculitis. Reproduced with permission from John Wiley & Sons, Inc. © Jennette JC, Falk RJ, Bacon PA, et al. 2012 revised international Chapel Hill consensus conference nomenclature of vasculitides. *Arthritis Rheum.* 2013;65(1):1–11.

Plasma exchange is commonly used in life-threatening scenarios, however the evidence for its use is not very robust. There is higher-quality evidence for renal disease than the pulmonary hemorrhage. Ongoing trial should provide more guidance soon.

CATASTROPHIC ANTIPHOSPHOLIPID SYNDROME (CAPS)

A rapidly progressive life-threatening disease that causes multiple-organ thromboses and dysfunction in the presence of antiphospholipid antibodies.

When to suspect: Rapid multiorgan thrombosis, especially in the setting of SLE, infections, or known APS. Elevated partial thromboplastin time (PTT) that does not correct with a 50:50 mixing study of patient plasma with normal plasma in the right clinical setting, in particular in the setting of a clot is also suggestive of the presence of an inhibitor and APS. Certain anticoagulant medications will alter the testing.

CAPS Features (Table 66.4)

It can be difficult to distinguish CAPS from other disease processes that can lead to multiple-organ thrombotic events such as HUS, TTP, and DIC.

CAPS Diagnostic Criteria (Table 66.5)

Management

High suspicion, early diagnosis, and aggressive therapy are essential

Treat the possible underlying infection

TABLE 66.2	Giant Cell Arteritis	
Risk Factors	Clinical Manifestations and When to Suspect	Treatment
• Age greater than 50, peak 70–80 • Scandinavian ethnicity, less common in Hispanics, Asians, and Mediterranean populations and least common in African Americans • Females have greater incidence than males • Polymyalgia rheumatica (PMR) • Family history	• Systemic symptoms including fever, weight loss, and fatigue • Presence of PMR • Headache • Jaw claudication • Cranial ischemic events including transient and permanent vision loss with classic ophthalmologic findings (anterior or posterior ischemic optic neuropathy or central retinal artery occlusion) • Large vessel vasculitis on imaging or pathology • Elevated ESR and CRP • Temporal artery tenderness or pulselessness • Imaging changes on MRI/MRA, ultrasonography, or PET imaging • Temporal artery biopsy with necrotizing arteritis or granulomatous inflammation with multinucleated giant cells	• High-dose steroids should be initiated early • If the suspicion is high the treatment with steroids should be initiated before the diagnosis is confirmed • If ischemic symptoms are present 1 mg/kg of prednisone or methylprednisolone daily should be started and pulse dose of methylprednisolone of 1 g/day x 3 days should be considered • If no ischemic symptoms are present lower initial doses of 40 mg/day prednisone can be considered • Start taper after 2–4 weeks • Consider low-dose daily aspirin 81–100 mg • In acute treatment failures consider cyclophosphamide • Consider tocilizumab as adjunct treatment to high-dose steroids based on the GiACTA study

- Anticoagulation with heparin
- Plasma exchange for 5 consecutive days with or without IVIG (400 mg/kg/day 5 days) after the plasma exchange has been completed.
- High doses of systemic glucocorticoids (pulse dose of methylprednisolone 1 for 3 days followed by oral or parenteral therapy equivalent to 1 mg/kg of pre sone per day, usually not exceeding 60 to 80 mg/kg).

TABLE 66.3	Clinical Features of ANCA-Associated Vasculitis		
	Granulomatosis with Polyangiitis (GPA) (Wegener's Granulomatosis)	Microscopic Polyangiitis	Eosinophilic Granulomatosis with Polyangiitis (EGPA) (Churg–Strauss Syndrome)
ANCA positive	80–90%	70%	50%
ANCA type	PR3 > MPO	MPO > PR3	MPO > PR3
Pulmonary	DAH, nodules, cavitary lesions, infiltrates	DAH	DAH, infiltrates, asthma
Renal	Segmental necrotizing glomerulonephritis	Segmental necrotizing glomerulonephritis	Segmental necrotizing glomerulonephritis
Ophthalmologic	Scleritis, episcleritis, uveitis	Rare: Scleritis, episcleritis, uveitis	Rare: Scleritis, episcleritis, uveitis
ENT	Saddle nose deformity, subglottic stenosis, hearing loss	Hearing loss	Allergic rhinitis, nasal polyps, hearing loss
Cardiac	Rare: Myocarditis, valvular lesions	Rare: Myocarditis	Myocarditis
Neurologic	CNS vasculitis, mononeuritis multiplex— occasional	CNS vasculitis, mononeuritis multiplex— common	CNS vasculitis, mononeuritis multiplex, very common
Pathology	Leukocytoclastic vasculitis, granulomas	Leukocytoclastic vasculitis	Leukocytoclastic vasculitis, eosinophilic granulomas/infiltrates

In refractory cases of CAPS in addition to standard therapy cyclophosphamide, rituximab and eculizumab have also been used.

Scleroderma Renal Crisis (Table 66.6)
Monoarthritis (Table 66.7)
Interpretation of Synovial Fluid Findings (Table 66.8)
Basic synovial fluid analysis includes:

Cell count with differential (EDTA-containing tube)
Gram stain and culture
Crystal analysis (often run from the cell count sample)

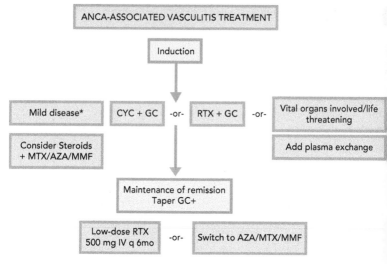

Figure 66.2. ANCA-associated vasculitis. *Not life or organ threatening disease.
MTX, methotrexate; AZA, azathioprine; MMF, mycophenolate; CYC, cyclophosphamide; RTX, rituximab;
GC, glucocorticoids.

TABLE 66.4	CAPS Features
Organ System Involved	**Clinical Features**
Heart	Cardiac valve thickening/Sterile endocarditis
Lungs	Pulmonary emboli, diffuse alveolar hemorrhage, ARDS
CNS	Cerebrovascular accidents
Viscera	Visceral ischemia
Other	Venous or arterial clot, especially atypical

TABLE 66.5	CAPS Diagnostic Criteria

Evidence of involvement of three or more organs, systems, or tissues
Manifestation development simultaneously or in less than 1 week
Histopathologic confirmation of small vessel occlusion in at least one organ or tissue
Laboratory confirmation of antiphospholipid antibodies (lupus anticoagulant,
 anticardiolipin antibodies, and/or anti–beta2-glycoprotein I antibodies)
Definite CAPS: All criteria met
Probable CAPS: Absence of second OR third criterion

TABLE 66.6	Scleroderma Renal Crisis

Risk Factors	Clinical Manifestations and When to Suspect	Management
• Diffuse skin involvement (up to 20%) • Palpable tendon friction rubs • Antibodies to RNA polymerase III • Use of systemic glucocorticoids	• Presence of scleroderma • Abrupt onset of severe hypertension • Acute onset, rapidly progressive renal failure • Microangiopathic hemolytic anemia and thrombocytopenia • Urinalysis can range from normal to mild proteinuria to abundant cells and casts (glomerulonephritis is not a feature)	• Antihypertensives, need to always include ACE inhibitors even in the setting of acute kidney injury and a rising creatinine • Supportive measures

TABLE 66.7	Arthrocentesis- Indications and Fluid Testing

Acute monoarthritis
Suspicion for infection, crystal-induced arthritis, or hemarthrosis
Joint effusion in the setting of trauma
Joint effusion with uncertain diagnosis

TABLE 66.8	Interpretation of Synovial Fluid Findings

	Non inflammatory	Inflammatory	Septic	Hemorrhagic
Appearance	Clear/Yellow/ Viscous	Cloudy/Yellow	Opaque/ Varies	Opaque/Red
WBC/ml	0–2000	>2000	>20,000	0–2000
PMNs	<25%	>50%	>75%	50–75%
Crystals	Absent	Present in gout and pseudogout	Absent	Absent
Comment	Normal/ Osteoarthritis	Gout, pseudogout, SLE, RA, spondyloarthropathy	Positive Gram stain and culture	High RBCs

GUIDANCE TO LABORATORY TEST INTERPRETATION AND KEY-ASSOCIATED FACTS

Systemic Lupus Erythematosus (SLE) (Table 66.9)
Systemic Sclerosis (SSc) (Scleroderma) (Table 66.10)
Antiphospholipid Antibody Syndrome (Table 66.11)
Vasculitis (Table 66.12)
Rheumatoid Arthritis (Table 66.13)
Myositis (Table 66.14)

TABLE 66.9	Systemic Lupus Erythematosus

Antinuclear Antibodies (ANA): If negative, extremely unlikely to have SLE. Positive test only useful if within the proper clinical scenario. Only 5% of the general population with positive ANA has SLE. Increased incidence with increased age, certain medications, malignancies, infections, and other autoimmune disorders.

Anti–Double Stranded DNA Antibodies (dsDNA): At moderate to high titers very specific for SLE.

Extractable Nuclear Antigen Antibodies (ENA):

Anti-Sm (Anti-Smith): Nearly 100% specific for SLE

Anti-Ro (SSA):
- Associated with Sjogren's syndrome (70%)
- Heart block in children with SSA-positive mothers
- Associated with subacute cutaneous lupus rash (SCLE)

Anti-La (SSB): Sjogren's syndrome

RNP: High titer anti–U1-ribonucleoprotein (RNP) antibodies in association with overlapping clinical features of SLE, systemic sclerosis (SSc), and polymyositis (PM) are seen in mixed connective tissue disease (MCTD)

Lupus Flare:
- Associated with elevated anti-dsDNA, low C3 and C4. These tests may correlate with disease activity, mainly with nephritis. Comparison to previous titers during low disease activity as well as disease flares can be helpful and can vary among different patients. Disease activity association with the anti-dsDNA, C3 and C4 tends to follow similar trends in individual patients.
- Urinalysis with urine microscopy and protein/creatinine ratio should be checked with suspected lupus nephritis.
- In anemic patients, hemolysis should be suspected and direct Coombs antibody test and evaluation for lupus-associated microangiopathic hemolytic anemia (MAHA) should be done.
- In thrombocytopenic patients ITP, TTP, and APS testing in addition to suspecting infectious and iatrogenic etiologies.
- In marked cytopenia of 2 or 3 cell lineages in the setting of SLE, especially if associated with a fever macrophage activation syndrome (MAS) should be suspected. MAS is also associated with elevated ferritin levels, elevated triglycerides, LFT elevations, elevated LDH and low haptoglobin, elevated soluble CD25 (sIL-2 receptor), abnormal PT/PTT and low fibrinogen and hemophagocytosis on bone marrow biopsy.

TABLE 66.10	Systemic Sclerosis (SSc) (Scleroderma)
Anti-Scl 70 (Topoisomerase)	**Diffuse** disease. Classically skin involvement proximal to the elbows. Can progress rapidly, can have severe ILD
Anticentromere antibody	**Limited** disease (CREST syndrome—Calcinosis, Raynaud's phenomenon, esophageal dysmotility, sclerodactyly, telangiectasias). Associated with pulmonary hypertension and digital ischemia
Anti-polymerase III	**Diffuse** disease, scleroderma renal crisis, GAVE (gastric antral vascular ectasia)
ANA	Present in 95% of systemic sclerosis, classically with nucleolar of centromere pattern

ANA is present in vast majority of systemic sclerosis patients (95%) and Raynaud's phenomenon is almost universal. The suspicion of systemic sclerosis should be dependent on the presence of both.

TABLE 66.11	Antiphospholipid Antibody Syndrome

IgG and IgM anticardiolipin antibodies (aCL)
IgG and IgM anti–beta2-glycoprotein (GP) I antibodies
Lupus anticoagulant testing
Additional testing: 50:50 plasma mixing study as described above under CAPS does not substitute for the formal testing but can provide a rapid test to increase the suspicion for the presence of the inhibitor

TABLE 66.12	Vasculitis
C-ANCA/P-ANCA	High titer anti-PR3 (proteinase 3) antibody is extremely specific (>95%)
Complement	Low serum complement levels are usually present in mixed cryoglobulinemia and SLE
Rheumatoid factor	High titers seen in rheumatoid arthritis/Sjögren's syndrome and cryoglobulinemia-associated vasculitis
Additional work up	Cryoglobulins, hepatitis B and C, serum protein electro-phoresis and immunofixation, antiglomerular basement membrane antibody
Strongly consider an angiographic study or biopsy if diagnosis not clear and with clinical suspicion of vasculitis

TABLE 66.13	Rheumatoid Arthritis	
RF (rheumatoid factor)	More sensitive (75%), less specific (75%)	
Anti-CCP antibody (anticyclic citrullinated peptide)	More specific (95%), less sensitive (65%)	

TABLE 66.14	Myositis
Creatine kinase (CK), aldolase, aspartate aminotransferase (AST), alanine aminotransferase (ALT), LDH (lactate dehydrogenase) (isolated elevation in aldolase may be suggestive of perimysial disease)
Anti-Jo-1 antibody (most common, more rapid result), and myositis-specific antibody panel (includes Jo-1)
EMG/NCS (electromyogram/nerve conduction studies)
Muscle biopsy, helpful if site identified with MRI/Ultrasound
Inflammatory arthritis, skin involvement, and interstitial lung disease (ILD) are also commonly present

SUGGESTED READINGS

Asherson RA, Cervera R, de Groot PG, et al. Catastrophic antiphospholipid syndrome: international consensus statement on classification criteria and treatment guidelines. *Lupus.* 200? 12(7):530–534.

Bernal-Macías S, Reyes-Beltrán B, Molano-González N, et al. Outcome of patients with autoimmune diseases in the intensive care unit: a mixed cluster analysis. *Lupus Sci Med.* 201? 2(1):e000122.

Buttgereit F, Dejaco C, Matteson EL, et al. "Polymyalgia rheumatica and giant cell arteritis: systematic review. *JAMA.* 2016;315(22):2442–2458.

Cartin Ceba R, Peikert T, Ashrani A, et al. Primary antiphospholipid syndrome-associated diffuse alveolar hemorrhage. *Arthritis Care Res (Hoboken).* 2014;66(2):301–310.

Cervera R, Bucciarelli S, Plasín MA, et al. Catastrophic antiphospholipid syndrome (CAPS descriptive analysis of a series of 280 patients from the "CAPS Registry. *J Autoimmun.* 200? 32(3):240–245.

Cervera R, Rodríguez-Pintó I, G Espinosa on behalf of the Task Force on Catastrophic Antiphospholipid Syndrom. Catastrophic antiphospholipid syndrome: task force report summary. *Lupus.* 2014;23(12):1283–1285.

Franks TJ, Koss MN. Pulmonary capillaritis. *Curr Opin Pulm Med.* 2000;6(5):430–435.

Gómez-Puerta JA, Hernández-Rodríguez J, López-Soto A, et al. Antineutrophil cytoplasm antibody-associated vasculitides and respiratory disease. *Chest.* 2009;136(4):1101–1111

Guillevin L, Bérezné A, Seror R, et al. Scleroderma renal crisis: a retrospective multicentre study on 91 patients and 427 controls. *Rheumatology (Oxford).* 2012;51(3):460–467.

Guillevin L, Pagnoux C, Karras A, et al. Rituximab versus azathioprine for maintenance ANCA-associated vasculitis. *N Engl J Med.* 2014;371(19):1771–1780.

Janssen NM, Karnad DR, Guntupalli KK. Rheumatologic diseases in the intensive care unit epidemiology, clinical approach, management, and outcome. *Crit Care Clin.* 2002;18(729–748.

ennette JC, Falk RJ, Bacon PA, et al. 2012 revised international chapel hill consensus conference nomenclature of vasculitides. *Arthritis Rheum.* 2013;65(1):1–11.

ones RB, Furuta S, Tervaert JW, et al. Rituximab versus cyclophosphamide in ANCA-associated renal vasculitis. *N Engl J Med.* 2010;363(3):211–220.

ara AR, Schwarz MI. Diffuse alveolar hemorrhage. *Chest.* 2010;137(5):1164–1171.

ichtenberger JP, Digumarthy SR, Abbott GF, et al. Diffuse pulmonary hemorrhage: clues to the diagnosis. *Curr Probl Diagn Radiol.* 2014;43(3):128–139.

IcCabe C, Jones Q, Nikolopoulou A, et al. Pulmonary-renal syndromes: an update for respiratory physicians. *Respir Med.* 2011;105(10):1413–1421.

ishimura K, Sugiyama D, Kogata Y, et al. Meta-analysis: diagnostic accuracy of anti–cyclic citrullinated peptide antibody and rheumatoid factor for rheumatoid arthritis. *Ann Intern Med.* 2007;146(11):797–808.

:o P, Stone JH. The antineutrophil cytoplasmic antibody-associated vasculitides. *Am J Med.* 2004;117(1):39–50.

obodin G, Hussein A, Rozenbaum M, et al. The emergency room in systemic rheumatic diseases. *Emerg Med J.* 2006;23(9):667–671.

one JH, Merkel PA, Spiera R, et al. Rituximab versus cyclophosphamide for ANCA-associated vasculitis. *N Engl J Med.* 2010;363(3):221–232.

one JH, Tuckwell K, Dimonaco S, et al. Efficacy and safety of tocilizumab in patients with giant cell arteritis: primary and secondary outcomes from a phase 3, randomized, double-blind, placebo-controlled trial. *Arthritis Rheumatol.* 2016;68(suppl 10):911.

Management of the Solid Organ Transplant Recipients in the ICU

Yuka Furuya and Chad A. Witt

INTRODUCTION

The number of solid organ transplants (SOTs) performed worldwide continues increase annually. In 2015, over 30,000 transplants were performed, with renal bei the most common (57.7%) followed by liver (23%), heart (9.1%), and lung (6.6 transplants. Moreover, the overall survival for most SOT recipients has been impro ing, owing to ongoing improvements in surgical techniques and longitudinal medi management of SOT recipients. As a result, it is increasingly likely to encounter SC recipients in various clinical settings including the ICU. Caring for SOT recipients the intensive care unit (ICU) presents a unique set of challenges. This chapter focu on caring for SOT recipients beyond the immediate perioperative period, includi infectious complications, an overview of immunosuppressive therapy and its pote tial complications, and common indications for admission to and consideratio relevant to the medical ICU.

INFECTIOUS COMPLICATIONS

Infectious complications are the leading cause for ICU admission after SC In general, the degree of immunosuppression is most intense in the first 6 12 months posttransplantation. SOT recipients may receive perioperative ind tion therapy with T-cell depleting agents (e.g., alemtuzumab, antithymocyte gl ulin), which can lead to profound and prolonged immunosuppression potenti lasting for several months. In the early (≤1 month) postoperative period, the of infection often involves the transplanted organ(e.g., mediastinitis in heart re ients, intra-abdominal infection in liver and kidney recipients, airway infecti pneumonia, or pleural infections in lung recipients). In addition, infections rel to the surgical site, wound dehiscence, or anastomotic leaks are often enco tered. Nosocomial infections with multidrug resistant (MDR) organisms suc MRSA, VRE, and MDR gram-negative organisms are also common. Donor recipient-derived infections such as CMV, EBV, and *Aspergillus* infections are traditionally seen early in the posttransplant course. However, with increa use of prophylaxis against infections such as CMV, *Pneumocystis jirovecii* *Aspergillus* spp., these infections can be seen later in the course after prophyl: antimicrobials are discontinued. Opportunistic infections such as CMV, toxo mosis, *Pneumocystis jirovecii*, *Cryptococcus*, mycobacteria, HSV, VZV, EBV, *List* and *Nocardia* tend to occur within the first 6 to 12 months posttransplanta

TABLE 67.1	Common Infectious and Noninfectious ICU Indications	
Infectious	Indications	Noninfectious
Viral or Fungal Pneumonia	**Acute respiratory failure**	Noncardiogenic Pulmonary Edema; Rejection (Lung recipient)
Bacterial Pneumonia;		
Fungemia	**Shock**	Rejection (Heart recipient)
Septic Shock		
BKVN (Kidney recipient)	**Acute kidney injury**	Calcineurin Inhibitor Toxicity; Rejection (Kidney recipient)
CNS Infections	**Altered mental status**	Posterior Reversible Encephalopathy Syndrome (PRES); Delirium

After 6 months, community-acquired infections including community-acquired pneumonia (CAP) and urinary tract infections (UTI) predominate. Opportunistic infections described above can also be seen in this period due to chronic suppression of T-cell immunity. Although highest early in the posttransplant course, the risk of infectious complications continues lifelong given the chronic, ongoing immunosuppression that SOT recipients require. Please refer to Chapter 40 for further reading on infections in SOT recipients. Table 67.1 summarizes common ICU indications of infectious and noninfectious etiology.

COMPLICATIONS OF IMMUNOSUPPRESSIVE THERAPY

Recent advances in immunosuppressive agents have resulted in greater tolerance and reduced systemic toxicity for SOT recipients. There are three major classes of maintenance immunosuppressive agents most commonly used in SOT: (1) corticosteroids, (2) antimetabolic agents, and (3) calcineurin inhibitors (CNIs) (Table 67.2). Over time, the use of mammalian target of rapamycin (mTOR) inhibitors is also increasing. Typically, immunosuppressive regimens include a combination of drugs from two to three different classes depending on the transplanted organ and how far the patient is out from the time of transplantation. In recent years, a combination of corticosteroid, mycophenolate, and tacrolimus is most commonly used. Antimicrobials and other commonly used medications in the ICU setting are known to interact with these immunosuppressive agents. A multidisciplinary approach in conjunction with clinical pharmacists is essential in the care of these complex patients. CNIs are widely utilized in the maintenance therapy of SOT recipients, and chronic kidney disease due to calcineurin inhibitor nephropathy (CIN) is prevalent. Drugs should be renally dosed, and other nephrotoxic drugs and iodinated contrast should be used with caution. Mild neurotoxicity manifested by tremor is common in patients on CNI.

Rarely, posterior reversible encephalopathy syndrome (PRES), a condition clinically characterized by encephalopathy, headaches, seizure, and visual disturbances, can occur in patients on immunosuppressive therapy, particularly CNIs. A

TABLE 67.2 Classes of Immunosuppressive Drugs

Class	Name	Mechanism of Action	Toxicity	Interactions	Notes	Monitoring
Corticosteroids	Prednisone, prednisolone, methylprednisolone	Multifactorial; Causes redistribution of leukocytes; Inhibit proliferation of T cells; Decrease synthesis of prostaglandins, proinflammatory cytokines, leukotrienes	Hyperglycemia, Hypertension, Osteopenia, Avascular necrosis of bone, Impaired wound healing, Adrenal suppression	No significant interactions	Wide range of side effects, in the acute setting most notably hyperglycemia and hypertension	None
Calcineurin Inhibitors	Tacrolimus	Binds to FKBP, forming a complex that inhibits calcineurin which leads to ↓ transcription of cytokines such as IL-2, IL-3, and IFN-γ	Renal dysfunction, Hypertension, Hyperkalemia, Hyperglycemia, Diabetes, Neurotoxicity (tremor, headaches), GI toxicity	Substrate and inhibitor of pGP and CYP3A4; Interacts with a wide array of drugs that induce or inhibit CYP3A4; Significant drug interaction with azoles dramatically increasing tacrolimus exposure	PO or Sublingual route preferred over IV to minimize renal toxicity	Trough level; Monitor renal function
	Cyclosporine	Same as above, binds to cyclophilin instead of FKBP	Renal dysfunction, Hirsutism, Tremor, Hyperlipidemia, Hyperplasia of gum, Hyperuricemia	Substrate and a strong inhibitor of pGP; Hepatically metabolized by CYP3A4; Interacts with a wide range of drugs, including CCB, antifungals, antibiotics, glucocorticoids, PI Grapefruit juice; Significant drug interaction with azoles dramatically increasing cyclosporine exposure	Sandimmune and Neoral differ in their pharmacokinetics and should NOT be used interchangeably	2-hr peak and/or trough level, monitor renal function

						Trough level
Inhibitors	everolimus	mTOR that is involved in cell cycle proliferation	...healing, anemia, leukopenia, thrombocytopenia, Hypokalemia, Oral ulcers, GI toxicity	...ssociate of pgP and CYP3A4; monitor carefully when coadministered with other CYP3A4 substrates. Concomitant administration with cyclosporine may aggravate renal dysfunction, myelosuppression and hyperlipidemia. Significant drug interaction with azoles dramatically increasing drug level	Not used early (<3 mo) in lung recipients due to airway dehiscence	
Antimetabolites	Mycophenolate mofetil and mycophenolic acid	Hydrolyzed to MPA, a selective inhibitor of IMPDH, an enzyme involved in synthesis of guanine nucleotide in lymphocytes	GI toxicity (nausea, diarrhea), leukopenia, anemia, thrombocytopenia	MPA is metabolized to inactive MPAG, which is renally excreted. Coadministration with antacids containing Mg or Al leads to ↓ absorption of MMF; Acyclovir and Ganciclovir may compete with MPAG for tubular secretion resulting in ↑ blood levels of both the antiviral and MPAG	Mycophenolic acid is enteric coated and may improve GI side effects compared to mycophenolate mofetil	CBC
	Azathioprine	Converted to 6-MP, which is converted to metabolites that inhibit purine synthesis, inhibiting cell proliferation	Bone marrow suppression, Leukopenia, Thrombocytopenia, Anemia, Hepatotoxicity, GI Toxicity, Alopecia, Pancreatitis	Partially metabolized by Xanthine Oxidase. Avoid concomitant use with Xanthine Oxidase inhibitor (e.g., Allopurinol) or dose ↓; Coadministration with ACEi may aggravate myelosuppressive effect	Low TPMT activity associated with higher risk of myelosuppression	CBC and LFTs

FKBP, FK506-binding protein; pGP, P-glycoprotein; NFAT, nuclear factor of activated T cells; CCB, calcium channel blockers; PI, protease inhibitors; Cr, creatinine; mTOR, mammalian target of rapamycin; MPA, mycophenolic acid; IMPDH, inosine monophosphate dehydrogenase; 6-MP, 6-mercaptopurine; MPAG, phenolic glucuronide TPMT, thiopurine methyltransferase

retrospective study from a large transplant center reported the rate of PRES to be 0.49% among all SOT recipients. While cyclosporine is the most commonly reported agent, there have been reports PRES associated with tacrolimus and the mTOR inhibitor sirolimus. Diagnosis is made both clinically and with supporting neuroradiographic findings of symmetric vasogenic edema in the white matter, typically seen in the posterior cerebral hemispheres on computed tomography (CT) or magnetic resonance imaging (MRI) of the brain. Supratherapeutic levels of CNI are often but not always observed, and the treatment usually involves cessation of the inciting agent and starting an alternative agent once the levels have come down. SOT recipients who develop PRES on one CNI will often tolerate the other CNI without difficulty. CNI-associated PRES resolves in about 90% of patients, with 10% of patients recovering with some residual neurologic sequelae. Maintaining a high index of suspicion is the key in early diagnosis and treatment.

Other nonimmunologic effects of chronic immunosuppression include higher risk for development of malignancies. In a large cohort study, the incidence of overall malignancy was two times that expected from an age and region adjusted cohort. In particular, malignancies associated with infectious etiology including Kaposi's sarcoma (HHV-8), liver cancer (HBV, HCV), non-Hodgkin's lymphoma (EBV), and vulvar cancer (HPV) had the highest increase in incidence.

ORGAN-SPECIFIC CONCERNS

The differential diagnosis of acute renal failure in renal transplant recipients include allograft rejection, drug toxicity (e.g., CNI, antibiotics), ATN (acute tubular necrosis), and BK virus nephropathy (BKVN). Differentiating between BKVN and allograft rejection is of particular importance since the treatment for each condition will drastically differ. In renal transplant recipients who present with hypertensive urgency or emergency, transplant renal artery stenosis (TRAS) should be in the differential diagnosis. TRAS is a well-recognized complication most commonly occurring during the first 6 months posttransplantation, but can present at any time. Arteriography remains the gold standard for diagnosis. However, given its invasive nature and substantial contrast load, MR or CT angiography, isotope renography, and renal Doppler ultrasonography are increasingly utilized. In addition, other factors contributing hypertension must be taken into account such as the use of CNI and glucocorticoid. ICU management should include assessment and stabilization of acute respiratory failure and control of blood pressure. Definitive treatment of TRAS involves angioplasty or surgical revision if percutaneous interventions fail.

Peritonitis or abdominal sources of sepsis in a liver transplant recipient should prompt an investigation into biliary duct complications, such as biliary leakage, stasis due to stenosis of the biliary duct, and cholangitis. Biliary leakage can be evaluated with cholangiogram or endoscopic retrograde cholangiography which allows for simultaneous intervention. Anastomotic stenosis usually occurs within the first year posttransplant. Nonanastomotic stenosis can be caused by hepatic artery thrombosis or recurrence of an underlying disease such as primary sclerosing cholangitis and can manifest later. Treatments include balloon dilation and stent placement.

Lung recipients with respiratory failure must be evaluated for both infectious complications, including bacterial, viral, and fungal pneumonia, as well as immune mediated allograft dysfunction. This workup often requires bronchoscopy with bronchoalveolar lavage and transbronchial biopsy. It is important to evaluate for and treat infections, given that the therapy for acute immune mediated graft dysfunction (including acute cellular rejection and antibody mediated rejection) generally involves high-dose immunosuppression, such as methylprednisolone 500 to 1000 mg for several days, antithymocyte globulin, and/or antibody-directed therapies including plasma exchange, rituximab, and bortezomib.

Heart transplant recipients with evidence of graft dysfunction need to be evaluated for acute rejection, antibody-mediated rejection, and coronary artery vasculopathy. This evaluation often starts with noninvasive testing such as echocardiography, but often endomyocardial biopsy is necessary to fully evaluate the patient.

Lastly, in both transplant recipients and potential candidates, blood transfusion may increase the risk of allosensitization and blood products should be used judiciously. In the United States, most blood products undergo leukoreduction. However, there are a minority of independent blood centers that have not implemented universal leukoreduction, and leukoreduced blood should be requested for SOT recipients. In addition, CMV seronegative blood products are available in some institutions for recipients who have received organs from CMV seronegative donors, although its advantage in preventing CMV transmission over leukoreduced blood is unclear. Irradiated blood products are generally not necessary as transfusion-associated graft-versus-host disease (GVHD) in SOT recipients is exceedingly rare. However the use of anti-CD52 antibody alemtuzumab as an induction agent is an exception, and the use of irradiated blood products until the recovery of lymphpenia is recommended.

SUGGESTED READINGS

Bartynski WS, Tan HP, Boardman JF, et al. Posterior reversible encephalopathy syndrome after solid organ transplantation. *AJNR Am J Neuroradiol.* 2008;29(5):924–930.
Retrospective study of SOT recipients with a diagnosis of PRES. Incidence of PRES among SOT recipients was found to be 0.49% (21 out of 4,222 SOT recipients). Liver recipients typically presented with PRES earlier post-transplant, and had a greater degree of brain edema compared with kidney recipients.

Bowden RA, Slichter SJ, Sayers M, et al. A comparison of filtered leukocyte-reduced and cytomegalovirus (CMV) seronegative blood products for the prevention of transfusion-associated CMV infection after marrow transplant. *Blood.* 1995;86(9):3598–3603.
A prospective, randomized trial in CMV seronegative bone marrow transplant recipients who received either filtered or CMV seronegative blood products. There were no significant differences in the incidence of CMV infection or CMV disease between the two groups.

Canet E, Zafrani L, Azoulay É. The critically ill kidney transplant recipient: a narrative review. *Chest.* 2016;149(6):1546–1555.
Review article on the ICU indications and management of renal transplant recipients. Focuses on cardiovascular events, infections, drug-related toxicity, ICU management and outcome.

Dummer JS, Hardy A, Poorsattar A, et al. Early infections in kidney, heart, and liver transplant recipients on cyclosporine. *Transplantation.* 1983;36(3):259–267.
Single center analysis of kidney, heart, and liver transplant recipients. This study found that renal transplant recipients receiving azathioprine had the more infections compared with liver, heart, and kidney recipients receiving cyclosporine. There was a preponderance of abdominal infections in liver recipients, intrathoracic in heart recipients, and urinary tract infections in kidney recipients.

Engels EA, Pfeiffer RM, Fraumeni JF, et al. Spectrum of cancer risk among US solid organ transplant recipients. *JAMA*. 2011;306(17):1891–1901.

> *Large cohort study linking SOT data with state and regional cancer registries. Found elevated risk in SOT recipients for 32 different malignancies. Most common malignancies with elevated risk were non-Hodgkin lymphoma, cancer of the lung, liver, and kidney.*

Organ Procurement and Transplantation Network (OPRN) and Scientific Registry of Transplant Recipients (SRTR). OPTN/SRTR 2014 Annual Data Report. Rockville, MD: Department of Health and Human Services, Health Resource and Services Administration; 2016.

> *An annual report by the OPTN and SRTR on organ-specific transplant data such as the number of patients on the waiting list, deceased donor and living donor organ donation statistics, number of transplants, immunosuppressive regimen used, and outcomes.*

Song T, Rao Z, Tan Q, et al. Calcineurin inhibitors associated posterior reversible encephalopathy syndrome in solid organ transplantation: report of 2 cases and literature review. *Medicine (Baltimore)*. 2016;95(14):e3173.

> *Case report and a comprehensive literature review of calcineurin inhibitor associated PRES. Found most common presenting symptoms included seizures (77.5%), encephalopathy (62%), headache (29.6%), and visual disturbances (22.5%).*

Transplant trends. UNOS (online, cited 2016 Sep 12). Available from: https://www.unos.org/data/transplant-trends/#transplants_by_organ_type+year+2015.

> *Provided by the United Network for Organ Sharing (UNOS), up-to-date data on solid organ transplantation performed in the United States can be found.*

Treleaven J, Gennery A, Marsh J, et al. Guidelines on the use of irradiated blood components prepared by the British Committee for Standards in Haematology blood transfusion task force. *Br J Haematol*. 2011;152(1):35–51.

> *Consensus guideline from the British Committee for Standards in Haematology (BCSH). Recommendations and review of evidence on topics, including the use of irradiated blood products and transfusion practices in hematopoietic and solid organ transplant recipients.*

68

Maternal–Fetal Critical Care

Lorene A. Temming, Nandini Raghuraman, and Shayna N. Conner

lthough less than 1% of pregnant patients will require admission to the intensive
are unit, the overall acuity of this patient population remains high. The incidence of
egnancy-related ICU admission is anticipated to increase over time given increasing
aternal age and a rise in medical comorbidities and cesarean deliveries. Over half of
CU admissions in pregnancy are directly related to obstetric conditions such as hyper-
nsive disorders from eclampsia/severe preeclampsia and hemorrhage. However, there
e many other conditions for which a critical care practitioner should be prepared.
itical care management in pregnancy must consider the health of both the mother
d the fetus. Optimal care of a critically ill patient in pregnancy must involve multi-
sciplinary team management. To fully understand how to take care of this vulnerable
tient population, it is important to understand the basic physiologic adaptations
at occur in the mother in response to the demands of pregnancy (Table 68.1).

XYGENATION AND RESPIRATORY SUPPORT URING PREGNANCY

rmal physiologic changes of pregnancy increase oxygen delivery to the placenta and
e fetus. Fetal oxygenation is dependent on maternal oxygen status. It is important
note that pregnancy is a chronically compensated state of respiratory alkalosis with
aternal pH of 7.40 to 7.47. Respiratory alkalosis is secondary to the increase in
nute ventilation, which leads to a decrease in $PaCO_2$ to approximately 30 mm Hg.
is is compensated for by increased renal excretion of bicarbonate (normal value in
gnancy: 18 to 22 mEq/L).

Pregnancy itself increases oxygen consumption by 15% to 20%. Pregnancy-
ociated anemia results in lower hemoglobin concentration and arterial oxygen
tent, however an increase in cardiac output during this time optimizes oxygen
ivery. Maintaining cardiac output is therefore pivotal to oxygen delivery in preg-
cy. Bearing in mind the physiologic changes in ventilation during pregnancy and
fetal oxygen dissociation curve, tighter parameters for oxygenation are required
maintain maternal and fetal well-being. Respiratory support in pregnancy should
aggressive, and the goal should be to maintain maternal SpO_2 ≥95% to 96% as
sustain adequate oxygen perfusion to the fetus. The same respiratory support
ices used in nonpregnant patients may be used in pregnant patients. Indications
intubation are similar to the general population with exception of a reduced
O_2 threshold. A PCO_2 above 35 mm Hg may be a signal of impending respi-
ry failure. When determining difficulty of intubation, airway edema related to

TABLE 68.1	Physiologic Changes of Pregnancy
Cardiovascular	
BP	Decreased (reaches a nadir in the second trimester)
Heart rate	Increased (17%)
Cardiac output	Increased (40%)
Stroke volume	Increased (25%)
Systemic vascular resistance	Decreased (20%)
Hematologic	
Blood volume	Increased (40–50%)
Coagulation factors	Increase in fibrinogen, vWF, clotting factors II, VII, VIII, IX, and X and protein C resistance. Decrease in protein S
Red blood cell mass	Increased
White blood cell count	Increased
Hemoglobin	Decreased
Platelets	Decreased (secondary to hemodilution)
Renal	
Glomerular filtration rate	Increased (50%)
Renal plasma flow	Increased (50–75%)
BUN and creatinine	Decreased
Urinary protein excretion	Increased
Pulmonary	
Tidal volume	Increased (40%)
Respiratory rate	Little to no change
Minute ventilation	Increased (40%)
Vital capacity	Unchanged
FEV_1	Unchanged
Residual volume	Decreased (20%)—secondary to elevated diaphragm
Functional residual capacity (FRC)	Decreased (20%)—secondary to elevated diaphragm
Inspiratory capacity	Increased (5–10%)—secondary to decreased FRC

pregnancy and decreased esophageal sphincter tone and slower gastric empty should be considered.

RESPIRATORY FAILURE

Diagnosis of respiratory distress may be difficult in the gravid patient, because al half of all pregnant women will have complaints of shortness of breath, fatigue, decreased exercise tolerance. A careful evaluation of these symptoms and assessm of vital signs is imperative to discern between normal pregnancy complaints respiratory compromise. The most common causes of respiratory failure in pregn are pulmonary embolus, pulmonary edema (secondary to preeclampsia, cardio opathy, or tocolysis), infection, and asthma. Clinical recognition and treatr of a pregnant patient in respiratory failure is extremely important because maternal oxygen status directly affects fetal oxygen status. Arterial blood gas (ABG) assessment can be key to determining the etiology and management of respiratory failure in pregnancy. A change in fetal heart rate pattern may also be one of the first signs of maternal respiratory failure. A general rule of thumb is to stabilize the maternal condition before considering delivery. If indicated, initiating mechanical ventilation in the mother will likely improve fetal condition.

Asthma Exacerbation: Up to 8% of pregnant women have a diagnosis of asthma and approximately 30% of these women will have exacerbations that require medical intervention. Although functional residual capacity is decreased in pregnancy, forced expiratory volume in 1 second (FEV_1) and peak expiratory flow should remain unchanged. Patients with asthma exacerbations will typically present with cough, shortness of breath, and wheezing. A preliminary assessment of peak expiratory flow/FEV_1, respiratory rate, oxygen saturation, ABG, and presence of wheezing on pulmonary auscultation are key to the diagnosis and management of an asthma exacerbation. A chest x-ray (CXR) should be considered to rule out other causes of respiratory difficulty. Concerning features of an exacerbation include peak expiratory flow <60% of baseline, PCO_2 >35 mm Hg, PO_2 <60 mm Hg, tachypnea >22/min, and tachycardia >120 bpm. Patients with these features should be promptly admitted and treated with oxygen, steroids, and/or nebulized beta agonists or anticholinergics. Fetal monitoring should be performed for pregnancies beyond 24 weeks. Intubation should be considered if the patient is unable to maintain 90% oxygen saturation despite supplemental oxygen, has a PCO_2 >40 mm Hg, increasing acidosis, or altered mental status (Algorithms 68.1 and 68.2).

AMNIOTIC FLUID EMBOLISM

Amniotic fluid embolism (AFE) is a rare but devastating obstetric disorder. Although uncommon with an incidence of about 1 in 20,000 deliveries, the maternal mortality rate can be as high as 60%. The pathophysiology of AFE is poorly understood. It appears to be due to an abnormal maternal immune response to fetal antigens, which is why AFE is sometimes referred to as an anaphylactoid syndrome of pregnancy. There are no known identifiable risk factors in pregnant women that predispose her to AFE. Classically a pregnant woman in labor, postcesarean delivery, postdilation and evacuation, or 30 minutes postpartum will present with a sudden onset of acute hypoxia, acute hypotension ± cardiac arrest, followed by fetal hypoxia (if patient is antepartum), and consumptive coagulopathy. Unfortunately, for women that suffer from an AFE in its classic form, maternal death is the most common outcome.

When a patient experiences hypoxia, hypotension, coagulopathy, or cardiopulmonary arrest immediately following cesarean, vaginal delivery, or pregnancy termination, AFE must be suspected. Clinical variations of the syndrome exist, and patients may not exhibit all symptoms. Differential diagnosis for these symptoms includes air embolus, anaphylaxis, myocardial infarction, peripartum cardiomyopathy, pulmonary embolus, transfusion reaction, and septic shock. The initial treatment for AFE is supportive care with oxygen and immediate, high-quality cardiopulmonary resuscitation as necessary. Large bore intravenous access and arterial line placement or pulmonary artery catheterization should be achieved for treatment and monitoring. If patients become hypotensive, they may require volume expansion to optimize preload, as well as inotropic support. Given the propensity for the development of acute

ALGORITHM 68.1 Differential Diagnosis for Respiratory Distress

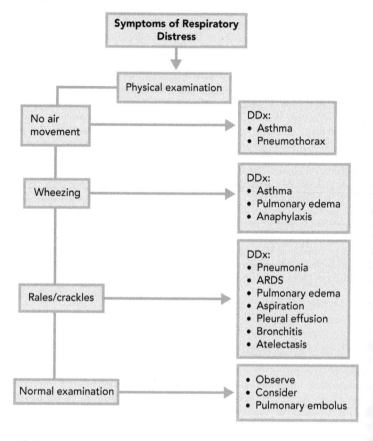

heart failure and cardiogenic pulmonary edema in AFE, care should be taken to avoid excessive fluid resuscitation. Given the similar pathophysiology to anaphylaxis, high doses of corticosteroids and epinephrine may be considered when AFE is suspected. When coagulopathy is suspected, massive transfusion protocol should be initiated to facilitate blood product support. Novel treatments for AFE, including extracorporeal membrane oxygenation, exchange transfusion, nitric oxide, and cardiopulmonary bypass or assist devices have shown benefit in case reports.

In antepartum cases of AFE, the fetal status must be followed closely. Initially, every attempt should be made to hemodynamically stabilize the mother, as this will serve to resuscitate the fetus and cesarean section on an unstable patient may contribute to mortality in the setting of AFE. Once the patient is stabilized, cesarean delivery should be performed to improve resuscitation of the mother and neonatal survival. If a patient progresses to frank cardiac arrest, the likelihood of maternal survival

ALGORITHM 68.2 Asthma

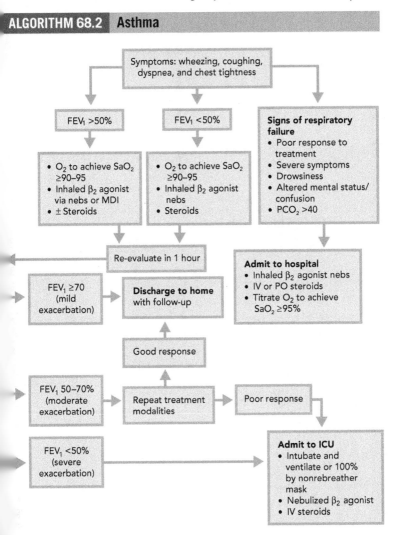

Symptoms: wheezing, coughing, dyspnea, and chest tightness

FEV₁ >50%
- O₂ to achieve SaO₂ ≥90–95
- Inhaled β₂ agonist via nebs or MDI
- ± Steroids

FEV₁ <50%
- O₂ to achieve SaO₂ ≥90–95
- Inhaled β₂ agonist nebs
- Steroids

Signs of respiratory failure
- Poor response to treatment
- Severe symptoms
- Drowsiness
- Altered mental status/confusion
- PCO₂ >40

Re-evaluate in 1 hour

Admit to hospital
- Inhaled β₂ agonist nebs
- IV or PO steroids
- Titrate O₂ to achieve SaO₂ ≥95%

FEV₁ ≥70 (mild exacerbation)

Discharge to home with follow-up

Good response

FEV₁ 50–70% (moderate exacerbation)

Repeat treatment modalities

Poor response

FEV₁ <50% (severe exacerbation)

Admit to ICU
- Intubate and ventilate or 100% by nonrebreather mask
- Nebulized β₂ agonist
- IV steroids

ceedingly low. Neonatal outcomes are directly correlated to the duration from arrest delivery, so perimortem cesarean delivery should be initiated within 4 minutes of liac arrest diagnosis in patients with suspected AFE (Algorithm 68.3).

LMONARY EDEMA IN PREGNANCY

gnant women are at increased risk of pulmonary edema due to an increase in plasma me and a decrease in colloid oncotic pressure. Pulmonary edema complicates

ALGORITHM 68.3   Amniotic Fluid Embolus

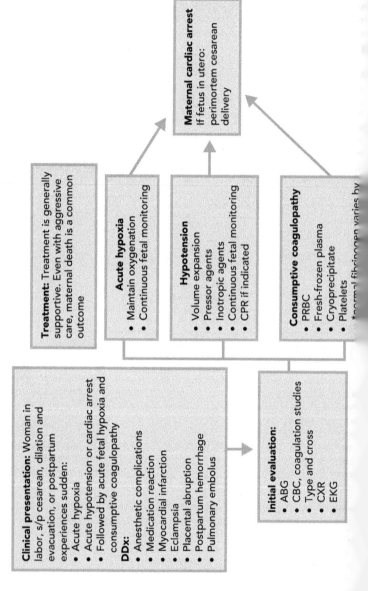

Clinical presentation: Woman in labor, s/p cesarean, dilation and evacuation, or postpartum experiences sudden:
- Acute hypoxia
- Acute hypotension or cardiac arrest
- Followed by acute fetal hypoxia and consumptive coagulopathy

DDx:
- Anesthetic complications
- Medication reaction
- Myocardial infarction
- Eclampsia
- Placental abruption
- Postpartum hemorrhage
- Pulmonary embolus

Initial evaluation:
- ABG
- CBC, coagulation studies
- Type and cross
- CXR
- EKG

Treatment: Treatment is generally supportive. Even with aggressive care, maternal death is a common outcome

Acute hypoxia
- Maintain oxygenation
- Continuous fetal monitoring

Hypotension
- Volume expansion
- Pressor agents
- Inotropic agents
- Continuous fetal monitoring
- CPR if indicated

Consumptive coagulopathy
- PRBC
- Fresh-frozen plasma
- Cryoprecipitate
- Platelets
- *normal fibrinogen varies by

Maternal cardiac arrest
If fetus in utero: perimortem cesarean delivery

approximately 1 in 1000 pregnancies. The most common causes of pulmonary edema in pregnancy are secondary to cardiogenic causes, tocolytic use, fluid overload, and preeclampsia. Historically, pulmonary edema caused by the use of beta agonists for tocolysis was common, but decreasing use of terbutaline and ritodrine for prolonged tocolysis has decreased the incidence of pulmonary edema in pregnancy. Currently, the most common cause of pulmonary edema in pregnancy is preeclampsia due to capillary permeability.

Patients with pulmonary edema often present with complaints of dyspnea, tachycardia oxygen desaturation, and tachypnea. On physical examination bilateral crackles should always be present and sometimes an S3 gallop may be auscultated. It is important to note that an S3 gallop can also be a normal manifestation in pregnancy, especially in the third trimester, secondary to increased blood volume. CXR will usually demonstrate bilateral diffuse interstitial opacities with a reticular pattern, more prominent in the lung bases. An enlarged heart size, presence of perihilar or "batwing" distribution of edema, pleural effusions, and Kerley B-lines are all suggestive of cardiogenic pulmonary edema. Noncardiogenic pulmonary edema more commonly shows a peripheral distribution of edema with normal heart size and normal central vasculature. Echocardiogram is useful in the setting of pulmonary edema to differentiate between cardiogenic and noncardiogenic pulmonary edema and to determine the type of cardiac dysfunction.

Management of pulmonary edema should begin with improving oxygenation by sitting the patient upright and administering oxygen with a goal of maintaining oxygen saturation >95%. Furosemide should be given intravenously with a goal of achieving approximately 2 L of diuresis over several hours. Additionally, 2 to 5 mg of intravenous morphine may cause venodilation and reduce patients' symptoms. After initial stabilization, management of underlying causes, including delivery for preeclampsia, medical therapy for hypertension or heart failure, and aggressive fluid management is indicated (Algorithm 68.4).

THROMBOEMBOLISM IN PREGNANCY

Venous thromboembolism (VTE) is a common complication of pregnancy, with pregnant women four to five times more likely to develop VTE than non-pregnant women. Pulmonary embolism (PE) is the leading cause of maternal mortality in the United States, accounting for 9% of all maternal deaths. Pregnancy-associated changes, including hypercoagulability, decreased mobility, increased venous stasis, and compression of the inferior vena cava by the uterus all contribute to the increased risk of VTE in pregnancy. The risk of thromboembolism, though present from the first trimester, increases throughout pregnancy and is highest in the postpartum period.

Deep Vein Thrombosis

Most pregnant women with deep vein thrombosis (DVT) present with pain or swelling in an extremity. DVT occurs more often in the deep proximal veins and more commonly in the left leg secondary to increased compression of the left iliac vein by the right iliac artery where they cross. The clinical diagnosis of DVT is challenging, and suspected DVT must be confirmed with objective testing given the long-term complications of anticoagulant therapy and workup. DVT should be suspected in those with a difference in calf circumference of >2 cm between the affected and

ALGORITHM 68.4 Differential Diagnosis for Pulmonary Edema in Pregnancy

Diagnosis of pulmonary edema made by physical examination and CXR

→ Calculate intake and output

→ If positive intake: treat for **fluid overload**

Is patient having elevated BPs with proteinuria?

→ Treat for **severe preeclampsia** and possible delivery

Does patient have an abnormal echocardiogram?

→ EF <45%: treat for **peripartum cardiomyopathy and possible delivery**

Is patient on tocolytic therapy?

→
- Discontinue tocolytic agent
- Place patient in semi-fowler position
- Administer O₂ via nonrebreather or with CPAP
- Intubation may be needed
- Furosemide: 20–40 mg IV, repeat if necessary
- Strict input and output and limit intravenous fluid infusion
- If no resolution of pulmonary edema seen within 12–24 hours, alternate causes for

ormal extremity. When suspected, the initial diagnostic test should be compression ultrasonography of the proximal veins of the lower extremities. If the test is negative, but iliac vein thrombosis is suspected, additional testing with magnetic resonance imaging is recommended. If either test is positive or equivocal, and the patient has clinical signs of DVT, proceed with treatment as described below. Of note, pregnancy is associated with an increase in D-dimer levels and they are not useful for predicting VTE in pregnancy.

Pulmonary Embolism

Sudden onset of shortness of breath, chest pain, tachypnea, and tachycardia are the most common clinical signs of PE in pregnancy. Although most women with PE have hypoxia, a normal oxygen saturation does not rule out a PE, and a high index of suspicion followed by objective testing is necessary to diagnose PE in pregnancy.

If a PE is suspected in a pregnant patient, initial workup should include compression ultrasonography of the lower extremities, an electrocardiogram (ECG), CXR, and ABG. If the patient has a lower extremity DVT, anticoagulation can be started without further testing. The most common ECG finding associated with PE is tachycardia, although signs of right heart strain and nonspecific T-wave inversions may also be seen. The ABG may be used to identify an abnormal alveolar–arterial oxygen gradient, which is typically >15 mm Hg in the setting of PE. However, a normal ECG and alveolar–arterial oxygen gradient do not exclude PE in pregnancy. The CXR may be used to eliminate other causes of the patients' symptoms and to help determine the best next diagnostic test.

Although computed tomographic angiography (CTA) is the gold standard for diagnosis outside of pregnancy, physiologic changes may make this test less reliable in pregnancy. A recent study illustrated that pregnant or immediately postpartum women with a normal CXR are more likely to have a diagnostic study with a ventilation–perfusion (VQ) scan, while CTA is a better initial test in those with an abnormal CXR. If results of a VQ scan after normal CXR are indeterminate, then CTA may be obtained (see Algorithm 68.5).

Treatment of Thromboembolism in Pregnancy

women with acute VTE in pregnancy are candidates for therapeutic anticoagulation, either with low–molecular-weight heparin (LMWH) or unfractionated heparin (UFH). Hospitalization is indicated in the case of hemodynamic instability, large clot burden, or maternal comorbidities. Consideration can be given to the use of IV unfractionated heparin for patients who are unstable with PE and when thrombolysis may be necessary. LMWH is dosed at 1 mg/kg twice daily due to altered metabolism in pregnancy, and should be followed to keep anti-Xa levels between 0.6 and 1 U/mL. UFH is typically initially dosed at 10,000 units or more every 12 hours to target aPTT to a therapeutic range of 1.5 to 2.5 times control range. Patients with a history of thrombosis or those who are at an increased risk of thrombosis during pregnancy and the postpartum period are candidates for prophylactic or therapeutic anticoagulation. This includes patients with inherited or acquired thrombophilias or patients who are otherwise on long-term anticoagulation. Decisions regarding dosing and duration of treatment should be made in conjunction with the patients' obstetrician.

ALGORITHM 68.5 Pulmonary Embolism (PE)

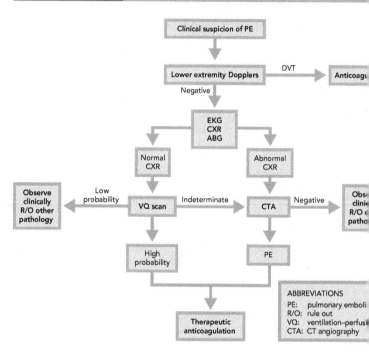

Clinical suspicion of PE

Lower extremity Dopplers → DVT → Anticoagu...

Negative

EKG
CXR
ABG

Normal CXR

Abnormal CXR

Observe clinically R/O other pathology ← Low probability — VQ scan — Indeterminate → CTA ← Negative → Obs... clini... R/O ... patho...

High probability

PE

Therapeutic anticoagulation

ABBREVIATIONS
PE: pulmonary emboli...
R/O: rule out
VQ: ventilation–perfusi...
CTA: CT angiography

ACUTE KIDNEY INJURY IN PREGNANCY

Acute kidney injury (AKI) in pregnancy is difficult to recognize without an u... standing of renal physiology changes in pregnancy. An increase in glome... filtration rate (GFR) in pregnancy results in a baseline decreased serum creat... such that nonpregnant "normal" values may represent significant kidney inju... pregnancy. The general approach to AKI is similar to that of a nonpregnant pa... In addition to prerenal, intrinsic, and obstructive causes, there are specific pregn... related conditions such as preeclampsia, HELLP, and acute fatty liver of pregr... that may result in AKI. Obtaining complete blood cell counts, liver function... urine and serum electrolytes and osmolality can be key in distinguishing etiolo... AKI in this setting. Preeclampsia and HELLP-related AKI is typically associated... hypertension and proteinuria. Acute fatty liver of pregnancy is typically assoc... with renal failure, as well as significant hepatic dysfunction including coagulop... and hypoglycemia. As with worsening AKI associated with severe preeclam... prompt delivery is indicated for maternal benefit. In these cases, careful fluid... agement is required as the need for renal perfusion must be balanced with the r... excess fluid administration in the setting of underlying endothelial injury. Rec... of renal function should be seen within a few days of delivery although a smal... centage of women will have long lasting renal dysfunction.

ALGORITHM 68.6 Acute Kidney Injury in Pregnancy

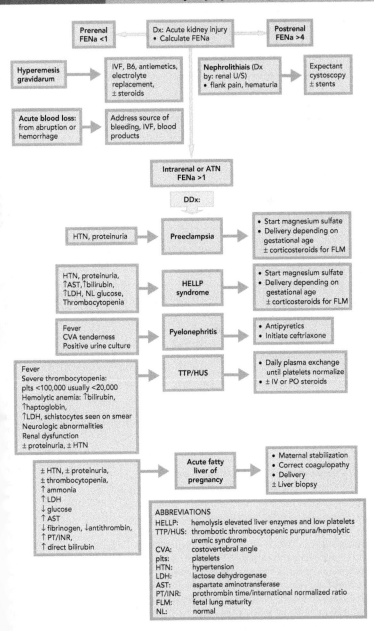

ALGORITHM 68.7 Management of Shock in Pregnancy

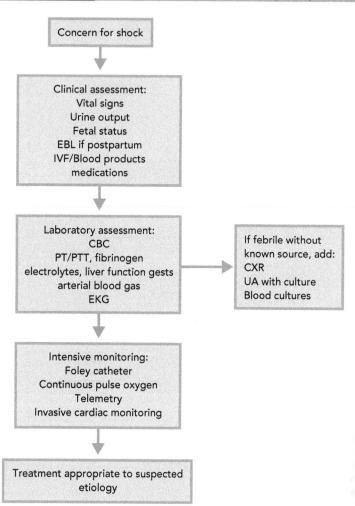

Concern for shock

↓

Clinical assessment:
Vital signs
Urine output
Fetal status
EBL if postpartum
IVF/Blood products
medications

↓

Laboratory assessment:
CBC
PT/PTT, fibrinogen
electrolytes, liver function gests
arterial blood gas
EKG

→ If febrile without
known source, add:
CXR
UA with culture
Blood cultures

↓

Intensive monitoring:
Foley catheter
Continuous pulse oxygen
Telemetry
Invasive cardiac monitoring

↓

Treatment appropriate to suspected
etiology

The diagnoses of thrombotic thrombocytopenic purpura (TTP) and hemolyt uremic syndrome (HUS) are rare in pregnancy. Often thought to be an imitator preeclampsia-related disorders, TTP/HUS can present with the similar findings hypertension, anemia, and thrombocytopenia, however the degree of renal dysfur tion as well as fever and neurologic abnormalities can be distinguishing features.

Treatment of AKI is similar to that in nonpregnant patients and involves care identification of the underlying cause of AKI. Supportive therapy and close attenti to fluid balance is essential to placental perfusion. The need for dialysis in pregnar

ALGORITHM 68.8 Differential Diagnosis of Shock in Pregnancy

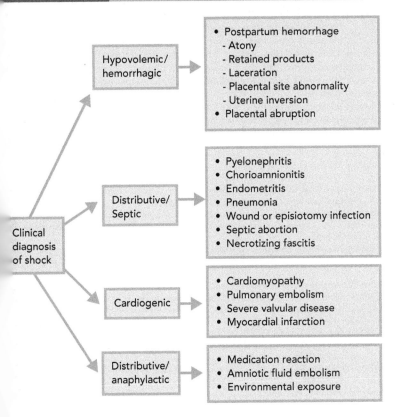

Clinical diagnosis of shock

Hypovolemic/ hemorrhagic
- Postpartum hemorrhage
  - Atony
  - Retained products
  - Laceration
  - Placental site abnormality
  - Uterine inversion
- Placental abruption

Distributive/ Septic
- Pyelonephritis
- Chorioamnionitis
- Endometritis
- Pneumonia
- Wound or episiotomy infection
- Septic abortion
- Necrotizing fasciitis

Cardiogenic
- Cardiomyopathy
- Pulmonary embolism
- Severe valvular disease
- Myocardial infarction

Distributive/ anaphylactic
- Medication reaction
- Amniotic fluid embolism
- Environmental exposure

the setting of AKI is rare. If dialysis is required, frequent exchanges may allow ideal fluid and blood pressure management. Electrolyte and acid–base management are generally unchanged from that of a nonpregnant patient. In the absence of chronic renal disease, worsening kidney function may be a consideration for delivery depending gestational age and etiology (Algorithm 68.6).

SHOCK IN PREGNANCY

Shock is a life-threatening condition associated with inadequate tissue perfusion, hypotension, altered mentation, decreased urine output, and abnormal laboratory values. The pathophysiology of shock in pregnancy falls into the same categories as the nonpregnant patient, including cardiogenic, hypovolemic, distributive, and obstructive shock.

The most common etiologies of shock in pregnancy are hypovolemic shock related to hemorrhage and distributive shock related to sepsis. Regardless of the cause, treatment of shock in pregnancy is similar to the treatment in nonpregnant patients. Clinicians should first attempt to identify and eliminate the originating cause, provide adequate fluid replacement, and improve cardiac function and circulation in order to restore tissue oxygenation. Aggressive resuscitation of the mother usually adequately resuscitates the fetus. Choice of antibiotics in septic shock should take fetal safety into consideration when alternative treatments are available. Blood component therapy using massive transfusion protocol as necessary is the foundation of therapy for hemorrhagic shock. Given the propensity of pregnant or postpartum patients to develop consumptive coagulopathy, care should be taken to provide adequate replacement with fresh-frozen plasma or cryoprecipitate. Normal fibrinogen levels for pregnancy vary by trimester and range from 300 to 600 mg/dL (Algorithms 68.7 and 68.8).

SUGGESTED READINGS

Bandi VD, Munnur U, Matthay MA. Acute lung injury and acute respiratory distress syndrome in pregnancy. *Crit Care Clin.* 2004;20(4):577–607.

Bates SM, Greer IA, Hirsh J, et al. Use of antithrombotic agents during pregnancy: the Seventh ACCP Conference on Antithrombotic and Thrombolytic Therapy. *Chest.* 2004;126 627S–644S.

Cahill AG, Stout MJ, Macones GA, et al. Diagnosing pulmonary embolism in pregnancy using computed-tomographic angiography or ventilation-perfusion. *Obstet Gynecol.* 2009;114 124–129.

Clark SL. Amniotic fluid embolism. *Clin Obstet Gynecol.* 2010;53(2):322–328.

Clark SL, Belfort MA, Dildy GA, et al. Maternal death in the 21st century: causes, prevention, and relationship to cesarean delivery. *Am J Obstet Gynecol.* 2008;199:36.e1–36.e5; discussion 91–2 e7–11.

Cunningham FG, Leveno KJ, Bloom SL, et al. Maternal physiology. In: Cunningham F, Leveno KJ, Bloom SL, et al., eds. *Williams Obstetrics.* New York: McGraw-Hill; 200 121–150.

Dildy GA, Phelan JP, Saade GR, et al., eds. *Critical Care Obstetrics.* 4th ed. Malden: Blackwell Science; 2004.

Foley MR, Strong TH, Garite TJ, eds. *Obstetric Intensive Care Manual.* New York: The McGraw Hill Companies, Inc.; 2004:390.

Heit JA, Kobbervig CE, James AH. Trends in the incidence of venous thromboembolism during pregnancy or postpartum: a 30-year population-based study. *Ann Intern Med.* 2005;143 697–706.

James A. Practice bulletin no. 123: thromboembolism in pregnancy. *Obstet Gynecol.* 2011 118:718–729.

Kim CS, Liu J, Kwon JY, et al. Venous air embolism during surgery, especially cesarean delivery. *J Korean Med Sci.* 2008;23(5):753–761.

Lombaard H, Soma-Pillay P, Farrell el-M. Managing acute collapse in pregnant women. *Best Pract Res Clin Obstet Gynaecol.* 2009;23(3):339–355.

Martin SR, Foley MR. Intensive care monitoring of the critically ill pregnant patient. In: Creasy RK, Resnik R, Iams JD, et al., eds. *Creasy and Resnik's Maternal-Fetal Medicine Principles and Practice.* 6th ed. Philadelphia, PA: Saunders Elsevier; 2009:1167–1194.

Martin JN Jr., Stedman CM. Imitators of preeclampsia and HELLP syndrome. *Obstet Gynecol Clin North Am.* 1991;18(2):181–198.

Nijkeuter M, Ginsberg JS, Huisman MV. Diagnosis of deep vein thrombosis and pulmonary embolism in pregnancy: a systematic review. *J Thromb Haemost* 2006;4:496–500.

Sciscione AC, Ivester T, Largoza M, et al. Acute pulmonary edema in pregnancy. *Obstet Gynecol* 2003;101(3):511–515.

Shaikh N, Ummunisa F. Acute management of vascular air embolism. *J Emerg Trauma Shock.* 2009;2(3):180–185.

Sheffield JS. Sepsis and septic shock in pregnancy. *Crit Care Clin.* 2004;20(4):651–660.

Sibai BM. Imitators of severe preeclampsia. *Obstet Gynecol.* 2007;109(4):956–966.

Society for Maternal-Fetal Medicine (SMFM). Pacheco LD, Saade G, Hankins GD, Clark SL. SMFM Clinical guidelines No. 9: amniotic fluid embolism: diagnosis and management. *Am J Obstet Gynecol.* 2016; pii: S0002-9378(16)00474-9.

Zeeman GG. Obstetric critical care: a blueprint for improved outcomes. *Crit Care Med.* 2006; 34(suppl 9):S208–S214.

Zeeman GG, Wendel GD Jr., Cunningham FG. A blueprint for obstetric critical care. *Am J Obstet Gynecol.* 2003;188(2):532–536.

69 Preeclampsia and Eclampsia

Molly J. Stout and Jessica M. Despotovic

Preeclampsia is a hypertensive disorder of pregnancy characterized by elevated blood pressure and evidence of end-organ dysfunction that typically occurs after 20 weeks of gestation. It can also occur in the early postpartum period. The classic definition of preeclampsia included the presence of hypertension and proteinuria. However, preeclampsia can be diagnosed in the absence of proteinuria if there is evidence of end-organ involvement, such as thrombocytopenia, renal insufficiency, impaired liver function, neurologic or visual disturbances or pulmonary edema. Preeclampsia complicates approximately 12% to 22% of all pregnancies and is directly responsible for 17% of maternal deaths in the United States. Risk factors for preeclampsia include history of preeclampsia in a prior pregnancy, nulliparity, age younger than 20 years or older than 35 years, multifetal gestations, in vitro fertilization, African American race, obesity, underlying chronic hypertension or chronic kidney disease, diabetes, thrombophilia, vascular and connective tissue disorders, and a family history of preeclampsia.

The exact pathophysiologic mechanism for preeclampsia is unknown but likely has to do with dysregulation of placental factors such as regulators of angiogenesis, growth factors, cytokines, and regulators of vascular tone ultimately leading to poor perfusion to many organs including the central nervous system (CNS), kidneys, as well as the fetoplacental unit. It is notable that the underlying physiology of preeclampsia has to do with placental trophoblastic tissue and can occur in the absence of a fetus, as seen in women with a hydatidiform mole.

DIAGNOSIS

Preeclampsia can manifest with wide-ranging severity of disease, from asymptomatic hypertension to life-threatening neurologic, renal, or coagulopathic abnormalities. Hypertension is defined at blood pressure ≥140 systolic or ≥90 diastolic on two occasions at least 4 hours apart in a woman with previously normal blood pressure. Severely elevated blood pressure ≥160 systolic or ≥110 diastolic confirmed within a few minutes (to expedite treatment) is also diagnostic. Proteinuria is defined urinary excretion of 300 mg of protein in a 24-hour urine collection, alternatively protein/creatinine (mg/dL) ratio of at least 0.3 is an acceptable equivalent.

Preeclampsia is a progressive disease and women must be monitored for the development of severe features (listed in Table 69.1) that when present increase the risk of morbidity and mortality. Severe, life-threatening complications are listed Table 69.2.

TABLE 69.1	Severe Features of Preeclampsia
Hypertension	Systolic blood pressure ≥160 or diastolic blood pressure ≥110 mm Hg (can be confirmed within a short interval to expedite treatment)
CNS	Neurologic or visual disturbances including headache
Thrombocytopenia	Platelet count ≤100,000/μL
Renal	Acute kidney insufficiency (serum creatinine concentration >1.1 mg/dL or doubling of serum creatinine)
Hepatic	Elevation in transaminases (to twice normal concentration), epigastric or right upper quadrant pain
Pulmonary	Pulmonary edema

CNS, central nervous system.

The syndrome of hemolysis, elevated liver enzymes, and low platelets (HELLP syndrome) is a life-threatening variant of severe preeclampsia. Women with HELLP syndrome may present with vague epigastric discomfort or mild nausea and vomiting. Notably, HELLP can be found in patients with minimal or absent hypertension and proteinuria. The laboratory findings in HELLP syndrome overlap with other life-threatening complications of pregnancy such as acute fatty liver of pregnancy and thrombotic thrombocytopenic purpura, which should be considered in the differential diagnosis. The main differential diagnosis of preeclampsia/eclampsia/HELLP syndrome is presented in Table 69.3, and several helpful laboratory tests are presented in Table 69.4. HELLP syndrome is associated with an increased risk for both maternal and fetal adverse outcomes including placental abruption, renal failure, recurrent preeclampsia, preterm delivery, and maternal or fetal death.

TABLE 69.2	End-Stage Complications in Patients with Preeclampsia/Eclampsia
System	Complications
CNS	Seizures, cerebrovascular hemorrhage, temporary cortical blindness
Cardiopulmonary	Critical hypertension, heart failure, cardiopulmonary arrest, pulmonary edema
Renal	Acute renal failure
Hepatic	Subcapsular hematoma, hepatic rupture with hemorrhage
Hematologic	Disseminated intravascular coagulation, hemolysis
Fetal	Fetal demise, placental abruption, intrauterine growth restriction, preterm delivery

CNS, central nervous system.

TABLE 69.3	Key Differential Diagnosis of Severe Preeclampsia/Eclampsia/HELLP

1. CNS
   a. Seizure disorder
   b. Hypertensive encephalopathy
   c. Cerebrovascular
      i. Intraventricular-intracerebral hemorrhage
      ii. Arterial embolism or thrombosis
      iii. Hypoxic ischemic encephalopathy
      iv. Angioma, atrioventricular malformation, or aneurysm
   d. Reversible posterior leukoencephalopathy syndrome
   e. Tumors
   f. Cerebral vasculitis
2. Thrombotic thrombocytopenic purpura
3. Acute fatty liver of pregnancy
4. Metabolic disease
   a. Hypoglycemia
   b. Hyponatremia

HELLP, hemolysis, elevated liver enzymes, and low platelets.
Modified with permission from differential diagnosis figure. Sibai BM. Diagnosis, prevention, and management of eclampsia. *Obstet Gynecol.* 2005;105:402–410.

Eclampsia is defined as preeclampsia with generalized tonic–clonic seizures and coma. Approximately 50% of all cases of eclampsia are diagnosed during the antepartum period, 20% present with an intrapartum event, and the remaining 30% are diagnosed during the postpartum period. Although most postpartum seizures occur in first 48 hours, cases have been reported as late as 3 weeks after delivery. Notably, near 15% of women with eclampsia initially present without hypertension and another 1 may lack proteinuria. Furthermore, the severity of hypertension and the amount proteinuria in a preeclamptic patient are poor predictors of progression to eclampsia.

Women with underlying chronic hypertension or proteinuria present a diagnostic challenge. Worsening hypertension relative to measurements early in pregnancy or hypertension that becomes refractory to antihypertensive medications can be used as diagnostic clues. In addition, worsening proteinuria from a baseline 24-hour urine protein obtained early in pregnancy can also be used. Certainly, any development end-organ damage or HELLP syndrome suggests superimposed preeclampsia.

PATHOPHYSIOLOGY BY ORGAN SYSTEM

Vascular

Hemoconcentration and hypertension are the main vascular changes in preeclampsia. Women with preeclampsia may not develop the normal hypervolemia of pregnancy. Vascular reactivity mediated by alterations in prostaglandins, prostacyclin, nitric oxide, and endothelins causes intense vasospasm and intravascular contraction. Alterations in plasma oncotic pressure and endothelial leak can cause third spacing fluid manifested as edema. Careful attention to fluid status is required, as aggressive resuscitation with crystalloids or colloids can often cause pulmonary edema.

TABLE 69.4	Imitators of Preeclampsia/HELLP: Laboratory Findings			
Laboratory Finding	Normal Pregnancy	Preeclampsia/ HELLP	TTP	AFLP
Hematocrit	↓ 4–7%	↑ with hemoconcentration ↓ with hemolysis	↓	↔
Platelet count	Slight ↓, but remains >150,000 μL	↓	↓	↔ to slight ↓
Fibrinogen	↑ (nl >300 mg/dL)	↔ or may ↓ with thrombocytopenia, DIC	↔	↓
PT and PTT	↔	↔ except in DIC	↔	↑
Serum creatinine	↓	↑	↑	↑
Serum uric acid	↓ 33%	↑	↑	↑
Urine protein	↑ but remains <300 mg/day Protein/creatinine ratio <0.19[a]	↑ >300 mg/day Protein/creatinine ratio >0.19[a]	↔ to ↑	↔
Hepatic transaminases	↔	↑	↔ to ↑	↑
WBC	Slight ↑	↔	↑	↑
LDH	↔	↑	↑	↑
Glucose	↔	↔	↔	↓
Ammonia	↔	↔	↔	↓
Bilirubin	↔	↑	↑	↑ (>5 mg/dL)

[a]Shown to correlate strongly with 24-hour urine protein quantity.

HELLP, hemolysis, elevated liver enzymes, and low platelets; TTP, thrombotic thrombocytopenic purpura; AFLP, acute fatty liver of pregnancy; DIC, disseminated intravascular coagulation; PT, prothrombin time; PTT, partial thromboplastin time; WBC, white blood cell; LDH, lactate dehydrogenase; nl, normal.

Modified with permission from Sibai BM. Imitators of severe preeclampsia/eclampsia. *Clin Perinatol.* 2004;31:835–852.

Hematologic

Hematocrit may be increased secondary to hemoconcentration. In the context of HELLP syndrome, hematocrit may be low due to hemolysis. Thrombocytopenia also characterizes HELLP syndrome.

Hepatic

Elevation of transaminases to at least twice normal concentration is a severe feature pre-eclampsia. Hepatic hemorrhage with hepatic capsule irritation may cause right upper quadrant pain. Hepatic rupture is rare but is associated with catastrophic outcome.

Central Nervous System

Eclampsia and intracranial hemorrhage are associated with increased maternal mortality. Temporary blindness, headache, blurred vision, scotomata, and hyperreflexia are also CNS signs and symptoms and are severe features of preeclampsia.

Renal

Normal pregnancy physiology involves an increased glomerular filtration rate and renal blood flow resulting in decreased serum creatinine (typically less than or equal to 0.8 mg/dL). Vasospasm in preeclampsia causes a reversal of this normal physiologic change, and oliguria and increased serum creatinine may occur. Renal dysfunction is typically defined as a serum creatinine >1.1 mg/dL or a doubling of baseline serum creatinine in the absence of other renal disease.

Fetal

Intrauterine growth restriction, oligohydramnios, and placental infarctions may be seen as manifestations of preeclampsia but are no longer criteria for diagnosis.

TREATMENT

The definitive treatment of preeclampsia with severe features, eclampsia, and HELLP syndrome is delivery. The decision to proceed with delivery must balance maternal and fetal risks. Close attention should be initially paid to the medical stability of the mother, with consideration of specific target organs (Algorithm 69.1). Magnesium sulfate is the preferred antiseizure drug in the setting of preeclampsia/eclampsia. It provided as an initial intravenous load of 4 to 6 g over 20 minutes, followed by continuous infusion of 2 g/hr. During seizures, the patient's airway should be protected and adequate oxygenation ensured. If seizures recur while the patient is receiving magnesium, a repeat (4 g) bolus of magnesium may be given. Other alternatives include intravenous administration of amobarbital or benzodiazepines (lorazepam or diazepam). Because magnesium undergoes renal clearance, frequent physical examination should be performed to screen for magnesium toxicity including arousability/neurologic status and deep tendon reflexes. Serum magnesium levels can be assessed in any woman with evidence of impaired renal function and the dose adjusted as needed to sustain blood level between 4 and 7 mEq/L (4.8 to 8.4 mg/dL, 2 to 4 mmol/L). Meticulous attention to pulmonary status and deep tendon reflexes on clinical examinations should be used in women on magnesium sulfate infusions to prevent magnesium intoxication which in the most severe form can cause cadiorespiratory collapse. Phenytoin may used in women with impaired renal function or compromised cardiopulmonary function. Seizure prophylaxis should continue for 24 hours after delivery and extended the patient does not demonstrate evidence of improvement.

Once maternal stabilization is accomplished, the well-being of the fetus should be assessed using heart rate monitoring and ultrasonography, as emergency cesarean delivery is often necessary when the fetal status worsens. The priority of maternal

Treatment Algorithm for Patients with Severe Preeclampsia/Eclampsia

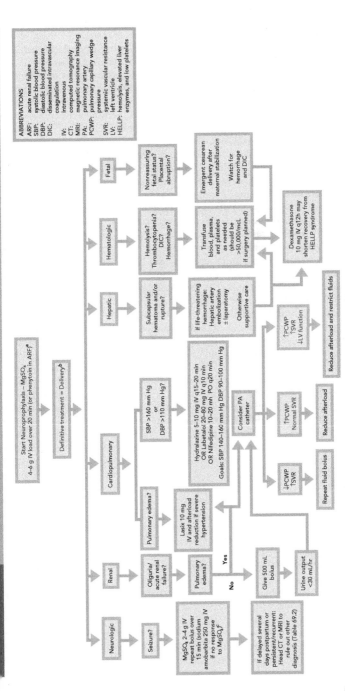

ABBREVIATIONS
ARF: acute renal failure
SBP: systolic blood pressure
DBP: diastolic blood pressure
DIC: disseminated intravascular coagulation
IV: intravenous
CT: computed tomography
MRI: magnetic resonance imaging
PA: pulmonary artery
PCWP: pulmonary capillary wedge pressure
SVR: systemic vascular resistance
LV: left ventricle
HELP: hemolysis, elevated liver enzymes, and low platelets

Start Neuroprophylaxis — MgSO₄
4–6 g IV load over 20 min (for phenytoin in ARF)ᵃ

Definitive treatment = Deliveryᵇ

Neurologic

Seizure?

MgSO₄ 2–4 g IV repeat bolus over 15 min (sodium amobarbital 250 mg IV if no response to MgSO₄)ᶜ

If delayed several days postpartum or persistent/recurrent: Head CT or MRI to rule out other diagnosis (Table 69.2)

Renal

Oliguria/acute renal failure?

Pulmonary edema?

No → Give 500 mL bolus → Urine output <30 mL/hr

Yes → Lasix 10 mg IV and afterload reduction if severe hypertension

Cardiopulmonary

Pulmonary edema?

SBP >160 mm Hg or DBP >110 mm Hg?

Hydralazine 5–10 mg IV q15–20 min OR Labetalol 20–80 mg IV q10 min OR Nifedipine 10–20 mh PO q20 min
Goals: SBP 140–160 mm Hg DBP 90–100 mm Hg

Consider PA catheter

↓PCWP ↑SVR → Repeat fluid bolus

↑PCWP Normal SVR → Reduce afterload

↑PCWP ↑SVR ↓LV function → Reduce afterload and restrict fluids

Hepatic

Subcapsular hematoma and/or rupture?

If life-threatening hemorrhage: Hepatic artery embolization ± laparotomy

Otherwise supportive care

Hematologic

Hemolysis? Thrombocytopenia? DIC? Hemorrhage?

Transfuse blood, plasma, and platelets as needed (should be >50,000/mcL if surgery planned)

Fetal

Nonreassuring fetal status? Placental abruption?

Emergent cesarean delivery after maternal stabilization

Watch for hemorrhage and DIC

Dexamethasone 10 mg IV q12h may shorten recovery from HELLP syndrome

ᵃThe loading dose of magnesium is followed by MgSO₄ 2 g/hr with adjustment for therapeutic magnesium levels (4–7 mEq/L, 4.8–8.4 mg/dL).
ᵇSee exception in the text for a very preterm fetus (<34 wk) in a stable preeclamptic patient.
ᶜConsider lorazepam or diazepam IV with careful attention to respiratory depression.

617

stabilization is particularly important during periods of maternal seizures, which may be associated with impaired fetal oxygenation and nonreassuring fetal status. However, fetal status often improves with stabilization of maternal status.

The predominant cause of fetal morbidity and mortality is prematurity. Preeclampsia without severe features may be expectantly managed to minimize the risk of prematurity and allow administration of corticosteroids for fetal lung maturity. However, severe preeclampsia involving eclampsia, persistent hypertension despite medical therapy, persistent CNS symptoms, pulmonary edema, HELLP syndrome, coagulopathy, abruptio placenta, and acute kidney insufficiency require expedited delivery. There are circumstances when severe preeclampsia can be expectantly managed but these patients should be followed by a multidisciplinary obstetric team. When preeclampsia with severe features presents in the postpartum period, magnesium sulfate may still be used to prevent eclamptic seizures. Similarly, if preeclampsia is diagnosed in association with molar pregnancy, uterine evacuation, and curettage are needed to remove retained placental fragments.

Unlike other hypertensive disorders, the course of preeclampsia/eclampsia is not influenced by antihypertensive therapy. Treatment with these medications is designed to prevent maternal stroke and congestive heart failure. Furthermore, the preeclamptic patient is often edematous secondary to extravasation of fluid into the interstitial tissues in the setting of capillary leakiness and reduced oncotic pressure. This results in reduced intravascular volume despite the increase in total whole-body water that characterizes the disease. Therefore, vasodilatation should be performed carefully, it may contribute to diminished organ perfusion, which may also impact uteroplacental perfusion and jeopardize the undelivered fetus. The use of furosemide should be reserved for the treatment of pulmonary edema. Antihypertensive drugs, including hydralazine, calcium channel blockers, or labetalol, are generally administered for the treatment of diastolic blood pressure levels of ≥ 110 mm Hg or systolic blood pressure levels ≥ 160 mm Hg. There is no clear evidence that one of these antihypertensive agents is superior to the others for improving maternal and/or fetal outcome. Although not routinely indicated, head imaging using computed tomography or magnetic resonance imaging of preeclamptic women may reveal reversible posterior leukoencephalopathy. Conditions that may prompt providers to obtain CNS imaging studies in order to rule out cerebrovascular hemorrhage or other diseases include lateralizing signs, prolonged unconsciousness, papilledema, seizures while on magnesium sulfate, delayed presentation >48 hours after delivery, or an uncertain diagnosis of eclampsia with suspicion of alternative etiologies for neurologic abnormalities.

Most women with preeclampsia/eclampsia are expected to have a full recovery after delivery and removal of trophoblastic tissue. It is rare for patients to develop chronic renal failure or permanent neurologic deficits following preeclampsia. The recovery phase is heralded by the onset of increased diuresis, which can be expected within 24 hours after delivery but, in rare cases, can be delayed up to 1 week postpartum. Because of the high incidence of preeclampsia in pregnancy, the severe sequelae of the disease are among the most common indications for admission of a pregnant or postpartum patient to an intensive care unit. With thorough, prompt, and coordinated care by perinatal and critical care specialists, most patients will recover from preeclampsia/eclampsia without residual disease. However, women with hypertensive disease of pregnancy are at increased risk for cardiovascular morbidity and mortality throughout their lifespan. These women should have yearly assessment of blood pressure, lipids, blood glucose, and body mass index.

New evidence suggests a benefit from the use of aspirin for the prevention of preeclampsia in women with certain characteristics as well as those with a history of preeclampsia in a prior pregnancy.

SUGGESTED READINGS

American College of Obstetricians and Gynecologists. *Diagnosis and Management of Preeclampsia and Eclampsia.* Washington, DC: American College of Obstetricians and Gynecologists; 2002. Practice Bulletin 33.

American College of Obstetricians and Gynecologists. *Hypertension in Pregnancy.* Washington, DC: American College of Obstetricians and Gynecologists; 2013.

American College of Obstetricians and Gynecologists. *Emergent Therapy for Acute-Onset, Severe Hypertension During Pregnancy and the Postpartum Period.* Washington, DC: American College of Obstetricians and Gynecologists; 2015. Committee Opinion 623.

Baxter JK, Weinstein L. HELLP syndrome: the state of the art. *Obstet Gynecol Surv.* 2004;59: 838–845.

    Review of the history, pathophysiology, clinical presentation, differential diagnosis, and management of HELLP syndrome.

Dekker G, Sibai B. Primary, secondary, and tertiary prevention of preeclampsia. *Lancet.* 2001;357: 209–215.

    Review of risk factors for preeclampsia, methods of early detection, and the failure of primary and secondary prevention of the disease, highlighting the need for proper antenatal care and timed delivery in tertiary prevention.

Duley L, Henderson-Smart DJ, Meher S. Drugs for treatment of very high blood pressure during pregnancy. *Cochrane Database Syst Rev.* 2006;3:CD001449.

    A review of 24 trials of medications used in the treatment of severe hypertension in pregnancy, demonstrating that hydralazine, labetalol, and calcium channel blockers are acceptable options.

Ehrhart CM, Barrilleaux PS, Rinehart BK, et al. Postpartum seizure prophylaxis: using maternal clinical parameters to guide therapy. *Obstet Gynecol.* 2003;101:66–69.

    Prospective clinical study demonstrating that clinical criteria could be used successfully to shorten the duration of postpartum magnesium sulfate administration for seizure prophylaxis in preeclamptic patients.

Lucas MJ, Leveno KJ, Cunningham FG. A comparison of magnesium sulfate with phenytoin for the prevention of eclampsia. *N Engl J Med.* 1995;333:201–205.

    A randomized clinical trial demonstrating the superiority of magnesium to phenytoin in the prevention of eclampsia.

Mabie WC. Management of acute severe hypertension and encephalopathy. *Clin Obstet Gynecol.* 1999;42:519–531.

    Review of the pathophysiology and management of preeclampsia, briefly discussing the similarities and differences between eclampsia and hypertensive encephalopathy.

Sibai BM. Imitators of severe preeclampsia/eclampsia. *Clin Perinatol.* 2004;31:835–852.

    Review of disorders which should be included in the differential diagnosis of severe preeclampsia, focusing on acute fatty liver of pregnancy and thrombotic microangiopathies.

Sibai BM. Diagnosis, prevention, and management of eclampsia. *Obstet Gynecol.* 2005;105: 402–410.

    Comprehensive review of eclampsia—timing of onset, cerebral pathology associated with the disease, differential diagnosis, maternal and perinatal outcomes, prevention, and management.

Sibai BM, Mercer BM, Schiff E, et al. Aggressive versus expectant management of severe preeclampsia at 28 to 32 weeks gestation: a randomized controlled trial. *Am J Obstet Gynecol.* 1994;171:818–822.

    A randomized trial demonstrating maternal and fetal safety with expectant management of severe preeclampsia less than 32 weeks, resulting in decreased neonatal morbidity.

Walker JJ. Preeclampsia. *Lancet.* 2000;356:1260–1265.

   Review of the pathophysiology, diagnosis, management, morbidity and mortality associated with preeclampsia.

Zeeman GG. Obstetric critical care: a blueprint for improved outcomes. *Crit Care Med.* 2006;34: S208–S214.

   Review of critical care issues in the obstetric patient and treatment options for preeclampsia and massive obstetric hemorrhage.

70

Trauma Care for the Intensive Care Unit

Nadia M. Obeid and Douglas J.E. Schuerer

are of the traumatically injured patient is a complex issue, given the multiple ptential systems that can be affected. This chapter reviews the initial evaluation and eatment of the trauma patient, then focuses on injuries that are most likely to cause arly intensive care unit (ICU) death in this population. In addition, we review the anagement of the common traumatic injuries most likely to result in ICU admis- on. Any critical care of the trauma patient must be in conjunction with the various ecialists who are needed for this patient population, including general surgery, urosurgery, orthopedic surgery, facial surgery, hand surgery, and rehabilitation edicine. This team approach is essential to ensure positive outcomes in the acutely jured patient. Another important factor in trauma care is that the trauma patient often younger than the typical ICU population and, despite frequently being tremely ill initially, most have a high potential for recovery. Because of the brevity this guide, it cannot be a thorough review of all traumatic injuries, but instead cuses on the most life-threatening ones that are related to eventual ICU care.

RAUMA EVALUATION

e basic tenets of the initial resuscitation and management of the injured patient are scribed in the Advanced Trauma Life Support course. The course was designed to teach physicians the basics of trauma care to better standardize and improve early inter- ations. Most trauma patients are initially evaluated in an emergency department, but sfers and other reasons may place a nonevaluated trauma patient directly in the ICU.

mary Survey

e primary survey is commonly remembered as the ABCDEs of trauma. It is per- ned rapidly but completely and systematically to avoid missing injuries.

way

ess for:

Dbstruction, including foreign bodies, facial fractures, or bleeding. Begin mea- sures to remove obstruction and establish airway.
?atency, which may be compromised because of head injury, intoxication, or welling.

   Note: Patients who are verbal without hoarseness or stridor usually have a patent ay, but this does not rule out future airway compromise. Maneuvers to obtain a definitive airway should begin immediately upon recognition of the problem an[d] before other lifesaving interventions.

Potential problems:

1. Swelling leading to delayed airway compromise.
2. Inability to obtain airway in a paralyzed patient; surgical airway a must.
3. Unknown laryngeal or tracheal disruption.

Breathing and Ventilation

Assess for:

1. Adequate chest wall excursion not limited by mental status, rib fractures, or pai[n.]
2. Loss of or diminished breath sounds on either side from pneumothorax, hemoth[o]rax, pulmonary contusion, or other lung pathology.
3. Evidence of bruising or laceration to the chest.
4. Deviated trachea from tension pneumothorax or neck hematoma.

Potential problems:

1. Airway compromise and ventilation failure may be difficult to discern from o[ne] another.
2. Massive pulmonary injuries may falsely seem to be airway-related because of sev[ere] dyspnea.
3. Airway placement may worsen some pulmonary issues because of positive press[ure] ventilation (worsening pneumothorax).

Circulation with Hemorrhage Control

Assess for:

1. Blood volume and cardiac output
    a. Mental status deteriorates with increasing amounts of blood loss and prog[res]sion of hemorrhagic shock.
    b. Ashen gray skin and poor capillary refill both imply poor circulation.
    c. Pulses are a marker of perfusion in the younger patient without vascular dise[ase.] Full and regular pulses are positive. Fast, thready, or diminished pulses li[kely] delineate poor global flow or decreased flow to the affected extremity. Irreg[ular] pulses may indicate blunt cardiac injury.
2. Bleeding
    a. External blood loss is recognized readily and is best stopped by direct press[ure.] Multiple layers of gauze make tamponade more difficult. Tourniquets sho[uld] not be used except in unusual circumstances.
    b. Occult bleeding from internal hemorrhage should be expected if patient [has] signs of shock.
    c. Potential sources are:
        i. Abdomen: bruising, tenderness, or distension.
        ii. Chest: decreased breath sounds, evidence of rib fractures.
        iii. Pelvis: unstable pelvis, pelvic bony pain.
        iv. Legs: femur fractures may have up to 1500 mL blood loss in the thigh.

Potential problems:

1. Patients on beta-blockade may not develop tachycardia as a response to blee[ding] or anemia.

2. Elderly patients have less reserve and may decompensate quickly.
3. Children have more reserve and will not show signs of shock until severely volume-depleted.
4. Multiple occult sources for blood loss may exist in any one patient.

Disability or Neurologic Status

Rapid neurologic examination:

1. Glasgow Coma Score total score (3 to 15)
   a. Eye opening (1 to 4)
   b. Motor response (1 to 6)
   c. Verbal response (1 to 5)
2. Pupillary size and reactivity
3. Lateralizing signs
4. Spinal injury level

Potential problems:

1. Intoxication masking or reproducing a closed head injury.
2. Lucid intervals can be seen before compromise from intracranial lesions.

Exposure/Environmental Control

1. All clothing and dressings need to be removed to inspect for injuries and examination.
2. After assessment, patient should be covered as quickly as possible and warmth maintained. Hypothermia worsens bleeding and outcomes in trauma.

Resuscitation: During and continuing after the primary survey, resuscitation should be performed while completing each portion of the survey.

. Airway: A definitive airway should be established if there is a loss of the airway for any reason. If there is doubt or worsening of swelling, the airway should always be obtained early when it is safest.
. Breathing and ventilation
   a. Add high-flow oxygen to all patients.
   b. If airway obtained, ensure continued ventilation with hand-bagging or a ventilator.
   c. Pneumothoraces and hemothoraces need to be released to permit adequate ventilation.
Circulation:
   a. Two large-bore intravenous (IV) lines should be obtained. If no peripheral IV access, consider a large-bore (not triple-lumen) catheter into a major vein.
   b. Adult intraosseous needles are available as well.
   c. Consider area of injury before placing IV access.

Adjuncts to the primary survey: Certain interventions are important in the resuscitation of the trauma patient. These are normally performed during the primary survey or immediately afterward.

Electrocardiographic monitoring: usually continuous on a monitor. Formal electrocardiogram may be needed if arrhythmias or possible ST segment changes present.

2. Pulse oximetry: helpful in assessing perfusion status and blood oxygenation trends.
3. Urinary catheter: assesses for blood and follow urine output. Risk of problems by not assessing for signs of urethral injury first (bruising at perineum, blood at meatus, high-riding prostate.)
4. Gastric catheter: assesses stomach contents for blood and evacuates stomach to lessen the risk of aspiration. Consider risk of intracranial injuries with nasogastric tube in patients with facial injuries.
5. Continuous blood pressure monitoring: may need arterial line if critically unstable, but this should not delay definitive care.
6. Chest plain films if major blunt or penetrating trauma; pelvic films if blunt trauma or penetrating wound to abdomen. Other films are determined after the secondary survey.

Secondary survey: The secondary survey is a thorough examination and assessment of the entire patient after the primary survey is complete and resuscitation is started. The following list is not exhaustive, but shows an example of what each body area examination should include.

1. History
   a. AMPLE History
      i. A—allergies
      ii. M—medications
      iii. P—past illness/pregnancy
      iv. L—last meal
      v. E—events of the injury
   b. Should include accident details or type of gun or knife used
2. Head: lacerations, bruises, eye injuries, vision
3. Maxillofacial: facial stepoffs, facial nerve injuries, intraoral mandible fractures
4. Neck: spine tenderness, trachea midline, hematomas
5. Chest: bruises, tenderness, change in breath sounds, crepitus, uneven chest excursion
6. Abdomen: bruising, tenderness, distention, evisceration of bowel or omentum
7. Perineum: vaginal tears, rectal tone, hematomas, blood at meatus, rectal bleeding and pregnancy test in female patients.
8. Limbs: distal pulses and capillary refill, tenderness, crepitus with movement, deformity of the limb
9. Neurologic: detailed neurologic examination, especially levels of injury if paralysis

Tertiary survey: Often patients admitted to the ICU have not been able to be fully assessed in the emergency department because of intoxication, head injury, or hemodynamic instability. It is therefore crucial that the ICU staff helps to perform continual reassessment similar to the secondary survey as the patient stabilizes and able to respond to the examiner. The tertiary survey must be done systematically as can often find undiagnosed fractures or other injuries.

Major Immediate Life-Threatening Conditions

After initial resuscitation, several immediately life-threatening conditions may present, but may not be diagnosed at the time of initial resuscitation. These may become clinically apparent once the patient has arrived in the ICU for continued care.

Tension Pneumothorax

Tension pneumothorax often presents in delayed fashion, especially if the patient is on positive pressure ventilation. Blunt or penetrating injury to the chest and line insertions during resuscitation are often the cause.

Diagnosis:
 Hypotension
 Distended neck veins
 Decreased breath sounds on one side
 Chest x-ray (only if stable)
Treatment:
 Needle decompression if unstable
 Chest tube with closed suction drainage after needle decompression

Cardiac Tamponade

Cardiac tamponade most often is seen after penetrating injury to the heart, but can also develop with blunt trauma from direct cardiac injury or fractures of the sternum or ribs.

Diagnosis:
 Hypotension
 Distended neck veins
 Equalization of pressures, if pulmonary artery catheter present
 Diminished heart sounds
 Echocardiography
Treatment:
 Pericardiocentesis—may be repeated
 Surgery is the definitive treatment

Blunt Cardiac Injury

Blunt trauma can cause several types of cardiac injury, including cardiac contusion, coronary artery dissection or transection, valve injury, chordae tendinae rupture, septal defects, and pericardial tamponade.

Diagnosis:
 Arrhythmias
 Unexplained hypotension despite adequate resuscitation
 Echocardiography
 Cardiac enzymes (creatine phosphokinase, troponin) have _no_ proven benefit
  in the diagnosis or treatment of blunt cardiac injury.
Treatment:
 Inotropic agents
 Supportive care
 Surgery
 Cardiac catheterization if coronary dissection

Massive Hemothorax

Massive hemothorax is a large collection of blood in the chest that can lead to hemorrhagic shock as well as tension-like physiology in the chest. It can be due to major pulmonary vascular injury or blunt aortic rupture.

Diagnosis:
  Hypotension
  Decreased breath sounds
  Chest x-ray
  Computed tomography (CT) scan of the chest with IV contrast if hem
    namically stable
Treatment:
  Chest tube
  Resuscitation
  Surgery

OTHER INJURIES REQUIRING ICU CARE

Hemorrhagic Shock

Hemorrhagic shock can quickly arise in the traumatically injured patient. A pa
may have one bleeding focus or many. Differentiating this from distributive or s
shock is also necessary, but shock secondary to continued bleeding should alway
considered and treated first.

Major causes:
  Liver or spleen injuries
  Massive hemothorax
  Exsanguinating peripheral arterial injuries
  Pelvic fractures
  Long-bone fractures
  Retroperitoneal hematomas
Diagnosis:
  Known or suspected bleeding diathesis
  Anemia
  Tamponade and tension pneumothorax ruled out
Treatment:
  Rapid transfusion of blood and products as needed
  Control of bleeding through surgery, splinting, or embolization

Distributive (Spinal) Shock

This type of shock develops after spinal cord injury and is due to the loss of syr
thetic innervation to the heart and distal vessels. It must be a diagnosis of exclu
after hemorrhagic and cardiogenic causes are ruled out.

Diagnosis:
  Known spinal cord injury
  Hypotension unresponsive to appropriate fluid resuscitation
Treatment:
  Vasopressors and inotropes as needed

Flail Chest

Flail chest is secondary to massive blunt injury to the chest causing fracture of at
three contiguous ribs in two or more places. It results in paradoxical movement o
chest wall during inspiration. Pulmonary contusions are often underlying the inj

Diagnosis:
   Chest x-ray
   CT scan of the chest
   Physical examination (paradoxical motion and extreme tenderness)
Treatment:
   Pain control—consider thoracic epidural
   Pulmonary toilet
   Intubation and ventilation if needed
   Surgical stabilization may be helpful if slow improvement

Pulmonary Contusion

Pulmonary contusion is a common finding in the ICU trauma patient and ranges from mild to severe. Treatment is supportive. Pulmonary contusions usually worsen over 48 hours before improving, and that time lag is important when making future treatment decisions regarding the pulmonary system. Although the trauma patient often has massive needs for resuscitation, in patients with isolated pulmonary contusion, care should be taken to avoid fluid overload.

Diagnosis:
   Chest x-ray
   CT scan of the chest
Treatment:
   Pulmonary toilet
   Oxygen
   Positive pressure ventilation if severe
   Intubation if needed
   Protective lung ventilation similar to patients with acute respiratory distress
      syndrome
   Consider placing affected side down if significant pulmonary hemorrhage

Spleen and Liver Injuries, Pelvic Hematomas

These are included together given the similarity of approach in these patients. For this group, the diagnosis is often known prior to ICU admission. The worst of these injuries that rendered the patient hemodynamically unstable have likely already been stabilized with packing or resection in the operative theater. Further management includes:

   Serial assessment of blood counts and bleeding parameters
   Continued resuscitation with appropriate fluids or products
   If further bleeding continues, the patient likely requires further intervention with
   interventional radiology or surgery.
   Need for pelvic stabilization to reduce venous bleeding in pelvic fractures
   Referral to interventional radiology for angiography/embolization should be considered in patients with pelvic fractures in the following situations:
   a. Hemodynamic instability or signs of ongoing bleeding, after nonpelvic sources
      ruled out
   b. Evidence of contrast extravasation on pelvic CT scan
   c. Repeat angiography with possible embolization should be considered for
      patients who have already undergone pelvic angiography with or without embo-
      lization, with signs of ongoing bleeding (after nonpelvic sources ruled out)

ALGORITHM 70.1 Barnes Jewish Hospital/Washington University Trauma Service Pelvic Ring Injury Protocol

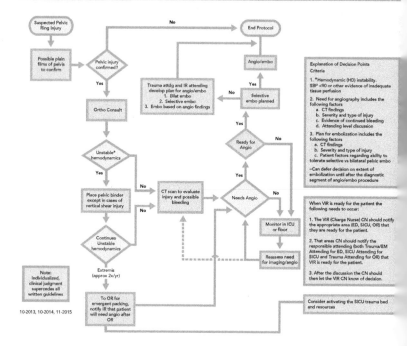

Several guidelines and treatment algorithms for the management of pelvic fracture hemorrhage have been established and updated. Algorithm 70.1 is the algorithm currently used in our institution.

Head Injury

Often patients with multiple injuries also have head injuries. Intracranial injury ca[...] is reviewed elsewhere, but treatment strategies for the multiply injured patient a[...] often different than those for isolated head injuries. The care of these patients mu[...] involve all of the specialty teams in the medical decision making.

Cervical Spine Injury

Trauma victims are often brought to the ICU with their C-collar still in place. T[...] collar should stay in place until an appropriate algorithm to exclude cervical spi[...] injury has been followed. However, leaving the collar in place for an unnecessar[...] prolonged period of time can lead to complications due to pressure wounds a[...] difficulty with airway management. Algorithm 70.2 is the algorithm curren[...] used in our institution. Recently updated evidence-based guidelines are availab[...] at https://www.east.org/education/practice-management-guidelines/cervical-spi[...] injuries-following-trauma.

ALGORITHM 70.2 Cervical Spine Evaluation Guideline for Trauma Patients

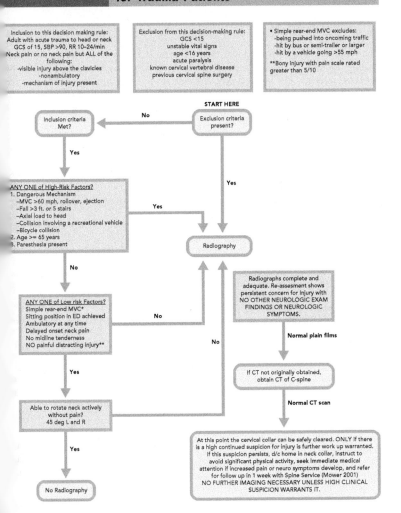

Inclusion to this decision making rule:
Adult with acute trauma to head or neck
GCS of 15, SBP >90, RR 10–24/min
Neck pain or no neck pain but ALL of the following:
-visible injury above the clavicles
-nonambulatory
-mechanism of injury present

Exclusion from this decision-making rule:
GCS <15
unstable vital signs
age <16 years
acute paralysis
known cervical vertebral disease
previous cervical spine surgery

• Simple rear-end MVC excludes:
-being pushed into oncoming traffic
-hit by bus or semi-trailer or larger
-hit by a vehicle going >55 mph
**Bony injury with pain scale rated greater than 5/10

START HERE

Exclusion criteria present? — No → Inclusion criteria Met?

Inclusion criteria Met? — Yes

Exclusion criteria present? — Yes → Radiography

ANY ONE of High-Risk Factors?
1. Dangerous Mechanism
   -MVC >60 mph, rollover, ejection
   -Fall >3 ft. or 5 stairs
   -Axial load to head
   -Collision involving a recreational vehicle
   -Bicycle collision
2. Age >= 65 years
3. Paresthesia present

ANY ONE of High-Risk Factors? — Yes → Radiography

ANY ONE of High-Risk Factors? — No

ANY ONE of Low risk Factors?
Simple rear-end MVC*
Sitting position in ED achieved
Ambulatory at any time
Delayed onset neck pain
No midline tenderness
NO painful distracting injury**

ANY ONE of Low risk Factors? — No → Radiography

Able to rotate neck actively without pain? 45 deg L and R

Able to rotate neck actively without pain? — No → Radiography

Able to rotate neck actively without pain? — Yes → No Radiography

Radiographs complete and adequate. Re-assessment shows persistent concern for injury with NO OTHER NEUROLOGIC EXAM FINDINGS OR NEUROLOGIC SYMPTOMS.

Normal plain films

If CT not originally obtained, obtain CT of C-spine

Normal CT scan

At this point the cervical collar can be safely cleared. ONLY if there is a high continued suspicion for injury is further work up warranted. If this suspicion persists, d/c home in neck collar, instruct to avoid significant physical activity, seek immediate medical attention if increased pain or neuro symptoms develop, and refer for follow up in 1 week with Spine Service (Mower 2001) NO FURTHER IMAGING NECESSARY UNLESS HIGH CLINICAL SUSPICION WARRANTS IT.

TER COMPLICATIONS

...ough the traumatically injured ICU patient is apt to develop any of the com-
...a ICU complications, pulmonary emboli and fat emboli are more common in
...population. Careful thromboembolic prophylaxis must be initiated as soon as
...ible with careful screening for deep venous thrombosis throughout the hospital
...rse. Fat emboli are associated with long-bone fractures, usually after repair, and

can cause severe lung disease, but are treated as most respiratory distress patients wit supportive care.

CONCLUSION

The traumatically injured patient often requires ICU care and monitoring. Reco nizing the most common life-threatening concerns quickly is important in the ca of these patients. The initial survey is important to systematically identify and tre those conditions as rapidly as possible. Continuous resuscitation is the key to t survival and ultimate recovery of these patients, as well as following and recognizi the endpoints of that resuscitation.

SUGGESTED READINGS

American College of Surgeons, Committee on Trauma. *Advanced Trauma Life Support for D tors.* 9th ed. Chicago: American College of Surgeons; 2012.

Carney N, Totten AM, O'Reilly C, et al. Guidelines for the management of severe traumatic br injury. 4th ed. *Neurosurgery.* 2017;80(1):6–15.

Dunham CM, Barraco RD, Clark DE, et al. Guideline for emergency tracheal intubation imm diately after traumatic injury. *J Trauma.* 2003;54:391–416.

> *Emergency tracheal intubation indicated for trauma patients with airway obstructi hypoventilation, severe hypoxemia, severe cognitive impairment (GCS ≤8), care arrest, or severe hemorrhagic shock. Emergent tracheal intubation in patients with sm inhalation injury and the presence of: airway obstruction, severe cognitive impairm major cutaneous burn (≥40%), moderate to severe facial/oropharyngeal burn, or mod ate to severe airway injury visualized on bronchoscopy.*

Management of pelvic fracture with hemodynamic instability. Available at: http://weste trauma.org/algorithms/algorithms.html

Management of pulmonary contusion and flail chest: an EAST practice managem guideline. Available at: https://www.east.org/education/practice-management-guideli pulmonary-contusion-and-flail-chest%2c-management-of.

Nonoperative management of blunt hepatic injury: an EAST practice management gu line. Available at: https://www.east.org/education/practice-management-guideli blunt-hepatic-injury%2c-selective-nonoperative-management-of.

Practice management guidelines for hemorrhage in pelvic fracture. Available https://www.east.org/education/practice-management-guidelines/pelvic-fract hemorrhageupdate-and-systematic-review.

Practice management guidelines for identification of cervical spine injuries follo trauma. Available at: https://www.east.org/education/practice-management-guideli cervical-spine-injuries-following-trauma.

Screening for blunt cardiac injury: an EAST practice management guideline. Avai' at: https://www.east.org/education/practice-management-guidelines/blunt-car injury%2c-screening-for.

Selective nonoperative management of blunt splenic injury: an EAST practice mar ment guideline. Available at: https://www.east.org/education/practice-managem guidelines/blunt-splenic-injury%2c-selective-nonoperative-management-of.

Schreiber MA, Meier EN, Tisherman SA, et al. A controlled resuscitation strategy is fea and safe in hypotensive trauma patients: results of a prospective randomized pilot *J Trauma Acute Care Surg.* 2015;78(4):687–695.

> *Prospective trial randomizing trauma patients with out-of-hospital SBP ≤90 to either trolled resuscitation (250 cc bolus for SBP <70 or no radial pulse, with addi boluses to maintain SBP ≥70 or radial pulse) or standard resuscitation (2 L*

initially, with additional boluses as needed to maintain SBP ≥110). Patients sustaining blunt trauma had lower 24-hour mortality with controlled versus standard resuscitation; no difference identified for penetrating trauma.

Schuerer DJ, Whinney RR, Freeman BD, et al. Evaluation of the applicability, efficacy, and safety of a thromboembolic event prophylaxis guideline designed for quality improvement of the traumatically injured patient. *J Trauma*. 2005;58:731–739.

Risk-stratified prophylaxis guideline for DVT/PE was developed and then implemented, with prospective data collection for trauma patients (general trauma and orthopedic trauma) admitted for >48 hours. Thromboembolic events were lower after implementation of the guideline, as well as for patients admitted to the ICU initially.

Simon BJ, Cushman J, Barraco RD, et al. Pain management guidelines for blunt thoracic trauma. *J Trauma*. 2005;59:1256–1257.

Literature review of multiple databases on pain management in blunt thoracic trauma, with the following evidence-based recommendations: epidural analgesia recommended over other modalities of pain control (i.e., opioids, NSAIDs, transdermal fentanyl); multimodal analgesia recommended, despite lack of high-quality evidence, with high value placed on patient preferences.

Tisherman SA, Barie P, Bokhari F, et al. Clinical practice guideline: endpoints of resuscitation. *J Trauma*. 2004;57:898–912.

A committee was formed to develop practice management guidelines with the following recommendations: standard hemodynamic parameters do not fully quantify severity of injury. Base deficit, lactate, or gastric pH should be used to identify patients needing ongoing resuscitation (level I), ability to achieve oxygen delivery parameters correlates with improved survival (level I), RVEDVI may be a better indicator of resuscitation (preload) than CVP or PCWP (level II), tissue O_2 and/or CO_2 may be used to identify patients needing further resuscitation and are at risk for MOF (level II), serum bicarbonate may be substituted for base deficit (level II), O_2 delivery should be increased during resuscitation to achieve a normal base deficit/lactate during the first 24 hours (level II).

71 The Acute Abdomen
Douglas J.E. Schuerer

Acute abdominal pathology is a common event in the intensive care unit (ICU) setting, but the diagnosis is often delayed because of the absence of typical signs and symptoms of peritonitis. Physical examination signs that define an acute abdomen such as global tenderness, rigidity, rebound, and guarding, are not always obvious in the ICU setting when a patient has multiple ongoing medical issues. A retrospective cohort study of medical ICU patients with abdominal pathology found surgical delay was more likely to occur in patients with altered mental states, absence of peritoneal signs, previous opioid analgesia, antibiotics, and mechanical ventilation. The delay in diagnosis and management of an acute abdomen is associated with increased mortality rates. Therefore, learning to identify an acute abdomen in a critically ill patient with masked physical symptoms is a life-saving skill.

PATIENT HISTORY

Obtaining a history from a patient in the ICU is frequently complicated by an altered mental state, chemical sedation, or intubation. A careful review of the patient's medical history, surgical history, allergies, and medications can provide a possible cause of the abdominal pathology. If the patient is alert, the description of the pain, including quality and radiation, may help to focus the differential diagnosis. Most often, a patient not alert and important medical history must be obtained from family members. One of the most important pieces of information influencing the differential diagnosis is whether or not the patient has recently had an operation. The temporal relationship of a change in abdominal examination from time of surgery can be suggestive of different pathologies. For example, a patient who recently underwent abdominal surgery (<3 days) is at greater risk for bleeding and anastomotic leaks, whereas a patient a week out from surgery is more likely to have an intra-abdominal abscess.

LABORATORY HISTORY

Laboratory tests are important adjuncts in the critical care setting, where most patients cannot provide an accurate history or description of their current physical symptoms. Following laboratory value trends can provide insight into an ongoing abdominal process. An increasing trend in the white blood cell (WBC) count is usually a signal of infection or inflammation but is fairly nonspecific after a recent surgical procedure or in a patient receiving steroids. Conversely, an extreme WBC (35,000 to 40,000 cells/mcL) can indicate a more severe infection, such as *Clostridium diffi-*

olitis, and the workup should be done accordingly. A normal or decreasing WBC count can be misleading; thus, it is important to obtain a differential cell count and evaluate for a left shift. A decreasing WBC to leukopenic levels with a large left shift is concerning for overwhelming sepsis.

Abnormal liver function tests including fractionated bilirubin, alkaline phosphatase, and transaminase levels may localize the pathology to the gallbladder, biliary system, or liver, but are rarely diagnostic. Instead, they help guide further diagnostic strategies like appropriate imaging. Of note, in the critically ill patient, an acute increase in bilirubin may signify acalculous cholecystitis. Elevated amylase and lipase levels hone the diagnosis to pancreatitis, but an isolated amylase elevation may indicate a perforated viscus or ischemic bowel. Concomitant increase in both bilirubin and amylase suggests obstruction at the distal common bile duct or pancreatic duct. Although an elevated lactate level (>4 mmol/L) may signal the emergent condition of mesenteric ischemia with necrotic bowel, it, less specifically, may be the result of acidemia, hypoxia, hypovolemia, anemia, or renal or liver failure. An arterial blood gas should be obtained to determine if acidosis or hypoxemia is present and to quantify the base deficit. Abdominal compartment syndrome should be suspected when acidosis, hypoxemia, oliguria, and a distended abdomen are present. Bladder pressure can be transduced; a pressure >30 mm Hg may require emergent surgical decompression. Urine analysis is not specific, but microscopic hematuria or pyuria can suggest a urinary tract infection or a lower abdomen/pelvic infection.

PHYSICAL EXAMINATION

The physical examination is less reliable in a patient receiving analgesics, sedatives, or steroids and must focus more on changing physical examination signs rather than the traditional signs of peritonitis. In a patient whose clinical course is declining, it is important that the abdominal examination is performed serially and a digital rectal examination is completed.

Because abdominal pain may be difficult to elucidate in the critically ill patient, nonspecific signs such as tachycardia, hypotension, and fever raise concern for occult abdominal pathology. A sudden change in ventilatory settings, overbreathing the ventilator, or increasing airway pressures may signal a patient's attempt to compensate for a metabolic acidosis or indicate an elevation in intra-abdominal compartment pressure. An increase in nasogastric output, abdominal distention, absence of bowel movements, or abrupt intolerance of enteral feeds is concerning for a bowel obstruction, mesenteric ischemia, or an acute ileus due to an intra-abdominal infection. Because the nursing staff spends more extended periods of time with the patient, it is important to communicate with them about changes in the patient's condition, including the quantity and quality of bowel movements (C. difficile colitis or intestinal ischemia), drain output (abdominal sepsis, leak, or fistula), and wound drainage (intra-abdominal abscess or wound dehiscence). For a patient who has recently undergone an abdominal procedure, nonspecific signs would be concerning for some type of anastomotic leak (intestinal, biliary, pancreatic). For a patient who is about a week out of surgery, intra-abdominal sepsis, ischemia, or abscess should be considered.

An acute abdomen in the ICU setting may be of medical or surgical consequence, although there are some diagnoses that overlap (Table 71.1). To assist in differentiating abdominal pain in the critically ill patient in the ICU, the abdomen is best divided into six regions to help evaluate the source of the abdominal pathology (Table 71.2).

TABLE 71.1	Medical Versus Surgical Causes of Acute Abdominal Pathology in the Intensive Care Unit
Medical	**Workup**
Acute renal failure (uremia)	↓ UOP, UA (casts), ↑ BUN and Cr, FeNa, renal ultrasound
Sickle cell crisis	↓ Hematocrit, peripheral blood smear
Adrenal insufficiency/ addisonian crisis	BMP (↑ K^+, ↓ Na^+, ↓ glucose), plasma cortisol and ACTH, cosyntropin stimulation test
Spontaneous bacterial peritonitis	Ultrasound, paracentesis with Gram stain and culture
Diabetic ketoacidosis	Glucose, UA, BMP (Na^+ and K^+ levels), ABG (acidosis)
Gastroenteritis/enterocolitis	WBC,[a] stool ova/parasites
Esophagitis	EGD, barium swallow, pH monitoring
Hepatitis	LFTs, hepatitis panel
Peptic ulcer disease/gastritis	EGD, barium swallow, pH monitoring, manometry
Nephrolithiasis/pyelonephritis	UA (pyuria, hematuria), renal ultrasound
Myocardial infarction	ECG, troponins
Pneumonia	Chest x-ray, sputum sample, WBC
Urinary tract infection	UA (bacteria, leukocyte esterase, nitrites)
Gynecologic disease	Pelvic examination, gonorrhea/chlamydia, ultrasound
Medical and Surgical	**Workup**
Diverticulitis/IBD	WBC, CT scan,[b] flexible sigmoidoscopy/colonoscopy
Clostridium difficile colitis	Stool toxin assay × 3, severely elevated WBC
Pancreatitis/pancreatic abscess	Amylase, lipase, ultrasound, CT scan to r/o necrosis
Intra-abdominal abscess	WBC, CT scan
Small/large bowel obstruction	WBC, lactate, plain film x-rays, CT scan
Choledocholithiasis	LFTs, RUQ ultrasound
Cholangitis	LFTs, WBC, RUQ ultrasound
Mallory–Weiss tear	EGD, hematocrit, coagulation studies
Surgical	**Workup**
Acute cholecystitis	WBC, LFTs, RUQ ultrasound
Acalculous cholecystitis	WBC, LFTs, RUQ ultrasound, HIDA scan
Perforated peptic or duodenal ulcer	Plain film x-rays (free air), upper GI series, CT scan
Acute appendicitis	WBC, CT scan with rectal contrast, ultrasound to r/o other pathology
Mesenteric ischemia and necrotic bowel	WBC, lactate, ABG (acidosis), CT scan
Colonic perforation	WBC, plain film x-rays (free air), CT scan
Ruptured or leaking abdominal aortic aneurysm	Hematocrit, coagulation studies, CT angio (only need IV contrast)
Toxic megacolon	*C. difficile* stool toxin assay × 3, WBC, plain film x-rays, CT scan
Sigmoid or cecal volvulus	Plain film x-rays, CT scan

TABLE 71.1	Medical Versus Surgical Causes of Acute Abdominal Pathology in the Intensive Care Unit (*Continued*)
Surgical	Workup
Boerhaave syndrome	Plain film x-rays, gastrografin swallow
Wound dehiscence	WBC, wound culture, ultrasound, CT scan
Anastomotic leak (intestinal, biliary, pancreatic)	WBC, CT scan (if patient had a recent surgical procedure)
Abdominal compartment syndrome	↓ UOP, WBC, lactate, ABG (acidosis), bladder pressures

UOP, urine output; UA, urinalysis; BUN, blood urea nitrogen; Cr, creatine; BMP, blood metabolic profile; ACTH, corticotropin; ABG, arterial blood gas; WBC, white blood cell; EGD, esophagogastro-duodenoscopy; ECG, electrocardiogram; CT, computed tomography; r/o, rule out; RUQ, right upper quadrant; HIDA, hepatobiliaryiminodiacetic acid; GI, gastrointestinal; IV, intravenous.
WBC should always be obtained with a differential cell count.
CT scan should always be obtained with IV and oral contrast unless contraindicaton exists, that is, abnormal renal function.

The actual explanation of all possible acute abdominal emergencies and their diagnosis and treatment is beyond the scope of this chapter. An algorithm is provided to help guide management decisions for those patients in the ICU who may be experiencing intra-abdominal pathology (Algorithm 71.1).

RADIOGRAPHIC EXAMINATION

Imaging the abdomen helps to confirm or exclude intra-abdominal catastrophe. Initially, three plain film views of the abdomen (kidney/ureter/bladder, upright chest, and lateral decubitus) should be obtained. Air in the biliary tree or intestines, known as *pneumatosis*, suggests necrotic bowel and indicates the need for an emergent surgical consultation. Free air in the peritoneum or retroperitoneum suggests an intestinal or gastric perforation. However, in a patient who has recently undergone laparotomy, free air should be interpreted with caution as it may be the result of the procedure itself.

Abdominal ultrasound is noninvasive and is the imaging modality of choice for a patient with right upper quadrant symptoms or concerning liver function tests. Ultrasound can elucidate gallbladder pathology by demonstrating pericholecystic fluid, wall thickening, gallstones, ductal dilatation, or a distended gallbladder, indicating calculous or acalculous cholecystitis. If the concern for acalculous cholecystitis is high, then a hepatobiliary iminodiacetic acid (HIDA) scan will confirm the diagnosis. Abdominal ultrasound can also identify fluid in other areas, particularly around the pancreas or in the pelvis. Although nonspecific, fluid in the pelvis can indicate intra-abdominal pathology or be a consequence of aggressive resuscitative efforts.

Computed tomographic scanning (CT scan) with contrast is useful in identifying bowel thickening secondary to edema, dilated and fluid-filled intestines, fat stranding, and pneumatosis, all imaging signs concerning for necrotic bowel and requiring immediate surgical evaluation. CT scan can also demonstrate a transition point in a bowel obstruction for easier surgical management. In a recent surgical patient with sudden clinical deterioration and a drop in hematocrit, a CT scan can

TABLE 71.2 Cause of Abdominal Pathology Based on Location

I. Right Upper Quadrant	II. Epigastrium	III. Left Upper Quadrant
Acute cholecystitis	Pancreatitis	Splenic hemorrhage or abscess
Alculous cholecystitis	Peptic ulcer disease/ gastritis	Peptic ulcer disease
Hepatitis	Perforated peptic or duodenal ulcer	Perforated peptic or duodenal ulcer
Choledocholithiasis	Mallory–Weiss tear	Pancreatitis
Cholangitis	Boerhaave syndrome	Pancreatic pseudocyst or abscess
Hepatic abscess	Esophagitis	Nephrolithiasis/pyelonephritis
Pancreatitis	Gastroenteritis	Pneumonia (left lower lobe)
Peptic ulcer disease/ gastritis	Myocardial infarction	
Nephrolithiasis/ pyelonephritis	Pneumonia	
Appendicitis (women in pregnancy)		
Myocardial infarction		
Pneumonia		

IV: Right Lower Quadrant	V. Periumbilical/Nonspecific	VI. Left Lower Quadrant
Acute appendicitis	Small/large bowel obstruction	Sigmoid diverticulitis
Small/large bowel obstruction	Mesenteric artery ischemia or occlusion	Sigmoid volvulus
Cecal perforation	Ruptured or leaking abdominal aortic aneurysm	Colonic perforation
Cecal volvulus	Early appendicitis	Small/large bowel obstruction
Cecal diverticulitis	*Clostridium difficile* colitis or toxic megacolon	Enterocolitis
Enterocolitis	Wound dehiscence	Inflammatory bowel disease
Inflammatory bowel disease	Abdominal compartment syndrome	Nephrolithiasis
Nephrolithiasis	Intra-abdominal abscess	Urinary tract infection
Urinary tract infection	Anastomotic leak (intestinal, biliary, pancreatic)	Gynecologic disease
Gynecologic disease		

Diagnosis and Management of Acute Abdominal Pathology in the Intensive Care Unit

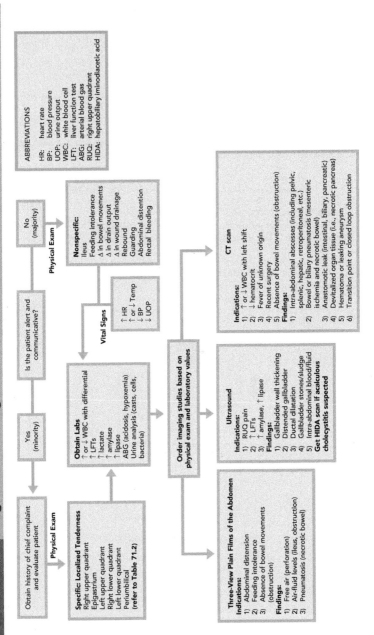

Obtain history of chief complaint and evaluate patient

Physical Exam

Is the patient alert and communicative?

Yes (minority)

No (majority)

Physical Exam

Specific: Localized Tenderness
Right upper quadrant
Epigastrium
Left upper quadrant
Right lower quadrant
Left lower quadrant
Periumbilical
(refer to Table 71.2)

Nonspecific:
Ileus
Feeding intolerance
Δ in bowel movements
Δ in drain output
Δ in wound drainage
Rebound
Guarding
Abdominal distention
Rectal bleeding

Obtain Labs
↑ or ↓ WBC with differential
↑ LFTs
↑ lactate
↑ amylase
↑ lipase
ABG (acidosis, hypoxemia)
Urine analysis (casts, cells, bacteria)

Vital Signs
↑ HR
↑ or ↓ Temp
↓ BP
↓ UOP

Order imaging studies based on physical exam and laboratory values

Three-View Plain Films of the Abdomen
Indications:
1) Abdominal distention
2) Feeding intolerance
3) Absence of bowel movements (obstruction)
Findings:
1) Free air (perforation)
2) Air-fluid levels (ileus, obstruction)
3) Pneumatosis (necrotic bowel)

Ultrasound
Indications:
1) RUQ pain
2) ↑ LFTs
3) ↑ amylase, ↑ lipase
Findings:
1) Gallbladder wall thickening
2) Distended gallbladder
3) Ductal dilatation
4) Gallbladder stones/sludge
5) Intra-abdominal blood/fluid
Get HIDA scan if acalculous cholecystitis suspected

CT scan
Indications:
1) ↑ or ↓ WBC with left shift
2) ↓ hematocrit
3) Fever of unknown origin
4) Recent surgery
5) Absence of bowel movements (obstruction)
Findings:
1) Intra-abdominal abscesses (including pelvic, splenic, hepatic, retroperitoneal, etc.)
2) Bowel or biliary pneumatosis (mesenteric ischemia and necrotic bowel)
3) Anastomotic leak (intestinal, biliary, pancreatic)
4) Devitalized organ tissue (i.e., necrotic pancreas)
5) Hematoma or leaking aneurysm
6) Transition point or closed loop obstruction

ABBREVIATIONS
HR: heart rate
BP: blood pressure
UOP: urine output
WBC: white blood cell
LFT: liver function test
ABG: arterial blood gas
RUQ: right upper quadrant
HIDA: hepatobiliary iminodiacetic acid

reveal an evolving hematoma or an acute bleed. Finally, CT scan is useful in ident
fying the location and size of intra-abdominal abscesses and in guiding managemen
by either percutaneous drainage or laparotomy and washout.

SUGGESTED READINGS

Fink MP. Acute abdominal pain. In: Kruse JA, Fink MP, Carlson RW, eds. *Saunders Manual*
Critical Care. Philadelphia, PA: Elsevier Science; 2003:439–445.
  Short review of important physical exam findings, laboratory values, and imaging studies
  the most common causes of an acute abdomen.
Gajic O, Urrutia LE, Sewani H, et al. Acute abdomen in the medical intensive care unit. *C*
Care Med. 2002;30:1187–1190.
  Retrospective cohort study in a tertiary care center's medical intensive care unit that evalua
  predictors of surgical delay for patients with an acute abdomen and the associat
  between surgical delay and increased mortality in those patients.
Martin RF, Rossi RL. The acute abdomen: an overview and algorithms. *Surg Clin North A*
1997;77:1227–1243.
  Basic overview of managing a patient with an acute abdomen.
Martin RF, Flynn P. The acute abdomen in the critically ill patient. *Surg Clin North Am.* 19
77:1455–1464.
  Overview of the diagnostic difficulties encountered in critically ill patient with an acute ab
  men in the ICU and possible management strategies.
Sosa JL, Reines HD. Evaluating the acute abdomen. In: Civetta JM, Taylor RW, Kirby RR, e
Critical Care. 3rd ed. Philadelphia, PA: Lippincott, Williams & Wilkins; 1997:1099–11
  Textbook chapter reviewing the general approach to a patient with an acute abdomen in
  ICU.

72

Management of the Organ Donor

Stephanie H. Chang and Varun Puri

The number of patients awaiting organ transplantation in the United States continues to rise, with the current UNOS registry showing over 120,000 patients on the waiting list. This increasing need is significantly greater than the number of available organs, leading to a vital shortage that results in the death of many patients awaiting organ transplantation. Different methods have been utilized in an effort to increase the number of available organs, such as widening the donor pool to include donations from extended criteria donors and after cardiac death. Standardized and aggressive donor management protocols have led to increased numbers of transplant organs from potential donors. Additionally, specialized donor centers have also resulted in increased organ transplantation.

ORGAN DONATION

The Health Care Financing Administration of the Department of Health and Human Services requires hospitals to contact the local organ-procurement organization when a patient whose death is imminent and is then deemed a suitable candidate for potential organ donation. The local organ-procurement organization, in conjunction with the intensive care unit (ICU) team, establishes if the patient meets the criteria of donor suitability. Table 72.1 summarizes various criteria for establishing the suitability for organ donation.

After consent is obtained from the family, blood tests and other noninvasive tests are ordered to evaluate if a patient is a potential donor. However, invasive procedures that may be required to further assess for organ donation should not be performed prior to the patient being declared brain dead. Brain death is established by performing two clinical examinations, apnea testing, and laboratory confirmation 24 to 48 hours apart by physicians trained in this area (specific criteria for brain death are covered in another chapter). If brain death cannot be established, the patient may be evaluated for potential donation after cardiac death (DCD). A summary of the process of consent for organ donation is presented in Table 72.2.

Certain patients require other invasive procedures to determine candidacy for potential organ donation. Some examples are cardiac catheterization to evaluate coronary artery disease, lymph node biopsies to assess lymphadenopathy and for more recipient matching, and other surgical procedures to rule out malignancy for incidental findings. If preoperative procedures need to be performed, they should be coordinated between the appropriate specialist (i.e., interventional cardiologist or surgeon) and the ICU team for optimal patient care.

TABLE 72.1	Criteria for Organ Donation

Donor age
- Absolute contraindication → age >80
- Organ-specific relative contraindication → lungs, kidneys, age >60

Lack of significant past medical history
- No malignancy with high potential for recurrent or metastatic disease
- No significant system-specific disease (e.g., cardiac, pulmonary, liver)
- No donor sepsis
- Cause of death not due to massive poisoning, with potential for transplanted organ nonfunction (acetaminophen, tricyclic antidepressants, carbon monoxide, cyanide, ethanol)

Relative contraindications
- No primary brain tumors—relative contraindication
- No significant infectious disease, including HIV[a], hepatitis[a], syphilis, toxoplasma. Routine serologic testing includes HIV, HTLV, hepatitis B, hepatitis C, CMV, syphilis, and toxoplasma.

HIV, human immunodeficiency virus; HTLV, human T-cell leukemia virus; CMV, cytomegalovirus.
[a]There are recently more HIV+ donor to HIV+ recipient transplants, and Hep C donor to Hep C recipient transplants.

Once a patient has been declared brain dead and deemed a suitable candidate for organ donation, the goals of ICU care focus on maintaining end-organ function and perfusion. Brain death can lead to widespread hemodynamic and metabolic dysfunction with deleterious effects on organs intended for transplantation. Several clinical problems apply to donors with brain death, as well as those that are deemed potential candidates for DCD, and these are discussed in the following sections and summarized in Algorithm 72.1. Increasingly, the transplant community has been considering organ transplants using organs donated after cardiac death in the absence of brain death. Newer techniques, such as pumps to maintain kidney perfusion or ex-vivo lung perfusion have allowed for increased organ utilization, especially in the DCD setting.

TABLE 72.2	Obtaining Consent for Organ Donation

- Contact local organ-procurement organization (OPO)
- In conjunction with OPO, obtain verbal consent to perform noninvasive testing (blood sampling, ECG, radiology studies) to determine suitability for organ donation
- Establish the diagnosis of brain death
- After brain death has been declared and in conjunction with OPO, obtain written family consent for donation.
- In the absence of brain death, consider the option of "Donation after Cardiac Death" or the so-called "Nonheartbeating Donor."

ALGORITHM 12.1 Management Goals of Organ Donor Patients

Primary Management Goals of the Organ Donor

Normalize blood pressure and intravascular volume
- Volume, dopamine, levophed, dobutamine to maintain SBP >90 (based on parameters like CO, SVR)
- Sodium nitroprusside to maintain DBP <100
- Hormone replacement therapy

Optimize lung function and ventilator parameters
- Bronchoscopy
- Pulmonary toilet
- Oral hygiene
- PEEP 5–10 cm H_2O
- Maintain pCO_2 at 40–45 mm Hg
- Maintain FIO_2 ≤60%

Correct acid/base and electrolyte imbalances
- Frequent monitoring of serum and urine electrolytes/osmolality
- Tight glycemic control
- Treatment of DI with hypotonic solution and vasopressin

Establish normothermia
- Prevent passive heat loss
- Warming blanket
- Heat ventilator circuit
- Use fluid warmer
- Heat ICU room

ABBREVIATIONS

SBP: systemic blood pressure
CO: cardiac output
SVR: systemic vascular resistance
DBP: diastolic blood pressure
PEEP: positive end-expiratory pressure
DI: diabetes insipidus
ICU: intensive care unit

DONOR MANAGEMENT PROTOCOLS

Normalize Hemodynamics

Brain death may cause cardiac dysfunction as well as vasodilation, leading to decreased end-organ perfusion in potential donors. Cardiovascular management in the potential donor is focused on preventing hypotension (mean arterial blood pressure [MAP] less than 60 mm Hg) and optimizing cardiac output.

Hypotension is frequently encountered in brain-dead patients, with initial treatment directed at volume expansion to a central venous pressure of greater than 12 mm Hg. Establishing normovolemia is critical in providing adequate blood pressure and end-organ perfusion. Crystalloid solutions, colloid solutions, and blood products (i.e., packed red blood cells, fresh-frozen plasma, etc.) may be required to establish normovolemia, especially in trauma victims who commonly have excessive volume loss due to hemorrhage.

Persistent hypotension in the setting of adequate resuscitation and CVP should lead to placement of a pulmonary artery catheter to assess cardiac output and systemic vascular resistance (SVR). Low SVR (less than 400 dynes/s/cm), or decreased cardiac contractility are common causes of refractory hypotension. In the setting of low SVR, vasoactive agents may be necessary to maintain end-organ perfusion. Common vasoactive agents are dopamine infusions (5 to 10 mcg/kg/min) or norepinephrine infusions (2 to 12 mcg/min), with target MAPs >60 mm Hg. Brain death leads to depressed cardiac function due to cardiac beta-receptor desensitization, and may exacerbate other causes of cardiac dysfunction in donors, such as cardiac arrest, blunt cardiac injury, or brainstem herniation. In the setting of decreased cardiac contractility, inotropic and chronotropic agents may be used to augment cardiac function with a target cardiac index greater than 2 L/min/m^2. Agents of choice include dopamine (5 to 10 mcg/kg/min) or dobutamine (2 to 5 mcg/kg/min).

In patients who continue to have hemodynamic instability after volume replacement, and treatment with vasoactive and inotropic therapy, hormone replacement therapy is a potential option. While the mechanics are poorly understood, hormone therapy seems to stabilize the hypothalamic–pituitary axis, which often becomes deregulated in brain-dead patients due to deficiencies in thyroid hormone and cortisol. Hypotensive donors receiving vasopressors greater than 10 mcg/kg/min should receive thyroid hormone (4.0 mcg), methylprednisolone (15 mg/kg), vasopressin (1 u), and insulin with continuous infusions administered until the time of procurement.

Significant hypertension is rarely encountered in brain-dead patients, and if present, is usually related to brainstem herniation. Hypertension with diastolic blood pressures greater than 100 mm Hg should be treated to avoid arrhythmias. Sodium nitroprusside is the treatment of choice. Prolonged nitroprusside treatment should be avoided because of cyanide toxicity.

Optimize Pulmonary Function

Pulmonary function is critical in all organ donors to help maintain adequate gas exchange, but is especially vital in potential lung donors. Common practices to help improve pulmonary function include frequent suctioning, chest percussion, and patient turning. Bronchodilator therapy can help airway clearance, prevention of atelectasis, and avoidance of pulmonary edema. Bronchoscopy is helpful both in a diagnostic setting, assessing if the patient is a potential lung donor, and in a therapeutic setting, optimizing pulmonary function by clearance of mucus plugs secretions. Additionally, good oral hygiene can help prevent ventilator-associated pneumonia.

Mechanical ventilation in patients should be tailored to prevent atelectasis, pneumonia, and pulmonary edema. Brain-dead patients may develop pulmonary edema that is attributable to systemic inflammatory and neurogenic responses. Positive end-expiratory pressure (PEEP) can be used with a target of 5 to 10 cm H_2O to offset this increased capillary permeability seen with pulmonary edema, as well as to maintain alveolar expansion. However, PEEP levels higher than 10 cm H_2O can result in impaired venous return, which negatively impacts cardiac output. Ventilator settings should be optimized to maintain arterial pCO_2 at 40 to 45 mm Hg and, whenever possible, at a fraction of inspired oxygen at ≤0.6 to minimize oxygen toxicity.

Hypervolemia should be avoided in patients who are potential lung donors. Judicious volume administration, often guided by CVP or pulmonary artery catheter information, to achieve end-organ perfusion should be balanced against the accumulation of extravascular fluid in the lungs.

Correct Acid–Base and Electrolyte Disturbances

Brain-dead patients can frequently develop polyuria, with urine outputs greater than 500 mL/hr. The causes of polyuria can be multifactorial, including physiologic, osmotic, chemical (furosemide) or hypothermic diuresis, as well as central diabetes insipidus. Uncontrolled diuresis can lead to profound electrolyte disturbances such as hypernatremia, hypokalemia, and hyperosmolality. In order to avoid cardiac dysfunction, electrolytes and serum osmolality should be frequently monitored and corrected to within a normal range. Protocol-driven continuous insulin infusions are also necessary to maintain tight glucose control, which prevents significant hyperglycemia-related osmotic diuresis.

When other causes of polyuria have been excluded, the likely diagnosis is diabetes insipidus (DI). DI can be established by three of the following criteria:

Urine output >500 mL/hr
Serum sodium >155 mEq/L
Urine-specific gravity <1.005
Serum osmolality >305 mOsm/L

DI is treated by rapid replacement of 50% of the free water deficit with hypotonic saline or 5% dextrose in water (D_5W). Frequent electrolyte and hemodynamic monitoring is essential to correct further imbalances. Refractory cases can be treated with intravenous vasopressin (initial dose: 10 units) or 1-desamino-8-D-arginine vasopressin (DDAVP), which are titrated to maintain a urine output of 150 to 300 mL/hr. Vasopressin functions by decreasing plasma hyperosmolality, increasing blood pressure, reducing inotrope requirements, and helping to maintain cardiac output.

Maintain Normothermia

Thermoregulation in healthy individuals is controlled by the hypothalamus. Hypothalamic dysfunction and decreased compensatory responses (i.e., shivering, vasoconstriction) in brain-dead patients often leads to hypothermia. Passive heat loss and treatment with unwarmed fluids and blood products also contribute to hypothermia in potential organ donors. Hypothermia should be managed aggressively to avoid the coagulopathy, cardiac dysfunction, arrhythmia, and leftward shift of the oxyhemoglobin dissociation curve. Additionally, severe hypothermia prevents the determination of brain death.

Measures to prevent hypothermia include warming the ICU room to >75°F, forced-air warming blankets, administration of warmed fluids, and warming of ventilator circuits.

SPECIALIZED DONOR CENTERS

Donor procurement is generally performed with transplant surgeons from differing recipient centers traveling to the organ donor's hospital, and often involves operating room staff that are not familiar with the steps to an organ procurement surgery. Given this complex nature of coordinating between multiple teams and hospitals, in addition to variability in donor management at individual hospitals, specialized donor centers have been created, with brain-dead potential donors being transferred to these facilities. These centers are used for donor workup and management of brain-dead donors, as well as having operating rooms and staff that are specially trained to help with organ procurements. The first organ procurement organization (OPO) center was started in St. Louis, and not only contains an operating room, tissue recovery room, cardiac cath lab, two-bed intensive care facility, and multiple nurse coordinators and scrub technicians, but also is located less than 2 miles from both transplant centers in the OPO area.

While very few specialized donor centers exist, they have been proven to be beneficial for multiple reasons. Cold ischemic time is greatly reduced, due to decreased need for fly out and due to the close proximity to both hospitals. Organ procurements at OPO centers have higher overall yield compared to organ procurements at hospitals (28% increase). Standard criteria and extended criteria donor organ yield was also higher than the national average (by 6% and 18% respectively). Additionally, these allow for more efficient procurements with decreased cost and decreased time spent by surgeons traveling for procurement.

SUMMARY

The focus of management for a potential organ donor is on preserving end-organ function and viability. Standardized aggressive donor management protocols and specialized donor centers have been shown to increase the rates of organ procurement. After consent is obtained and the patient meets selection for donation, care should be focused on maintaining normothermia and hemodynamic stability, restoring intravascular volume, optimizing lung function, and correcting acid–base and electrolyte disturbance. Management of these systems minimizes the deleterious effects of brain death on organs suitable for transplant, while specialized donor centers cut down on cold ischemic time, both of which potentially improve long-term allograft function. Many of the steps outlined in this chapter are also suitable for preserving the viability of organs procured from DCD in the absence of brain death. However, specialized donor centers are only viable options for brain-dead donors.

SUGGESTED READINGS

Arbour R. Clinical management of the organ donor. *AACN Clin Issues.* 2005;16(4):551–580.
  An expanded and detailed guide for managing organ donors.
Doyle M, Subramanian V, Vachharajani N, et al. Organ donor recovery performed at an organ procurement organization-based facility is an effective way to minimize organ recovery costs and increase organ yield. *J Am Coll Surg.* 2016; 222(4):591–600.
  An article looking at improved organ recovery at specialized organ donor facilities.

Doyle MB, Vachharajani N, Wellen JR, et al. A novel organ donor facility: A decade of experience with liver donors. *Am J Transplant.* 2014;14(3):615–620.

The first article to detail how to set up specialized donor centers, as well as its impact on cost effectiveness.

Dubose J, Salim A. Aggressive organ donor management protocol. *J Intensive Care Med.* 2008;23(6): 367–375.

A review of protocol driven approaches to management of organ donors.

Tutsogiannis DJ, Pagliarello G, Doig C, et al. Medical management to optimize donor organ potential: review of the literature. *Can J Anaesth.* 2006;53(8):820–830.

A lengthy review article discussing the evidence supporting management strategies for potential organ donors.

Ratschke J, Wilhelm MJ, Kusaka M, et al. Brain death and its influence on donor organ quality and outcome after transplantation. *Transplantation.* 1999;67(3):343–348.

A study that evaluates the influence of the duration of brain death on the eventual outcome of the transplantation procedure.

Whiting JF, Delmonico F, Morrissey P, et al. Clinical results of an organ procurement organization effort to increase utilization of donors after cardiac death. *Transplantation.* 2006;81(10): 1368–1371.

A study that reviews the impact of increased use of DCD donors on the outcomes of transplantation.

Wood KE, Becker BN, McCartney JG, et al. Care of the potential organ donor. *N Engl J Med.* 2004; 351(26):2730–2739.

A detailed review article on care of the potential organ donor.

73

Nutrition in the Intensive Care Unit

Beth E. Taylor and Julianne S. Dean

The metabolic response to critical illness is characterized by changes in carbohydra, fat, and amino acid metabolism. These metabolic changes cause an important sh from an anabolic state to a catabolic state characterized by severe macromolecu breakdown of essential proteins, fats, and carbohydrates. Given improvements ICU care over the past decade more patients are surviving their ICU stay, but exp rience the consequences of a prolonged catabolic state, developing weakness a other neuromuscular abnormalities likely due to a rapid protein loss during the fi 10 days of admission. This translates into increased time on mechanical ventilatio infectious complications, length of ICU and hospital stay and mortality risk, a decreased physical independence and quality of life. Nutrition therapy strategies t target provision of appropriate macro- and micronutrients individualized to patie by risk stratification, has the potential to favorably impact the nutritional status improve the recovery of critically ill patients.

Nutrition risk includes variables related to the metabolic state of a patient, s as disease severity, that may lead to a rapid decline in a patient's nutrition sta resulting in adverse outcomes. A previously well-nourished patient may be identif at high nutrition risk based on the extent of injuries or disease severity upon adm sion to the ICU. Currently two tools exist to make this determination, the NRS 20 and NUTRIC score (Table 73.1). Patients diagnosed with severe acute malnutri are also likely to benefit more from nutrition therapy than well-nourished patie (Table 73.1). Patients initially identified as low risk who are then exposed to ongo stress and inflammation via a prolonged ICU stay, may transition to a high risk malnourished state.

Patients diagnosed with moderate to severe malnutrition or identified as h nutrition risk should undergo a complete nutrition assessment with the goal of e nutrition intervention. The components of the nutrition assessment include a nutriti focused physical exam, diet history (specifically recent intake to determine risk refeeding syndrome), biochemical data (complete metabolic panel, magnesi phosphorus, CBC, and other patient specific values), anthropometrics (hei weight, recent weight changes) functional status, and social history. The pati ideal body weight (IBW) and body mass index (BMI) should be determined to with energy and protein needs calculation (Table 73.2). Plasma albumin and p bumin are reflective of critical illness, not nutritional status. Both are affected plethora of factors. Levels are increased by corticosteroids, insulin, thyroid horm and dehydration. In contrast, inflammatory mediators, severe liver and renal dis malabsorption, and intravascular volume overload decrease levels.

TABLE 73.1	Parameters for High Nutrition Risk and Severe Acute Malnutrition	
Severe Acute Malnutrition *(At least two of following are present)*	**NRS 2002** *Total score* *≥5 = High Risk*	**NUTRIC Score** *Total score* *≥5 = High Risk*
Energy intake ≤50% of need for 5 days or more	Energy intake for 7 days: 1 point: <50–75% 2 points: 25–50% 3 points: 0–25%	Age (years) 0 point: <50 1 point: 50–74 2 points: >75
Weight loss: >2% in 1 week, >5% in 1 month, >7.5% in 3 months	Weight loss 1 point: >5% in 3 months 2 points: >5% in 2 months (BMI 18.5–20.5) 3 points: >5% in 1 month (BMI < 18.5)	APACHE II 0 point: <15 1 point: 15–19 2 points: 20–27 3 points: ≥28
Moderate fat loss muscle wasting and/or peripheral edema	Diagnosis 1 point: chronic condition 2 points: acute condition 3 points: head injury, BMT, ICU patient	SOFA 0 point: <6 1 point: 6–9 2 points: ≥10 No. of comorbidities 0 point: 0–1 1 point: ≥2 Days from hospital to ICU admit 0 point: 0–1 1 point: ≥1
Decreased functional status		

A nutrition-focused physical examination consists of a review of oral health, skin turgor and rashes, and assessment for muscle mass wasting and fat loss. Identification of sarcopenic patients in the ICU is challenging. New technology with serial ultrasound measurements shows promise as a simplistic bedside tool that can be used by the dietitian or other nonphysician personnel to determine muscle wasting. However, validation trials are still required. Very few equations have been studied exclusively in the critically ill patient for energy requirements. The two most popular,

TABLE 73.2	Body Mass Index and Ideal Body Weight Calculations
Body Mass Index	**Ideal Body Weight**
Weight (lbs) × 704/in² Weight (kg)/m²	Men: 106 lbs for first 5 ft plus 6 lbs for each inch above 5 ft Women: 100 lbs for the first 5 ft plus 5 lbs for each inch above 5 ft

TABLE 73.3	Weight-Based Energy Needs
BMI (kg/m^2)	Energy (Kcal/kg/day)^a
<15	35–45
15–19	30–35
20–24	25–30
25–29	20–25
30–50	11–14
>50	22–25/kg ideal body weight

^{a}kg, actual weight or estimated dry weight unless otherwise specified.

the Ireton-Jones and Penn State equations are cumbersome to complete, prompting guidelines to support the use of more simplistic weight-based formulas (Table 73.3). The lower range in each category should be considered in insulin-resistant patients to decrease the risk of hyperglycemia and infection associated with overfeeding in diabetic and elderly patients. In the critically ill obese patient (BMI ≥30), hypocaloric high protein feeding is recommended.

Protein needs should be determined using either the patient's actual body weight (majority), estimated dry weight (fluid fluctuation conditions, e.g., ascites), or IBW (morbid obesity). Data suggest protein is the macronutrient of primary importance in critical illness to maintain muscle mass and function, as well as supporting numerous metabolic pathways. Increased protein intake in ICU patients has been associated with a decline in mortality. The increased metabolic rate associated with critical illness along with other potential factors including diagnosis, burns, wounds, temporary open abdomen closure, sepsis, and continuous renal replacement therapy for acute kidney injury (AKI) may significantly increase the requirements for protein (Table 73.4). Once the decision to begin nutrition therapy has been made, the optimal delivery route needs to be determined and feeding initiated (Algorithm 73.1). At present, the general consensus is to feed enterally whenever possible. Early enteral nutrition (EN) has nutritional and nonnutritional benefits. It protects gut mucosal integrity by maintaining villous height and supporting IgA producing immunocytes which comprise the gut-associated lymphoid tissue (GALT). Loss of integrity in the intestinal lumen may lead to the migration of bacteria to the portal and systemic circulation, thereby increasing the risk of systemic infection and potential for multiorgan dysfunction syndrome (MODS). If the use of EN is not feasible, parenteral nutrition (PN) should be considered, starting within 5 to 7 days in low nutrition risk patients or as soon as possible in patients with evidence of severe acute malnutrition or high nutrition risk. Each route has advantages and disadvantages along with contraindications (Table 73.5).

If initiating EN, either gastric or small bowel feeding is acceptable, with the majority of ICU patients able to be fed gastrically. In critically ill patients with gastric feeding intolerance (patient complaints of pain, vomiting, or abdominal distention), placement of a small bowel feeding tube should be considered. Daily surveillance of gastric residual volume (GRV) is no longer recommended as it does not correlate with aspiration risk or clinical outcomes. However, use of GRV has been shown to inhibit adequate nutrient delivery with frequent EN interruptions. Patients who may benefit from early placement of a postpyloric feeding tube are presented in Table 73.6.

TABLE 73.4	Recommended Daily Protein Intake[a]
Clinical Condition	Protein Needs (g/kg ABW/day)[b]
Medical ICU	1.2–2.0
Surgical/Neurology ICU	1.2–2.0
Acute kidney injury	
No dialysis	1.0–1.5
HD/SLED	1.5–2.0
CRRT	2.0–2.5
Hepatic failure	1.2–2.0[c]
Trauma	
General	1.5–2.0
Traumatic brain injury	1.5–2.5
Open abdomen	1.5–2.0 (+15 g/L/exudate)
Burn	1.5–2.0
Sepsis	1.2–2.0
BMI 30–40	2.0–2.5[d]
BMI >40	2.5[d]

[a] Clinical conditions are not additive; to calculate needs, use value that prescribes the highest protein needs.
[b] ABW, actual body weight.
[c] Use dry weight.
[d] Use ideal body weight.

patients at risk for bowel ischemia, EN should be held in the setting of escalating/multiple pressors and hemodynamic instability. If trophic or trickle feeds (generally defined as ≤20 mL/hr or 50 mL bolus every 4 hours) are started in patients on stable pressor dosing, gastric feeds should be initiated with frequent abdominal exams. In this instance, GRV may be used to determine gastric emptying of EN. The short-term addition (24 to 72 hours) of prokinetic agents such as metoclopramide and erythromycin have been shown to temporarily improve gastric emptying and EN tolerance, however longer use may lead to drug-induced complications. Regardless of the site of feeding, the recommendations to troubleshoot complications are the same (Table 73.7).

The appropriate type of tube feeding formula to use in the critically ill patients is still up for debate. Based on the current evidence, standard polymeric formulas are recommended unless symptoms of malabsorption are present, and then a semielemental peptide-based product should be initiated. Studies using immune-modulating formulas (those enriched with glutamine, arginine, omega-3 fatty acids, antioxidants, nucleotides) have been found to be associated with improved clinical outcomes in trauma and postoperative patients. In severe acute pancreatitis, early EN with a polymeric formula in concert with ongoing resuscitation is suggested. No benefit of immune-modulating formulas has been established in patients with severe sepsis or general medical ICU patients. The evidence does not mandate the use of fish oil and/or antioxidants in the acute respiratory distress syndrome (ARDS) or severe acute

ALGORITHM 73.1 Determination of Route and Initiation of Feeding

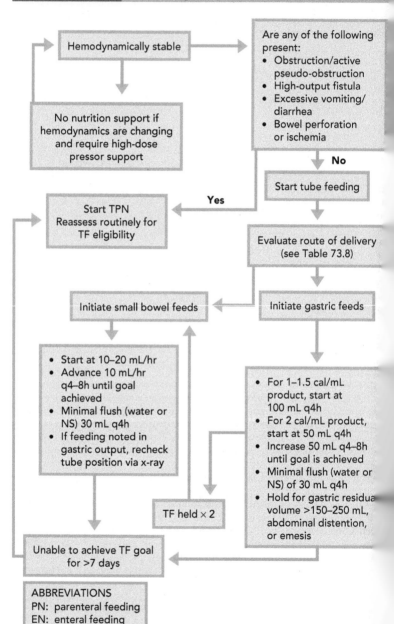

Hemodynamically stable

No nutrition support if hemodynamics are changing and require high-dose pressor support

Are any of the following present:
- Obstruction/active pseudo-obstruction
- High-output fistula
- Excessive vomiting/ diarrhea
- Bowel perforation or ischemia

No

Start tube feeding

Yes

Start TPN
Reassess routinely for TF eligibility

Evaluate route of delivery (see Table 73.8)

Initiate small bowel feeds

Initiate gastric feeds

- Start at 10–20 mL/hr
- Advance 10 mL/hr q4–8h until goal achieved
- Minimal flush (water or NS) 30 mL q4h
- If feeding noted in gastric output, recheck tube position via x-ray

- For 1–1.5 cal/mL product, start at 100 mL q4h
- For 2 cal/mL product, start at 50 mL q4h
- Increase 50 mL q4–8h until goal is achieved
- Minimal flush (water or NS) of 30 mL q4h
- Hold for gastric residual volume >150–250 mL, abdominal distention, or emesis

TF held × 2

Unable to achieve TF goal for >7 days

ABBREVIATIONS
PN: parenteral feeding
EN: enteral feeding

TABLE 73.5	Advantages and Disadvantages of Enteral and Parenteral Nutrition	
Type of Feeding	Advantages	Disadvantages
Enteral nutrition	Preserves gut mucosal integrity Less costly than TPN May blunt hypermetabolic response	Requires functional GI tract More time to reach goal calories Multiple contraindications (e.g., obstruction, fistula)
Parenteral nutrition	Does not require functioning GI tract Full therapy in <24 hours	Intestinal atrophy Requires central IV access Increased rate of infectious complications

...ung injury populations. At present, no recommendation can currently be made for ...se of probiotics in the general ICU population because of the lack of consistent outcome effect and heterogeneity of the bacterial strains studied. Insoluble fiber should ...e avoided in all critically ill patients and soluble fiber should only be used in resuscitated, hemodynamically stable patients with intractable diarrhea. Both forms should ...e avoided in any patient with severe dysmotility or at risk of bowel ischemia. A large ...ulticenter observational study highlighted that the majority of ICU patients receive ...ell below the prescribed amount of EN. Steps should be taken (volume-based feeding protocols, early placement of small bowel tubes) to avoid interruptions to EN or ...o provide adequate amounts in spite of them.

Critically ill patients presenting with injuries (traumatic brain injury) or conditions (severe dysphagia due to cerebral vascular accident) that will require >4 weeks ...f EN therapy will benefit from early placement of long-term feeding access. For ...onditions requiring <4 weeks of therapy, placement of short-term feeding access via ...e nose or mouth should be instituted. Several options of both short- and long-term ...ccess and their associated risks are reviewed in Table 73.8.

PN must be administered via a designated port of a central venous catheter ...o avoid potential complications associated with incompatibilities with intravenous ...edication administration. In the absence of signs or symptoms of bacteremia, a

TABLE 73.6	Gastric and Small Bowel Feeding Indications
Gastric Feeding	Small Bowel Feeding

Majority of ICU patients
Short gut
	Delayed gastric emptying
	Postoperative gastric ileus
	Proven intolerance to gastric feeding
	Severe acute pancreatitis
	   Intolerant to gastric feeds
	   Requiring gastric decompression

, intensive care unit

TABLE 73.7	Troubleshooting Tube Feeding Complications

Residuals: Should not be routinely used. If used, a volume of 500 mL should be correlated with clinical signs of intolerance: abdominal distention, fullness, discomfort, or presence of emesis. If present consider:

- Repeat radiograph to confirm position of tube or check pH of contents.
- Start a prokinetic agent: IV metoclopramide 10 mg q 6 hours (if no renal failure present), for no greater than 72 hours.
- Change to a more calorically dense product to decrease total volume infused.
- Order a small bowel feeding tube.

Diarrhea: Quantify amount of stool. May have 4–5 loose stools per day on EN. If present consider:

- Review medications. Diarrhea may be secondary to an enteral medication. Try changing medication route to IV.
- Rule out the presence of *Clostridium difficile.*
- Try adding a soluble fiber to feeds (10–20 g in divided doses over 24 hours) if patient fully resuscitated and without risk of bowel ischemia. (no fiber on GI surgery patients for 1 week).
- Once infectious cause is ruled out, use an antidiarrheal agent (loperamide 2–4 mg q6h).
- KEEP FEEDING.

Constipation: Difficulty passing or no bowel movement >3 days after feedings are at goal.

- Start bowel regimen per hospital protocol.
- Check for signs of dehydration, such as hypernatremia, prerenal azotemia, oliguria, low skin turgor, orthostatic hypotension.
- Order KUB to rule out obstruction
- Increase amount of free water.
- Rectal examination with disimpaction.
- Once obstruction is ruled out; consider suppository and/or enema as PRN

IV, intravenous; TID, three times a day; KUB, kidney/ureter/bladder x-ray; PRN, as needed; BID, two times a day.

newly placed catheter is not required as long as a designated port is available with the existing access. PN via a peripheral intravenous line is not appropriate for the critically ill patient. Subclavian lines are preferred because of the ease in maintaining an occlusive dressing and the lower rate of infections. The least desirable is a femoral line that has been associated with a higher incidence of venous thrombosis. The choice of catheter type depends on the reason for PN, expected duration of PN, and the patient's overall status (Table 73.9).

The practitioner prescribing and monitoring the patient on PN must be knowledgeable regarding safety of final macronutrient concentrations, the form in which electrolytes are provided, and conditions or other medical treatments precipitating change in the macro- or micronutrient prescription (Table 73.10). Clinicians often underestimate the importance of nutrition therapy in the ICU patient population, understanding the massive catabolic state that exists and adverse outcomes associated

| TABLE 73.8 | Short- and Long-Term Enteral Feeding Access |

- **Salem sump nasogastric or orogastric:** a short-term feeding tube generally placed by the bedside nurse for decompression that may be used for feeding. The patient must have a functioning GI tract, adequate gastric-emptying, and low risk of aspiration. Nasally placed tubes carry the risk of sinusitis and nasal necrosis.
- **Nasoenteric feeding tube** for gastric or small bowel placement: a short-term, softer, more flexible tube with less risk of causing sinusitis or nasal necrosis, this tube may also be placed orally. Generally placed in patients for comfort. Small bowel tubes are placed in patients with poor gastric-emptying and have a high risk of reflux.
- **G-tube**[a] for surgical or percutaneous endoscopic gastrostomy: a long-term feeding tube for patients with a functioning GI tract and adequate gastric-emptying. G-tubes have a lower risk of aspiration when compared with above-the-diaphragm feeding access.

  J-tube[a] for surgical or percutaneous endoscopic jejunostomy: a long-term feeding tube indicated for patients with a functioning GI tract, poor gastric-emptying, and a high risk for reflux and aspiration.

  G-J tube[a]: a long-term feeding tube placed percutaneously or at time of laparotomy in patients for feeding into the distal duodenum with a gastric port for decompression.

gastrointestinal.
[a] tubes that transverse the two epithelial barriers of the skin and mucosa of the GI tract carry the risk of hemorrhage and infection at the incision site as well as peritonitis and risk of dislodgment.

| ABLE 73.9 | Catheter Selection for Total Parenteral Nutrition |

Triple/quad lumen catheter: used for in-hospital patients on total parenteral nutrition (TPN). The distal port is preferred for the infusion of TPN solution to maintain sterility and avoid contamination. Blood is drawn through the medial port and other infusions are performed through the proximal port(s).

PICC (peripheral inserted central catheter): PICC lines are placed via the brachiocephalic vein. PICC lines have a long catheter (60 cm) with the tip positioned in the superior vena cava.

Tunneled catheter: This is a silastic catheter (single-, double-, or triple-lumen) that is tunneled subcutaneously several centimeters from the insertion site before exiting the skin. If no infection is present, these catheters can stay in place indefinitely.

Hohn: A percutaneously placed catheter used for patients requiring 6 months or less of TPN or IV medication. The distal port (red) is preferred for the infusion of TPN solution to maintain sterility and avoid contamination.

Implanted venous access device: This is a subcutaneously implanted chamber attached to a silastic central venous catheter, either single- or double-lumen. Because the reservoir is implanted in the SQ, it must be accessed with a needle for drawing blood or administering TPN or other IV infusions. These catheters are generally reserved for patients receiving chemotherapy who require periodic infusions.

travenous.

TABLE 73.10	Electrolytes Administered via the Total Parenteral Nutrition Solution	
Suggested Electrolytes (per liter)	Conditions That May Require Alteration of Amount Provided	Electrolyte Carriers
Sodium 60–150 mEq	• Renal function • Fluid status • GI losses • Traumatic brain injury	NaCl Na acetate $NaPO_4$
Potassium 40–120 mEq	• Renal function • GI losses • Metabolic acidosis • Refeeding	KCl K acetate KPO_4
Phosphate 10–30 mM	• Renal function • Refeeding • Bone disease • Hypercalcemia • Rapid healing[a] • Hepatic function	$NaPO_4$ KPO_4
Chloride 60–120 mEq	• Renal function • GI losses (gastric) • Acid-base status	NaCl KCl
Acetate 10–40 mEq	• Renal function • GI losses (small bowel) • Acid-base status • Hepatic function	Na acetate K acetate
Calcium 4.5–.2 mEq	• Hyperparathyroidism • Malignancy • Bone disease • Immobilization • Acute pancreatitis • Renal function	Ca gluconate $CaCl_2$
Magnesium 8.1–24.3 mEq	• Renal function • Refeeding • Hypokalemia	Mg sulfate

GI, gastrointestinal.
[a]Rapid healing examples are burn, and young trauma patients who have rapid tissue generatic

with long-term exposure underscores the need for early and precise nutrition the
Early nutrition therapy in patients identified to be severely malnourished or at
nutrition risk may have the most impact on the recovery of critical illness. A c
cated nutrition specialist as part of the multidisciplinary team is imperative to er
that patients are identified for appropriate and timely provision of nutrition the
and ongoing monitoring of the effects of that therapy.

SUGGESTED READINGS

Alberda C, Gramlich L, Jones N, et al. The relationship between nutritional intake and clinical outcomes in critically ill patients: results of an international multicenter observational study. *Intensive Care Med.* 2009;35:1821–1827.

  Caloric intake in ICU patients approximates 60% of the prescribed nutritional support, thus many patients are underfed and in patients with the lowest BMI and severe malnutrition, this underfeeding could be impacting outcomes.

Crook M. Refeeding syndrome: problems with definitions and management. *Nutrition.* 2014; 30(11–12):1448–1455.

  Reviews symptoms and management of refeeding syndrome, including the role of nutrition.

Kondrup J. Nutrition-risk scoring systems in the intensive care unit. *Curr Opin Clin Nutr Metab Care.* 2014;17:177–182.

  Overview of nutrition risk scoring systems and current support for their use in the ICU.

Kudsk KA. Effect of route and type of nutrition on intestine-derived inflammatory responses. *Am J Surg.* 2003;185:16–21.

  This review article looked at the effects on the gastrointestinal tract from lack of feeding. Findings included an increase in proinflammatory markers and showed that the addition of glutamine reverses many of the defects seen in starvation in the critically ill.

Lee ZY, Barakatun-Nisak MY, Noor Airini, et al. Enhanced protein-energy provision via the enteral route in critically ill patients (PEP uP Protocol): a review of the evidence. *Nutr Clin Pract.* 2016;31:68–79.

  An example of an enteral volume-based feeding protocol and the impact on delivery.

Marik PE, Zaloga G. Immunonutrition in high-risk surgical patients: A systematic review and analysis of the literature. *J Parenter Enter Nutr.* 2010;34:378–386.

  In surgery patients immunonutrition is associated with a reduction in risk of acquired infection and wound complications and a shorter LOS. However, there was not a mortality advantage.

Needham DM, Dinglas VD, Bienvenu OJ, et al. One year outcomes in patients with acute lung injury randomized to initial trophic or full enteral feeding: prospective follow-up of EDEN randomized trial. *BMJ.* 2013;346:f1532.

  Enteral feeding whether at low or full rate provides some degree of benefit in certain ICU patients.

Paris MT, Mourtzakis M, Day A, et al. Validation of bedside ultrasound of muscle layer thickness of the quadriceps in the critically ill patient (VALIDUM Study). *JPEN J Parenter Enter Nutr.* 2017;41(2):171–180.

  Introduction of how US guided imagery may be used to assess muscle mass in ICU patients.

Taylor BE, McClave SA, Martindale RG, et al. Guidelines for the provision and assessment of nutrition therapy in the adult critically ill patient: Society of Critical Care Medicine and American Society for Parenteral and Enteral Nutrition. *JPEN J Parenter Enteral Nutr.* 2016;40(2):159–211.

  Evidence-based practice and consensus guideline for nutrition therapy in all ICU patients. Reviews differences in several subsets of patients.

74 Arterial Catheterization

Adam Anderson

Arterial catheterization is common in intensive care medicine. Indications for placing an arterial line include direct arterial hemodynamic monitoring, frequent arterial blood gas measurements in patients with respiratory insufficiency, and less commonly for placement of an intra-aortic balloon pump or direct arterial administration of drugs (e.g., thrombolytics). Noninvasive arterial oxygen saturation may be inaccurate in unstable patients, and frequent direct measurement of the arterial pH, bicarbonate and partial pressures of oxygen and carbon dioxide is often needed in patients on ventilator support or with impending respiratory collapse. In unstable patients, non invasive blood pressure monitors may be imprecise necessitating the use of arterial lines for accurate hemodynamic monitoring.

Equipment required for catheterization includes maximal sterile barrier pre cautions, an intravascular catheter, suture or affixation device, noncompliant tubing flush device with pressurized flush solution, transducer, and electronic monitoring equipment including a connecting cable and a monitor with an amplifier and display screen. Real-time ultrasonography is recommended to increase success rate of vessel cannulation. The tubing is connected to the transducer, which in turn is connected to the electronic monitor via a connecting cable. The noncompliant tubing transmits the pressure waveform from the artery to the transducer, which converts the pressure waveform to an electrical waveform. The electric waveform is amplified and dis played on the oscilloscope screen. The flush device allows continuous fluid infusion to prevent thrombus formation and is pressurized to prevent backup of high-pressure arterial blood into the tubing.

The most common site selected for arterial catheterization is the radial artery followed by the femoral artery. Less common sites include the dorsalis pedis, brachial and axillary arteries. Although both radial and femoral sites are acceptable and have a similar complication profile, the radial site is preferred with a lower infection risk

The radial and ulnar arteries are the distal branches of the brachial artery and are located on the lateral and medial sides of the wrists in anatomic position, respectively. They are connected by the deep and superficial palmar arches in the hand. The arterial anastomoses are taken into consideration when a radial line is placed, as potential complication of radial artery catheterization is thrombosis. If thrombus occurs, collateral circulation from the ulnar artery through the palmar arches typically ensures adequate blood flow to the hand. Peripheral vascular disease that occludes the palmar arches could interrupt blood flow to the hand if radial artery thrombus occurs

The Allen test can identify patients who have compromised collateral palmar circulation. The test is performed by raising the patient's arm to 45 degrees, with the examiner compressing the radial and ulnar arteries with both hands. The patient is asked to repeatedly open and close the hand to drain the blood. Once pallor develops, one artery is released and the time to palmar flushing is timed. Less than 7 seconds is considered positive, 8 to 14 seconds is equivocal, and 15 or more seconds is considered a negative test and evidence for a lack of adequate collateral circulation. The test is repeated with the other artery. Results may be difficult to interpret for patients on vasopressors and those unable to cooperate. Thus, many have abandoned the routine performance of the Allen test.

Three types of arterial catheters are commonly used. The simplest utilizes a similar angiocatheter to a peripheral intravenous (IV) without guidewire assistance. Guidewire kits offer either a preloaded system or a separate guidewire using the Seldinger technique. No method has shown superiority, and kit selection is based on provider preference and availability. Catheter gauge and length vary on the basis of arterial site.

STEPS FOR RADIAL ARTERY CANNULATION

1. Position the supine patient's hand with 30 to 60 degrees of extension by propping the dorsal wrist surface on a rolled towel or other supporting structure with the ventral surface up.
2. Remove all objects from the wrist and cleanse the skin with an antiseptic solution such as chlorhexidine or Betadine.
3. Create a sterile field by draping the wrist and donning a sterile gown and gloves (a reasonable rule is to gown and mask when placing objects in a patient that will remain in place and act as a potential source of infection).
4. Palpate the radial artery on the patient's ventral wrist with the first two fingers of the nondominant hand 3 to 4 cm proximal to the crease at the base of the thenar eminence. If employing ultrasonography, use a sterile sleeve and identify pertinent structures including the radial artery.
5. For conscious patients, infiltrate a liberal volume (>2 mL) of local anesthetic.
6. With the dominant hand, hold the catheter like a pencil between the first and second fingers.
7. While palpating gently, or visualizing with the ultrasound probe, with the nondominant hand, enter the skin at a 30- to 45-degree angle with the catheter tip just caudad to the fingertips of the nondominant hand. Pressing too firmly on the radial artery can occlude flow and make cannulation difficult.
8. Advance the catheter toward the artery until a flash of blood enters the catheter tip.
9. If using a simple catheter-over-needle configuration, advance the tip of the needle slightly further into the artery to ensure that the tip of the catheter is in the arterial lumen (note: go to step 12 if using a device with a wire).
10. While holding the needle steady, advance the catheter gently forward into the artery lumen with a slight twisting motion.
11. Remove the needle; correct placement should result in pulsatile blood flow (if using a catheter without a wire, go to step 15).
12. If using a kit with a guidewire, when the flash of blood occurs, hold the needle steady and advance the guidewire into the arterial lumen, which should meet little resistance. Ultrasonography, if available, should document the intraluminal guidewire.

13. If using a preloaded guidewire, advance the catheter over the wire and into the arterial lumen. If using a separate guidewire, remove the needle while leaving the guidewire in place and replace with a catheter.
14. Remove the needle and wire; correct placement should result in pulsatile blood flow
15. Connect the catheter to the transducer tubing and flush device.
16. Secure the catheter to the skin with suture or adhesive device.
17. Cleanse the skin and catheter with antiseptic solution and cover with sterile dressing.

TIPS

If the initial attempt is unsuccessful, reposition the catheter and try again. A less steep angle may decrease the chance of traversing the artery. If further attempts are unsuccessful, try advancing the needle through the artery when the initial flash of blood is seen in the catheter tip. Next, slowly withdraw the catheter until a flash of blood again occurs and attempt to advance a guidewire through the catheter and into the arterial lumen. Once the guidewire is in place, the catheter can be advanced. Deliberate palpation of the artery, focused technique, and real-time ultrasonography will aid in a successful result. The artery often is transfixed initially with no blood flow. Thus, the catheter should always be withdrawn slowly as success can be achieved while withdrawing the catheter.

For femoral artery cannulation, a kit similar to a central venous catheterization kit is often used. The femoral artery lies in the femoral triangle bordered superiorly by the inguinal ligament, laterally by the sartorius muscle, and medially by the adductor longus muscle (see Figure 75.5). From the lateral to medial positions in the triangle is the femoral nerve, femoral artery, and femoral vein. The site should be cleaned and prepared in a sterile fashion. Similar to the radial artery, the femoral artery is palpated with the nondominant hand or with ultrasonography guidance. Cannulation of the artery is performed in the same manner as venous cannulation (see Chapter 75), but when blood returns into the syringe and it is disconnected from the needle, pulsatile blood confirms arterial placement (although it may be nonpulsatile during cardiac arrest).

Complications of arterial line placement are listed in Table 74.1. Clinically significant complications are relatively uncommon, but can be life-threatening.

TABLE 74.1	Complications of Arterial Cannulation
Thrombosis	
Local or systemic infection	
Hematoma	
Pseudoaneurysm	
Hemorrhage	
Significant blood loss from frequent blood testing	
Heparin-induced thrombocytopenia (for heparin-flushed lines)	
Retroperitoneal hematoma (femoral lines)	
Limb ischemia	
Peripheral neuropathy	
Insertion site pain	

Thrombosis is the most common complication. Infection can also occur with arterial line placement. Risk can be minimized with careful sterile technique during catheter placement, routine catheter care, and radial artery preference. Catheter dressings should be changed approximately every 48 hours. Careful sterile technique should be used when drawing blood samples from the catheter. In part because of higher pressure blood flow, arterial lines are less likely to become infected than central venous lines. For febrile patients, arterial lines do not necessarily need to be removed unless no other infectious source is identified. However, catheters should be removed as soon as they are no longer needed.

SUGGESTED READINGS

DeFer TM, Knoche EM, LaRossa GN, et al. *Guide to Procedures. The Washington Manual Internship Survival Guide.* 4th ed. Philadelphia, PA: Lippincott Williams and Wilkins; 2013:215–221.

Garland A. Arterial lines in the ICU: a call for rigorous controlled trials. *Chest.* 2014;146(5): 1155–1158.

Miller AG, Bardin AJ. Review of ultrasound-guided radial artery catheter placement. *Respir Care.* 2016;61(3):383–388.

O'Horo JC, Maki DG, Krugg AE, et al. Arterial catheters as a source of bloodstream infection: a systematic review and meta-analysis. *Crit Care Med.* 2014;42(6):1334–1339.

Shiloh AL, Eisen LA. Ultrasound-guided arterial catheterization: a narrative review. *Intensive Care Med.* 2010;36(2):214–221.

75 Central Venous Catheterization

Rachel McDonald and Adam Anderson

Central venous catheterization is commonly performed in the intensive care unit when peripheral access is inadequate. Indications for central venous catheterization include administration of noxious medications, hemodynamic monitoring, therapies requiring rapid blood flow rates (hemodialysis, plasmapheresis), insertion of invasive devices, rapid large-volume fluid or blood product administration, and emergency venous access. Noxious medications that require infusion into large central veins include vasopressors, chemotherapy, and total parenteral nutrition (TPN). Hemodynamic monitoring and invasive devices requiring central access include monitoring of central venous pressure, measurement of central venous hemoglobin saturation, and insertion of pulmonary artery catheters or transvenous pacemakers. Contraindications for central venous catheterization include known thrombosis of the target vessel and infection over the site of entry. There is no definitive cut-off for the insertion of a central venous catheter in coagulopathic or thrombocytopenic patients; however, the subclavian site is generally avoided in coagulopathic patients due to inability to monitor for bleeding or adequately compress the site should bleeding occur. Use of a micropuncture kit or correction of the coagulopathy with fresh-frozen plasma and platelet transfusion may be useful prior to the procedure.

Complications of central venous catheterization include mechanical complications (arterial puncture, pneumothorax, hemothorax, air embolus, retroperitoneal hemorrhage), infectious complications (central venous catheter-associated bacteremia, cellulitis), and catheter-associated thrombosis or stenosis. Although conflicting data exist, general consensus is that the risk of infection is least with subclavian cannulation and highest with femoral cannulation. In addition to avoiding the femoral site due to infectious complications, the Centers for Disease Control and Prevention (CDC) guidelines for cannulation site selection recommend avoiding femoral cannulation in adult patients because of increased rates of venous thrombosis and restriction of patient mobility. Subclavian cannulation should be avoided in patients with coagulopathies for the aforementioned reasons or in patients with advanced kidney disease due to the risk of subclavian stenosis.

The use of ultrasound guidance to aid in the placement of central venous catheters has been shown to decrease complication rates, decrease the number of attempts necessary to cannulate the vein, and decrease the amount of time necessary to perform the procedure. Ultrasound is used both to identify the location of the target vein and its accompanying artery and to assess the vein for thrombosis or stenosis. In general, the internal jugular vein is typically anterolateral to the carotid artery, and the femoral vein is medial to the femoral artery. The vein can further be identified ultrasound by its compressibility. Veins should be completely compressible (the anterior and posterior walls of the vessel should approximate) with pressure applied with the ultrasound probe. If the vein is not compressible, there should be suspicion for a venous thrombosis. Veins can also be identified using spectral color or pulsed wave Doppler, as flow in arteries is typically pulsatile and flow in veins is not. However, this can be misleading in certain clinical conditions, such as in patients with severe tricuspid regurgitation.

Before performing central venous catheterization, obtain informed consent based on the policies of each institution. All present must agree on the patient identification, the procedure being performed, and the site of the procedure. Sterile precautions must be observed, including hand hygiene, full sterile drape, sterile gloves, sterile gown, mask with face shield, and hair covers. All present in the room should wear masks and hair covers. It is helpful to have a nonsterile assistant present during the procedure.

The following guidelines are for the placement of central venous catheters using commercially available kits via Seldinger's guidewire technique.

INTERNAL JUGULAR CENTRAL VENOUS CATHETER PLACEMENT

(Note: ultrasound guidance is preferred.)

1. Place the patient in Trendelenburg position, and have the patient turn his or her head 45 degrees to the direction opposite the site of catheter placement.
2. If ultrasound is available, use ultrasound to identify the vascular structures prior to sterilizing the procedure site. Evaluate the vein for patency and compressibility as described above to ensure that there are no contraindications to catheterization (e.g., venous thrombosis or stenosis).
3. Prepare the ultrasound for sterile use by applying nonsterile gel to the ultrasound transducer. (Alternatively, this may be performed by a nonsterile assistant.)
4. Don sterile gown, sterile gloves, mask with face shield, and hair cover.
5. Prepare the skin with antiseptic solution (e.g., chlorhexidine or Betadine).
6. Use a sterile full-body drape with a site hole or surgical towels to cover the body, head, and face, exposing only the necessary skin.
7. Flush all ports of the catheter to ensure appropriate functioning. (If ultrasound is not available, proceed step 14.)
8. With help from a nonsterile assistant, lower the ultrasound transducer into the sterile plastic sheath. Make sure to avoid contact between the transducer and the outer surface of the plastic sheath. The nonsterile assistant should then pull the plastic sheath to cover the length of the transducer probe that will come into contact with the sterile field.
9. Place sterile gel on the procedure site. Confirm location of the vessels using ultrasound again.
10. Once the site is confirmed, anesthetize the skin and subcutaneous tissue.
11. Use ultrasound to maintain a transverse view of the vein and artery. While holding the ultrasound probe over the vein with the nondominant hand, use the dominant hand to hold the introducer needle.
12. Enter the skin with the introducer needle, bevel up, just cephalad to the ultrasound transducer at a 45-degree angle.

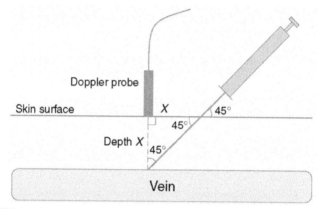

Figure 75.1. Needle insertion using ultrasound guidance. (From DeFer TM. *The Washington Manual Interns Survival Guide.* 4th ed. Philadelphia, PA: Wolter Kluwer Health/Lippincott Williams & Wilkins; 2013.)

13. With the ultrasound transducer, locate the tip of the introducer needle. Move ultrasound transducer and introducer needle together in order to visualize the of the introducer needle throughout its approach to the target vein, aspirati while advancing. Once the vein is cannulated, dark blood will enter the syrin (Skip to step 18 if using direct ultrasound guidance.) (Fig. 75.1)

14. Identify the triangle formed by the two heads of the sternocleidomastoid mus and the sternum, and palpate the carotid pulse (Fig. 75.2).

15. Anesthetize the skin and subcutaneous tissue.

16. Palpate the carotid pulse. Lateral to the carotid pulse, advance the 22-gau needle (finder needle), bevel up, at a 30- to 45-degree angle to the patie directed at the ipsilateral nipple while aspirating. If no venous blood retur noted, withdraw the needle and change the angle to a more lateral and then m medial position. Maintain palpation of the carotid pulse. When venous bloo aspirated, make note of the angle and depth of the finder needle, and rem the finder needle. *If the carotid artery is entered (bright red and/or pulsatile blo remove the needle and hold pressure.*

17. At the same site and angle as the internal jugular vein was entered with the fin needle, insert the introducer needle until free flow of dark venous blood is no (Fig. 75.3).

18. Securely hold the needle, remove the syringe (placing a finger over the ne hub to reduce the risk of air embolism), and insert the guidewire. The guidev should advance with little resistance. Always maintain control of the guidew

19. While holding the guidewire, remove the introducer needle. Once the introd needle is outside the patient's skin, hold the guidewire at the entry site and s the needle off the guidewire.

20. Use ultrasound to confirm correct placement of the guidewire within the lu of the target vein. Obtain a transverse view of the internal jugular vein, identify the wire within the lumen of the vein. Trace the tract of the guide from the skin insertion site into the insertion into the vein. Move the u sound transducer in the caudal direction to follow the course of the guide

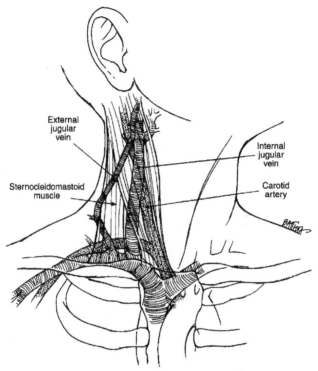

Figure 75.2. Internal jugular vein anatomy. (From Lin TL, Mohart JM, Sakurai KA. *The Washington Manual Internship Survival Guide.* 2nd ed. Philadelphia, PA: Lippincott Williams & Wilkins; 2001:191.)

toward the superior vena cava. Continue moving the transducer caudally confirming the guidewire remains within the lumen of the vein for its entire course through the neck. The ultrasound transducer probe can then be rotated 90 degrees to confirm the guidewire is within the lumen of the vein in the longitudinal axis (Fig. 75.4).

1. Using a scalpel, make a small incision in the skin at the entry site. Ensure that the cutting edge of the scalpel is facing away from the guidewire and perform a stabbing motion to make the incision.
2. Pass the dilator over the guidewire, dilate the tract to the depth of the target vein, and remove the dilator.
3. Ensure that the distal port of the catheter is open. Pass the catheter over the guidewire. When the catheter is near the entry site, feed the guidewire out until it emerges from the distal port on the catheter. Grasp the guidewire distally, and insert the catheter to the desired depth (15 to 16 cm for the right subclavian vein, 18 to 20 cm for the left subclavian vein, 16 to 17 cm for the right IJ vein, 17 to 18 cm for the left IJ vein).
4. Hold the catheter in place, and withdraw the guidewire. Ensure that the guidewire is intact once it is completely removed.

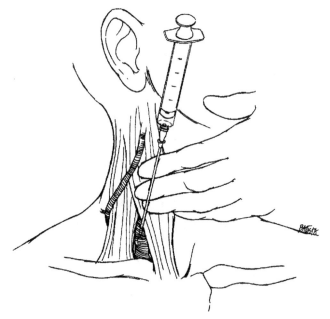

Figure 75.3. Cannulation of the internal jugular vein. (From Lin TL, Mohart JM, Sakurai KA. *The Washington Manual Internship Survival Guide*. 2nd ed. Philadelphia, PA: Lippincott Williams & Wilkins; 2001:192.)

25. Flush all ports to ensure that they are functioning properly, and place caps on all ports.
26. Secure the catheter with suture or a commercially available sutureless kit.
27. Cleanse the site with antiseptic solution and place a sterile dressing.
28. Obtain a chest radiograph for placement and to evaluate for pneumothorax. The tip of the catheter should reside in the superior vena cava.

FEMORAL CENTRAL VENOUS CATHETER PLACEMENT

(Note: ultrasound guidance if preferred.)

1. Place the patient in the supine position, with the ipsilateral thigh slightly abducted and externally rotated.
2. If using ultrasound, follow steps 2 to 13, followed by steps 18 to 27 from internal jugular venous catheter placement. Remember when locating the femoral vein with ultrasound that the femoral vein typical lies medial to femoral artery. If ultrasound is unavailable, follow steps 4 to 7 from internal jugular venous catheter placement above, followed by the steps below.
3. Palpate the femoral arterial pulse inferior to the inguinal ligament. The femoral vein is medial to the femoral artery (Fig. 75.5). With the introducer needle bevel up, enter the skin 1 cm medial to the pulse, inferior to the inguinal ligament, at a 30- to 45-degree angle (Fig. 75.6). Continue to aspirate as the needle is advanced

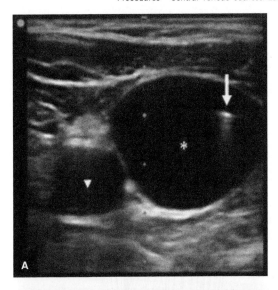

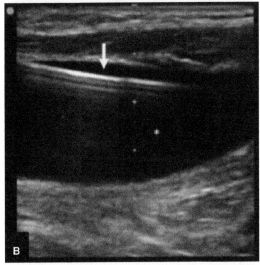

Figure 75.4. Internal jugular vein with verification of guidewire placement. **A:** Transverse view. **B:** Longitudinal view. Arrowhead: carotid artery, Asterisk: internal jugular vein, White arrow: guidewire within internal jugular vein.

until the return of venous blood. If the needle is advanced 5 cm with no return of venous blood, withdraw while continuing to aspirate, angle more medially, and try again. *If the femoral artery is entered (bright red and/or pulsatile blood), hold pressure.*

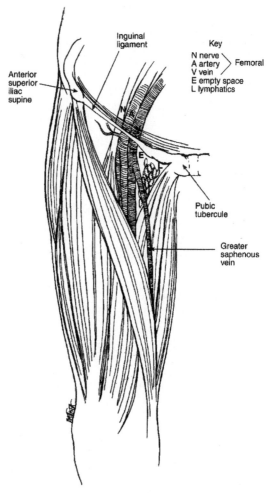

Figure 75.5. Femoral vein anatomy. (From Lin TL, Mohart JM, Sakurai KA. *The Washington Manual Intern Survival Guide.* 2nd ed. Philadelphia, PA: Lippincott Williams & Wilkins; 2001:183.)

4. Follow steps 18 through 27 for internal jugular central venous catheter placeme For the femoral site, the entire length of the catheter is inserted (20 cm) secured in place.

SUBCLAVIAN CENTRAL VENOUS CATHETER PLACEMEN

1. Place the patient in Trendelenburg position, and place a towel roll between scapulae. Keep the head in neutral position or toward the side of line placem to help direct the guidewire inferiorly.

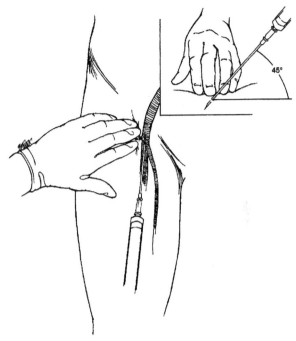

gure 75.6. Femoral vein cannulation. (From Lin TL, Mohart JM, Sakurai KA. *The Washington Manual ternship Survival Guide.* 2nd ed. Philadelphia, PA: Lippincott Williams & Wilkins; 2001:197.)

Don sterile gown, sterile gloves, mask with face shield, and hair cover.

Prepare the skin with antiseptic solution (e.g., chlorhexidine or Betadine).

Use a sterile full-body drape with a site hole or surgical towels to cover the body, head, and face, exposing only the necessary skin.

Flush all ports of the catheter to ensure appropriate functioning.

Place the index finger of the nondominant hand at the sternal notch and the thumb of the same hand on the clavicle where it bends over the first rib (approximately where the lateral third and medial two-thirds of the clavicle meet). The subclavian vein should traverse a line between the index finger and the thumb (Fig. 75.7).

Anesthetize the skin and subcutaneous tissue just inferior to the clavicle and lateral to the thumb.

With the introducer needle, bevel up, enter the skin lateral to the thumb and inferior to the clavicle (~2 cm inferior and 2 cm lateral to the bend in the clavicle). Aim at the index finger (sternal notch), aspirating while advancing. It is imperative to keep the needle parallel to the floor during advancement. If the clavicle is contacted, depress the entire needle with the thumb until it passes under the clavicle, rather than changing the angle of approach. Dark blood will enter the syringe when the vein is cannulated. If there is no blood return after advancing the needle 5 cm, withdraw the needle while continuing to aspirate (frequently the vein has been

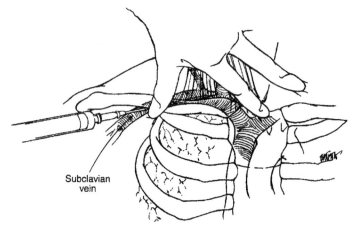

Figure 75.7. Subclavian vein anatomy and cannulation. (From Lin TL, Mohart JM, Sakurai KA. *The Washington Manual Internship Survival Guide.* 2nd ed. Philadelphia, PA: Lippincott Williams & Wilkins; 2001:195.)

pierced, and successful blood flow will be obtained during withdrawal). Redirect the needle more cephalad, and try again. Multiple repeated attempts are not recommended. Once appropriate venous return is noted, rotate the bevel of the needle 90 degrees inferior (bevel now pointing toward the patient's feet).

9. Follow steps 18 through 28 for internal jugular central venous catheter placement.

SUGGESTED READINGS

Hind D, Calvert N, McWilliams R, et al. Ultrasonic locating devices for central venous cannulation: meta-analysis. *BMJ.* 2003;327:361.

Marik PE, Flemmer M, Harrison W. The risk of catheter-related bloodstream infection with femoral venous catheters as compared to subclavian and internal jugular venous catheters: a systematic review of the literature and meta-analysis. *Crit Care Med.* 2012;40(8):2479–2485.

McGee DC, Gould MK. Preventing complications of central venous catheterization. *N Engl J Med.* 2003;348:1123–1133.

O'Grady N, Alexander M, Burns L, et al. Guidelines for the prevention of intravascular catheter-related infections. *Clin Infect Dis.* 2011;52(9):e162–e193. Centers for Disease Control and Prevention. https://www.cdc.gov/hicpac/pdf/guidelines/bsi-guidelines-2011.pdf

Parienti JJ, Mongardon N, Megarbane B, et al. Intravascular complications of central venous catheterization by insertion site. *N Engl J Med.* 2015;373(13):1220–1229.

76 Endotracheal Intubation

Adam Anderson

ndotracheal intubation maintains airway patency, assures delivery of mechanical
entilator defined breaths, facilitates pulmonary toilet, and helps prevent aspiration.
sual indications for endotracheal intubation include airway obstruction, encepha-
pathy, respiratory failure, and cardiopulmonary arrest.

Risks include trauma to the oropharynx, hypoxemia from prolonged attempts,
mesis with aspiration of gastric contents, unrecognized misplacement of the endo-
acheal tube, and death. The incidence of complications increases when an inad-
quately trained or inexperienced provider attempts intubation. These providers
ould attempt to achieve adequate ventilation and oxygenation using bag-valve-
ask devices or other airway devices that do not require visualization of the vocal
rds.

EQUIRED PREPARATIONS

sessment of the airway anatomy facilitates recognition of potentially difficult intu-
tions. An abbreviated assessment should be performed even in emergent cases. A
mmonly utilized assessment tool follows the "LEMON" mnemonic (Table 76.1).
nicians should pay particular attention to dentition and dental appliances, the
bility of the tongue and its size relative to the oropharynx or Mallampati score
g. 76.1), range of extension and flexion of the cervical spine, mobility of the jaw,
d presence of stridor. A difficult intubation may be anticipated in patients with
ck necks, narrow mouth openings, facial hair, large tongues, and limited motion
he cervical spine.

Successful intubation requires overcoming the normal barriers to objects entering
trachea, including reflexes arising from laryngeal stimulation, the mal-alignment
he major axes of the upper airway, and the anatomic barriers of the tongue and
glottis. Endotracheal intubation is an inherently uncomfortable procedure, and
n patients with decreased mental status may cough and resist attempts at intuba-
n. In addition, laryngeal stimulation increases sympathetic tone with consequent
reases in blood pressure, heart rate, and intracranial pressure.

Judicious use of appropriate medications can blunt the potential adverse phys-
gic effects while providing analgesia, sedation, and amnesia. Decisions regarding
of specific agents are based on knowledge of their advantages and disadvan-
s relative to the patient's clinical status and comorbidities (Table 76.2). Only
titioners skilled in endotracheal intubation should administer paralytic agents.
id-sequence intubation (RSI) is employed when airway control is emergent, the

TABLE 76.1 | **LEMON Airway Assessment**

- **L**ook externally
  - General impression of difficulty airway (anatomy, habitus, dentition, tongue, trauma, facial hair)
- **E**valuate (3-3-2 rule) Patient should have at least:
  - 3 finger breadths between incisors with mouth opening
  - 3 finger breadths within the thyromental distance
  - 2 finger breadths between hyoid and thyroid cartilage
- **M**allampati Score (Fig. 76.1)
  - Mallampati I and II predict easy laryngoscopy
  - Mallampati III predicts a difficult laryngoscopy
  - Mallampati IV predicts a very difficult laryngoscopy
- **O**bstruction/**O**besity
  - Supraglottic mass, secretions, blood or redundant tissue
- **N**eck Mobility
  - Spinal disease or C-collar immobilization

airway is predicted to not be difficult, and gastric insufflation is contraindicated. R includes simultaneous administration of a paralytic and a laryngoscopy attempt pr to bag-valve mask ventilation. Vasopressors should be readily available in the event hemodynamic decompensation.

All necessary equipment should be immediately available prior to intubati attempts (Table 76.3).

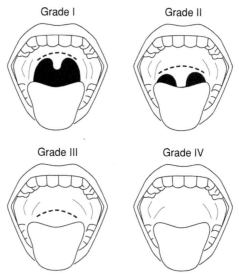

Figure 76.1. Mallampati classification. (From WK Health.)

TABLE 76.2	Agents Used for Intubation				
Agent	Action	IV Dose	Onset	Duration	Comments
Etomidate	Sedation	Stable: 0.3 mg/kg Unstable: 0.15 mg/kg	15–45 s	3–12 min	• Inhibits cortisol synthesis • Decreases focal seizure threshold • Hemodynamically neutral
Fentanyl	Analgesia	2 mcg/kg slow IV over 2 min	15 s	0.5–1 hr	• Hypotension, bradycardia with large doses • Used mostly at lower doses as an adjunctive agent
Ketamine	Sedation Amnesia Analgesia	1–3 mg/kg	30 s	5–10 min	• Bronchodilator • Increases HR, BP • Use adjuvant benzodiazepine **Caution:** elevated BP or ICP
Midazolam	Sedation Amnesia	0.02–0.08 mg/kg (~1–5 mg in 70 kg adult)	30–60 s	15–30 min	• Hypotension • Beneficial in seizure
Propofol	Sedation Amnesia	Stable: 1–1.5 mg/kg Unstable: 0.5 mg/kg	30–60 s	5–10 min	• Beneficial in seizure **Contraindication:** Egg allergy **Caution:** Hypotension, bradycardia
Succinyl-choline	Paralytic	1–1.5 mg/kg	30–60 s	5–15 min	**Contraindication:** Hyperkalemia, history of malignant hyperthermia, myopathy, neuropathy
Rocuro-nium	Paralytic	1 mg/kg	45–60 s	30–45 min	**Caution:** Concern for difficult intubation or bag-valve-mask ventilation

g: microgram; HR: heart rate; BP: blood pressure; ICP: intracranial pressure.

TABLE 76.3	Necessary Equipment Prior to Laryngoscopy Attempt

- Suction equipment
- Endotracheal tube
  - Usually 7.0–8.5 for adult patients
  - Test balloon prior to attempt
  - Stylet
  - Lubricant
- Syringe for balloon inflation
- Supraglottic device
- Bag-valve-mask connected to 15 L/min oxygen
- PEEP valve for bag-valve-mask
- Laryngoscope with blade loaded and alternate sizes available
- Oropharyngeal or nasopharyngeal airway
- End-tidal carbon dioxide detector (favor continuous over colorimetric)
- Tracheal tube introducer (e.g., Bougie)
- Monitor with pulse oximetry, blood pressure, heart rate, cardiac rhythm
- Medications (analgesia, sedative, paralytic, vasopressor)
- Tape or endotracheal tube holder

HOW TO INTUBATE

The "sniffing" position, achieved by flexing the neck approximately 30 degrees an extending the head at the atlanto-occipital joint to 20 degrees, helps align the ora laryngeal, and pharyngeal axes (Fig. 76.2). Placement of towels under the occipu supports maintenance of this position. Pre-oxygenation is achieved using a high flow oxygen system for at least 3 minutes prior to induction. An oropharygne airway, nasopharyngeal airway, or jaw thrust is frequently required after induction t maintain upper airway patency. Apneic oxygenation via a nasal cannula is typical continued during laryngoscopy to decrease the risk of desaturation.

The laryngoscope is used to displace the tongue and lift the epiglottis awa from the glottic opening. Laryngoscope blades vary in size and shape. Blade siz range from 0 to 4 with higher the number corresponding to larger blades. The curve (MacIntosh) blade has a broad, flat surface, and tall flange. Straight blades inclu Miller, Wisconsin, and Phillips. The straight blades vary with regard to their widt presence and size of flange, and shape of distal end. Curved blades apply upwa traction to the base of the tongue at the vallecula, indirectly lifting the epiglottis wh straight blades lift the epiglottis directly (Figs. 76.3 and 76.4). Choice of speci equipment should be left to the individual practitioner. In general, straight blad allow visualization of a larger portion of the vocal cords as the epiglottis is remov from the field of view. It may be difficult to control a large tongue with a Mil blade, which is relatively narrow. Video laryngoscopy should be utilized for nov users. Similar to direct laryngoscopy, several shapes and sizes of video laryngosco blades are available.

As with any procedure, a verbal time-out to identify medication strategy, hea care team roles, and airway algorithm is recommended. With the patient in the "sniffir

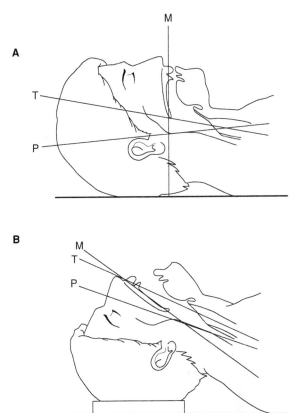

Figure 76.2. Anatomic axes for endotracheal intubation. **A:** With the head in the neutral position, the axis of the mouth (M), the axis of the trachea (T), and the axis of the pharynx (P) are not aligned with one another. If the head is extended at the atlanto-occipital joints, the axis of the mouth is correctly placed. If the back of the head is raised off the table with a pillow, thus flexing the cervical vertebral column, the axes of the trachea and pharynx are brought in line with the axis of the mouth. (From Snell R. *Clinical Anatomy*. 7th ed. Philadelphia, PA: Lippincott, Williams & Wilkins; 2003.)

position, the laryngoscope is held in the left hand and the blade is inserted into the right side of the mouth to the base of the tongue. The blade is then moved to the midline sweeping the tongue to the left. The laryngoscope handle and blade should align with the nasal septum. The tip of straight blades is advanced to the epiglottis, while the tip of curved blades is placed in the vallecula.

The vocal cords are exposed by elevating the epiglottis through a lifting motion using the arm and shoulder in a plane 45 degrees from the horizontal. The wrist must be kept stiff to avoid a prying motion that uses the teeth as a fulcrum. Once the vocal cords are visualized, the endotracheal tube is advanced from the right side of the mouth with the tip directed so that it intersects the tip of the laryngoscope blade at the level of the glottis allowing the operator to view the entry of the tube

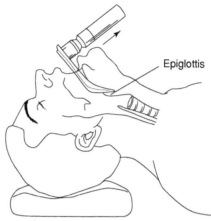

Figure 76.3. Intubation with a Macintosh blade. Blade is used anterior to the epiglottis. (From Blackbourne LH. *Advanced Surgical Recall.* 2nd ed. Baltimore, MD: Lippincott Williams & Wilkins; 2004.)

into the trachea (Fig. 76.5). The tube is advanced through the vocal cords until the cuff disappears. The stylet is removed and cuff inflated with sufficient air to prevent leakage during ventilation with a bag valve. The endotracheal tube must be held firmly in place at all times to prevent displacement. Attempts at intubation should take no longer than 1 minute. In patients where there is difficulty intubating the trachea, repeated attempts increase the risk of trauma and hypoxemia. A supraglottic airway device offers a temporary airway while a more skilled provider is contacted for assistance.

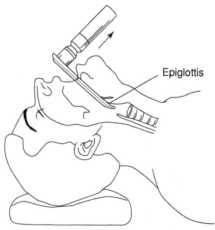

Figure 76.4. Intubation with a Miller blade. Blade is used to hold the epiglottis (posterior to the epiglottis). (From Blackbourne LH. *Advanced Surgical Recall.* 2nd ed. Baltimore, MD: Lippincott Williams & Wilkins; 2004.)

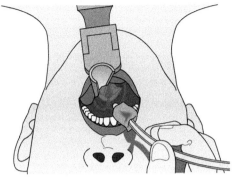

Figure 76.5. Endotracheal intubation-intubating. Illustration showing correct method for intubating victim during endotracheal intubation. (From *LifeART Image* copyright (c) 2007 Lippincott Williams & Wilkins. All rights reserved.)

ADDITIONAL TECHNIQUES

Cricoid pressure (Sellick maneuver) may decrease the risk of aspiration by compressing the esophagus between the cricoid cartilage and the vertebral column. Pressure should be applied prior to intubation attempts and maintained until confirmation of correct endotracheal tube placement. Bimanual laryngoscopy using the right hand to manipulate the thyroid cartilage or hyoid bone may improve visualization of the vocal cords. An assistant must apply identical pressure to facilitate optimal visualization. Alternatively, the "BURP" maneuver (backward, upward, rightward pressure) can be employed, though typically with less success than bimanual laryngoscopy.

Alternate approaches to endotracheal intubation via direct laryngoscopy include video laryngoscopy, optical stylets, supraglottic airways, laryngeal tube airways, fiberoptic intubation, and percutaneous tracheostomy. Supraglottic and laryngeal tube airways are placed blindly into the upper airway and form a seal over the laryngeal inlet to ventilate and oxygenate patients while partially occluding the esophagus allowing for directed ventilation into the trachea.

CONFIRMATION

Correct tube placement is established via visualization of endotracheal tube through the vocal cords, condensation within the endotracheal tube, visualization of chest expansion, and auscultation over the epigastrium and lung fields during ventilation. Continuous end-tidal carbon dioxide (CO_2) confirmation is preferred, although colorimetric end-tidal CO_2 detection devices may be used. A chest radiograph should be reviewed to document appropriate endotracheal tube placement.

Upon confirmation of placement, the endotracheal tube is secured firmly in place with either tape or a commercial device. Initial ventilator management is an integral component to any airway and should not be overlooked, especially if paralytics were administered. Regardless of outcome, a debriefing session for feedback of team members is recommended to improve future attempts.

SUGGESTED READINGS

Butler KH, Clyne B. Management of the difficult airway: alternative techniques and adjuncts. *Emerg Med Clin N Am.* 2003;21:259–289.

How to recognize patients at high risk for difficult tracheal intubation and alternative techniques available to the practitioner.

Mechlin MW, Hurford WE. Emergency tracheal intubation: techniques and outcomes. *Respir Care.* 2014;59(6):881–892.

Overview of techniques and medication selection for endotracheal intubation.

Reynolds SF, Heffner J. Airway management of the critically ill patient: rapid-sequence intubation. *Chest.* 2005;127(4):1397–1412.

Overview of airway management with algorithmic approaches.

77 Percutaneous Tracheostomy

Alexander C. Chen and Kevin Haas

Tracheostomy is a technique for creating an artificial airway between the neck surface and cervical trachea. There are two main tracheostomy techniques. The surgical approach uses surgical dissection to form the tract between the neck surface and the trachea. More recently, a percutaneous approach has been developed. Variations on this approach use the Seldinger technique to form the tract between the neck surface and the trachea. Although not suitable for all patients, the percutaneous approach has potential advantages over the surgical approach in appropriately selected intensive care unit (ICU) patients. A meta-analysis showed a lower rate of peristomal bleeding and postoperative infection with percutaneous tracheostomy. In addition, because percutaneous tracheostomies are commonly performed in the patient's ICU room, the risk of adverse events associated with transporting critically ill patients is reduced, and scheduling flexibility is increased. Lastly, some research supports percutaneous tracheostomies as the more cost-effective tracheostomy approach for ICU patients.

The remainder of this chapter will focus on percutaneous tracheostomies.

INDICATIONS

Upper airway obstruction. A surgical approach is often more appropriate for upper airway obstruction due to tumor.
Need for long-term mechanical ventilation.
Access for frequent suctioning and other airway care.
Treatment of severe obstructive sleep apnea when continuous positive airway pressure is ineffective or not tolerated.

CONTRAINDICATIONS

Contraindications unique to the percutaneous approach include difficult-to-palpate neck anatomy or history of prior neck surgery or radiation. Patients with high ventilatory and oxygenation requirements may be better served by a surgical approach because of the reduced ability to ventilate around the bronchoscope and likelihood of greater positive end-expiratory pressure loss during the procedure. Coagulopathies should be corrected prior to proceeding, although there are no well-validated thresholds. One center described a low rate of complications for percutaneous tracheostomy in the setting of significant thrombocytopenia as long as platelets were administered before the procedure. Hypotension can be worsened because of the significant amount of sedatives commonly needed to perform the procedure, making hypovolemia and hypotension relative contraindications.

TIMING OF TRACHEOSTOMY PROCEDURE IN CRITICALLY ILL PATIENTS

Most patients receive tracheostomies in the ICU because of difficulty weaning from the ventilator or because they cannot protect and clear their own airways. Potential advantages of tracheostomy over prolonged endotracheal intubation include greater comfort, decreased sedation requirements, enhanced ability to participate in rehabilitation, and facilitated weaning. Optimal timing for tracheostomy in ICU patients is controversial. If prolonged intubation is predicted at admission, a tracheostomy on day 1 or 2 may be appropriate. In most patients, a tracheostomy is considered after 1 to 2 weeks of endotracheal intubation. The preponderance of evidence supports earlier tracheostomy over prolonged endotracheal intubation, and a recent meta-analysis including 12 studies suggested that early tracheostomy is associated with more ventilator-free days, shorter ICU stays, decreased sedation requirements, and improved long-term mortality when compared to late tracheostomy.

PROCEDURE FOR PERCUTANEOUS TRACHEOSTOMY

Approaches differ slightly on the basis of operator preferences and the particular brand of percutaneous tracheostomy kit used. The following description describes the Ciaglia technique modified by the use of a single dilator with a hydrophilic coating.

1. Explain procedure including risks and benefits. Obtain consent.
2. A team approach makes the procedure more efficient and optimizes patient safety. The bronchoscopist is responsible for bronchoscopic guidance and maintenance of the airway. The bronchoscopist should be skilled in airway management in case of accidental extubation during the procedure. Video bronchoscopy is advantageous because it allows the operator to see the interior of the trachea continuously during the procedure. The nurse assists with intravenous anesthesia during the procedure. A respiratory therapist makes appropriate changes to the ventilator throughout the procedure. The operator performs the procedure and communicates to other members of the team to ensure coordination.
3. Increase FiO_2 to 100%.
4. Monitor blood pressure every 3 to 5 minutes; monitor other variables, including heart rate, pulse oximetry, and airway pressure, continuously.
5. A variety of anesthetic regimens can be used, although combinations of a benzodiazepine and short-acting narcotic or propofol work well. Traditionally, after deep sedation is achieved, a paralytic is administered to prevent coughing. Currently, we perform most of our procedures without a paralytic and have not had significant problems with this approach.
6. A small pad is placed under the shoulders to slightly extend the neck. The skin is prepared with chlorhexidine and a large surgical drape is used to completely cover the patient, with a small opening at the neck. The operator scrubs and dons a hat, protective eyewear, a mask, and sterile gloves and gown.
7. The operator selects the appropriate incision site by palpating the thyroid and cricoid cartilages and the sternal notch. Typically, the space between the

and second, or second and third cartilaginous rings can be approached with an incision halfway between the cricoid cartilage and the sternal notch.

8. After creating a skin wheal with lidocaine, the needle is raised to form a 90-degree angle with the trachea. The tract is anesthetized and the needle is advanced slowly while continuously aspirating. Air bubbles will appear when the needle penetrates the trachea.

9. A 1.5- to 2-cm incision through the skin and superficial subcutaneous tissue is made either horizontally or vertically.

10. A small, curved Kelley clamp is used to dissect a tract down to the trachea.

11. The bronchoscopist carefully withdraws the endotracheal tube over the bronchoscope until the tip lies just below the vocal cords and the tracheal lumen is visible. Firm pressure is applied to the trachea with the Kelly clamp to confirm placement between the appropriate cartilaginous rings.

12. Under continuous bronchoscopic visualization, the catheter-over-needle apparatus is advanced through the skin incision, between the selected tracheal rings, and into the trachea under continuous bronchoscopic surveillance. The catheter is advanced off the needle into the trachea while the needle is withdrawn.

13. The guidewire is threaded through the catheter toward the carina.

14. The catheter is removed, leaving the guidewire in place.

15. A punch dilator is advanced through the trachea and then removed.

16. Next, the curved dilator is inserted over the wire into the trachea. Remove dilator.

17. Load tracheostomy tube onto dilator and advance over guidewire. Percutaneous tracheostomy tubes have tapered ends that allow for easier tracheal insertion.

18. Next, the bronchoscopist removes the bronchoscope from the endotracheal tube and quickly inspects through the tracheostomy tube to ensure proper placement. The patient is reconnected to mechanical ventilation through the tracheostomy tube.

19. The bronchoscopist can inspect the trachea above the tracheostomy tube to rule out active bleeding, suction blood and secretions, confirm the tracheostomy ballon is completely in the airway, and then remove the endotracheal tube.

20. The tracheostomy tube is sewed into place, secured with tracheostomy ties, and dressed appropriately.

21. The tracheostomy tube is changed on day 10 to 14.

COMPLICATIONS

Percutaneous tracheostomy complications are typically divided into early and late categories. More common early complications include transient hypotension and minor bleeding during the procedure. Massive hemorrhage from damage to the innominate vessels has been described but is exceedingly rare. Pneumothoraces and cardiac arrests are uncommon early complications. Fractured tracheal rings occur frequently, although the clinical significance of this complication is unknown. Late complications include stomal infections, bleeding, accidental decannulation, and tracheal stenosis. Bronchoscopic visualization reduces, although does not eliminate, other described complications such as posterior tracheal perforation. Although still under investigation, there is growing evidence that ultrasound-guided percutenous tracheosomy may improve the safety of the procedure.

Tracheal stenosis rates vary widely in the literature, with some reports finding them to be rare and others finding them to be more common in patients undergoing percutaneous tracheostomies compared with those who undergo surgical tracheostomies.

The use of different techniques and study population selection may explain some of the discrepancies in the literature. When stenosis develops in patients who have undergone percutaneous tracheostomy, they tend to be subglottic in location and may be more challenging to correct surgically.

SUGGESTED READINGS

Ahrens T, Kollef MH. Early tracheostomy. Has its time arrived? *Crit Care Med*. 2004;32:1796–1797.
Discusses controversies surrounding timing of tracheostomies.

Alansari M, Alotair H, Al Aseri Z, et al. Use of ultrasound guidance to improve the safety of percutaneous dilational tracheostomy: a literature review. *Crit Care*. 2015;19:229.

Barba CA, Angood PB, Kauder DR, et al. Bronchoscopic guidance makes percutaneous tracheostomy a safe, cost-effective, and easy-to-tech procedure. *Surgery*. 1995;118:879–883.
Experience comparing percutaneous and surgical tracheostomies in 48 trauma patients. Percutaneous approach found to be easy to learn and perform and to be cost-effective.

Beiderlinden M, Walz MK, Sander A, et al. Complications of bronchoscopically guided percutaneous dilational tracheostomy: beyond the learning curve. *Intensive Care Med*. 2002;28:59–62.
Reviews complications in 136 percutaneous tracheostomies in a mixed surgical and medical ICU setting. Other than clinically relevant bleeding episodes in 2.9% of patients complications were rare.

Ciaglia P, Firsching R, Syniec C. Elective percutaneous dilational tracheostomy. A new simple bedside procedure; preliminary report. *Chest*. 1985;87:715–719.
Description of percutaneous technique in 134 patients.

Freeman BD, Isabella K, Lin N, et al. A meta-analysis of prospective trials comparing percutaneous and surgical tracheostomy in critically ill patients. *Chest*. 2000;118:1412–1418.
Meta-analysis reviewing studies that compared surgical to percutaneous tracheostomies. It found a lower incidence of peristomal infection, postoperative bleeding, and overall postoperative complication rate with the percutaneous compared with the surgical approach.

Hosokawa K, Nishimura M, Egi M, et al. Timing of tracheotomy in ICU patients: a systematic review of randomized controlled trials. *Crit Care*. 2015;19:424.

Putensen C, Theuerkauf N, Guenther U, et al. Percutaneous and surgical tracheostomy in critically ill adult patients: a meta-analysis. *Crit Care*. 2014;18:544.

Raghuraman G, Rajan S, Marzouk JK, et al. Is tracheal stenosis caused by percutaneous tracheostomy different from that by surgical tracheostomy? *Chest*. 2005;127:879–885.

Rajajee V, Williamson CA, West BT, et al. Impact of real-time ultrasound guidance on complications of percutaneous dilational tracheostomy: a propsensity score analysis. *Crit Care*. 2015;19:198.

78 Chest Tube Insertion

A. Cole Burks and Alexander C. Chen

DEFINITION

Thoracostomy refers to the insertion of a hollow, flexible tube into the pleural space.

INDICATIONS

Drainage of air or fluid from the pleural space.
Administration of therapeutic pleural agents such as sclerosants.

CONTRAINDICATIONS

Bleeding diatheses (prothrombin time or partial thromboplastin time greater than two times normal, platelets <50,000, or creatine level >6) should be corrected in nonemergent settings.
A history of thoracic surgery or pleurodesis on the side of proposed chest tube insertion requires additional caution, as lung tissue can become adherent to the chest wall after these procedures, resulting in lung injury or hemorrhage during insertion. Image guidance or operating room placement may be required.

IMAGING

Confirmation of the suspected pleural process prior to tube placement is imperative to avoid inadvertent damage to lung or other organs and the attendant morbidity and mortality. In patients with cystic or emphysematous lung disease, large bullae can mimic pneumothoraces on standard upright radiographs. Tumors with associated atelectasis can be mistaken for pleural effusions. In the postoperative setting, diaphragmatic paralysis or injury with resultant diaphragmatic elevation on routine chest radiograph may be confused with significant pleural effusion. Attempted chest tube placement can cause significant morbidity in these situations. Lateral decubitus films may help confirm the existence of free-flowing air or fluid. If any doubt exists, or in difficult cases, chest computed tomography or ultrasound imaging should be performed.

SITE SELECTION

Physical examination findings consistent with a pleural effusion include decreased breath sounds on auscultation, dullness to percussion, loss of tactile fremitus, and asymmetric chest wall expansion with inspiration. Physical examination findings consistent with pneumothoraces include hyperresonance and decreased breath sounds. In tension pneumothoraces, shift of mediastinal structures may be observed.

2. For free-flowing air or fluid, chest tubes are traditionally placed in the "Triangle of Safety," delineated by the lateral border of the pectoris major or anterior axillary line (anteriorly), the lateral border of the latissimus dorsi or middle axillary line (posteriorly), and the fifth intercostal space (inferiorly). Alternatively, the second interspace in the midclavicular line can be used for drainage of pneumothoraces with small, percutaneous catheters.

3. Loculated air or fluid collections often require image guidance by ultrasound or fluoroscopy for optimal tube placement. A good understanding of the overlying anatomy is required in this situation to prevent damage to anatomic structures during tube insertion.

4. Avoid any overlying cutaneous abnormalities such as cellulitis, candidiasis, burns, or other wounds.

CHOOSING THE OPTIMAL TUBE SIZE AND APPROACH

The blunt dissection and guidewire (also known as Seldinger) methods are the two most commonly used techniques for tube thoracostomy (Table 78.1). Different indications dictate the appropriate tube size and approach (see Chapter 16 for more information).

TABLE 78.1	Chest Tube Size and Insertion Method by Indication	
Indications	Tube Size	Insertion Method
Simple pneumothorax—including primary, secondary, traumatic, and iatrogenic	8–14 French	Image-guided guidewire
Loculated pneumothorax	8–14 French	Real-time image-guided guidewire
Pneumothorax—positive pressure ventilation	20–28 French	Either image-guided guidewire OR blunt dissection
Bronchopleural fistula	28 French or greater	Blunt dissection
Malignant effusion	8–14 French	Image-guided guidewire
Complicated parapneumonic Effusion—pH <7.2[a]	8–14 French 20 French or greater	Image-guided guidewire Either image-guided guidewire OR blunt dissection
Empyema[a]	8–14 French 20 French or greater	Image-guided guidewire Either image-guided guidewire OR blunt dissection
Hemothorax	Greater than 32 French	Blunt dissection

[a]Based on clinical situation and expertise with available procedures.

on pleural disease and indications for chest tube insertion). Chest tube sizes are reported in French (F), where 3 F equals one millimeter (mm) of outer diameter, so that 24 F tube equals 8 mm.

Traditionally, large bore chest tubes (LBCT)—greater than 20 F—were used for most pleural diseases requiring drainage. Increasing data suggest that small bore chest tubes (SBCT)—8 to 14 F—are less painful and easier to place with few complications. SBCT are equally as efficacious in pneumothoraces (primary, secondary, traumatic, and iatrogenic) and malignant pleural effusions. Recent data suggests that these smaller caliber chest tubes may be as effective as larger chest tubes for managing infected pleural spaces.

Indications for LBCT include bronchopleural fistulae, pneumothorax in mechanically ventilated patients, and hemothorax. An SBCT often are not sufficient to adequately drain the air from the space in bronchopleural fistulae because the amount of air leak is too large. The same is often true in patients on positive pressure ventilation. A 20 to 28 F tube is preferred in these instances and can be placed either by the guidewire technique or by blunt dissection depending on the degree of air leak and the clinical situation. Hemothoraces (pleural fluid hematocrit at least 50% of peripheral blood hematocrit) require at least a 32 F tube to prevent tube blockage and allow adequate drainage.

Loculated air or fluid collections are often more readily approached by a real-time, image-guided, guidewire approach. Anatomically, free flowing air will accumulate anteriorly and apically in the supine position, therefore, chest tubes placed for simple pneumothoraces are typically placed in an anteroapical direction. In contrast, fluid accumulates in the posterior and basal diaphragmatic gutters, and as such, chest tubes placed for effusions are placed in a inferoposterior direction.

Procedure Steps

Blunt Dissection Approach

1. Explain benefits, risks, alternatives, and obtain consent.
2. Gather necessary equipment (Table 78.2). Kits prepared ahead of time can simplify this process.
3. Typically, the patient is placed in a semirecumbent position with the head and shoulders about 30 degrees off the bed. The ipsilateral arm is placed above the head for exposure of the axilla and to increase the distance between ribs.

TABLE 78.2	Materials Necessary for Blunt Dissection Thoracostomy	
Sterile gloves	60-mL syringe	Kelly clamps × 2
Mask	25-Ga needle[b]	Sterile dressing
Antiseptic solution[a]	22-Ga × 1.5-in needle[c]	Silk sutures
Sterile drape or towels	Scalpel with no. 11 blade	Sterile specimen cups
1% Lidocaine w/o epinephrine (50-mL bottle)	Chest tube	Pleural drainage system
50-mL syringe	Sterile gauze	

[a] Chlorhexidine or Betadine.
[b] anesthetize skin.
[c] anesthetize tract and pleura.

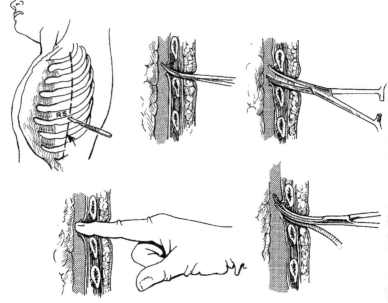

Figure 78.1. Chest tube insertion procedure (see text for details).

4. Clean the area with antiseptic and sterilely drape.
5. After appropriate site and corresponding inferior rib identification, infiltrat subcutaneous tissue with 1% lidocaine without epinephrine (Fig. 78.1).
   a. Next, inject lidocaine down to the appropriate rib. Move needle superiorl over the rib in a stepwise fashion, aspirating as you advance, stopping to inje lidocaine every 1 to 2 mm.
   b. Confirm entry into the pleural space with aspiration of air for pneumothorac or fluid for effusions by aspirating the syringe as it is advanced.
   c. Next, withdraw the syringe while aspirating until no air or fluid return an inject lidocaine to generously anesthetize the parietal pleura. Typically, th equivalent of 25 to 40 mL of 1% lidocaine should achieve adequate loc anesthesia.
6. Make a skin incision through the subcutaneous tissue that is wide enough insert a finger (1 to 2 cm).
7. Using medium-sized Kelly clamps, bluntly dissect to the top of the selected r This is done by applying forward pressure with the clamps while opening, relaxi forward pressure while closing, and repeating as necessary. Once the rib reached, continue with blunt dissection over the top of the rib. A rush of air fluid signals entry into the pleural space. When entering the pleural space, use not push too far, so as to prevent lung injury.
8. Place finger through tract into the pleural space, sweep circumferentially arou the entry site to confirm the lack of adherent lung in the direction of chest tu placement.

9. Clamp the end of the chest tube with a Kelly clamp and guide into the pleural space. Direction is generally anteroapical for drainage of air and inferoposterior for drainage of fluid. Depending on body wall size, insert to 10 to 12 cm at the skin.

10. Attach external end of tube to the drainage system. Drainage of air or fluid as well as evidence of respiratory variation suggest proper placement into the pleural space.

11. Securely suture tube to prevent dislodgment. Some operators place a mattress suture at the time of the insertion, leaving the ends loose, which they use to close the incision at the time of tube removal.

12. Using occlusive gauze to seal the skin around the tube is controversial. Some authors argue that this leads to skin breakdown.

13. Dress area with a generous amount of gauze and tape.

14. Check chest x-ray for proper placement.

15. Check on chest tube output, signs of respiratory variation, and the presence of air leaks at least daily. Evaluate site for bleeding or signs of infection.

Guidewire Approach

Note: this approach may vary slightly, depending on kit used.

1. Obtain consent, position patient, obtain materials as per Table 78.2 and the guidewire insertion kit and prepare area as for blunt dissection approach. Multiple companies make preassembled kits containing most of the necessary materials; check kit labeling to ensure all materials are available.

2. Anesthetize rib and pleural space in the selected interspace using same technique described above.

3. Insert the introducer needle just superior to the appropriate rib. Stop just past the point where fluid or air is aspirated.

4. Remove syringe and cover needle opening with finger to prevent excessive air entry. Introduce wire into pleural space. Remove needle from patient, leaving guidewire in pleural space.

5. Make a small skin nick at the wire entry site to allow introduction of dilators and chest tube.

6. Using sequential dilators, dilate tract into pleural space. Generally, tactile feedback is present when the dilator has punctured through the parietal pleura (can be described as a giving way, or "pop.") Dilators should be advanced only a small amount (1 cm) beyond this point to ensure proper tract formation, while using caution to avoid further advancement potential harm to the lung.

7. Introduce chest tube over the wire into the pleural space. Confirm that all openings are in the pleural space (depending on body wall size, typically at 8 to 12 cm at the skin). Remove wire.

8. Connect chest tube to drainage system.

9. Suture tube in place and dress with gauze and tape.

10. Check chest x-ray for proper placement.

DRAINAGE SYSTEMS

The most common drainage system for hospitalized patient is the three-bottle drainage system. The functions of the three-bottle system are most commonly incorporated into one container today. The first column serves as a drainage repository, collecting fluid that drains from the pleural space. The second column serves as a water seal, which prevents retrograde air entry into the pleural space. The third column allows fo adjustment of the negative pressure applied to the pleural space.

GUIDELINES FOR CHEST TUBE REMOVAL

There is considerable practice variation involved in chest tube removal. The mos important requirement is for the resolution of the initial indication for placement. Fo pneumothoraces, this generally means a fully expanded lung with resolution of the a leak, and for pleural fluid, this implies a maximum drainage of 100 to 150 mL/da There is no consensus regarding timing of pulling during respiratory cycle, no regarding the practice of tube clamping, placing on water seal, or continuing suctio until removal.

Our approach is to remove from suction, that is, place on water seal once th indication for placement has resolved. We then perform a follow-up chest x-ray 1 to 24 hours later. If there is no significant air leak or reaccumulation of air or flui the tube is removed. In difficult cases, the tube can be clamped for 2 to 4 hours, wi careful monitoring and a repeat chest x-ray to confirm stability.

Removal Steps

1. Gather materials—suture removal kit, gauze, 1.0 silk suture, needle driver, sc sors, 10-mL 1% lidocaine without epi, 10-mL syringe with 25-g needle, tape.
2. Patients can be given a small amount of narcotic prior to removal where clinica indicated.
3. Remove sutures
4. Have patient make a full inspiration and pull tube out quickly while occluding track with gauze in your other hand.
5. Approximate the wound.
   a. For LBCT: Approximate the incision either by tying a previously placed m tress suture or by placing new suture.
   b. For SBCT: A simple occlusive dressing should suffice.
6. A follow-up chest x-ray should be taken 12 to 24 hours later (or sooner, if cli cally indicated) to rule out recurrence of pneumothorax or pleural fluid.

COMPLICATIONS

Complications from chest tube placement are less well studied than complicati associated with other common thoracic procedures. The site of placement (en gency department, intensive care unit, floor, or operating room) and circumsta of placement (emergent or elective) are undoubtedly important. One study looke complications from chest tubes inserted by pulmonary fellows with attending su vision. Many, although not all, of the patients were in the intensive care unit. largest number of chest tube placements in the study were for ventilator-associate iatrogenic pneumothoraces. Problems were stratified as early (first 24 hours) or and by size of the chest tube placed (less than or equal to 14 French or larger). E complications included the tube not being placed in the pleural space, nonfuncti tubes, and laceration of the lung. Late complications included nonfunctional t a site infection, and a leak around tube. All complications were more common small tubes (36%) versus larger tubes (9%).

Other possible complications include hemothoraces from intercostal vessel injury or intra-abdominal placement. Infections associated with tube placement are uncommon. Prophylactic antibiotic use is supported by one meta-analysis in trauma patients, but is probably not justified in other clinical situations.

SUGGESTED READINGS

Bell RL, Ovandia P, Abdullah F, et al. Chest tube removal: end-inspiration or end-expiration? *J Trauma.* 2001;50:674–677.
Patients randomized to end-inspiration or end-expiration removal of tube. No significant difference in outcomes found.

Collop NA, Kim S, Sahn SA. Analysis of tube thoracostomy performed by pulmonologists at a teaching hospital. *Chest.* 1997;112:709–713.
Study of 126 tube thoracostomies performed by a pulmonary division at an academic medical center. Reviews indications and complications.

Fallon WF, Wears RL. Prophylactic antibiotics for the prevention of infectious complications including empyema following tube thoracoscopy for trauma: results of a meta-analysis. *J Trauma.* 1992;33:110–117.
Showed a benefit for prophylactic antibiotics in trauma patients requiring chest tube placement.

Martino K, Merrit S, Boyakye K, et al. Prospective randomized trial of thoracostomy removal algorithms. *J Trauma.* 1999;46:369–371.
205 patients requiring chest tube insertion for blunt and penetrating trauma. When removal of the chest tube was indicated, patients were randomized to a water seal waiting period or to immediate removal of the chest tube. It appeared that a short period of time on water seal might allow for the detection of occult air leaks.

McVay PA, Toy PTCY. Lack of increased bleeding after paracentesis and thoracentesis in patients with mild coagulation abnormalities. *Transfusion.* 1991;31:164–171.
Retrospective study of 608 patients undergoing thoracentesis or paracentesis. Argues that prophylactic plasma and platelet transfusions are unnecessary for patients with mild to moderate coagulopathies.

Rahman NM, Maskell NA, Davies CW, et al. The relationship between chest tube size and clinical outcome in pleural infection. *Chest.* 2010;137:536–543.
405 patients with pleural infections treated with various sized chest tubes and either guide-wire or surgical technique. Showed no difference in clinical outcome between smaller caliber chest tubes and larger caliber chest tubes.

Silverman SG, Mueller PR, Saini S, et al. Thoracic empyema: management with image-guided catheter drainage. *Radiology.* 1988;169:5–9.
43 patients treated with imaged guided catheters for empyemas. Proved successful by pre-defined criteria in 72% of patients.

79 Paracentesis

Rachel McDonald and Adam Anderson

Paracentesis is a procedure frequently performed in the intensive care unit for diagnostic and therapeutic purposes. Diagnostic paracentesis should be performed in patients with suspected spontaneous bacterial peritonitis (SBP) or ascites of unknown cause. In patients with significant shortness of breath or abdominal discomfort, therapeutic paracentesis may alleviate symptoms. The complications of paracentesis are rare and usually without clinical consequence. Ascitic fluid leak can occur if a large bore needle has been used, a large skin incision is made, or if a Z-track technique has not been performed. A repeat paracentesis to relieve tension in the abdomen may be required to control ascitic fluid leak if the ascitic fluid cannot be decreased with diuretic treatment. Perforation can occur if the needle punctures the bowel wall. Even if perforation does occur, it rarely results in clinically significant secondary peritonitis. Bleeding due to inadvertent puncturing of an artery or vein is an uncommon complication, but can be potentially fatal. Selecting a paracentesis site that avoids the inferior epigastric vessels decreases the risk of bleeding. The risk of bleeding may also be increased in patients with renal disease. Treatment is usually supportive, and rarely requires further intervention.

Many patients undergoing paracentesis (especially those with underlying liver disease) are coagulopathic and thrombocytopenic at the time of the procedure. It has been shown in such patients that there is no need to correct the coagulopathy or transfuse platelets prior to the procedure. Paracentesis should not be performed in patients with disseminated intravascular coagulation. Additionally, in patients with small bowel obstruction, a nasogastric tube should be placed prior to the procedure. In patients who have undergone prior abdominal surgery, the area of the surgical scar should be avoided, as this may be associated with bowel tethering to the abdominal wall by adhesions. Patients with urinary retention should undergo bladder catheterization prior to paracentesis.

The most common sites of paracentesis are the abdominal left lower quadrant, suprapubic, or right lower quadrant regions. Physical examination, particularly percussion and examining for shifting dullness, can help determine the ideal site. When available, ultrasound should be used to aid in selecting the ideal procedure site. When performing a paracentesis, the catheter should not be inserted through infected skin.

Once the site of the procedure has been determined and all present agree on the identification of the patient, the site, and the procedure being performed, one can proceed with paracentesis.

PERFORMANCE OF PARACENTESIS

Note: Ultrasound guidance, if available, is the preferred method

1. Use ultrasound to identify a site where ascitic fluid is present and there is an absence of bowel or solid organs and mark the site.
2. At a minimum, sterile gloves and a mask with face shield are worn. Additional sterile equipment should be used according to hospital policy.
3. The patient should be placed supine with the head of the bed slightly elevated.
4. The site is prepared with antiseptic solution (e.g., chlorhexidine or Betadine), and a sterile drape is placed.
5. Using a 22- or 25-gauge needle, local anesthesia with 1% lidocaine is injected, starting with a subcutaneous wheel followed by deeper anesthesia. While injecting the deeper tissues, maintain continuous negative pressure on the syringe, and inject lidocaine periodically. Maintain an angle of entry perpendicular to the abdominal wall.
6. When ascitic fluid is obtained, inject lidocaine around the peritoneum.
7. Ideally, a catheter specifically designed for paracentesis (e.g., Caldwell needle) should be used, although a large-bore intravenous catheter may be used. Attach a 10-mL syringe to the catheter.
8. Using a scalpel, make a small incision in the skin at the insertion site to facilitate insertion of the paracentesis catheter.
9. Using the Z-tract technique, pull the skin 2 cm caudad prior to inserting the catheter. This theoretically causes the tract to close, and thus reduces the rate of leakage when the catheter is withdrawn.
10. Insert the catheter slowly, with continued negative pressure on the syringe. When ascitic fluid is obtained, stop advancing the needle/catheter system, advance the catheter over the needle, and remove the needle.
11. Obtain an adequate amount of ascitic fluid for diagnostic studies (typically at least 25 mL). Culture bottles should be inoculated at the bedside to increase yield.
12. If a therapeutic paracentesis is being performed, tubing should be connected from the catheter to the vacuum bottle.

DIAGNOSTIC CONSIDERATIONS

Diagnostic studies performed on ascitic fluid are determined by the clinical situation (Table 79.1). Other less common diagnostic studies include triglycerides (chylous ascites), amylase (pancreatic ascites), mycobacterial culture (tuberculous ascites) and bilirubin (bile leak). If there is concern for SBP, fluid should be sent for cell count and culture. Cell count demonstrating >250 polymorphonuclear cells/mm^3 without secondary source of infection (e.g., perforated viscous) or a grossly bloody tap suggests SBP. The definitive diagnosis is based on positive culture results. In patients with findings suggestive or diagnostic of SBP, empiric treatment should be initiated with third-generation cephalosporin (ceftriaxone or cefotaxime) or a fluoroquinolone (ciprofloxacin or levofloxacin) pending culture results and sensitivities.

The routine use of albumin infusion (6 to 8 g albumin/L fluid removed) for large-volume paracentesis (5 L or more) is controversial but has been shown

TABLE 79.1	Common Clinical Situations and Pertinent Studies for Ascitic Fluid	
Clinical Situation	Studies	Comments
Concern for SBP	• Cell count • Culture (blood culture bottles inoculated at bedside)	• >250 cells/mm^3 consistent with SBP • Culture definitive for diagnosis • Treat with third-generation cephalosporin or fluoroquinolone
Determining if ascites is secondary to portal hypertension	• Serum albumin • Ascites albumin • Total protein	• SAAG ≥1.1 g/dL (portal hypertension): cirrhosis, alcohol hepatitis, cardiac ascites, portal-vein thrombosis, Budd–Chiari syndrome, liver metastases. TP ≥2.5 g/dL: cardiac ascites. TP <2.5 g/dL: cirrhotic ascites • SAAG <1.1 g/dL: peritoneal carcinomatosis, tuberculous peritonitis, pancreatic ascites, nephrotic syndrome, serositis
Concern for malignant ascites	• Cytology	• Sensitivity can be increased by sending three samples, and examining samples promptly

SBP, spontaneous bacterial peritonitis; SAAG, serum ascites albumin gradient = (serum albumin) (ascites albumin); TP, total protein.

to decrease circulatory dysfunction and the potential precipitation of hepatorenal syndrome.

SUGGESTED READINGS

Bernardi M, Caraceni P, Navickis RJ, et al. Albumin infusion in patients undergoing large volume paracentesis: a meta-analysis of randomized trials. *Hepatology.* 2012;55(: 1172–1181.

DeFer TM, Knoche EM, LaRossa GN, et al. *Guide to procedures.* The Washington Manual Internship Survival Guide. 4th ed. Philadelphia, PA: Lippincott Williams & Wilki: 2013:215–221.

Runyon BA. Management of adult patients with ascites. *Hepatology.* 2004;39:841–856.

Thomsen TW, Shaffer RW, White B, et al. Paracentesis. *N Engl J Med.* 2006;355:e21.

Lumbar Puncture

Jennifer Alexander-Brett

The lumbar puncture (LP) is commonly performed in the intensive care unit to obtain cerebrospinal fluid (CSF) for diagnostic purposes. This chapter will discuss the indications, technique, complications, and common pitfalls of performing an LP in adults.

INDICATIONS AND CONTRAINDICATIONS

It is useful to remember the old adage, "If you consider an LP, you should do it." Delay in the diagnosis of meningitis leads to inappropriate treatment and difficulty in later establishing the diagnosis when the patient fails to improve. Likewise, prompt diagnosis of subarachnoid hemorrhage results in early treatment of aneurysms and prevention of rebleeding. Table 80.1 lists common indications for LP.

There are fewer contraindications to LP. Coagulopathy is an important contraindication because an LP may cause an epidural hematoma leading to compression of the cauda equina. No studies have established useful cutoffs, but an international normalized ratio >1.4, partial thromboplastin time >50, and/or platelet count 100,000/mm^3 are commonly corrected with fresh-frozen plasma and/or platelet transfusions prior to an LP. Those targets can be lowered in the setting of hematologic disorders and thrombocytopenia resistant to correction, and the risk to benefit should be assessed individually. In the setting of altered mental status, papilledema, focal neurologic deficit, or if there is suspicion for subarachnoid hemorrhage, a head computed tomography scan should be obtained prior to LP. Signs of herniation and large posterior fossa masses preclude an LP because the pressure drop following CSF removal can precipitate tonsillar herniation.

Other contraindications to LP include local skin infections, known spinal cord tumors, and very recent surgical instrumentation. Prior to performing an LP, informed consent must be obtained according to the policy at each institution.

TECHNIQUE

Collect the Supplies

Gather the following: sterile 20-gauge or smaller spinal needle with a stylet, a sterile 25-gauge needle and syringe for local anesthesia, topical antiseptic, sterile drape and gauze, 1% to 2% lidocaine solution, a sterile manometer, sterile surgical gloves, and tubes for collection of the fluid. With more experience, a smaller gauge spinal needle,

TABLE 80.1	Common Indications for Lumbar Puncture

- Diagnosis of bacterial, viral, fungal, parasitic, or mycobacterial meningitis
- Diagnosis of carcinomatosis meningitis
- Diagnosis of subarachnoid hemorrhage
- Assessing central nervous system and meningeal inflammation for diagnosis of conditions, including multiple sclerosis, Devic disease, and neurosarcoidosis
- Measuring CSF protein levels for the diagnosis of Guillain–Barré syndrome
- Measuring intracranial pressure for diagnosis of pseudotumorcerebri
- Removing CSF for treatment of pseudotumorcerebri or normal-pressure hydrocephalus

CSF, cerebrospinal fluid.

preferably a Sprotte needle, helps reduce post-LP headaches. In morbidly obese patients, a needle longer than the standard 3.5 in may be necessary.

Position the Patient

Lateral decubitus positioning is required to accurately measure the intracranial CSF pressure. The patient is positioned such that the hips and shoulders are squarely above one another, the back is parallel to the wall, and the patient is curled up with the knees and chin tucked deeply into the torso (Fig. 80.1). In other cases, a sitting position aids in determining the midline of the spine, increases the space between spinous processes, and may increase filling of the lumbar cistern, thus improving the chance of successful LP. In this position, the patient is positioned such that the back is straight and arched outward, with the chin tucked deeply into the chest. Ultimately, the choice of positioning should be determined by the indications for the LP, patient comfort, and operator experience.

Find the L4–5 Space

In most adults, the spinal cord ends at L1, and in a few adults it ends at L2. Therefore, the L3–4, L4–5, and L5–S1 spaces represent safe and effective locations to insert a spinal needle. In most adults, a line (Tuffier line, Fig. 80.1) drawn across the top of both iliac crests crosses the L4 spinous process or the L4–5 space. Use the spinous

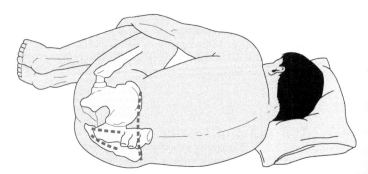

Figure 80.1. Positioning the patient. Tuffier line is indicated by the *dashed line*. (From Taylor C, Lillis C, LeMone P. *Fundamentals of Nursing.* 2nd ed. Philadelphia, PA: JB Lippincott; 1993:543, with permission.)

space on or immediately below the Tuffier line. Attention to superficial anatomy helps ensure appropriate placement of the spinal needle.

Scrub and Anesthetize the Space

Scrub the location with antiseptic solution (e.g., chlorhexidine or Betadine). There are now adequate data that chlorhexidine is a safe alternative to Betadine and it does not significantly increase the risk of neurologic complications. Using sterile gloves, place a sterile drape at the selected location with the lumbar space above it exposed. Lidocaine is injected subcutaneously and about 2 cm deep along the expected track of the spinal needle.

Insert the Spinal Needle

The spinal needle with its stylet in place should then be introduced through the skin in a tract that is angled toward the navel or about 15 degrees cephalad. The needle must be entered at midline and orthogonal to the plane of the back. The bevel should initially be perpendicular to the long axis of the body to minimize tearing of the dura and the subsequent post-LP headaches.

Advance the Spinal Needle

After penetrating the skin and subcutaneous fat, the needle should traverse the supraspinatus ligament, the interspinous ligaments, the ligamentum flavum, the epidural space, and finally the dura (Fig. 80.2). Severe pain may indicate being away from the

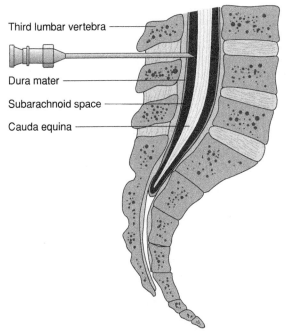

Third lumbar vertebra

Dura mater

Subarachnoid space

Cauda equina

Figure 80.2. The ideal tract of the spinal needle. (From Taylor C, Lillis CA, LeMone P. *Fundamentals of Nursing.* 2nd ed. Philadelphia, PA: JB Lippincott; 1993:543, with permission.)

midline. Once the needle has been inserted about 3 to 4 cm, or if a "pop" or sudden loss of resistance is experienced, remove the stylet to check for CSF. If no CSF is obtained, replace the stylet and advance the needle another 2 to 3 mm and remove the stylet again to check for CSF. Once the lumbar cistern has been entered, CSF should flow freely through the spinal needle, and the stylet can be replaced to limit CSF leakage until it can be collected or a manometer can be attached to measure CSF pressure. Hitting bone while inserting the needle indicates either incorrect angling of the needle or the skin has been entered away from the midline. When this occurs, retract the needle to the subcutaneous tissue, reposition its angle so that it is closer to being 15 degrees or less cephalad and more directed toward the midline, and then enter again. This procedure can be repeated a few times until a tract free of bone is achieved. After several attempts at the first lumbar space, using the L3–4 space (the space immediately above the Tuffier line) is permissible, but using any higher space risks inserting the needle into the tip of the spinal cord.

On occasion, the LP needle is inserted to the hub without obtaining CSF. This problem can be avoided by using a needle that is sufficiently long, ensuring a correct entry point and angle, and occasionally by sitting up the patient. Fluoroscopic or ultrasound guidance may be necessary in obese or uncooperative patients.

Measure CSF Pressure and Collect Fluid

Once the needle has entered the lumbar cistern, a manometer can be used to measure "opening" CSF pressure. This measurement is accurate only when the patient is in the lateral decubitus position and relaxed enough to allow visible respiratory excursion of the CSF in the manometer. Normal pressure is 8 to 22 cm H_2O, although it can be slightly higher in normal obese patients or in patients on positive pressure ventilation. The fluid in the manometer should be collected for CSF analysis. Sufficient CSF should be collected for all of the necessary tests, and additional fluid should be collected and saved in case further testing is desired. If the opening pressure is >50 cm H_2O, the minimum amount of fluid necessary should be collected. Fluid analyses are listed in Table 80.2. If the CSF appears bloody initially and later it clears, this suggests a "traumatic" tap, whereby the needle had punctured a vein en route to the lumbar cistern. Xanthochromia, or a yellowish tint to the fluid, indicates either blood products >12 to 24 hours old in the subarachnoid space or greatly elevated protein levels. Careful replacement of the stylet before and after collection helps avoid excessive CSF leak. After CSF collection, a closing pressure can be measured if necessary. Replace the stylet before removing the needle. Samples collected should be sent for cell count with differential, chemistry, and Gram stain/culture; additional studies may be included based on suspected underlying diagnosis (Table 80.2). Of note, samples should be analyzed as soon as possible after collection, as cell counts are prone to decline markedly over the course of hours.

COMPLICATIONS

Following the LP procedure, the patient should be placed in the supine position for 1 hour. This helps reduce post dural-puncture headaches immediately after and, though probably does not prevent post-LP headaches due to a dural tear and persistent CSF leakage. The latter can be reduced by appropriate spinal needle selection and proper technique. Fluids, caffeine, acetaminophen, and nonsteroidal anti-inflammatory drugs are effective in most cases of post-LP headaches. Characteristically, the head

TABLE 80.2	Common Tests for CSF Analysis (to Be Ordered Based on Clinical Concern)

- Complete cell count and differential
- CSF glucose and protein levels
- Gram stain and bacterial, fungal, and mycobacterial cultures
- Cytology and wet mount inspection
- Spectrophotometer analysis for xanthochromia
- IgG and albumin levels, serum IgG and albumin levels to determine the IgG index: (CSF–IgG/CSF–albumin)/(Serum–IgG/Serum–albumin)
- Oligoclonal bands
- PCR tests for a variety of pathogens, including HSV, VZV, EBV, CMV, enteroviruses, TB, arboviruses, and toxoplasmosis
- Other tests for pathogens, including cryptococcal antigen testing, syphilis (VDRL or FTA-ABS), cysticercosis, histoplasmosis, coccidioidomycosis, and malaria

IgG, immunoglobulin G; PCR, polymerase chain reaction; HSV, herpes simplex virus; VZV, varicella-zoster virus; EBV, Epstein–Barr virus; CMV, cytomegalovirus; TB, tuberculosis; VDRL, Venereal Disease Research Laboratory; FTA-ABS, fluorescent treponemal antibody-absorption.

worsens with sitting up or standing and resolves when lying down. If the headaches persist longer than 5 days, an epidural blood patch may be required.

Rarely, the patient may complain of paresthesias or pain referred to one leg. During the procedure, this indicates impingement of a nerve root, and the spinal needle should be retracted, repositioned further toward the midline, and then reinserted. Careful controlled insertion of the needle helps avoid such nerve damage. When symptoms of cord compression occur following the procedure, there is concern for an intraspinal epidermoid tumor or an epidural hematoma. In both cases, obtaining a magnetic resonance image or computed tomography is mandatory, and neurosurgical consultation is warranted if any such mass is discovered.

Other rare complications include cerebral herniation syndromes and spontaneous rupture of a subarachnoid arterial aneurysm. These can be avoided by careful physical examination and, when indicated, brain imaging prior to the LP.

SUGGESTED READINGS

Boon JM, Abrahams PH, Meiring JH, et al. Lumbar puncture: anatomical review of a clinical skill. *Clin Anat.* 2004;17:544–553.
   This comprehensive article reviews the relevant anatomy for performing a lumber puncture. It is well written and is advised particularly when one is having trouble successfully performing the procedure.
Ellenby MS, Tegtmeyer K, Lai S, et al. Videos in clinical medicine. Lumbar puncture. *N Engl J Med.* 2006;355:e12.
   A video and accompanying article that demonstrates the proper method of performing a lumber puncture. This is highly recommended to everyone who has never performed this procedure before.

81 Thoracentesis

A. Cole Burks and Alexander C. Chen

DEFINITION

Thoracentesis—inserting a needle and/or catheter into the pleural space for aspiration of air or fluid.

INDICATIONS

1. To evaluate pleural effusions of unknown etiology.
2. To exclude empyema or complicated parapneumonic effusions in febrile patient with pleural effusions.
3. Therapeutic removal of air or fluid from the pleural space.

RELATIVE CONTRAINDICATIONS

1. Uncooperative patient.
2. Cutaneous abnormality such as an infection at the proposed sampling site.

Note. There are no data to confirm that uncorrected bleeding diathesis (prothrombin time or partial thromboplastin time greater than two times normal, INR >1.5 platelets <50,000, or a creatine level >6) increases the risk of hemorrhagic complications. However, one must consider the risks and benefits for each procedure before proceeding without correcting coagulopathy or thrombocytopenia.

HISTORY

1. Patients with risk factors or a history suggestive of bleeding problems should have coagulation factors measured.
2. Screen for allergies to local anesthetics.
3. The urgency of the procedure (i.e., the benefits of rapid diagnosis and treatment of empyema/parapneumonic effusion or relief of tension pneumothorax) can help guide the need to forgo correction of coagulopathy or thrombocytopenia holding of anticoagulant medications.

SITE SELECTION

1. Physical examination findings consistent with pleural effusions include decreased breath sounds, dullness to percussion, loss of tactile fremitus, and asymmetric diaphragmatic excursion.

TABLE 81.1	Materials Necessary for Thoracentesis	
Sterile gloves	60-mL syringe	Green top blood tube[d]
Mask	25-Ga needle[b]	Sterile dressing
Antiseptic solution[a]	22-Ga x 1.5 in needle[c]	Lavender top tube[e]
Sterile drape or towels	Scalpel with No. 11 blade	Sterile specimen cups[f]
1% Lidocaine w/o Epinephrine	Pleural catheter	Fluid collection bag
10-mL syringe	Sterile gauze	

Chlorhexadine or Betadine. [b]To anesthetize skin. [c]To anesthetize tract and pleura. [d]For chemical analysis. [e]For cell count. [f]For cultures and cytology.

- A lateral decubitus film, ultrasound, or computed tomography scan of the chest can exclude alternative diagnoses that mimic pleural fluid on standard PA and lateral chest radiographs.
- Using ultrasound for site selection is recommended by the British Thoracic Society guidelines on pleural procedures and is now widely considered standard of care in America. Ultrasound-guided thoracentesis can be performed safely in patients on mechanical ventilation.
- Radiographic and physical examination can be used for site selection if ultrasound is not available, but at least 1 cm of fluid should layer out on a lateral decubitus film in order to safely sample an effusion without ultrasound guidance. Ultrasound guidance is recommended if two unsuccessful, or "dry taps" are performed.

PROCEDURE

- Explain the procedure, risks, benefits, alternatives; answer questions and obtain consent.
- There are a number of commercially available procedure kits that simplify the gathering of needed equipment (Table 81.1 lists necessary equipment for thoracentesis).
- Sit patient up with arms draped forward over a bedside table or procedure stand to maximize the intercostal space and amount of fluid in the posterior gutter. If the patient is intubated (or unable to sit up), our preference is to roll the patient so that the intended side for thoracentesis is up.
- With ultrasound guidance, identify the diaphragm between the mid-scapular line and the posterior axillary line and go one rib space up. Mark a site where at least 1.5 cm of fluid is between the chest wall and the underlying lung (Fig. 81.1).
- If ultrasound is not available, percuss down the chest until an area of dullness is reached and go one interspace below the area of dullness. Avoid the paraspinal area to avoid intercostal vessels. Do not go below the ninth rib interspace to avoid splenic or hepatic laceration (Fig. 81.2).
- Don a mask and sterile gloves.
- Cleanse the chosen site with an appropriate antiseptic (chlorhexadine or betadine).
- Cover surrounding area with sterile drape or towels.
- Use a 25-gauge needle attached to the 10-mL syringe filled with lidocaine to create a skin wheal over the top of the appropriate rib.

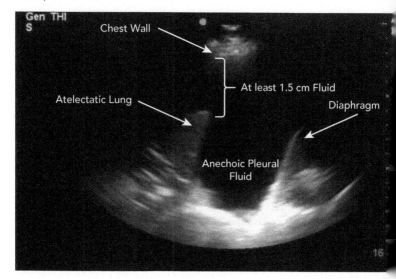

Figure 81.1. Ultrasound image depicting diaphragm and 1.5 cm of fluid between chest wall and underlying lung.

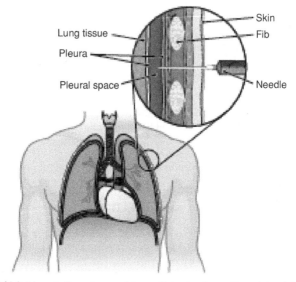

Figure 81.2. Schematic illustrating appropriate needle location for sampling and pleural effusion.

10. Use a 22-gauge needle to go through the wheal while aspirating. It is important to keep the needle perpendicular to the skin surface at all times. Advance by a few millimeters at a time, injecting lidocaine with each stop, until fluid is aspirated. At this point, withdraw slowly until flow of fluid stops and inject the remainder of lidocaine to properly anesthetize the pleura. Remember, the skin, top of the rib, and parietal pleura require the most anesthetic.

11. If using a needle without a catheter device, insert needle into previously anesthetized tract until fluid is aspirated. Collect fluid for studies.

12. If using a needle with a catheter device, first make a skin nick with a scalpel. Insert the needle and catheter device through the skin nick and advance while aspirating, making certain to keep the device perpendicular to the skin surface and in line with the anesthetized tract. After fluid is aspirated, advance needle and catheter 2 to 3 mm further into the pleural space and then advance the catheter off the needle into the pleural space while preventing the needle from advancing further. Remove the needle, leaving the catheter in place.

13. Using a large syringe, remove fluid for studies. Samples for chemical evaluation are typically sent in a mint green top blood tube, and cell counts in a lavender top blood tube. Cytology and microbiology samples for study can be sent in small, sterile containers. Although submission of large amounts of cytology fluid is commonly advocated, the yield for diagnosis appears to be independent of the fluid amount submitted. (See Chapter 16 "Pleural Disorders in the Intensive Care Unit" for further guidance on fluid analysis.)

14. If performing a therapeutic procedure, connect the catheter to a syringe and collection bag system. Vacuum bottles or wall suction devices **should not** be used for thoracentesis, as this has been associated with an increased risk for pneumothorax and may increase risk for re-expansion pulmonary edema (REPE).

15. Cough is expected as the underlying atelectatic lung re-expands. Shoulder/scapular pain or unilateral posterior chest pain is thought to likely be due to catheter-induced irritation of the diaphragm or pleura. Slowing the rate of fluid removal or temporarily stopping the procedure until the pain improves is acceptable.

16. It is generally recommended that the procedure be stopped when the patient develops symptoms of intractable cough or anterior chest/neck discomfort (as these are thought to be signs of increasingly negative pleural pressures) or after approximately 1,500 mL of pleural fluid is removed to avoid REPE. Alternatively, one can monitor pleural manometry, if available, and keep pleural pressures less than -20 cm H_2O.

17. Remove the catheter during exhalation, as this is when intrathoracic pressure is positive, decreasing the likelihood of entrainment of air, that is, pneumothorax. Cover site with a sterile dressing.

18. Chest x-rays are commonly performed to exclude pneumothorax, but data suggest that they may not be needed unless there are concerning symptoms or problems with the procedure that suggests that the lung may have been punctured.

COMPLICATIONS

Complications can be separated into major complications, such as pneumothorax, significant bleeding or REPE, and minor complications, such as pain or failed procedure/dry tap.

Operator experience and ultrasound guidance play a significant role in the risk of complications, emphasizing the importance of having the proper background knowledge and experience in the performance of the procedure.

REPE is a feared, but rare complication of therapeutic thoracentesis. The pathophysiology is unclear, but has been hypothesized to be due to excessive negative pleural pressure during pleural drainage procedures. Symptoms include anterior chest or neck pain/pressure and intractable cough. Therapy is supportive.

Factors that affect hemorrhagic complications are number of needle passes and location on the chest (decreasing risk the further from the spine the site is). Although guidelines recommend correcting thrombocytopenia (platelets <50,000) or coagulopathy (INR >1.5), there are little data to support this practice, and growing literature suggests it is unnecessary. We recommend taking into account the risk to benefit ratio for each case individually when considering correcting bleeding risk.

SUGGESTED READINGS

Bartter T, Mayo PD, Pratter MR, et al. Lower risk and higher yield for thoracentesis when performed by experienced operators. *Chest.* 1993;103:1873–1876 .
  Prospective study involving 50 consecutive thoracenteses performed by pulmonary fellows or attendings. Showed significantly lower rates of major complications compared to similar studies of procedure performed by non-pulmonary housestaff.
Collins TR, Sahn SA. Thoracentesis: clinical value, complications, technical problems, and patient experience. *Chest.* 1987;91:817–822.
  Prospective study of 129 thoracenteses primarily performed by medical housestaff and students.
Havelock T, Teoh R, Laws D, et al. Pleural procedures and thoracic ultrasound: British Thoracic Society pleural disease guideline 2010. *Thorax.* 2010;65(Suppl 2):ii61–ii76.
Hibbert RM, Atwell TD, Lekah A, et al. Safety of ultrasound-guided thoracentesis in patients with abnormal preprocedural coagulation parameters. *Chest.* 2013;144(2):456–463.
  Retrospective cohort study of 1,009 thoracenteses done in patients with either thrombocytopenia or coagulopathy. Suggests that attempting to correct an abnormal INR or platelet level before the procedure is unlikely to confer a reduced risk of hemorrhagic complications.
Jones PW, Moyers JP, Rogers JT, et al. Ultrasound-guided thoracentesis: is it a safer method? *Chest.* 2003;123:418–423.
  Prospective descriptive study of 941 thoracenteses in 605 patients. Showed a low rate of complications when thoracentesis was performed under ultrasound by experienced operators. Also showed low incidence of re-expansion pulmonary edema regardless of the amount of fluid removed.
McVay PA, Toy PT. Lack of increased bleeding after paracentesis and thoracentesis in patients with mild coagulation abnormalities. *Transfusion.* 1991;31:164–171.
  Retrospective study of 608 patients undergoing thoracentesis or paracentesis. Argues that prophylactic plasma and platelet transfusions are unnecessary for patients with mild moderate coagulopathies.
Petersen WG, Zimmerman R. Limited utility of chest radiograph after thoracentesis. *Chest.* 2000;117:1038–1042.
  Prospective, cohort involving 251 thoracenteses. Showed that clinically significant pneumothoraces were always associated with symptoms or aspiration of air.
Puchalski JT, Argento AC, Murphy TE, et al. The safety of thoracentesis in patients with uncorrected bleeding risk. *Ann Am Thorac Soc.* 2013;10(4):336–341.
  Prospective study of 312 patients undergoing thoracentesis. Implies that thoracentesis may be safely performed without prior correction of coagulopathy, thrombocytopenia, or medication induced bleeding risk.
Seneff MG, Corwin RW, Gold LH, et al. Complications associated with thoracentesis. *Chest.* 1986;90:97–100.
  Prospective study of 125 procedures primarily performed by housestaff.

82

Pulmonary Artery Catheterization

Warren Isakow

ince its inception in the 1970s, the clinical use of the pulmonary artery catheter PAC) has been controversial. The PAC provides direct pressure measurements from he right atrium (RA), right ventricle (RV), pulmonary arteries (PAs), and pulmonary apillary wedge pressure (PCWP) as well as a means of measuring cardiac output CO) by thermodilution. The PAC rapidly gained favor when it was recognized how naccurate physician assessments of these parameters were. Use of the catheter became idespread, and bedside management was often influenced by the hemodynamic arameters; however, no clinical validation of the benefit of this approach had been erformed.

A number of subsequent trials in different patient populations, including surgi-l patients, patients with acute myocardial infarction, congestive heart failure, and ute lung injury, have shown no benefits, and possibly increased risk, from use of a AC. A study by the acute respiratory distress syndrome clinical trials network found differences in outcomes of patients with this syndrome who had their fluid balance ided by use of a central line with central venous pressure monitoring or use of a AC. Routine use of the PAC should be avoided, but it still has a role in patients with lmonary arterial hypertension and congenital heart disease, and in patients with mplex fluid management issues. In addition, as new therapies emerge, information treatment benefits may require invasive assessment of hemodynamic parameters.

Newer, noninvasive techniques to assess hemodynamic parameters are being ined and are reducing dependence on the PAC. The clinician using the PAC needs ask how the information obtained from a PAC will change management of a cific patient, and be alert to possibly the greatest danger of the device: misinterpre-ion of its hemodynamic measurements. The PAC should be used for the shortest ne possible and with the understanding that it is unlikely to alter the clinical course a patient with multiple complex medical problems (Table 82.1).

ROCEDURE TECHNIQUE

e easiest insertion sites are normally the right internal jugular (RIJ) vein or the subclavian vein; however, femoral or even brachial vein sites can be used. Prior tarting the procedure, an evaluation of any contraindications to the procedure uld be made. In cases with suspected RV dysfunction, pulmonary arterial hyper-ion, tricuspid regurgitation, or RA enlargement, consideration should be given to ing the PAC with fluoroscopic guidance, as direct visualization enhances ability ass the PAC in difficult cases.

TABLE 82.1	Contraindications to, Indications for, and Complications of Pulmonary Artery Catheter Placement
Relative Contraindications	**Complications**
Left bundle branch block	Complications related to introducer placement:
Severe coagulopathy	• Pneumothorax
	• Hemothorax
	• Hematoma at site of insertion
	• Infection at insertion site
Indications (Controversial)	
Diagnosis and management of shock states	Complications related to PAC use:
Oliguric acute renal failure	• Arrhythmias
Assessment of volume status	• Right bundle branch block
Titration of therapy for cardiogenic shock	• Complete heart block
Diagnosis of PAH	(pre-existing left heart block)
Vasodilator testing in PAH	• Catheter thrombosis
Diagnosis of multiple cardiac disorders includ-	• Pulmonary embolism
ing pericardial constriction, VSD, RV infarction	• Pulmonary infarct
Perioperative management of major	• Line sepsis
procedures	• Pulmonary artery rupture
	• Pulmonary artery pseudoaneurysm
	• Valvular damage
	• Cardiac perforation
	• Catheter kinking

PAC, pulmonary artery catheter; PAH, pulmonary arterial hypertension; VSD, ventricular septal defe
RV, right ventricle.

The intravenous lines, pressure bags, transducers, and zeroing apparatus sho
all be assembled and ready prior to the sterile insertion of the PAC. It is useful
have an assistant or nurse available for the procedure. A sterile procedural field sho
be used, with strict attention to handwashing, mask and cap usage, sterile gl
and gown use, as well as full-length drapes. The introducer catheter is inserted i
similar manner to a central venous catheter using the Seldinger technique. The in
ducer catheter is slightly different in that the dilator is advanced through the introdu
rather than as a separate piece of equipment, as occurs with a regular central ven
catheter insertion. Additionally, the guidewire and dilator are removed togethe
the conclusion of the introducer insertion, which leaves the introducer alone in
vessel.

The PAC (see Fig. 82.1) should have all ports flushed and the balloon chec
for leaks prior to insertion. In addition, the operator should check that the ball
tip does not protrude beyond the inflated balloon as this can increase the ris
vascular rupture. All ports of the PAC should be attached to the pressure transdu
and flushed prior to insertion. Waving of the catheter tip prior to insertion with
ification of a waveform on the monitor confirms that the catheter ports are corre
attached. Prior to starting the procedure, a final check to verify that the prote

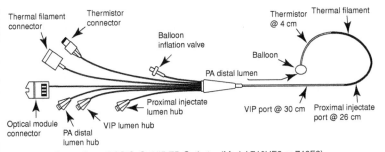

Swan–Ganz CCO/SvO$_2$/VIP TD Catheter (Model 746HF8 or 746F8)

Figure 82.1. Pulmonary artery catheter. (From Clark SL, Phelan JP. *Critical Care Obstetrics*. 2nd ed. Boston, MA: Blackwell Scientific; 1990:63, with permission.)

catheter sheath has been inserted over the catheter should be performed. The catheter should be oriented prior to insertion to match the natural curve in the catheter to the projected course through the vasculature.

The PAC is advanced through the introducer, and when the catheter tip is in the RA, the balloon should be inflated gently. The distance from the insertion site to the RA will vary depending on site, but is usually 15 to 20 cm from the RIJ or left subclavian sites. Once the balloon is inflated and the lock on the inflating syringe has been activated, the catheter is advanced and the waveforms on the monitor are inspected. The RA waveform will increase in amplitude as the RV is entered, which normally occurs at approximately 30 cm (from an RIJ approach). The passage of the catheter through the RV is arrhythmogenic and should not be of prolonged duration. Conversion of the RV waveform to a PA waveform, as the catheter tip traverses the pulmonary valve, is identified by an increase in the diastolic pressure and the development of a dicrotic notch in the tracing (often at 40 cm). Difficulty in traversing the pulmonary valve is not uncommon in patients with pulmonary arterial hypertension from any cause and, if excessive catheter length has been advanced without this transition occurring, the most likely explanation is that the catheter is coiled in the enlarged RV. If this occurs, the balloon should be deflated and the catheter should be withdrawn until an RA tracing is obtained, after which the balloon should be inflated and the procedure attempted again. The PCWP tracing is identified by loss of the arterial tracing to a flatter tracing of lower amplitude than the PA diastolic pressure (often at 50 cm). (See Fig. 82.2 for the pressure tracings obtained as the catheter advances.)

At this point, the balloon should be deflated and the PA waveform should be observed. Gentle reinflation of the balloon while feeling for increased resistance and monitoring the waveform for overwedging is crucial. The 1.5-mL balloon should be fully inflated when a wedge tracing is obtained. If a wedge tracing is obtained and the balloon is only partially inflated, this signifies that the catheter tip is too distal and increases the risk of PA rupture by full inflation of the balloon. With this scenario, the catheter should be gently withdrawn 1 to 2 cm with the balloon deflated, and the balloon inflation procedure performed again to obtain a wedge tracing optimally at full balloon inflation. If there is no wedge tracing obtained with full inflation of the balloon, the catheter should be advanced with the balloon inflated till a wedge tracing is obtained. The catheter should never be withdrawn with the balloon inflated and

Catheter position	Waveform	Normal pressure range (mm Hg)

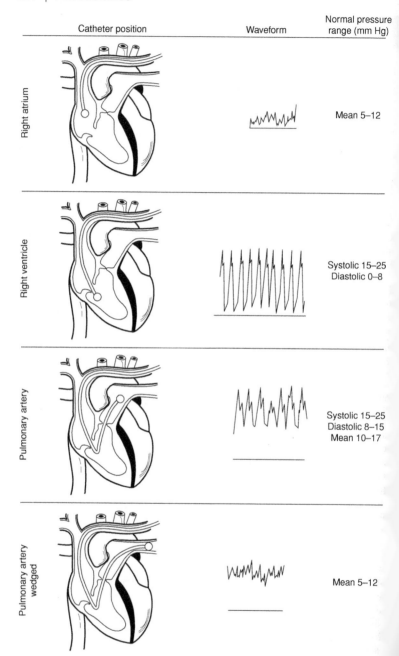

Right atrium — Mean 5–12

Right ventricle — Systolic 15–25 Diastolic 0–8

Pulmonary artery — Systolic 15–25 Diastolic 8–15 Mean 10–17

Pulmonary artery wedged — Mean 5–12

Figure 82.2. Pulmonary artery catheter placement. Catheter position, corresponding waveforms, and pressures are shown. (From Clark SL, Phelan JP. *Critical Care Obstetrics.* 2nd ed. Boston, MA: Blackwell Scienti 1990:67, with permission.)

TABLE 82.2	Examples of Hemodynamic Parameters Obtained by a Pulmonary Artery Catheter in Different Clinical Situations					
CVP (mm Hg)	RV Pressures (mm Hg)	PA Pressures (mm Hg)	PAOP (mm Hg)	CO (L/min)	SVR (dynes/ s/cm⁻⁵)	Diagnosis
4	17–30/ 0–6	15–30/ 5–13	2–12	3—7	900–1200	Normal
10	48/12	48/30	28	2.2	3200	Cardiogenic shock
4	26/4	26/8	6	7	700	Sepsis
14	26/14	26/14	14	3.0	3000	Cardiac tamponade
16	80/30	80/40	8	3.5	1400	Pulmonary arterial hypertension
14	45/12	45/18	6	3	2800	Pulmonary embolism (acute)
2	30/2	30/12	3	2.5	2500	Hypovolemic shock

/P, central venous pressure; RV, right ventricle; PA, pulmonary artery; PAOP, pulmonary arterial
clusion pressure; CO, cardiac output; SVR, systemic vascular resistance.

ould never be advanced without the balloon inflated, as this can result in perfora-
n of the heart or a PA.

Once insertion is completed, the distance of insertion from the introducer site
ould be noted and recorded as a reference point. The catheter should be secured
h tape and a sterile dressing and a chest x-ray should be obtained to verify catheter
urse, tip position, and to rule out any complications from the procedure, such as a
eumothorax. As the catheter warms up in the patient's body, it tends to soften and
grate distally, which increases the risk of overwedging, pulmonary infarction, and
rupture with balloon inflation, so this should be re-evaluated with a daily chest
ay as well as bedside by cautious inflation of the balloon and inspection of the
veforms (Table 82.2).

rdiac Output Determination

ce the PAC has been verified to be correctly placed, hemodynamic data can be
ained. The catheter system must be opened to the air to set the zero point as
nospheric pressure and the catheter transducer must be referenced to the level of
heart. The CO is determined by both thermodilution and the Fick calculation.
thermodilution, a known volume (usually 5 to 10 mL) of cold saline is injected
ough the proximal port of the PAC. The distal port has a thermistor which records
change in temperature of the blood over time and displays this as the thermo-
tion curve. The area under the thermodilution curve is proportional to the CO

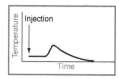

Normal thermodilution curve
With an accurate monitoring system and a patient who has adequate CO, the thermodilution curve begins with a smooth, rapid upstroke and is followed by a smooth, gradual downslope. The curve shown at left indicates that the injectant instillation time was within the recommended 4 seconds and that the temperature curve returned to baseline.

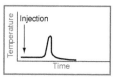

Low CO curve
A thermodilution curve representing low CO shows a rapid, smooth upstroke (from proper injection technique). However, because the heart is ejecting blood less efficiently from the ventricles, the injectant warms slowly and takes longer to be ejected from the ventricle. Consequently, the curve takes longer to return to baseline. This slow return produces a larger area under the curve, corresponding to low CO.

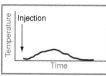

High CO curve
Again, the curve has a rapid, smooth upstroke from proper injection technique. However, because the ventricles are ejecting blood too forcefully, the injectant moves through the heart quickly and the curve returns to baseline more rapidly. The smaller area under the curve suggests higher CO.

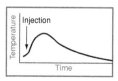

Curve reflecting poor technique
This curve results from an uneven and too slow (taking more than 4 seconds) administration of injectant. The uneven and slower than normal upstroke and the larger area under the curve erroneously indicate low CO. A kinked catheter, unsteady hands during the injection, or improper placement of the injectant lumen in the introducer sheath may also cause this type of curve.

Figure 82.3. Cardiac output measurement. Analyzing thermodilution curves.

(pulmonary artery flow rate) as long as there is not an intracardiac shunt (falsely elevated CO) or tricuspid regurgitation (falsely low CO). Normally, three thermodilution curves with minimal variance (less than 10%) are used to determine the mean CO utilizing the Stewart Hamilton equation. Figure 82.3 shows various thermodilution curves.

The Fick equation can also be used to calculate the CO. The Fick principle is

$$CO = \frac{Oxygen\ consumption}{Arteriovenous\ oxygen\ content\ difference \times 10}$$

Oxygen consumption is normally assumed and is calculated by using a value for O_2 consumption at rest of 110 to 125 mL/min/m^2 depending on age and sex. The arteriovenous oxygen content calculation requires a simultaneous arterial blood gas (SaO_2) and sampling of blood from the distal port of the PAC (SvO_2) and calculated as follows:

Arteriovenous oxygen content difference = 1.34 × hemoglobin concentration × (SaO_2 − SvO_2).

Pressure measurements are all measured at end-exhalation, when intrathoracic pressure most approaches atmospheric pressure. Use of a mainstream end-tidal CO_2 detector is useful to determine this point in intubated patients. In nonintubated patients, review of the hemodynamic tracings can identify fluctuations in pressure associated with normal respiration and end-exhalation can be identified. Utilization of all the hemodynamic data obtained from the catheter, together with knowledge of the patients clinical scenario, can greatly aid in interpretation of the data.

The PAC has a unique ability to identify diverse etiologies of shock, including hypovolemia, cardiogenic, and distributive/septic shock. In addition, patients with predominantly right ventricular dysfunction and patients with pericardial tamponade can be identified. Use of continuous oximetry during catheter insertion can also identify stepups in oxygen saturations which can help diagnose intracardiac left to right shunts.

Titration of inotropes, fluids, and vasodilators can be performed with serial measurements from the PAC to optimize tissue oxygen delivery and hemodynamics.

SUGGESTED READINGS

Binanay C, Califf RM, Hasselblad V, et al. Evaluation study of congestive heart failure and pulmonary artery catheterization effectiveness: the ESCAPE trial. *JAMA.* 2005;294(13):1625–1633.

Randomized controlled trial in 433 patients with severe symptomatic heart failure where therapy guided by a PAC did not affect mortality or hospitalization but did increase adverse events.

Cohen MG, Kelly RV, Kong DF, et al. Pulmonary artery catheterization in acute coronary syndromes: insights from the GUSTO 2b and GUSTO 3 trials. *Am J Med.* 2005;118:482–488.

Retrospective study of 26,437 patients experiencing acute coronary syndromes. 735 patients had PAC inserted and these patients had higher mortality even after adjustments for baseline patient differences. This did not apply to patients who were in cardiogenic shock.

Connors AF Jr., Speroff T, Dawson NV, et al. The effectiveness of right heart catheterization in the initial care of critically ill patients. SUPPORT Investigators. *JAMA.* 1996;276:889–897.

Observational study of 5735 critically ill patients, where after adjustment for treatment selection bias, PAC use was associated with increased mortality and increased resource utilization.

Eisenberg PR, Jaffe AS, Schuster DP. Clinical evaluation compared to pulmonary artery catheterization in the hemodynamic assessment of critically ill patients. *Crit Care Med.* 1984;12(7):549–553.

Prospective study in 103 patients which emphasized the difficulty of accurately predicting hemodynamics based on clinical evaluation. The study found that planned therapy was changed in 58% of the cases after insertion of a PAC, with unanticipated therapy added in 30% of the cases.

Harvey S, Harrison DA, Singer M, et al. Assessment of the clinical effectiveness of pulmonary artery catheters in management of patients in intensive care (PAC-Man): a randomized controlled trial. *Lancet.* 2005;366(9484):472–477.

Large multi-center randomized controlled study in UK ICU's which noted no difference in outcomes when a PAC was used to manage critically ill patients. 46 of 486 patients had a complication from PAC insertion, none of which were fatal.

Rhodes A, Cusack RJ, Newman PJ, et al. A randomized, controlled trial of the pulmonary artery catheter in critically ill patients. *Intensive Care Med.* 2002;28(3):256–264.

Single center randomized trial in 201 critically ill patients did not show a mortality difference between the PAC and control groups.

Richard C, Warsjawski J, Anguel N, et al. Early use of the pulmonary artery catheter and outcomes in patients with shock and acute respiratory distress syndrome: a randomized controlled trial. *JAMA.* 2003;290(20):2713–2720.

Multicenter randomized study of 676 patients with septic shock, ARDS or both, where clinical management with a PAC did not affect morbidity or mortality.

Sandham JD, Hull RD, Brant RF, et al. A randomized, controlled trial of the use of pulmonary-artery catheters in high-risk surgical patients. *N Engl J Med.* 2003;348:5–14.

Randomized trial in 1,994 elderly, high risk surgical patients, found no benefit to PAC directed therapy over standard care and a higher rate of pulmonary embolism in the PAC group.

Steingrub JS, Celoria G, Vickers-Lahti M, et al. Therapeutic impact of pulmonary artery catheterization in a medical/surgical ICU. *Chest.* 1991;99(6):1451–1455.

> *An expert panel rated the performance of housestaff/attending interpretation of hemodynamic data in 154 medical/surgical patients. Most housestaff/attending performance was judged appropriate and the study suggested that information derived from a PAC was instrumental in managing patients who were unresponsive to initial therapy.*

Swan HJ, Ganz W, Forrester J, et al. Catheterization of the heart in man with use of a flow-directed balloon-tipped catheter. *N Engl J Med.* 1970;283:447–451.

> *The landmark initial description of the technique.*

The National Heart, Lung, and Blood Institute Acute Respiratory Distress Syndrome (ARDS) Clinical Trials Network. Wheeler AP, Bernard GR, et al. Pulmonary-artery versus central venous catheter to guide treatment of acute lung injury. *N Engl J Med.* 2006;354(21):2213–2224.

> *Randomized multi-center trial in 1000 patients with acute lung injury which had an explicit fluid management algorithm. PAC use did not improve survival or organ function and was associated with more complications than therapy guided by a regular central line.*

83 Alternative Hemodynamic Monitoring

Warren Isakow

No hemodynamic monitoring technique can improve patient outcomes by simply being utilized. The ideal hemodynamic monitor should provide accurate and reproducible measurements of clinically relevant variables that are able to guide therapy, should be easy to use with rapid response times, be operator independent and cause no harm. The perfect system does not exist and different approaches may be required in a single patient during different phases of their illness. There are several noninvasive or minimally invasive techniques that measure cardiac output (CO). These methods include esophageal Doppler, transpulmonary thermodilution, pulse contour analysis, partial carbon dioxide (CO_2) rebreathing, and thoracic electrical bioimpedance and bioreactance. The focus of this chapter is to describe these techniques, both their advantages, and limitations with a special focus on the esophageal Doppler.

ESOPHAGEAL DOPPLER

The esophageal Doppler has been utilized in a variety of situations including trauma patients, medical ICUs, intraoperative assessment, and for postoperative care.

Measurement of CO with the esophageal Doppler is based on measuring the velocity of blood flow through the descending aorta. The technique involves placing a transducer into the esophagus and rotating the probe to achieve an optimal signal. Blood flow velocity is measured by changes in the frequency of reflected sound waves. Stroke volume (SV) is estimated from the derivation of a velocity time integral (VTI) multiplied by aortic cross-sectional area (Fig. 83.1). Once SV is calculated, the CO is determined (CO = heart rate × SV).

In addition to SV and CO, the esophageal Doppler provides a measure of preload termed corrected flow time (FTc). FTc is systolic flow time corrected for heart rate; it is represented on the monitor display as the waveform's base. Normal values range between 330 and 360 ms. Achieving the longest possible FTc for a patient, correlates well with finding the optimal level of left ventricular filling or preload. The maximum or peak velocity is the waveform's height and can serve as a measure of contractility. The normal range for peak velocity declines with age.

Preload	⟹ Flow time	Peak velocity by age	
Contractility	⟹ Peak velocity	20 yrs	90–120 cm/s
Afterload	⟹ Velocity and flow time	50 yrs	70–100 cm/s
		70 yrs	50–80 cm/s

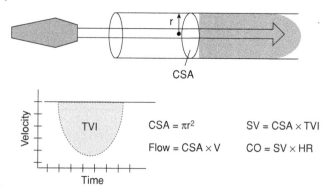

Figure 83.1. Schematic representation of the method for determining volumetric flow. This method is applicable for any laminar flow for which the cross-sectional area (*CSA*) of the flow chamber can be determined. The product of cross-sectional area and the time velocity integral (*TVI*) is stroke volume (*SV*). Cardiac output (*CO*) can be calculated as the product of stroke volume and heart rate. See text for further details.

Following both the FTc and peak velocity helps to optimize resuscitation efforts in a wide spectrum of patients and clinical situations. For example, in hypovolemic shock the monitor displays a narrow waveform base with a corresponding decrease in FT (<330 ms) and relatively normal peak velocity. The administration of fluid would widen the waveform base, or lengthen the FTc. If the underlying condition is myocardial depression, the initial waveform shows a low peak velocity and normal FTc. Inotropic therapy improves the peak velocity or contractility in such a situation (Fig. 83.2).

The major advantage of the esophageal Doppler is the ability to rapidly obtain a set of hemodynamic numbers which are generally easy to interpret. The probe is placed orally and advanced until approximately the midthoracic area, 35 to 40 cm. It is possible to leave the esophageal Doppler in place as long as 72 hours, but it is important to test the position of the probe to ensure the optimal signal. The device is safe to use in most patients including patients with coagulopathies. Probe placement in patients with known varices is a relative contraindication.

One drawback to this technique is its limitation to sedated and mechanically ventilated patients. There are also several assumptions in the calculation of SV and CO that affect its ability to give precise measurements. The SV is estimated from the proportion of blood flow that reaches the descending aorta. It is assumed that there is constant 70/30 division of flow between the descending aorta (70%) and the brachiocephalic arteries supplying the head and neck as well as the upper extremities (30%). The cross-sectional area of the aorta is estimated based on a nomogram utilizing characteristics of the patient (age, gender, and weight). Therefore, if significant aortic pathology (aneurysm or dilation) is present, the absolute derived values may not be accurate. The mathematical model also assumes that the aorta is cylindrical with constant laminar flow running parallel to the esophagus. In reality, flow may be turbulent due to arrhythmia, anemia, or aortic valve disease. The presence of any of these factors makes it difficult to obtain a consistent signal and the presence of severe kyphoscoliosis can alter the angle of interrogation of the probe so that it is not optimally positioned to measure flow in the descending area. If this angle between the probe and the flow down the descending aorta is greater than 15 to 30 degrees, measurements will be inaccurate

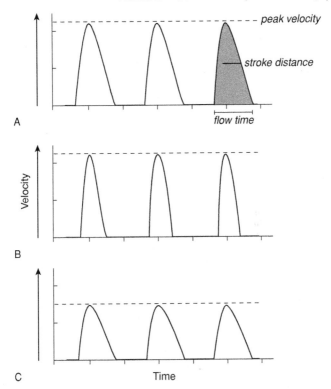

Figure 83.2. Schematic diagram of esophageal Doppler waveforms obtained during (**A**) normovolemia, (**B**) hypovolemia, and (**C**) left ventricular failure. The primary measurements obtained during esophageal Doppler monitoring are stroke distance (the area under the waveform during systole), the peak velocity, and the ejection time during systole ("*flow time*"). Note that during hypovolemia and heart failure, stroke distance is decreased. In addition, ideally, during hypovolemia, flow time is decreased but peak velocity is maintained, whereas during heart failure, flow time is normal but peak velocity is reduced. (From Isakow W, Schuster DP. Extravascular lung water measurements and hemodynamic monitoring in the critically ill: bedside alternatives to the pulmonary artery catheter. *Am J Physiol Lung Cell Mol Physiol.* 2006;291(6):L1118–L1131, used with permission.)

Esophageal Doppler monitoring is most useful when the device is used to obtain serial measurements to detect trends and response to therapy. Absolute values are not as important as trend analysis and this concept is explained in Chapter 84 (Functional Hemodynamic Monitoring). Improved outcomes utilizing esophageal Doppler–guided management have been shown in surgical patients undergoing orthopedic procedures but there is a lack of outcome data in most ICU patients.

TRANSPULMONARY THERMODILUTION

In contrast to the pulmonary artery (PA) thermodilution technique, transpulmonary thermodilution measures CO by detecting a cold bolus within the peripheral arterial system. The cold injectate is administered through a central venous catheter and

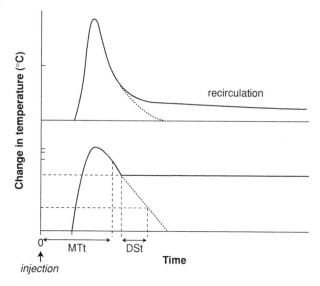

Figure 83.3. Diagrammatic representation of temperature-time curve during a thermodilution measurement plotted on linear-linear (**top**) and log-linear scales (**bottom**). The dotted lines in each case represent what the curve would have looked like in the absence of recirculation of the thermal indicator. Note that the decay of the thermal curve becomes linear when graphed on the semi-log scale (bottom). Also shown are typical points used to measure the mean transit time (*MTt*) and the downslope time (*DSt*). (From Isakow W, Schuster DP. Extravascular lung water measurements and hemodynamic monitoring in the critically ill: bedside alternatives to the pulmonary artery catheter. *Am J Physiol Lung Cell Mol Physiol.* 2006;291(6):L1118–L1131; used with permission.)

detected by a thermistor-tipped arterial catheter placed into the radial, axillary, or femoral artery. CO is calculated by the Stewart–Hamilton equation similar to PA thermodilution (Chapter 82). The benefit with the transpulmonary technique is the ability to obtain CO readings as well as other markers of preload (global end-diastolic volume [GEDV], intrathoracic blood volume [ITBV]), and extravascular lung water (EVLW), without a PA catheter.

Transpulmonary CO values are generally greater than the PA thermodilution values. It has been proposed that there is an unaccounted loss of cold indicator in the lung which would explain the difference as well as overcorrection for recirculation artifact.

Thermodilution measurements can be used not only to measure flow, but also to measure the volume through which flow is measured (i.e., from the point of injection to the point of detection). Figure 83.3 depicts a typical thermodilution curve utilizing transpulmonary thermodilution and explains the concept of mean transit time and downslope time. The derived volumes can be seen graphically in Figure 83.4:

- Intrathoracic thermal volume (ITTV) = CO × Mean transit time of the thermal indicator
- Pulmonary thermal volume (PTV) = CO × Downslope time of the thermal indicator
- Global end-diastolic volume (GEDV) = ITTV − PTV and provides a preload marker of moderate strength.

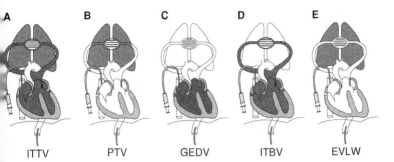

Figure 83.4. Schematic diagrams of different volumes that can be measured (*dark shaded areas*) with the transpulmonary thermodilution technique. ITTV, intrathoracic thermal volume; PTV, pulmonary thermal volume; GEDV, global end-diastolic volume; ITBV, intrathoracic blood volume; EVLW, extravascular lung water. (From Isakow W, Schuster DP. Extravascular lung water measurements and hemodynamic monitoring the critically ill: bedside alternatives to the pulmonary artery catheter. *Am J Physiol Lung Cell Mol Physiol.* 2006;291(6):L1118–L1131, used with permission.)

Intrathoracic blood volume (ITBV) = $1.25 \times$ GEDV $- 28.4$ (mL)
Extravascular lung water (EVLW) = ITTV $-$ ITBV and may be used to help guide fluid administration or distinguish between hydrostatic pulmonary edema and acute lung injury

The clinical utility of EVLW is not clear. Increases in EVLW may be used as an indication of early pulmonary edema. It has been found that mortality is greater when EVLW rises above 15 mL/kg. However, currently there is no established protocol using EVLW in patients with sepsis or ALI/ARDS. The value for EVLW is subject to error in certain situations. It is found to be overestimated in cases of severe lung injury. It is underestimated in patients with acute pulmonary embolism where the loss of perfusion affects the ability of the thermal indicator to detect all areas of lung water.

PULSE CONTOUR ANALYSIS

Pulse contour methods use the arterial pressure waveform to predict vascular flow and calculate SV. Most devices require calibration to provide a correction factor for differences in the arterial system. Indeed there are several assumptions necessary to derive the aortic pressure waveform from the shape of the peripheral pulse. Therefore, most models use either transpulmonary thermodilution or lithium dilution techniques as a reference point to derive CO. Current systems available include: PiCCO (Pulsion Medical Systems, Munich, Germany), PulseCO (LiDCO Ltd, Cambridge, UK), and Flo Trac/Vigileo (Edwards LifeSciences, Irvine, California, USA). Thermodilution is used in the PiCCO device, lithium is the indicator for PulseCO, while the Flo Trac/Vigileo device does not require any dilution technique.

Pulse contour analysis requires arterial line placement, and for the PiCCO or PulseCO devices a central venous catheter must be placed for calibration. Each device uses a different mathematical model of pressure and flow that must account for the changes in aortic impedance, arterial compliance, and systemic resistance. Calibration is generally needed to derive the correction factors for these mathematical algorithms. The Flo Trac/Vigileo uses demographic data to extrapolate its correction factor.

Pulse contour analysis provides continuous CO monitoring in contrast to the PAC thermodilution technique which is intermittent.

The CO provided by the pulse contour analysis is subject to error as well. These devices are limited by dynamic changes in vascular resistance which would require recalibration. It is generally recommended to recalibrate the PiCCO and PulseCO devices every 8 hours. The Flo Trac/Vigileo does not require calibration but may not be reliable in patients with reduced peripheral resistance such as in sepsis. Performance is also affected by the presence of aortic regurgitation, aortic aneurysm, and dampened waveforms. The PulseCO system cannot be used in patients taking lithium therapy or paralytics because this alters the sensor's ability to detect the indicator. Such limitations should be taken into account when deciding which hemodynamic monitoring device to use. These devices can provide useful information like pulse pressure variation and SV variation in patients who are totally mechanically ventilated (no spontaneous respiratory effort), in normal sinus rhythm and on a ventilator with adequate tidal volumes. This concept is explained in Chapter 84.

PARTIAL CARBON DIOXIDE REBREATHING

This technique relies on a modified Fick principle to calculate CO. The Fick equation is based on the belief that oxygen uptake from the lung is completely transferred into the bloodstream. Therefore, CO is calculated as a ratio between oxygen consumption and the arteriovenous difference in oxygen content. In the partial CO_2 rebreathing technique, the Fick principle is applied to CO_2 instead of oxygen. Several devices are necessary to obtain the appropriate measurements. These consist of a CO_2 infrared sensor, an air-flow or pressure pneumotachometer, a pulse oximeter, and a disposable rebreathing loop. No central lines are required to measure CO_2 content. The value for venous CO_2 is eliminated from the equation by measuring CO_2 under normal and rebreathing conditions.

The modified Fick equation requires an estimate of venous CO_2, arterial CO_2 content, and an adjustment for the slope of the CO_2 dissociation curve. The venous content is represented by the change in CO_2 during normal (N) minute ventilation versus rebreathing (R) conditions. Arterial CO_2 is estimated from end-tidal CO_2 at the end of both maneuvers multiplied by the slope (S) of the CO_2 dissociation curve.

$$CO = \frac{vCO_2(N) - vCO_2(R)}{S \times \Delta etCO_2}$$

Intrapulmonary shunt can affect this equation by changing the blood flow participating in gas exchange. The degree of shunting in severe lung injury may not be easily estimated and adjusted by the system. Some devices incorporate peripheral oxygen saturation and PaO_2 on blood gases to account for shunting. Nonetheless underlying lung disease, varying tidal volumes, and hemodynamic instability can alter the precision of this technique which is not recommended or widely used.

THORACIC BIOIMPEDANCE

In thoracic bioimpedance, SV is estimated from changes in the electrical resistance over time as a low magnitude, high-frequency current is applied. The patient does detect the low level of current, and this technique is considered the least invasive of the available devices. It requires placement of six electrodes: two on the upper chest wall or neck, and four on the lower. The electrical current follows the path of least resistance, which is aortic blood flow. As the left heart contracts, there is a change in aortic blood volume and therefore a decrease in impedance. For the calculation of SV, the amount of electrically participating tissue is estimated from gender, height, and weight of the patient. The surrounding tissue fluid volume becomes important in the precision of impedance measurements.

The change in surrounding tissue fluid volume and the effect of respiration on pulmonary blood volume must be accounted for in the calculation of aortic blood flow. This technique is sensitive to acute changes in tissue water content such as pulmonary edema, effusions, and anasarca. The electrodes cannot be moved during the measurement because it is a calculation of change over time. The calculation also depends on a constant R-R interval, therefore arrhythmias will cause error in measurement of SV and CO. Measurements are also affected by temperature and humidity. There is very limited use of thoracic bioimpedance in the ICU population due to the factors noted above and devices using bioreactance are felt to be more reliable.

THORACIC BIOREACTANCE

The most widely used device is the NICOM (Cheetah Medical, Portland, Oregon) device which measures bioreactance or the phase shift in voltage across the thorax. This device measures thoracic impedance and tracks changes in amplitude and direction (measured in degrees) of the impedance. Pulsatile blood flow causes these phase shifts in impedance and the vast majority of thoracic pulsatile flow is generated by aortic blood flow. The NICOM device incorporates a sensitive phase shift detector and therefore noninvasively measures aortic flow. The system is totally noninvasive and consists of a high-frequency sine wave generator (75 kHz) and four dual electrode stickers which establish electrical contact with the thorax. Two stickers are placed on each side of the thorax and CO is determined separately from each side of the body with the final noninvasive CO averaged from these two values. Bioreactance-based measurements are more accurate than bioimpedance techniques as they do not measure static impedance and also do not depend on the distance between the electrodes. Signals are averaged over 1 minute so this technology can be used in patients with cardiac arrhythmias. Validation studies of the NICOM have shown good correlation between NICOM-derived CO compared to CO obtained by thermodilution techniques and with the esophageal Doppler. There are conflicting data whether NICOM can track changes in CO to functional challenges like fluid boluses and passive leg raises in different ICU populations. NICOM is not reliable when electrocautery is being simultaneously applied for greater than 20 s/min. This technique is noninvasive, can be used in ventilated and nonventilated patients as well as patients with cardiac arrhythmias.

CONCLUSION

The decision to use one form of hemodynamic monitoring over the other depends on the understanding of the limitations of each device and assessing each patient's unique situation. At Washington University, the esophageal Doppler is often used for its easy placement in critically ill, ventilated patients, ease of interpretation, and quick results. It provides intermittent CO monitoring as well as hemodynamic indices of cardiac preload, contractility and afterload. Regardless of the method chosen, the clinical picture, physical examination findings and all other available data should be integrated to adequately determine a patient's hemodynamic status.

SUGGESTED READINGS

Brown LM, Liu KD, Matthay MA. Measurement of extravascular lung water using the single indicator method in patients: research and potential clinical value. *Am J Physiol Lung Cell Mol Physiol.* 2009;297(4):L547–L558.

Reviews the accuracy of single indicator methods, limitations of measuring EVLW, and clinical trials using EVLW as a predictor of response to therapy or disease progression.

Funk DJ, Moretti EW, Gan TJ. Minimally invasive cardiac output monitoring in the perioperative setting. *Anesth Analg.* 2009;108(3):887–897.

Provides more in depth review of the evidence to support the use of esophageal Doppler, thoracic electrical bioimpedance, pulse contour, and transpulmonary thermodilution techniques. This article also gives more detail to the theory of thoracic bioimpedance.

Isakow W, Schuster DP. Extravascular lung water measurements and hemodynamic monitoring in the critically ill: bedside alternatives to the pulmonary artery catheter. *Am J Physiol Lung Cell Mol Physiol.* 2006;291(6):L1118–L1131.

A comprehensive review of the theoretical, validation, and empirical databases for transpulmonary thermodilution and esophageal Doppler measurements.

Marik PE. Noninvasive cardiac output monitors: a state-of-the-art review. *J Cardiothorac Vasc Anesth.* 2013;27(1):121–134.

Excellent review article which covers the theoretical basis of many noninvasive techniques, their limitations and clinical validation data.

Morgan P, Al-Subaie N, Rhodes A. Minimally invasive cardiac output monitoring. *Curr Opin Crit Care.* 2008;14(3):322–326.

Reports the evidence to support using pulse contour techniques and a closer look at the different commercially available devices.

Young BP, Low LL. Noninvasive monitoring cardiac output using partial CO_2 rebreathing. *Crit Care Clin.* 2010;26(2):383–392.

This article reviews the use of partial carbon dioxide rebreathing devices to determine cardiac output and their application for hemodynamic monitoring in the ICU and operating room.

84 Functional Hemodynamic Monitoring

Warren Isakow

Hemodynamic instability is very common in the ICU. Clinical impressions regarding patient's hemodynamic profile can often be erroneous resulting in potentially harmful interventions. The need for accurate hemodynamic information to guide patient care resulted in the widespread use of the pulmonary artery catheter (PAC). The lack of benefit observed in prospective randomized controlled trials and the inherent invasiveness of the PAC has renewed interest in alternative modes of hemodynamic monitoring and the assessment of volume responsiveness.

Basic principles of hemodynamic optimization focus on improving oxygen delivery to the tissues by restoring adequate circulating volume, restoring perfusion by optimizing cardiac output (CO) and mean arterial pressure (MAP), and ensuring an adequate oxygen carrying capacity (optimal hemoglobin and hemoglobin saturation with oxygen).

Volume responsiveness refers to the increase in CO or stroke volume (SV) that occurs in response to a fluid challenge.

STATIC MARKERS OF VOLUME RESPONSIVENESS

Figs. 84.1 and 84.2 explain the concept of volume responsiveness by depicting the Frank–Starling curve of a normal heart. Clinicians have generally utilized static hemodynamic values, most commonly intravascular pressures, to predict which patients will benefit from fluid challenges. Table 84.1 summarizes the static markers commonly used in ICUs to help predict volume responsiveness.

CENTRAL VENOUS PRESSURE

Figure 84.3 shows a normal central venous pressure (CVP) tracing. CVP tracings in disease states are often characteristic:

- In atrial fibrillation, the a wave is lost.
- In states of atrioventricular dissociation, large cannon a waves may occur as the atrium contracts against a closed tricuspid valve.
- In patients with tricuspid regurgitation, a large fused cv wave is seen.
- Tricuspid stenosis results in giant a-waves and a reduced y descent.
- In constrictive pericarditis, the y descent is prominent and becomes steeper during inspiration
- In cardiac tamponade, the x descent is preserved and the y descent is attenuated.

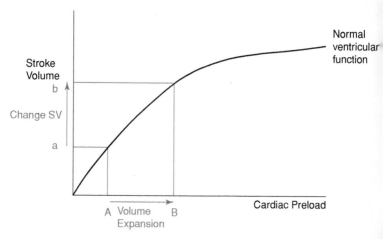

Figure 84.1. Volume responsive: Increase in stroke volume in response to a fluid challenge in a patient w normal biventricular function and on the steep portion (low preload) of the Frank–Starling curve.

CVP is used extensively in ICUs to make clinical decisions regarding volu status due to the high prevalence of central lines and the ease of acquisition from existing catheter. However, there is no association between CVP and circulating blo volume. The CVP is the intravascular pressure in the major thoracic veins, measu relative to atmospheric pressure. It provides an estimate of right atrial pressure as i ideally measured at the junction of the superior vena cava and the right atrium. Th are many factors that affect the CVP including blood volume, vascular tone, ri

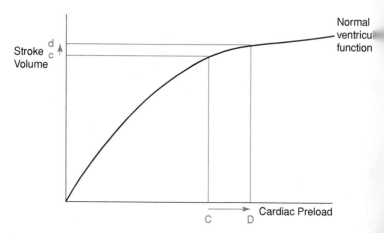

Figure 84.2. Volume unresponsive: Minimal augmentation of stroke volume despite volume expansi a patient with normal biventricular function on the flat portion (high preload) of the Frank–Starling c

TABLE 84.1	Static Markers of Volume Responsiveness			
Parameter	Required Elements	Invasiveness	Values	Comments
Central venous pressure (CVP)	Central venous line	+	Normal: 1–8 cm H_2O Target: 8–12 cm H_2O during sepsis	Most frequently used parameter due to ease of attainment. Predictive power of a single CVP value to predict volume responsiveness is in the 50% range.
Pulmonary artery occlusion pressure (PAOP)	Central access with a 8.5-French introducer catheter to insert the PAC	+++	Normal: 4–12 cm H_2O	Approximates LAP and LVEDP. Used as a surrogate for LVEDP assuming a linear pressure/volume relationship in the left ventricle. Single PAOP reading has a positive predictive value in the 50% range for assessing volume responsiveness. May be useful diagnostically when all parameters obtained from the PAC are evaluated.
Global end diastolic volume index (GEDVI)	Central venous catheter and thermistor-tipped femoral arterial line to perform transpulmonary thermodilution. (PiCCO system)	++	Normal: 680–800 mL/m^2	GEDVI is a moderate predictor of volume responsiveness. When utilized with SVV obtained from the PiCCO system, may improve ability to detect volume responsiveness.
Left ventricular end diastolic area (LVEDA)	Transesophageal echocardiography	++	LVED diameter: 49 ± 4 mm LVED volume: 102 ± 20 mL	Requires expertise and not available routinely in most ICUs. LVEDV is approximated using LVEDA by assuming ventricular geometry. Overall, LVEDA alone is a poor predictor of volume responsiveness.

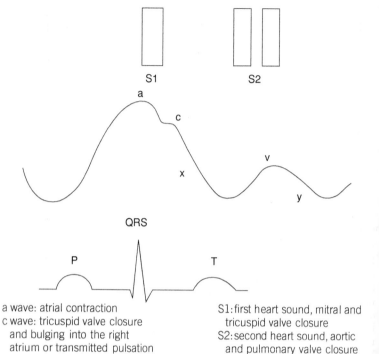

a wave: atrial contraction
c wave: tricuspid valve closure
   and bulging into the right
   atrium or transmitted pulsation
   from the carotid artery
x descent: atrial relaxation
v wave: atrial filling
y wave: atrial emptying

S1: first heart sound, mitral and
   tricuspid valve closure
S2: second heart sound, aortic
   and pulmonary valve closure
P wave: atrial depolarization
QRS complex: ventricular
   depolarization
T wave: ventricular repolarization

Figure 84.3. Normal CVP tracing a wave: atrial contraction c wave: tricuspid valve closure and bulging in
the right atrium or transmitted pulsation from the carotid artery x descent: atrial relaxation v wave: atr
filling y wave: atrial emptying S1: first heart sound, mitral and tricuspid valve closure S2: second heart sour
aortic and pulmonary valve closure P wave: atrial depolarization QRS complex: ventricular depolarization
wave: ventricular repolarization.

ventricular function and compliance, tricuspid valve disease, cardiac rhythm, intr
thoracic pressure (respiratory efforts and PEEP) as well as patient position. The abil
of any CVP value to accurately predict volume responsiveness is in the 56% range.
decrease in CVP is a relatively late sign of intravascular volume depletion particula
in patients with intact vascular tone. For all these reasons, CVP alone should not
utilized to guide fluid management decisions, but should be combined with knowled
of the patients underlying pathophysiology and additional hemodynamic parameter

DYNAMIC MARKERS OF VOLUME RESPONSIVENESS

A dynamic assessment of volume responsiveness is possible at the bedside and esse
tially consists of challenging the patients Frank–Starling curve. The principle is

induce a change in preload and monitor the response by documenting changes in the SV, CO, or other surrogates.

Commonly used techniques of inducing a change in preload are:

- Infusing a fluid bolus,
- Passive leg raising which autotransfuses about 200 to 300 mL of blood in the lower extremities back into the central circulation,
- Utilizing the natural cyclic changes that occur in right ventricular SV, left ventricular preload and ultimately left ventricular SV due to mechanical ventilation–induced changes in right ventricular preload. Large mechanical ventilation–induced changes in left ventricular SV will occur in patients with biventricular preload reserve with no change occurring if one or both of the ventricles is preload independent. To utilize this technique, that patient needs to be in normal sinus rhythm, totally mechanically ventilated with no spontaneous breathing attempts and the tidal volume needs to be adequate (normally 8 to 10 mL/kg).

Commonly used techniques of detecting a change in preload induced by one of the challenges above are:

Dynamic real-time monitoring of SV or CO utilizing esophageal or suprasternal Doppler, bedside echocardiography, or any other technique which can detect changes in CO/SV. If the SV or CO increases by more than 15% with a fluid challenge or in response to a passive leg raise maneuver, the patient is volume responsive. If the response is in the 10% to 15% range, the patient is likely volume responsive and if associated with evidence of end-organ hypoperfusion, the patient may benefit from fluid loading. If the change in SV or CO is less than 10%, the patient is likely not volume responsive and is functioning on the flatter portion of their Frank–Starling curve.

Dynamic changes in descending aortic blood flow velocity utilizing esophageal Doppler. A similar cutoff of 10% to 15% is used for volume responsiveness if this technique is used.

Measuring arterial pulse contour analysis and pulse pressure or stroke volume variation. A pulse pressure variation (PPV) or stroke volume variation (SVV) of greater than 10% to 12% predict volume responsiveness with high sensitivity and specificity (Fig. 84.4).

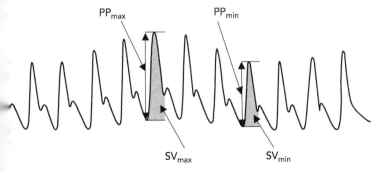

Figure 84.4. Arterial pressure tracing showing the presence of pulse pressure variation (PPV) and stroke volume variation (SVV).

Pulse pressure variation $= 100 \times (PP_{max} - PP_{min})/(PP_{max} + PP_{min})/2$

Stroke volume variation $= 100 \times (SV_{max} - SV_{min})/(SV_{max} + SV_{min})/2$

Functional hemodynamic monitoring and the assessment of volume responsiveness should only be used if a patient has:

* hemodynamic instability (MAP <65 mm Hg),
* evidence of tissue hypoperfusion (urine output <20 mL/hr, anxiety, confusion, lethargy, HR >100 b/min, lactate >2.2 mmol/L).

These criteria should be met before embarking on fluid challenges as many individuals in an ICU may be fluid responsive, but may not be in need of fluid administration. It is the clinical scenario which determines the need for utilizing any hemodynamic monitoring and intervention strategy.

Once the patient is deemed to be hemodynamically unstable, the next step in the evaluation is determination of preload responsiveness using one of the dynamic markers noted above with adequate fluid boluses. If the patient is preload responsive, serial fluid boluses and serial evaluations of continuing preload responsiveness should be performed until the patient is no longer hemodynamically unstable or no longer preload responsive. The septic patient who is persistently hypotensive and no longer preload responsive will require vasopressors titrated. In addition, further diagnostic workup with bedside echocardiography should be performed to identify cardiogenic dysfunction which would benefit from inotropic support or to identify another cause (pericardial tamponade, right ventricular dysfunction in acute pulmonary embolism, etc.).

ScvO₂ MONITORING

ScvO₂ is often used in the ICU as a surrogate of the true SvO₂ and reflects the balance between oxygen delivery and demand. A normal SvO₂ is between 65% and 75% and studies in critically ill patients which simultaneously measured the variables, show that the ScvO₂ is about 5% to 7% higher than the SvO₂ but that the variables track in the same direction with changes in a patient's condition. The ScvO₂ is therefore useful for trend analysis. The determinants of the ScvO₂ are shown in Figure 84.5.

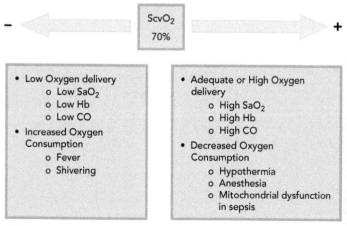

Figure 84.5. Variables affecting the ScvO₂.

SUGGESTED READINGS

Durairaj L, Schmidt G. Fluid therapy in resuscitated sepsis. *Chest.* 2008;133:252–263.
  An excellent review of fluid therapy as well as the static and dynamic predictors of volume responsiveness in the ICU.

Marik PE, Baram M, Vahid B. Does central venous pressure predict fluid responsiveness? A systematic review of the literature and the tale of the seven mares. *Chest.* 2008;134:172–178.
  A literature review of the utility of the CVP as a marker of volume responsiveness.

Monnet X, Rienzo M, Osman D. Passive leg raising predicts fluid responsiveness in the critically ill. *Crit Care Med.* 2006;34:1402–1407.
  A study utilizing esophageal Doppler monitoring of aortic blood flow together with passive leg raising to predict volume responsiveness. A leg raise induced increase of aortic blood flow ≥10% predicted fluid responsiveness with a sensitivity of 97% and a specificity of 94%.

Monnet X, Teboul JL. Volume responsiveness. *Curr Opin Crit Care.* 2007;13:549–553.
  A review of volume responsiveness focusing on the effect of respiratory variation on hemodynamic signals.

Osman D, Ridel C, Ray P, et al. Cardiac filling pressures are not appropriate to predict hemodynamic response to volume challenge. *Crit Care Med.* 2007;35:64–68.
  A retrospective study in a medical ICU showing that a CVP of <8 mm Hg and a PAOP of <12 mm Hg predicted volume responsiveness with a positive predictive value of only 47% and 54% respectively.

Rivers EP, Ander DS, Powell D. Central venous oxygen saturation monitoring in the critically ill patient. *Curr Opin Crit Care.* 2001;7:204–211.
  Excellent review article on $ScvO_2$ monitoring, including pathophysiologic aspects, clinical use, and comparison to SvO_2.

Teboul JL, Saugel B, Cecconi M, et al. Less invasive hemodynamic monitoring in critically ill patients. *Intensive Care Med.* 2016;42(9):1350–1359.
  Excellent review article covering multiple modalities of monitoring and emphasizing choosing appropriate monitoring based on patient clinical response and severity of illness.

Thiel SW, Kollef MH, Isakow W. Noninvasive stroke volume measurement and passive leg raising predict volume responsiveness in medical ICU patients: an observational cohort study. *Crit Care.* 2009;13(4):R111.
  A prospective study in medical ICU patients which revealed that a totally noninvasive suprasternal Doppler probe and passive leg raising was able to predict volume responsiveness with a sensitivity of 80% and specificity of 92%. The CVP in this study was not able to differentiate between volume responders and nonresponders.

85 Pericardiocentesis

Warren Isakow

Pericardiocentesis is indicated in the emergent setting by intensivists to treat cardiac tamponade, and more commonly by cardiologists as a diagnostic or therapeutic procedure for pericardial effusions. The procedure entails insertion of a needle into the pericardial sac, followed by insertion of a guidewire, successive dilations, and placement of a pericardial drainage catheter. In the acute situation of cardiac tamponade, the fluid may be bloody, purulent, inflammatory, or rarely transudative. Ideally, to reduce the risk of complications, the procedure should be performed using real-time echocardiography or fluoroscopy. The overall risk of pericardiocentesis using echocardiographic guidance is approximately 1.3% to 1.6% of procedures. This increases to 20.9% in emergent situations, without echocardiography. This chapter reviews the indications for immediate pericardiocentesis, in the situation of a patient in extremis, and the key steps necessary to aspirate fluid at the bedside.

Pericardiocentesis is performed in the critical care setting to relieve tamponade. Tamponade is a condition in which fluid accumulates in the pericardial space and prevents filling of the cardiac chambers. It is a clinical diagnosis classically marked by hypotension, jugular venous distension, and muffled heart sounds. These clinical signs, known as Beck's triad, are a result of decreased stroke volume and impaired venous return from the pressure effect of fluid in the pericardial sac. Additional signs of tamponade include the presence of pulsus paradoxus (a decrease in systolic pressure >10 mm Hg during inspiration), electrical alternans, and low voltage on electrocardiography.

It is recommended to perform a transthoracic echocardiogram to confirm the presence of an effusion and an ideal window for needle insertion, before proceeding to pericardiocentesis. In the postcardiac surgery patient, a transesophageal echocardiogram may be preferred because of the possibility of a loculated, posterior effusion (Fig. 85.1).

The amount of fluid necessary to cause tamponade varies and depends on the rapidity of fluid accumulation. In cases of malignant effusions, the fluid may collect gradually and stretch the pericardial sac to the point that it contains over 1 L of fluid before creating tamponade. In contrast, trauma may quickly lead to tamponade with only 100 to 200 mL of fluid or blood. A list of possible causes of cardiac tamponade in the ICU is found in Table 85.1. The most common cause of tamponade is malignancy. The decision to perform a bedside pericardiocentesis is based on hemodynamic instability and the development of obstructive shock. Intubation should

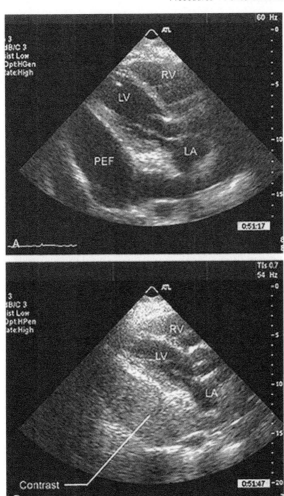

ure 85.1. Parasternal long-axis echocardiogram recorded in a patient with a large posterior pericardial
sion (PEF). Pericardiocentesis is being undertaken with echocardiographic guidance. **A:** There is a large
terior pericardial fluid collection. **B:** Agitated saline has been injected via the pericardiocentesis needle.
re is now echo contrast in the previously clear pericardial space confirming that the pericardiocentesis needle is
he pericardium. LA, left atrium; LV, left ventricle; RV, right ventricle. (Reprinted with permission from
scucci M. *Grossman & Baims Cardiac Catheterization, Angiography and Intervention.* 8th ed. Philadelphia, PA:
ters Kluwer; 2013.)

| TABLE 85.1 | Causes of Cardiac Tamponade in the ICU |

Neoplasm
Infectious pericarditis (viral, bacterial, tubercular, parasitic)
Uremia
Postmyocardial infarction with ventricular rupture
Complication of a catheter-based procedure (pacemaker lead insertion, central line placement, or coronary catherization)
Compressive hematoma after cardiothoracic surgery
Traumatic hemopericardium
Systemic autoimmune diseases (systemic lupus erythematosus, rheumatoid arthritis)
Aortic dissection
Drugs (hydralazine, procainamide, isoniazid, minoxidil, anticoagulation treatment)
Idiopathic

avoided if possible because it will worsen shock caused by tamponade. Vasopresso have limited capacity to improve organ perfusion in this setting.

The safety of the procedure is dramatically improved with the use of echocard ography to guide needle placement and by personnel with experience in performi the procedure (Fig. 85.2). Complications include myocardial injury and lacer tion, ventricular perforation, coronary artery laceration, pneumothorax, ventricu arrhythmias, infection, peritoneal puncture, liver laceration, air embolism, injury the stomach, vascular injury (internal mammary artery), failed drainage, and dea The incidence of such complications is approximately 1.3% to 1.6% with transth racic echocardiographic guidance, but can be as high as 20.9% without imaging gu ance (Fig. 85.3). Major complications such as ventricular rupture and death are ra

There are only a few relative contraindications for pericardiocentesis. Th include coagulopathy (INR >1.4), thrombocytopenia (platelets <50,000), and sm effusions located in a posterior, loculated space. Aortic dissection associated w hemopericardium is an absolute contraindication and patients with this conditi should have immediate surgery. A surgical procedure such as subxiphoid pericardi tomy is preferred in cases where effusions are likely malignant and time is availa (Fig. 85.4). The surgical approach allows for a pericardial window, which reduces rate of recurrence. Leaving a catheter in place for prolonged drainage after peri diocentesis has a similar rate of recurrence as placing a pericardial window. Cath drainage is typically left in place for 24 to 48 hours as the rate of fluid output dim ishes to less than 25 mL per day.

The following steps outline the procedure, which is ideally performed with r time ultrasound guidance.

STEPS FOR BEDSIDE PERICARDIOCENTESIS

1. *Gather the necessary equipment*, which is available at most centers in a prep aged pericardiocentesis kit. Equipment includes, but is not limited to:
   a. Antiseptic (betadine or chlorhexidine gluconate)
   b. Local anesthetic (lidocaine 1%)

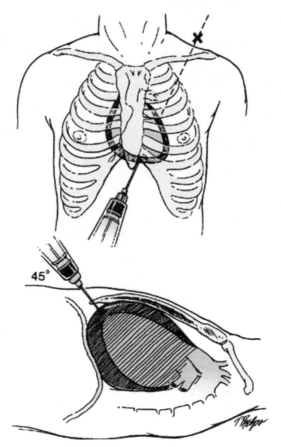

Figure 85.2. Pericardiocentesis. (Reprinted with permission from Nichols DG, Yaster M, Lappe DG, Haller JA, eds. *Golden Hour: The Handbook of Pediatric Advanced Life Support.* 2nd ed. St. Louis, MO: Yearbook; 1996.)

   c. Sterile drapes, gown, cap, and face mask
   d. Syringes, 20 mL and 60 mL
   e. Scalpel, no. 11
   f. Needles, 18 ga, 1.5 in; 25 ga, 5/8 in
   g. Spinal needle, 18 ga, 7.5 to 12 cm
   h. Guidewire
   i. Pericardiocentesis catheter

2. *Patient positioning:* Ensure the patient is on cardiac monitoring with supplemental oxygen. If time permits, decompress the stomach with a nasogastric tube. Place the head of the bed at a 45-degree angle to cause fluid to collect inferiorly and to bring the heart closer to the anterior chest wall.

3. *Identify insertion site:* Locate the patient's xiphoid process and left costal margin by palpation. The most common sites of needle insertion are marked by black

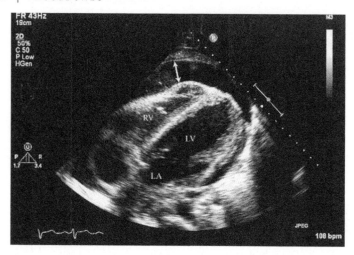

Figure 85.3. Echocardiogram recorded from the subcostal position in a patient with a moderate pericardial effusion. Note the approximate 1.5-cm distance between the pericardium and right ventricular free wall (*arrows*), implying a significant distance between the pericardium and the heart, which may confer a decreased risk of pericardiocentesis if approached from the subcostal position. (Reprinted with permission from Armstrong WF, Ryan T. *Feigenbaum's Echocardiography.* 7th ed. Philadelphia, PA: Wolters Kluwer; 2009.)

dots below. When using echocardiographic guidance, the ultrasound probe can identify the safest site for needle insertion. This is generally the subxiphoid site; however parasternal and apical approaches are also possible, depending on where the pericardial collection width is greatest.

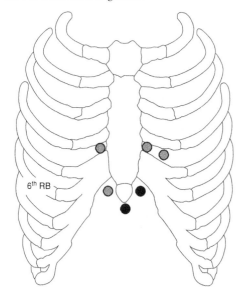

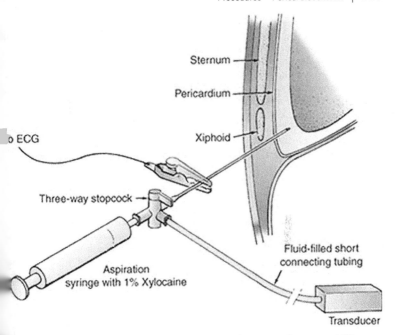

Figure 85.4. Diagram showing the subxiphoid approach to pericardiocentesis with pressure and ST segment monitoring. A hollow, thin-walled, 18-gauge needle is connected via a three-way stopcock to an aspiration syringe filled with 1% Xylocaine and to a short length of fluid-filled tubing connected to a pressure transducer. A sterile V lead of an electrocardiographic recorder may be attached to the metal needle hub. The needle is advanced until pericardial fluid is aspirated or an injury current appears on the V-lead electrocardiographic recording. Once fluid is aspirated, the stopcock is turned so that needle-tip pressure is displayed against simultaneously measured right atrial pressure from a right heart catheter. When needle-tip position within the pericardial space is confirmed, a J-tipped guidewire is passed through the needle into the pericardial space, the needle is removed, and a catheter with end and side holes is advanced over the guidewire and subsequently connected via the three-way stopcock to both the transducer and the syringe. This permits, first, thorough drainage of the pericardial effusion using a catheter rather than a sharp needle and, second, documentation that tamponade physiology is relieved when right atrial pressure falls and intrapericardial pressure is restored to level at or below zero. (Reprinted with permission from Moscucci M. *Grossman & Baims Cardiac Catheterization, Angiography and Intervention.* 8th ed. Philadelphia, PA: Wolters Kluwer; 2013.)

Prep site: Use sterile technique with antiseptic solution, drapes, and anesthetize the skin with lidocaine if time allows.

Needle insertion: First make a small incision at the insertion site with the scalpel. Fill the 20-mL syringe with 10 mL of sterile saline, evacuate the air, and attach to the 18-gauge needle. As the needle is advanced, place constant suction on the syringe. Stop to inject saline (0.5 to 1 mL) intermittently to prevent tissue from clogging the needle.

Needle angle: The needle should be advanced toward the left shoulder at a 30- to 45-degree angle to the abdominal wall. The needle is slowly advanced past the posterior rib border of the left costal margin, then flattened to a 15-degree angle.

7. *Needle advancement:* Continue advancing the needle until pericardial fluid is returned. ST segment elevation or abrupt ECG changes indicate myocardial injury. In this case, the needle should be slowly withdrawn back.

8. *Aspiration:* Remove the 20-mL syringe and replace with the larger available syringe to continue to aspirate as much fluid as possible. In shock due to tamponade, removal of as little as 50 mL of fluid can cause rapid improvement in cardiac output. If time is available and echocardiographic guidance is being utilized injection of agitated saline into the pericardial space can confirm the correct positioning of the needle tip, prior to guidewire insertion. If a bloody aspirate i obtained, it can be injected into a dish and observed for clotting. Pericardial fluid with blood will often not clot, blood aspirated from the ventricle will clot.

9. *Pericardial drain placement:* Pericardial drains help prevent reaccumulation o fluid in the next 1 to 2 days. First insert the guidewire found in the pericardio centesis kit into the needle. Remove the needle over the wire, and keep the wir in hand to avoid losing its place. Slide a 6- to 8-French dilator over the wire t form a tract. A larger skin incision may be needed to advance the dilator. Remov the dilator, and then advance the drainage catheter over the guidewire into th pericardial space. The guidewire is removed and discarded leaving the cathete available for draining the effusion. Suture in place and cover with sterile dressing Fluid can be removed through a three-way stopcock until the patient is hemody namically stable.

10. *Continued catheter drainage:* There are two options for continued drainage of th pericardial fluid. The catheter may be directly connected to tubing and placed o a suction bulb; or the tubing can be left to gravity drainage. To maintain patenc the tubing should be flushed with saline every 1 to 2 hours. Another alternative to fill the tubing and catheter with urokinase. In this case, the tubing must the be opened every 2 to 4 hours to drain for 1 hour.

11. *Diagnostic studies:* There are several possible studies to obtain depending on t clinical situation. The fluid may be sent for cell count with differential, glucos protein, Gram stain, culture (aerobic, anaerobic, AFB), hematocrit, lactate deh drogenase, cytology, tumor markers, hematocrit, rheumatoid factor (RF), a antinuclear antibody (ANA).

12. A postprocedure CXR should be performed to evaluate positioning of the dra and rule out a pneumothorax. A repeat transthoracic echocardiogram shou reveal resolution of the effusion.

SUGGESTED READINGS

Fitch MT, Nicks BA, Pariyadath M, et al. Emergency Pericardiocentesis. Videos in Clin. Medicine. *N Engl J Med.* 2012;366:e7.
  Video presentation which covers the procedure in detail, including risks.
Gluer R, Murdoch D, Haqqani HM, et al. Pericardiocentesis- How to do it. *Heart Lung C* 2015;24(6):621–625.
  Thorough review of the procedure with excellent images.
Imazio M, Brucato A, Trinchero R, et al. Diagnosis and management of pericardial diseases. *Rev Cardiol.* 2009;6:743–751.
  Review of pericardial disease with focus on management of acute and chronic pericarditis.
Loukas M, Walters A, Boon JM, et al. Pericardiocentesis: a clinical anatomy review. *Clin A* 2012;25:872–881.
  Anatomic review of the procedure and potential complications based on anatomic location

Maisch B, Seferovic PM, Ristic AD, et al. Guidelines on the diagnosis and management of pericardial diseases executive summary; The Task force on the diagnosis and management of pericardial diseases of the European society of cardiology. *Eur Heart J.* 2004;25:587.
Provides a review of the evidence used to create the current guidelines on managing constrictive pericarditis, tamponade, and acute pericarditis.
Spodick DH. Acute cardiac tamponade. *N Engl J Med.* 2003;349:684–690.
In depth review of causes, diagnosis, and management of cardiac tamponade.

86 ECLS

Patrick R. Aguilar

Although not technologically novel, extracorporeal life support (ECLS) represents an area of intense recent development in the care of critically ill patients. A variety of modalities exist to provide various levels of support to patients with cardiac and respiratory failure. Here, the discussion will focus on understanding the functionality of and evidence for the use of ECLS, selecting which level of support is appropriate in a given clinical situation, considering which candidates are most likely to benefit from ECLS, and reviewing the basic management of the patient on ECLS.

ECLS FUNCTION

Four components make up the most basic ECLS circuit: a drainage cannula, a pump, an oxygenator, and a return cannula. Blood exits the body via a drainage cannula. The drainage cannula is connected to a pump, which propels the blood forward to the oxygenator where gas exchange occurs. From there, the blood flows back into the body via a return cannula.

The size and position of the cannulas vary depending on intention and will be discussed later. Two basic types of pump are currently in use for ECLS. Roller-head pumps apply a mechanical force to the tubing, propelling blood forward. The function of these devices is similar to that seen in dialysis and apheresis machines. Centrifugal pumps, more commonly used for their improved durability and lower degree of heat generation and hemolysis, utilize impellers which sit in a plastic casing and come into direct contact with the blood. These impellers spin at a rate driven by a motorized magnet which sits inside the metal structure of the pump. In either circumstance, the number of rotations per minute can be adjusted to optimize flow rates through the oxygenator. Cannula size, volume status, and cardiac contractility, among other factors, affect the efficiency of flow in relation to pump activity.

A variety of oxygenators exist. Membrane oxygenators used in ECLS differ from those used in cardiopulmonary bypass in that the former lack a blood–air interface, do not pool blood, and therefore require lower degrees of anticoagulation. ECLS oxygenators generally function by passing blood through hollow fibers. Gas, of varying oxygen concentrations, passes across the fibers allowing blood to be oxygenated and carbon dioxide (CO_2) to be eliminated.

CO_2 elimination in ECLS is highly efficient and is generally controlled by the speed of gas transfer through the oxygenator, which is known as the "sweep speed." This can be increased to eliminate more CO_2 and decreased to reduce elimination. Oxygen exchange is less efficient and is controlled primarily by two variables: rate of blood flow through the oxygenator and fraction of delivered oxygen in the oxygenator

(FDO$_2$). A blender on the oxygenator allows for the gas to be composed of more (or less) oxygen as dictated by the clinical situation, ranging from an FDO$_2$ of 21% to 100%. The rate of blood flow through the oxygenator depends on multiple variables described above.

Many other components can be added into the circuit, depending on the clinical need. In most circumstances, a device is used to flow heated water through the oxygenator in a manner that maintains the temperature of the blood without actually having contact between the blood and the heated water. In the absence of such a device, the volume of blood outside of the body (sometimes as much as 4 to 5 L per minute) may be cooled to ambient temperatures.

Access sites along the cannula tubing can be included to facilitate blood draws or allow addition of a second extracorporeal device such as continuous renal replacement therapy or apheresis. These access sites can be convenient but have the potential to increase the potential for clot formation owing to turbulence at the stopcock sites. These access points can also be sites of bacterial contamination or entrainment of air into the circuit. Importantly, all access to the circuit should be located proximal to the oxygenator to allow for any entrained air or clots to be sent to the oxygenator rather than directly into the patient's circulation. Pressure and saturation monitoring devices can also be attached at various points along the circuit to assist with clinical decision making and mechanical optimization.

ECLS MODES

ECLS comprises three distinct modes of support: extracorporeal CO$_2$ removal (ECCO2R), venovenous extracorporeal membrane oxygenation (VV-ECMO) and venoarterial ECMO (VA-ECMO). The primary difference between these modes rests in the physiologic functionality being supported by the circuit.

ECCO2R

In ECCO2R, smaller cannulas are utilized to drain and return blood from the body. This allows for a lower rate of vascular complications, a lesser need for anticoagulation, and better patient tolerance of the cannulas. Importantly, the lower blood flows generated through the cannulas in this circumstance are generally insufficient to provide more than a modest degree of support in oxygenation. The efficiency of carbon dioxide elimination, however, enables excellent control of hypercapnia, even with relatively low blood flow rates. A recent systematic review demonstrated that the majority of patients treated with ECCO2R for exacerbations of chronic obstructive pulmonary disease (COPD) were able to either avoid endotracheal intubation or be weaned more quickly from mechanical ventilation after application of ECCO2R. No randomized controlled trials have been done to evaluate the impact of ECCO2R on mortality in any context. However, one retrospective analysis demonstrated a clinically and statistically significant improvement in ICU and hospital lengths of stay associated with the use of ECCO2R in exacerbations of COPD. While the impact of this technology on outcomes in acute respiratory distress syndrome (ARDS) has yet to be established, multiple proof-of-concept studies have demonstrated efficacy of ECCO2R in supporting CO$_2$ elimination in patients with ARDS and thus facilitating ultraprotective ventilation strategies. ECCO2R is not yet widely commercially available and multiple clinical trials are attempting to define the role it may play in supporting critically ill patients with respiratory failure.

VV-ECMO

VV-ECMO involves the use of larger cannulas and higher blood flow rates to provid support for oxygenation. The volume of blood flow that is necessary to achieve this en is variable and depends primarily on the size of the patient. Cannula placement can b adjusted to accomplish different therapeutic goals. Conventionally, a drainage cannul is positioned with its tip in the intrahepatic inferior vena cava (IVC) via the femor vein. This placement location is preferred to more distal locations on the basis of th relative collapsibility of positions lower in the IVC. This collapsibility would be asso ciated with an unacceptable impact on blood flow rates. A return cannula is general placed in the right atrium via the internal jugular vein. Blood is returned there from the oxygenator. Although relatively easy to place urgently in a patient who is critical ill, this cannulation strategy has a number of complications. First, the proximity of th return cannula to the negative pressure generated at the tip of the drainage cannula ca cause recirculation, a situation in which oxygenated blood is returned to the circu rather than circulated through the body. This can be affected by the speed of the pum (and thus the degree of negative pressure at the drainage cannula tip), the volume st tus of the patient, and the proximity of the two cannulas to each other. Additionall patients are necessarily immobile as a result of the femoral cannulation site. To addr these issues, some centers have used cannulation of the subclavian vein in place of o of the other cannulation sites. More recently, single-site, dual lumen cannulas have be developed. These are slightly more technically difficult to place and often require flu roscopic and/or echocardiographic guidance. The drainage lumen is positioned in t IVC and the return lumen sits adjacent to the tricuspid valve, ideally with flow aim directly into the right ventricle. These devices allow for greater mobility, althou movement of the catheter can result in changes in flow and improper directionality the return lumen. Regardless of cannulation strategy, the blood flow rate is occasion insufficient to meet the oxygenation needs of the patient. In those circumstances, extra drainage cannula can be placed at another site to allow for higher flows.

The pool of evidence regarding VV-ECMO is significantly more robu although it has yet to clearly establish the proper role for this technology in patie with respiratory failure. Early studies, such as that funded by the NIH in the 197 failed to demonstrate a mortality benefit of ECLS in this context. This study wa randomized controlled trial comparing patients treated with ECLS to those trea with conventional ventilation alone. Although no mortality benefit was observ several issues confound the interpretation of these results. Importantly, out of patients with acute respiratory failure, the total survival was just under 9%. Mana ment of respiratory failure in that era did not adhere to the current understandin best practices, possibly explaining the substantial mortality observed across the stu Additionally, given the vast technical difficulties associated with the use of ECLS is important to recognize that provision of this therapy at any two centers (part larly those with less experience), may be sufficiently different as to generate diffe results. Finally, ECLS in these patients was initiated several days into their acute re ratory failure, though duration of mechanical ventilation prior to initiation of EC has been shown to impact outcomes after ECLS. Despite the skepticism that n rally followed that trial, ECLS utilization continued over the ensuing three deca In particular, pediatric and neonatal applications drove advances in the techno of various components of the ECLS circuit. Changes in pump mechanics as we the plastic composition of the circuit tubing and oxygenator membranes drasti impacted the tolerance, performance, and functionality of ECLS over this time.

The CESAR trial, published in 2009, demonstrated a mortality benefit associated with referral to a center with experience in the provision of ECLS. While this was not, itself, a positive result for the impact of ECLS on disease, it revived interest in the technology among many adult intensivists. The same year, pandemic H1N1 influenza was associated with a substantial burden of disease and mortality, particularly among younger patients. A cohort study and propensity-matched analysis of ECLS use in French ICUs during this time demonstrated no mortality benefit in the matched cohort of patients treated with ECLS compared with those treated with mechanical ventilation alone. However, severely hypoxemic and younger patients treated with ECLS were unable to be matched with similar patients treated without ECLS. This group was not included in the propensity score analysis but, when reviewed individually, did have a lower mortality than the cohort as a whole.

VV-ECMO use has been widely reported in a variety of causes of the ARDS including pulmonary contusions and ARDS following trauma, inhalation injuries, and drowning. Beyond ARDS, VV-ECMO has also been studied in a number of other contexts. In particular, there are many reports of the use of ECLS to support patients awaiting lung transplantation. Additionally, VV-ECMO has been used in cases of status asthmaticus, severe pneumonia, pulmonary hypertension, pulmonary vasculitis and hemorrhage, exacerbations of chronic pulmonary diseases, and surgical airway reconstruction in patients who were unable to be otherwise supported during the procedure.

Unfortunately, there is not clarity on the proprietary role of VV-ECMO in the treatment of patients with respiratory failure. However, the EOLIA trial (clinicaltrials. gov NCT01470703) is currently enrolling patients in a randomized, controlled-trial comparing early initiation of ECLS to management with conventional mechanical ventilation. This trial and others like it are desperately needed to help delineate the appropriate role of ECLS in this context.

VA-ECMO

VA-ECMO represents the most intensive level of extracorporeal support for cardiopulmonary function. Large cannulas are used to generate sufficient blood flows to support oxygenation and CO2 elimination. The placement of the return cannula in the arterial system also allows for support of hemodynamics for patients with hypotension. Cannulas are conventionally placed in the femoral vein and femoral artery though many options for variability in this cannulation strategy. In particular, the counter-current return of oxygenated blood into the femoral artery does not always enable oxygenated blood return to reach the apex of the aortic arch or the ostia of the coronary arteries. In that event, oxygenated blood passes through the abdominal visceral and lower extremity circulation before returning to the heart, passing through the lungs, and ultimately reaching the coronary arteries, upper extremities, and brain. To correct this and allow for oxygenated blood return to directly reach these critical structures, the return cannula can be placed in the subclavian artery. Additionally, extra return cannulas can be placed in the venous system to allow oxygenated blood return to the right side of the heart. Finally, in some patients central VA-ECMO provided by utilizing a thoracotomy to place cannulas in various positions within the heart and central vasculature. This allows for increased flows and cannula stability but is obviously substantially more technically difficult and attended by significantly higher rates of complication and morbidity. However, the cannulation strategy is structured, the rate of blood flow can be adjusted to provide a variable degree of hemodynamic support. Full-dose anticoagulation is necessary in this context to prevent the development of clots in the arterial system, which can embolize to critical structures and cause significant ischemic damage.

VA-ECMO is utilized in a variety of shock circumstances. In cardiogenic shock, use of VA-ECMO is associated with outcomes that are superior to historical index values. VA-ECMO has been reported as a mechanism of support in cardiogenic shock from various forms of cardiomyopathy, fulminant myocarditis, and obstructive shock from valvular disease or pulmonary emboli. Additionally, many centers perform extracorporeal resuscitation (e-CPR) in instances where conventional cardiopulmonary resuscitation and advanced cardiac life support measures have failed. Although mortality is very high with this intervention, it represents an area of intense research as it potentially offers a significant benefit for patients who have a near-certain mortality otherwise. As with VV-ECMO, randomized clinical trial results are lacking in this context. However, as centers enhance their use of this technology, there will be many opportunities for collaboration in developing a more robust understanding of the best practices associated with VA-ECMO.

PATIENT SELECTION

ECLS should be considered in patients who have respiratory, cardiac, or combined respiratory and cardiac failure that is advanced, life-threatening, and refractory to less invasive measures of support. In keeping with the paucity of evidence described in the use of ECLS above, there is a poor understanding of who most benefits from this technology from a patient selection standpoint. ECLS is expensive, resource intense, and fraught with complications (described below). The database of the Extracorporeal Life Support Organization has been utilized to assess predictors of mortality on ECLS. These predictors can be analyzed using the SAVE and RESP risk assessment tools, referenced below. For patients placed on VV-ECMO, renal failure, advanced age, immunocompromised status, and associated nonpulmonary infection were among the variables associated with impaired hospital survival. Among those treated with VA-ECMO, chronic renal failure, lower serum bicarbonate level, lower pulse pressure, and congenital heart disease were associated with increased mortality. Longer duration of pre-ECLS mechanical ventilation and prior cardiac arrest were associated with increased mortality on both modes of ECLS.

In general, patients with acute, treatment refractory cardiac or pulmonary disease should be considered for ECLS when they have good premorbid functional status and generally good physiologic function outside of their acute illness. Consideration of ECLS should occur early in the course of disease and involve a collaborative team of physicians, surgeons, nurses, and respiratory therapists who are familiar with the technology. The RESP and SAVE scores referenced above provide a useful understanding of factors associated with greater likelihood of survival on ECMO. However, a comprehensive decision involving risk and benefit analysis for each particular patient must be undertaken prior to initiating ECLS.

COMPLICATIONS

Complications specific to ECLS can involve mechanical issues related to the ECMO device, vascular damage from the cannulas, and complications associated with anticoagulation. According to the most recent report of the Extracorporeal Life Support Organization registry, among adults treated with ECMO for respiratory failure, pump malfunction occurred in 2.1% of patients, oxygenator failure (typically due to clot aggregation in the oxygenator) occurred in 16.1% of patients, and cannula site bleeding occurred in 17.2% of patients. The most feared complication, intracranial hemorrhage, occurred in 3.9% of patients and was fatal in 17% of affected patients. In a separate report, ischemic stroke was reported to occur in 2% of patients on VV-ECMO. GI bleeding has been reported to occur in as many as 13.6% of patients treated with ECLS and is associated with an increased mortality. Infectious complications are similar to those seen in other settings involving central venous access, though there may be a slight increase in incidence of fungemia among patients on ECLS. Long-term outcomes after ECLS, including potential functional and psychological outcomes, are poorly understood and represent an area of active research.

MANAGEMENT OF PATIENTS ON ECLS

The comprehensive management of patients on ECLS is complex and should be undertaken by clinicians with experience and dexterity in dealing with this particular patient population. The optimal mode of mechanical ventilation on ECLS is controversial. Some centers engage in a practice of "lung rest," in which patients may be removed from the ventilator entirely. Others provide aggressive lung recruitment with higher pressures to attempt to encourage improved pulmonary functionality. Whatever mode of ventilation is selected should represent the clinician's best effort at preventing furthering lung injury while ECLS is continued. ECLS does not represent a therapeutic intervention aimed at treating the underlying disease. Instead, it provides support for the patient while the underlying disease is separately treated. An important principle, therefore, is to avoid exacerbating organ injury while providing support.

Anticoagulation remains a complex problem in ECLS. It is difficult to balance preventing thrombosis in the ECLS circuit while avoiding bleeding complications in the patient. A wide array of tests can be used to monitor levels of anticoagulation. Decisions about which to use should be made in the context of the specific center treating the patient with awareness of their particular laboratory's strengths and weaknesses.

Some patients are stable enough to ambulate on ECLS. Physical therapy is an important part of ICU care for all critically ill patients. Many centers employ ambulation programs or bedside physical therapy to try and maintain strength and stamina while patients are on ECLS. Analgesia should be provided as needed but sedation should be limited to whatever is necessary to ensure safety and comfort without preventing rehabilitation, whether it includes ambulation or not.

SEPARATING FROM ECLS

Patients are supported with the appropriate mode of ECLS for the duration of the time needed to support recovery. In some cases, organ recovery is not achieved despite aggressive measures to treat the underlying cause of dysfunction. Those represent ethically challenging cases as patients may be awake and seem stable on full support. In those instances, open and honest discussions regarding the propriety of continued support should involve patients and families with the aim of reaching the decision most consistent with their goals. In patients who do recover, ECLS can be weaned by way of decreasing blood flow rate through the oxygenator, the FDO2, and the sweep speed until organ recovery is sufficiently achieved to allow for adequate functionality on appropriate levels of ventilatory and hemodynamic support in the absence of a meaningful contribution from the ECLS circuit. At that point, the cannulas can be removed and usual critical care can continue to be provided.

SUGGESTED READINGS

Braune S, Burchardi H, Engel M, et al. The use of extracorporeal carbon dioxide removal to avoid intubation in patients failing non-invasive ventilation—a cost analysis. *BMC Anesthesio* 2015;15:160–167.

Brenner K, Abrams DC, Agerstrand CL, et al. Extracorporeal carbon dioxide removal for refractory status asthmaticus: experience in distinct exacerbation phenotypes. *Perfusion.* 2014;29(1) 26–28.

Brodie D, Bachetta M. Extracorporeal membrane oxygenation for ARDS in adults. *N Engl J Me* 2011;365:1905–1914.

Diaz-Guzman E, Hoopes CW, Zwischenberger JB. The evolution of extracorporeal life suppo as a bridge to lung transplantation. *ASAIO Journal.* 2013;59:3–10.

Fanelli V, Ranieri MV, Mancebo J, et al. Feasibility and safety of low-flow extracorporeal carbo dioxide removal to facilitate ultra-protective ventilation in patients with moderate acu respiratory distress syndrome. *Crit Care.* 2016;10(20):36–43.

Hryniewicz K, Sandoval Y, Samara M, et al. Percutaneous venoarterial extracorporeal membrar oxygenation for refractory cardiogenic shock is associated with improved short- and lon term survival. *ASAIO J.* 2016;62(4):397–402.

Lorusso R, Centofanti P, Gelsomino S, et al. Venoarterial extracorporeal membrane oxygenatic for acute fulminant myocarditis in adult patients: a 5-year multi-institutional experienc *Ann Thorac Surg.* 2016;101(3):919–926.

Luyt CE, Bréchot N, Demondion P, et al. Brain injury during venovenous extracorporeal mer brane oxygenation. 2016;42(5):897–907.

Mazzeffi M, Kiefer J, Greenwood J, et al. Epidemiology of gastrointestinal bleeding in adv patients on extracorporeal life support. *Intens Care Med.* 2015;41(11):2015.

Paden ML, Conrad SA, Rycus PT, et al. Extracorporeal life support organization registry rep 2012. *ASAIO J.* 2013;59:202–210.

Pham T, Combes A, Rozé H, et al. Extracorporeal membrane oxygenation for pandemic influer A (H1N1)-induced acute respiratory distress syndrome: a cohort study and propensi matched analysis. *Am J Resp Crit Care.* 2013;187(3):276–285.

Schmidt M, Burrell A, Roberts L, et al. Predicting survival after ECMO for refractory cardioge shock: the survival after veno-arterial-ECMO (SAVE) score. *Eur Heart J.* 2015;36(3 2246–2256.

Schmidt M, Bailey M, Sheldrake J, et al. Predicting survival after extracorporeal membr. oxygenation for severe acute respiratory failure. The respiratory extracorporeal membr oxygenation survival prediction (RESP) score. *Am J Respir Crit Care Med.* 2014;189(1 1374–1382.

Sklar MC, Beloncle F, Katsios CM, et al. Extracorporeal carbon dioxide removal in patie with chronic obstructive pulmonary disease: a systematic review. *Intensive Care Med.* 20 41(10):1752–1762.

Zapol WM, Snider MT, Hill JD, et al. Extracorporeal membrane oxygenation in severe ac respiratory failure. A randomized prospective study. *JAMA.* 1979;242(20):2193–2196

87

Basic Critical Care Ultrasound

Amy Cacace and Warren Isakow

INTRODUCTION TO CRITICAL CARE ULTRASOUND

Critical Care Ultrasound refers to clinician-performed and interpreted bedside ultrasound to help diagnose and manage critically ill patients with cardiopulmonary failure. Comparable to the physical examination, it is a noninvasive, rapid, and repeatable exam performed by the provider directly caring for the patient and is designed to answer specific clinical questions. The results are immediately available to guide time-sensitive decision-making. Multiple focused examinations are performed serially to document clinical responses to specific interventions. It differs from standard echocardiography and ultrasonography, which provide delayed, comprehensive, and mostly single examinations for diagnostic purposes, which are interpreted by physicians who are disassociated from the clinical care of the patient.

Ultrasound is an ideal modality for bedside use in the ICU and should be used diagnostically as well as for procedural guidance. Ultrasound involves no ionizing radiation, avoids patient transportation, and is repeatable. It functions as an extension of the physical examination. Barriers to the use of ultrasound in the critically ill include inadequate training, cost of equipment, difficulty achieving adequate ultrasound windows in ill patients for various reasons (obesity, dressings, incisions), and the risk of transmitting infections if a cleaning protocol of the probes and device is not followed.

Appropriate clinical application of the technology is dependent on the knowledge and skill of the operator/interpreter. Expertise in Critical Care Ultrasound requires a combination of didactic training, as well as many hours of bedside scanning and image interpretation sessions to review common pathologies. Critical Care Ultrasound is best learned at the bedside from a mentor who is an expert in the field. Societal guidelines have been published which define minimum criteria for achieving initial competence in Critical Care and Focused Cardiac Ultrasonography. The reader is encouraged to review these documents.

This chapter is a *brief* introduction to basic critical care diagnostic ultrasound. Topics include lung, cardiac, and abdominal ultrasound, and their application in the evaluation of patients with acute respiratory failure and shock (Table 87.1).

Basic Ultrasound Physics

Ultrasound refers to sound waves with a frequency of >20 kHz, which is too high for the human ear to hear. These high frequency waves are used to generate images of internal organs and can also detect blood flow velocities. Sound waves (vibrations)

TABLE 87.1 Comparison of Bedside Ultrasonography with Common Diagnostic Modalities Used in the Intensive Care Unit

Modes of Assessment	Immediately Available	Easily Repeatable	Specific/ Sensitive	Noninvasive/ Safe	Interpreted by Bedside Provider
History and Physical	Yes	Yes	+/–	Yes	Yes
Chest X-ray	No	No	+/–	+/–	+/–
Chest CT Scan	No	No	Yes	+/–	+/–
Esophageal Doppler	No	+/–	+/–	+/–	Yes
Pulmonary Artery Catheter	No	Yes	+/–	+/–	Yes
Formal Echo	No	No	Yes	Yes	+/–
Bedside Ultrasound	Yes	Yes	+/–	Yes	Yes

are transmitted through different media (solid, liquid, or gas) and are governed by the following relationship: propagation velocity = frequency × wavelength. In body tissues, sound waves propagate at approximately 1500 meters per second. Therefore, if the frequency of the waves is 1000 Hz (cycles per second), the wavelength is 1.5 m which is obviously inadequate for human ultrasound imaging since many of the tissues of interest are only millimeters thick.

Therefore, extremely high frequency sound waves are utilized in medical ultrasound (in the range of 2 to 15 MHz). Ultrasound waves with higher frequency will deliver higher resolution images but this needs to be balanced with the ability of the ultrasound waves to penetrate into the body. Lower frequency ultrasound waves tend to be less attenuated by tissue and so penetrate further.

Ultrasound waves are generated by a piezoelectric crystal transducer within an ultrasound probe. Electrical energy is converted by the crystals into movement and vibrations which set up the ultrasound waves which propagate into the surrounding. The unique properties of each crystal will determine the frequency of the wave generated. The transducer probes generate the sound waves but also receive returning waves from the tissues. Pulses of sound waves are generated by the transducer and then received back. It is this pulsed natured of the signal and the time delay between generation and reception which allows for the ultrasound machine to derive the distance of the structure of interest from the probe. Thousands of pulses per second are possible with modern machines. The returning waves are converted back to an electrical signal which is amplified and processed to generate the final image which will provide information about depth and tissue characteristics of the structures encountered by the sound waves. Modern transducer probes often have these crystals arranged, electronically steered or phased arrays, to generate a complete image from multiple wavelets that are generated in a series of radial lines.

The echogenicity of a particular tissue is determined by the degree of reflection of the ultrasound waves at tissue interfaces. If most of the waves are reflected back at a tissue interface, the tissue will appear very bright or echogenic. An example of this is bone which reflects most ultrasound waves and will not allow for visualization of the structures deeper to the bone. If most of the waves penetrate through the interface without reflection of the waves, the tissue will appear darker or black (hypoechoic) and this is typically seen with fluids. Varying degrees of gray are therefore seen with tissue imaging, dependent on the properties of the tissue.

The Ultrasound Machine

Modes

2D or B-mode (brightness mode): Standard, familiar, default mode which generates slice images. The machine processes the returning sound waves and displays structures as a gray scale cross-sectional image.

M-mode (motion mode): Plots motion over time. This mode provides excellent temporal resolution and is useful for visualizing moving structures and measuring cavity dimensions.

Doppler: The Doppler effect, first described by Christian Doppler in 1843, refers to a frequency change that occurs in the echo signal when an object moves toward or away from the source of the ultrasound waves. If a wave source is moving toward an observer, the waves are compressed causing a decrease in the wavelength. The opposite applies if the wave source is moving away from the observer.

- **Continuous Wave Doppler** utilizes a continuous cycle of ultrasound waves with simultaneous acquisition of the returning echoes. The ultrasound machine analyses the complex mix of returning echoes and Doppler shifts and generates a spectral Doppler layout from which it is able to discern the direction of flow as well as the peak velocity and mean velocity. CW Doppler is used routinely to measure high velocity flows in the heart, across valves and is useful for estimating pulmonary artery pressures.
- **Pulse Wave Doppler** allows for discrimination for where a particular Doppler shift signal arises from an ultrasound beam axis (the sample volume). PW Doppler is utilized in assessing blood velocity at a specific location of interest and is best used with low velocity flows as it is susceptible to a phenomenon called aliasing (Nyquist limit). We routinely use PW Doppler to assess the velocity of blood in the aortic outflow tract to estimate stroke volume.
- **Color Doppler** is a form of pulsed wave Doppler utilizing a grid with multiple interrogation points (pixels) and is generally used superimposed on the 2D image as a way to determine direction and velocity of flow in a large sample area.

Limitations of Doppler: the major limitation of Doppler is the need to align the ultrasound beam with the direction of the blood flow. This angle should at a maximum be 15 degrees to ensure accuracy.

Adjustable Settings

Gain: adjustments in gain allow for the operator to change the brightness and should be set to allow the maximum contrast resolution for the area of interest. Many machines have total gain, near gain, and far gain settings and users should try et uniform gain across the image. Excessive gain should be avoided.

Depth: the depth should be adjusted so that the area of interest is viewed in the middle of the ultrasound screen. Appropriate depth settings can often improve resolution.

Transducers

- Transducers vary by frequency and footprint (Table 87.2).
- **Frequency:** number of cycles of compressions and rarefactions that occur in 1 second, and is inversely proportional to wavelength.
  - Higher frequency transducers generate higher resolution images, but do not penetrate deeply into tissues. These are typically used to visualize superficial structures like vessels and nerves and are used for procedures like central line insertion. Most linear vascular probes have a frequency of 5 to 10 MHz.
  - Lower frequency transducers (1.0 to 5.0 MHz) are commonly used as phased array probes for cardiac, lung, and abdominal imaging as they provide more penetration to visualize deeper structures.
- **Footprint:** size and shape of probe area in contact with skin.

Standard Transducer Movements

- **Slide/Move:** movement of ultrasound footprint across skin surface (example: sliding probe vertically down anterior chest to evaluate lung slide between different rib spaces).
- **Rotate:** turning clockwise or counterclockwise without angling or changing the location on the body, in order to obtain an orthogonal plane (e.g., moving from a parasternal long axis to a parasternal short axis).
- **Tilt/Rock:** angling the transducer on its long axis on the same tomographic plane (e.g., when the inferior vena cava is visualized horizontally across the screen with the probe placed perpendicular to the abdomen, rocking the probe upward will demonstrate the inferior vena cava entering the right atrium).
- **Angle:** angling the transducer without moving it, in order to view adjacent tomographic planes (e.g., angling the probe side to side to appreciate the aorta running laterally to the inferior vena cava).

LUNG ULTRASOUND AND THE EVALUATION OF ACUTE RESPIRATORY FAILURE

Key Points

- Air has classically been considered the enemy of ultrasound as its reflective properties inhibit the ultrasound signal from reaching underlying structures.
- Lung ultrasound is therefore generally restricted to patterns seen at the pleural surface.
- Greater than 90% of etiologies of acute respiratory failure involve the pleural surface and cause ultrasound artifacts.
- These artifacts create specific patterns that correlate to traditional physical exam findings. These artifacts or lung ultrasound signatures, define lung ultrasound. They include lung slide, A-lines, B-lines, consolidation, and effusion.
- Lung ultrasound is superior compared to chest x-ray, and comparable to CT in the detection of pneumothorax, normal aeration patterns, interstitial syndrome, consolidation, and pleural effusion.
- The Bedside Lung Ultrasound in Emergency protocol (BLUE) is a rapid noninvasive exam which provides a decision tree framework to help delineate the most likely etiology in patients with acute respiratory failure (Fig. 87.1).

TABLE 37.2 | Characteristics, Uses and Advantages of Three Commonly Used Transducers

	Linear	Phased Array	Curvilinear
Footprint			
Frequency	5–10 MHz	1–5 MHz	2–5 MHz
Depth	9 cm	35 cm	30 cm
Uses	Vascular, lung, superficial structures	Cardiac, abdominal, lung, pleura, IVC	Abdominal, FAST exam
Advantages	Higher resolution	Small footprint fits between rib spaces	Large footprint with wide field of view

IVC, inferior vena cava; FAST, Focused Assessment with Sonography for Trauma.

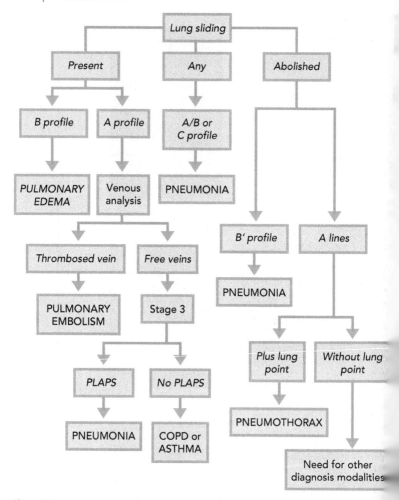

Figure 87.1. A decision tree utilizing lung ultrasonography to guide diagnosis of severe dyspnea.

Performing the Exam

Probe Selection (Fig. 87.2)

- **Phased array probe**
  - Set the depth to 15 cm to evaluate for consolidation, pleural effusions, and identify the diaphragm.
  - Able to appreciate lung slide, however provides less resolution of the pleural surface compared to linear probes. Decreasing the gain setting will often make the pleural line more apparent.
  - Has the advantage of not needing to switch transducers to perform a rapid and sequential lung, cardiac, and abdominal exam in a deteriorating patient.

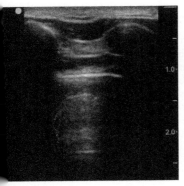
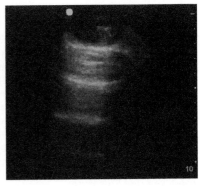

Figure 87.2. Comparison of normal lung ultrasound using a linear probe (**left**) and a phased array probe (**right**). Notice the higher resolution with the linear probe, however only able to penetrate a few centimeters.

High frequency, linear probe
- Has better resolution of superficial structures, making it easier to evaluate the pleural interface, including detecting lung slide and lung point.

Micro convex probe
- Small footprint allows for easy visualization between rib spaces.
- Frequencies between 5 and 8 mHz.

Machine Settings

- **Basic/abdominal setting:** avoid machine's advanced settings (i.e., cardiac presets) which diminish the artifacts that define lung ultrasound.

Probe Positioning (Fig. 87.3)

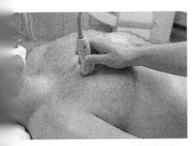
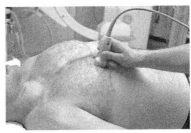

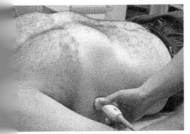

Figure 87.3. To evaluate for A lines, B lines, and lung slide, place the transducer on the anterior chest perpendicular to the chest wall and slide between the rib spaces with the indicator at 12 o'clock. To evaluate for pleural effusions, atelectasis/consolidation, and subdiaphragmatic structures, place the transducer in the mid-axillary line with the indicator at 12 o'clock. Slide the transducer superiorly and inferiorly until the diaphragm is identified. To completely evaluate this area, may need to move the transducer more posteriorly while angling upward toward the horizon.

- **Sagittal/longitudinal,** indicator pointing to 12 o'clock, **perpendicular** to chest wall.
- *Bilateral anterior chest*—examine artifacts between multiple rib spaces over the anterior chest, starting apically and moving down.
  - Convention is to include both adjacent rib shadows on the image to assess the underlying pleura and lung.
  - Multiple parallel and vertical scan lines are recommended.
- *Bilateral posterior and lateral axillary position*—obtain image in the mid-axillary and posterior axillary lines, identify the diaphragm, evaluate for atelectasis and pleural fluid, and assess subdiaphragmatic structures (liver/spleen). To do this correctly, the operator often needs to start very posteriorly and angle the probe toward the horizon.

The Five Lung Signatures

1. Lung Slide

Characteristics

- Horizontal hyperechoic line approximately 0.5 cm deep to the origin of rib shadow
- Dynamic finding, variably described as shimmering, sparkling, glimmering, twinkling appearance.
- Represents the movement of the visceral on the parietal pleura. Is often more apparent at the lung base than at the apex of the lung.
- Presence of lung slide rules out pneumothorax at the point of interrogation.
- Lung pulse is not the same as lung slide, but refers to pulsation of the pleural line interface with each cardiac pulsation, and is also able to rule out a pneumothorax when seen.
- Utilizing M mode, normal lung slide results in a finding described as the "sand beach sign." This provides evidence of movement of the underlying lung, underneath the pleural line (the sand on a beach) as opposed to the relatively stationary superficial soft tissue structures (seen as "waves" on M mode imaging). If a pneumothorax is present, the M mode finding is referred to as the stratosphere sign or barcode sign and consists of multiple horizontal lines on the screen without the haziness generated by lung motion (Fig. 87.4).
- Lung POINT: sign referring to the point or edge of a pneumothorax. Sliding lung is seen coming in and out of the ultrasound image as the patient breaths, and is juxtaposed to an area with absent lung slide. This finding is very specific for pneumothorax but not very sensitive, as it is not always seen and depends on pneumothorax location related to probe position.

Differential Diagnosis for Loss of Lung Slide

- Pneumothorax
- Severe pneumonia or ARDS with significant loss of lung compliance
- Prolonged apnea
- Prior history of pleurodesis
- Examination on the left side with right mainstem intubation
- Ventilatory modes without significant tidal volumes (high frequency oscillation)
- Bullous lung disease
- Adhesions
- Pulmonary contusions

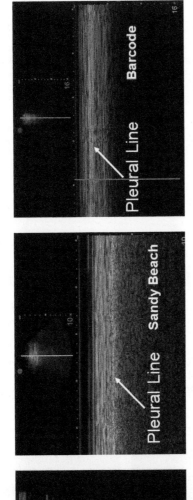

Figure 87.4. Lung slide represents the movement between the visceral and parietal pleura and is displayed as a bright, shimmering line between rib shadows (**left**). Movement beneath the pleural line can be assessed using M-mode. If the lung is in contact and moving below the pleural line, a grainy or sandy pattern is seen (**middle**). If there is no movement or the lung is not in direct contact with the parietal pleura, then a linear pattern is represented (**right**). These patterns are referred to as the sandy beach and stratosphere/barcode signs respectively.

2. A Lines

Characteristics

- A lines are a reverberation artifact, with serial repetitions of the pleural line.
- A lines are horizontal lines and are each separated by an equal distance (this is a reverberation artifact of the original distance from the probe to the pleural line).
- A lines are the normal expected pattern and represent aerated lung.

Differential Dx

- Normal lung, COPD/asthma, pneumothorax (A lines with absent lung slide), pulmonary embolism (without a pulmonary infarct).

3. B Lines

Characteristics

- Vertical, hyperechoic, dominant lines.
- Originate at the pleural surface and extend to the bottom of the screen without fading.
- Efface A lines where the two intersect.
- Move in synchrony with lung slide.
- Their presence excludes pneumothorax.
- Represents thickened subpleural interlobular septae surrounded by air-filled alveoli.
- The more B lines and the closer they are together, generally signifies a more severe involvement of the interlobular septae and progressive alveolar involvement.

Differential Diagnosis

- ARDS, cardiogenic pulmonary edema both interstitial and alveolar, pneumonia, lung contusion, interstitial lung disease.
- Multiple anterior and symmetric B lines: Generally signifies cardiogenic pulmonary edema.
- Asymmetric B lines interspersed with normal areas of A lines: noncardiogenic edema/ARDS, pneumonia (Fig. 87.5).

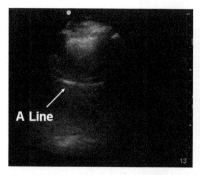 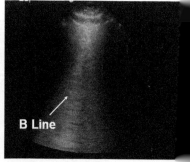

Figure 87.5. A lines, created by reflections of the pleural line, are equidistant horizontal lines (**left**). B lines dominant, bright vertical lines that move with the pleura, extend to the bottom of the screen, and repres thickened, fluid-filled interlobular septae (**right**).

4. Consolidation

Characteristics
- The lung is no longer air filled and so no A or B lines are seen. The consolidated lung appears like any other solid organ ("hepatization" of the lung).
- Best seen in lateral views just above the diaphragm.
- Often associated with effusions.
- Air bronchograms may be seen in the consolidated lung:
  - They appear as a hyperechoic artifact which moves with respiration and represents the movement of air within bronchi of the consolidated lung, suggesting preserved patency of the proximal airway.
  - Dynamic air bronchograms can differentiate pneumonia (present) from simple atelectasis (absent).

Differential Dx
  - Atelectasis, pneumonia, ARDS, tumor or mass, lung contusion.

. Pleural Effusion

Characteristics
- Pleural fluid is anechoic (black) on ultrasound.
- Most effusions are free flowing and so the patient should be positioned to optimize the view.
- Ultrasound can detect very small pleural effusions, before they are seen on a CXR.
- There should be at least 1 cm of pleural fluid before an attempt at thoracentesis is performed.
- Ultrasound of pleural fluid reveals it to be dynamic, meaning there is movement with respiration.
- It is always important to define the boundaries of the pleural fluid:
  - The boundaries of the pleural space consist of the chest wall, the diaphragm, and the lung.
  - This is a routine but extremely important component of pleural ultrasound, to avoid misidentifying the diaphragm and confusing it with the perirenal fascia.
  - Misidentification of the diaphragm can result in major injury if a thoracentesis is attempted with resultant subdiaphragmatic injury to the liver or spleen.
- Fluid characteristics:
  - Simple fluid is anechoic.
  - Exudates may not be anechoic and may have what appears to be swirling debris within the fluid (plankton sign)
  - Complex effusions may have multiple fibrous strands and septations within the effusion which are often not seen with CT.
    - This may signify loculation of the fluid and could be due to a parapneumonic effusion, empyema, or a resolving hemothorax (Fig. 87.6).

Approach to Acute Respiratory Failure

An algorithmic approach using a combination of lung ultrasound, coupled with a lower extremity venous exam is recommended when utilizing ultrasound to help determine an etiology for acute respiratory failure. In clinical practice, the history, exam findings, laboratory data, and basic imaging are combined with the knowledge of the bedside ultrasound exam to help determine what the most likely etiology for

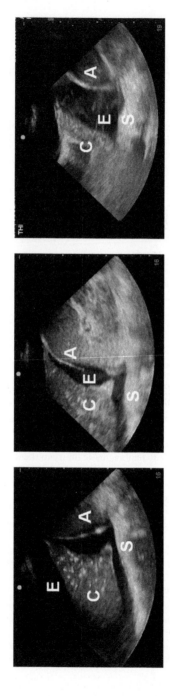

Figure 87.6. Three examples of lung consolidation and effusions. A consolidated lung has a similar echogenicity to the abdominal organs. Effusions are anechoic or black. Notice the echogenic material in the pleural fluid in the image on the right. This can be seen in complex effusions and suggests the need for a chest-tube. The diaphragm is visualized as a hyperechoic line above the abdominal structures. The spine can be seen posteriorly. C, consolidation; E, effusion; A, abdominal structures; S, spine.

respiratory failure is. This algorithm is known as the BLUE protocol (Fig. 87.1) and is reviewed conceptually below by a simple approach to bedside lung ultrasound.

- Is there a pneumothorax? Is lung slide present?
  - If NO, pneumothorax is possible. Is there Lung point present to confirm a pneumothorax? Are B lines or lung pulse present which will rule out a pneumothorax at the probe position?
  - Consider other causes of loss of lung slide as noted in the chapter above.
- Are the lungs normally aerated (dry) as signified by an A-line predominant pattern?
  - Yes, most likely diagnosis is COPD/Asthma, pulmonary embolism (proceed to evaluate the lower extremities for DVT).
- Is there an interstitial or alveolar process (wet) as signified by B lines?
  - Are the B lines diffuse, bilateral, and symmetric?
    - suggestive of cardiogenic pulmonary edema.
  - Are the B lines occasional, asymmetric, and interspersed with normal areas of A lines?
    - suggestive of noncardiogenic edema or pneumonia.
- Is there an asymmetric A/B profile (one lung has A pattern, the other has B pattern)?
  - Suggestive of pneumonia which may be confirmed by the finding of lung consolidation and dynamic air bronchograms.
- Is a pleural effusion present and does it appear to be simple or complex? Is it safe to proceed with thoracentesis?

FOCUSED ECHOCARDIOGRAPHY

Key Points

Bedside echocardiography is goal-directed and problem-oriented.
- Why is my patient hypotensive? What is the cause of hemodynamic instability?
- Is there a pericardial effusion? Is there tamponade physiology?
- Is the left ventricular function normal? Hyperdynamic? Moderately or severely depressed?
- What is the right ventricular size and function? Are there signs of RV strain?
- Are there any gross valvular or wall motion abnormalities?
- Is the IVC normal? Distended? Collapsible?
- Can more fluid be tolerated?

A phased array probe is used with the machine on cardiac setting (indicator on right side of screen).

Five standard views are obtained with the patient in a supine position.

Complements, does not replace, standard comprehensive echocardiography.

Should be viewed as an extension of the physical exam- findings should support clinical suspicion and help narrow differential diagnosis.

Limitations

Limited quantitative measurements and poorer image quality with portable bedside machines compared to comprehensive echocardiography.

Some significant findings are difficult to appreciate, including subtle wall motion abnormalities, valvular vegetations, and right ventricular hypertrophy.

Obtaining greater than two cardiac views may not be possible due to patient body habitus, COPD/lung disease, bandages, and positioning.

Misinterpretation of findings occur when the image is foreshortened or off axis, when less than two views are obtained, or when image quality is poor; *and* the interpreter is not conscious of these exam limitations.

- Referral for standard, comprehensive echocardiography should be considered in situations where findings are inconclusive or fall beyond the scope of the point-of-care exam.

Image Acquisition and Interpretation

Image window: position on patient's chest (parasternal, apical, and subcostal) (Fig. 87.7).

Image plane: Three standard image planes defined by the American Society of Echocardiography—long axis, short axis, and four chamber.

- Long Axis (sagittal plane): vertical bisection through left ventricular apex and center of aortic valve.
- Short Axis (transverse plane): perpendicular to long axis, cross sections of ventricles.
- Four Chamber (coronal plane): left ventricular apex to base, bisecting mitral and tricuspid valves.

1. Parasternal Long Axis (PLAX)

Image Acquisition

- Indicator toward patient's right shoulder (11 o'clock).
- Probe just left of sternum (between 2nd and 5th rib space).

Image Optimization

- Slide up and down along the left aspect of the sternum to locate the best viewing window.
- Stay close to the sternum to avoid lung interference.
- Find the interspace in which the inferior aspect of the septum is horizontal.
- Rotate so that mitral and aortic valves are in the same plane.
- The left ventricle should be seen in its longest axis and the aortic valve cusps should be symmetric.
- Tilt away from sternum so that the mitral and aortic valves are in the center of the screen.
- The apex should not be visualized.
- Adjust depth so descending aorta in view (14 to 16 cm) (Fig. 87.8).

Normal Structure and Function

- Right ventricular outflow tract, aortic outflow tract, and left atrium approximate the same size.
- LV systolic function: visualize myocardial thickening, symmetrical inward endocardial movement, anterior leaflet of mitral valve approximates the septum (<1 cm).
- Mitral and aortic valves: leaflets come together with normal opening and closing.

Is There a Pericardial Effusion?

- Appears as anechoic space between the myocardium and pericardium.
- Nonloculated effusions generally collect posteriorly in dependent areas.
- Anterior fat pad can be misinterpreted as an anterior effusion since it is located between myocardium and pericardium.
- Ascites and left-sided pleural effusions can be mistaken for pericardial effusions.
- Use the descending aorta to differentiate between a pericardial and pleural effusion. Pericardial effusions taper anterior to the descending aorta, pleural effusions extend posterior to the descending aorta.

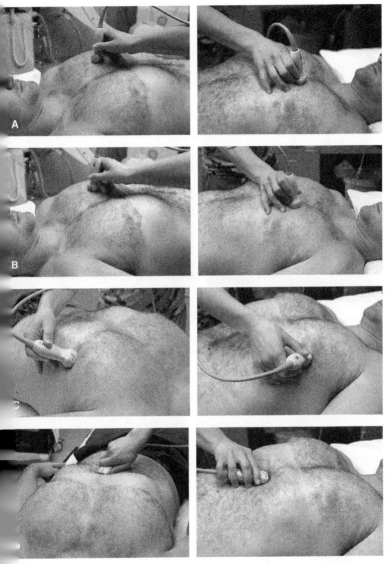

Figure 87.7. Cardiac exam probe positions. **A:** Parasternal long axis. **B:** Parasternal short axis. **C:** Apical long **D:** Subcostal long axis. (*continued*)

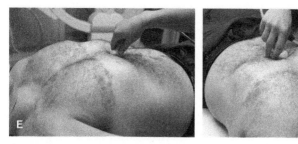

Figure 87.7. (*Continued*) **E:** Subcostal IVC.

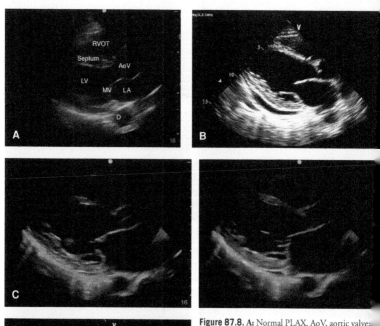

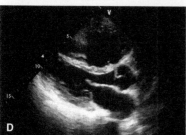

Figure 87.8. A: Normal PLAX. AoV, aortic valve; descending aorta; LA, left atrium; LV, left ventri MV, mitral valve. **B:** Circumferential pericardial e sion. The posterior aspect lies between the poste wall of the left ventricle and pericardium. Notice pericardial fluid is superior to the descending ac **C:** Severe left ventricular dysfunction in dias (**left**) and systole (**right**). Notice how the ante leaflet of the mitral valve barely opens and does approximate the septum. The cavity is dilated the walls hardly move inward during contract **D:** Right ventricular overload causing septal devia toward the left ventricle.

Is There LV Dysfunction?

- Dilated chamber, decreased myocardial thickening.
- Diminished MV opening, anterior leaflet >1cm from septum.

Is the LV Hyperdynamic?

- Small chamber size with anterior mitral valve leaflet contacting the septum.
- End diastolic cavity obliteration.

Is the RV Overloaded?

- Right ventricular outflow tract larger than the aorta and left atrium.
- Paradoxic septal motion.

Pitfalls of PLAX

- Only visualizing RV outflow tract, so unless severely abnormal, unable to evaluate RV size.
- May overestimate LV function in underresuscitated septic or hypovolemic patients. Off-axis views lead to underestimation of LV size and overestimation of function. Inaccurate assessment of MV or AV function:
  - normal appearing valves may have significant regurgitation.
  - vegetations may be subtle and can be missed by bedside ultrasound.
  - heavily calcified appearing AV may not be hemodynamically significant.

. Parasternal Short Axis (PSAX)

Image Acquisition

From a good parasternal long axis view, rotate the probe clockwise 60 to 90 degrees, until the left ventricle is circular.

Image Optimization

Center the left ventricle in the screen between the rib shadows.
Find the midventricular level by tilting the probe along the right shoulder–left hip axis until the papillary muscles are visualized (they will come into view just below the mitral valve, which looks like a fish-mouth).
Papillary muscles at 4 and 7 o'clock positions.

Normal Structure and Function

Circular LV with small, crescent-shaped RV.
LV systolic function: endocardium moves symmetrically toward center, equal ventricular thickening, papillary muscles approximate during end systole (Fig. 87.9).

Is There LV Dysfunction?

Dilated cavity with decreased contraction.
Obvious wall motion abnormalities or akinesis which may be global or in a specific coronary artery distribution.

Is There RV Overload?

Large, ovoid-shaped RV.
Septum moves toward LV cavity during early systole, progressing to septal flattening "D-shaped" LV.

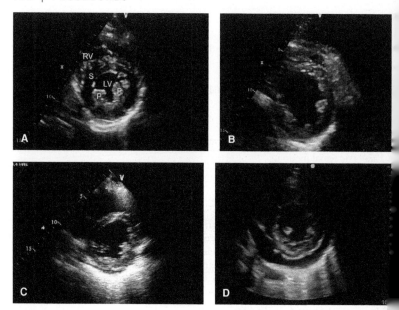

Figure 87.9. A: Normal PSAX during systole. RV, right ventricle; S, septum; LV, left ventricle; P, papillar muscle. **B:** Severe left ventricular dysfunction during systole. **C:** Right ventricular overload with flattening o the septum. **D:** Pericardial effusion.

Is the LV Hyperdynamic?

- Small LV cavity with touching papillary muscles.

Pitfalls of PSAX

- Off-axis evaluation, in which the LV appears elliptical, causes inaccurate assessmer of segmental wall movements and septal motion.

3. Apical Four Chamber (A4C)

Image Acquisition

- Probe placed over the cardiac apex at the point of maximal apical pulsation.
- Indicator is facing between the patient's axilla and the bed (about 2 to 3 o'clock).
- Probe is positioned in line with the long axis of the heart and tilted upward towa the base.
- Depth approximately 14 to 18 cm to image the entire heart, including the atria.

Image Optimization

- Deep inhalation may help bring the heart closer to the probe and improve the vie
- Positioning the patient with a left lateral tilt of the thorax often improves the vie
- Locate the apex of heart made up by the left and right ventricles and center at t top of the screen.
- Slide/rock the transducer until the interventricular septum is centered horizonta in the image and ventricles are fully visualized in their longest axis.

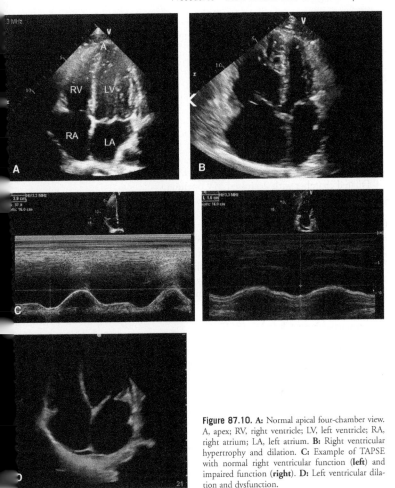

Figure 87.10. A: Normal apical four-chamber view. A, apex; RV, right ventricle; LV, left ventricle; RA, right atrium; LA, left atrium. **B:** Right ventricular hypertrophy and dilation. **C:** Example of TAPSE with normal right ventricular function (**left**) and impaired function (**right**). **D:** Left ventricular dilation and dysfunction.

Rotate until both mitral and tricuspid valves are seen in the same plane.
Angle transducer superiorly to appreciate the entire heart, including the atria Fig. 87.10).

rmal Structure and Function

RV is triangular and 2/3 the size of the LV. The majority of the apex is created by he LV.
V function: systolic shortening occurs in the long axis. Visual tricuspid annular lane systolic excursion (TAPSE) refers to the distance that the lateral annulus of he tricuspid valve moves during systole (M-mode, normal 15 to 20 mm).
litral and tricuspid valves: open and close normally.

Is the RV Dilated?

* Moderate dilation: RV 60% to 100% of LV.
* Severe dilation: RV larger than LV.
* Paradoxic septal movement present.

Is There RV Dysfunction?

* Decreased free wall motion.
* TAPSE <15 mm.
* McConnell's sign denotes hypokinesis or akinesis of the mid RV free wall and hyperkinesis of the apex.

Is There LV Dysfunction?

* Dilated chamber with decreased MV opening.
* Wall motion abnormalities which can be global or in a specific coronary distribution.

Pitfalls of A4C

* Challenging view to obtain in a critically ill supine patient.
* Off-axis imaging: inaccurate assessment of LV/RV function and size.
* Endocardium not always visualized, limiting assessment of LV function.
* It can be difficult to differentiate between acute and chronic RV volume/pressure overload. Chronic RV dilation is normally associated with hypertrophy of the RV free wall.

4. Subcostal Four Chamber (S4C)

Image Acquisition

* Gently place the probe under the xiphoid process flat against the patient's abdomen with the indicator pointing toward 3 o'clock.
* The probe is held differently to the other positions, with the hand overlying the probe (Fig. 87.7).

Image Optimization

* Apply pressure to keep the probe under the rib cage and tilt upward, bringing the handle of the probe toward the patient's abdomen.
* Direct the beam anteriorly until the heart comes into view, some gentle pressure may be required.
* If bowel gas is obscuring view, move the probe slightly to the left (patient's right) and use the liver as an acoustic window.
* Rotate the probe until the entire LV, including the apex, is visualized (Fig. 87.1).

Normal Structure and Function

* Compare size of chambers, LV/RV gross ventricular function, septal motion.

Is There Tamponade?

* Does the pericardial effusion cause RA or RV free wall collapse during systole/diastole respectively?

Is There RV Overload?

* RV size, visual TAPSE, septal abnormalities.

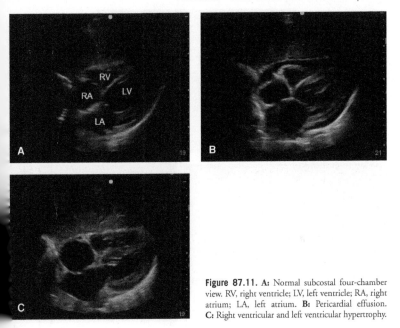

Figure 87.11. A: Normal subcostal four-chamber view. RV, right ventricle; LV, left ventricle; RA, right atrium; LA, left atrium. **B:** Pericardial effusion. **C:** Right ventricular and left ventricular hypertrophy.

Pitfalls of S4C

Off-axis imaging will lead to inaccurate assessment of LV/RV size and function.
Difficult to obtain in obese, muscular, or postsurgical patients.
Some patients unable to tolerate the pressure needed to obtain image.
Bowel gas or abdominal distention can be challenging.

Subcostal Inferior Vena Cava (SIVC)

Image Acquisition

Place the probe in the midline, on abdominal preset, with the indicator facing the patient's head.
Angle or slide the transducer until the IVC is seen horizontally across the screen.

Image Optimization

Rock the probe slightly inferiorly and tilt toward patient's left until IVC is seen entering RA.
Rotate until IVC traverses horizontally and the hepatic vein is visualized entering the IVC (Fig. 87.12).

Normal Anatomy and Function

Normal IVC size is between 1.5 and 2.5 cm with some variation with respiration.
Increasing age, respiratory effort and positive pressure ventilation all affect IVC diameter.

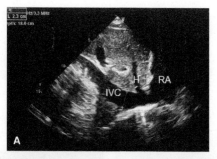

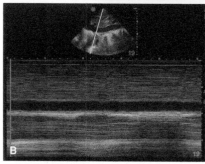
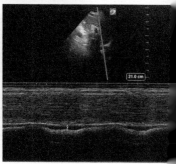

Figure 87.12. A: Subcostal inferior vena cava (IVC) view. H, hepatic vein; RA, right atrium. **B:** M-mode through the inferior vena cava. Dilated IVC without respiratory variation (**left**) compared to small, complete collapsing IVC (**right**).

Use of IVC Diameter to Assess Preload

- We caution against solely using IVC diameter to assess a patient's volume status and prefer more functional hemodynamic monitoring with response in SV to fluid challenges or a passive leg raise.
- At extremes, IVC diameter can be useful to assess preload responsiveness:
  - If IVC diameter is <1.0 cm, patient is likely preload responsive, particularly they are on positive pressure ventilation.
  - If IVC diameter is <1.5 cm and exhibits >50% collapsibility, likely preload respon sive.
  - If IVC diameter is >1.5 cm but still has >50% collapsibility, patient may be pre load responsive but need to use other measures of preload responsiveness.
  - If IVC diameter is >1.7 cm and exhibits <50% collapsibility, patient unlikely be preload responsive.

Pitfalls of SIVC

- Limited use in patients on positive pressure ventilation or in respiratory distress.
- Useful at extremes.
- Aorta can be misidentified as the IVC, especially in a severely hypovolemic patient in which the IVC may be very small or completely collapsed. Always identify bo the IVC and the aorta to ensure that you are truly assessing the IVC and not m taking it for the aorta.

Measuring Stroke Volume by Bedside Echocardiography

- The volume of blood traveling through a particular chamber of interest is determined by the following relationship:
  - Volume = Time period of flow × mean Velocity of flow × Cross Sectional Area of the chamber
- With pulsatile blood flow, when velocity of flow is frequently changing, a velocity time integral is used (VTI):
  - Volume = VTI × CSA
- VTI is also referred to as the stroke distance in some texts.
- The standard location to measure stroke volume is in the left ventricular outflow tract (LVOT)

This simple maneuver requires two standard echocardiographic views.

Firstly, the LVOT diameter is measured in the PLAX view at the level of the aortic valve, during systole with the valve wide open.

A caliper is used to measure the diameter of the LVOT at this point. Normal LVOT diameters vary from 1.8 to 2.2 cm.
Once the LVOT diameter is obtained, it is halved to obtain the radius of the LVOT. The cross-sectional area of the LVOT is then obtained by using the following equation:
- CSA = Π r² (Π is 3.14)

The **second view** is an apical five-chamber view which is a standard apical four-chamber view with a slight upward tilt of the ultrasound beam angle to visualize the LVOT. Pulsed wave Doppler is then used to obtain a sample from the LVOT, just below the level of the aortic valve.

The pulse wave Doppler profile at that point is obtained and the VTI value is calculated as the area under the VTI envelope using standard ultrasound machine calculations.
A normal LVOT VTI is 18 to 22 cm.

Stroke volume is obtained by multiplying the VTI by the CSA.

Serial assessments of VTI are easily obtainable without the need to keep measuring the LVOT diameter and so serial VTI measurements can be used as a surrogate for stroke volume to assess response to fluid loading or inotropic support (Fig. 87.13).

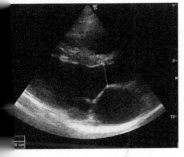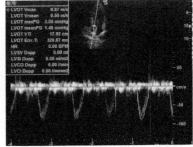

Figure 87.13. LVOT diameter and LVOT VTI to calculate stoke volume. In this example, stroke volume is cross-sectional area multiplied by LVOT VTI. LVOT diameter is 2 cm, so cross-sectional area equals LVOT VTI is calculated to be 17.92. Stroke volume therefore equals 56 mL.

SHOCK

Shock is common in the ICU and associated with high morbidity and mortality. It requires rapid recognition, evaluation, and treatment. Unfortunately, the etiology is not always clear by history and physical exam alone. Point of care ultrasound by an experienced user can quickly and accurately differentiate between distributive, hypovolemic, obstructive, and cardiogenic shock. A focused cardiac, lung, and inferior vena cava exam takes less than 5 minutes. We often combine this with a DVT screen of the lower extremities (Table 87.3).

1. Using the phased array probe in the abdominal mode, scan the anterior lung fields looking for lung slide, A lines, and B lines.
   - Lung slide? yes/no
   - A, B, or A/B pattern
2. Switch to the cardiac presets and perform a focused cardiac exam evaluating overall left ventricular size and function, right ventricular size and function, and presence of pericardial effusion.
   - Pericardial effusion? yes/no
   - LV function: hyperdynamic? normal? mod/severely depressed?
   - RV size: <2/3 LV? normal septal movement?
3. Finally, evaluate the inferior vena cava. A fixed, dilated IVC versus a small, collapsing IVC can help support or rule-out certain diagnoses.
   - Fixed and dilated >2.5 cm, no respiratory variation
   - Small and collapsing <1.5 cm, >50% variation with respiration

TABLE 87.3	Ultrasound Findings in Different Etiologies of Shock			
	Anterior Lung Exam	Focused Cardiac	IVC	Pitfalls
Pneumothorax	Loss of lung slide No B lines + A lines		Fixed, dilated	Loss of lung slide not specific for PTX
Tamponade		Pericardial effusion	Fixed, dilated	Difficult to assess hemodynamic significance
Hypovolemic/ Distributive	Predominantly A-lines	Hyperdynamic LV	Small, collapsing	Other conditions (i.e., RV failure) will appear to have hyperdynamic LV
Acute decompensated LV failure	Bilateral B-lines	Depressed LV function	Fixed, dilated	Significant valvular pathologies may not be appreciated
RV pressure/ volume overload	A-lines	Large RV, abnormal septal kinetics	Fixed, dilated	Difficult to differentiate between acute and chronic RV failure

Pneumothorax

The presence of lung slide, lung pulse, or B lines **rules-out** pneumothorax. Evaluate multiple areas on the anterior chest of a supine patient to rule-out pneumothorax. Absence of lung slide suggests pneumothorax, however this is not a specific finding. Loss of lung slide is also seen with severe pneumonia/ARDS, prior pleurodesis, bullous lung disease, examination on the left with a right mainstem intubation, and prolonged apnea. Lung point confirms the diagnosis of pneumothorax, however, if concerned for tension pneumothorax, do not spend extra time searching for this finding.

Tamponade

Presence of pericardial effusions are often easily identified; however, assessing hemodynamic importance can be difficult. **Hemodynamically significant pericardial effusions will always be associated with a fixed and dilated IVC.** The presence of RV collapse during diastole or RA collapse in systole supports hemodynamic significance. Any questionable pericardial effusion warrants cardiology consultation, and if time allows, evaluation with a more comprehensive echocardiographic exam evaluating for respiratory variation in mitral valve inflow velocities and pulmonary vein inflow velocities.

Acute LV Failure

LV dysfunction as a cause of acute hypotension requires more than just depressed LV function on cardiac ultrasound. Gross visualization of LV contraction and anterior mitral valve excursion are the recommended initial techniques to evaluate overall LV function. Attention should be focused on whether the decrease in LV function is segmental and in a coronary distribution, global or classic for stress-induced cardiomyopathy (apical ballooning and basilar hyperkinesis). Findings should be confirmed in at least two different cardiac views. Acutely decompensated LV failure may have additional ultrasound findings associated with increased CVP including bilateral B lines and a fixed, dilated IVC. If, after full clinical assessment, LV dysfunction is considered to be the cause of the hypotension and poor perfusion (i.e., cardiogenic shock), early initiation of Dobutamine or mechanical support should be considered. Repeated exams showing improved LV function and decreased B line severity as well as improving stroke volume can be used to guide interventions such as inotropy, diuresis, and/or afterload reduction.

Hypovolemic/Septic Shock

Both distributive and hypovolemic shock will appear similarly on bedside ultrasound. These patients will have a hyperdynamic LV, predominantly A-line pattern on lung exam, and collapsible IVC. Many times, the LV cavity is obliterated during systole and the endocardial borders appear to be "kissing." Attention to technique is important as off-axis views may make the LV cavity appear underfilled. It is important to keep in mind other states that will make the LV appear hyperdynamic. These include LV hypertrophy, mitral regurgitation, supraventricular arrhythmias, and decompensated RV failure. Once a hyperdynamic state is observed, other ultrasound findings may be helpful in differentiating between hypovolemia and sepsis. Free fluid in the abdomen can suggest hypovolemia related to acute bleeding or decompensated cirrhosis. Ultrasonographic evidence of an infection, including abscess, hydronephrosis or lung consolidation, may suggest sepsis as primary cause. Additional imaging and laboratory testing is often required for a final diagnosis.

RV Pressure/Volume Overload

The pulmonary circulation in health is normally a low pressure, high capacitance system and the thin-walled RV will dilate with substantial and sustained acute increases in pressure (acute cor pulmonale). The vast majority of patients with PE as a cause of shock will have features of RV dysfunction on point-of-care ultrasound.

RV size and function are best evaluated in A4C, S4C, or PSAX by direct comparison with the LV. In the A4C view, the RV should be triangular and <60% of the LV. As the RV enlarges, it's shape becomes more ovoid and it may progress to being the dominant chamber at the apex. Normally, the majority of the apex is made-up by the LV.

Septal bowing, bouncing, or paradoxical movement suggests pressure/volume overload of the RV. This is best appreciated in the PSAX view. Septal changes range from septal bouncing to complete flattening (D-shaped LV).

RV function can be assessed by measuring longitudinal movement of the RV free wall at the level of the tricuspid annulus (TAPSE). TAPSE is obtained by utilizing M-mode through the intersection of the RV free wall and tricuspid annulus and measuring the distance traveled. This can also be assessed visually in the S4C view. In addition, to assess chronicity of any process affecting the RV, the RV free wall can be evaluated with regards to its thickness. A previously healthy RV free wall should not exceed 5 mm in thickness. If the RV free wall is thickened, this would be suggestive of a more chronic process which has allowed the RV to hypertrophy over time. Another clue to a chronic process would be elevation of the pulmonary artery pressure, which is easily obtained utilizing continuous wave Doppler analysis of the tricuspid regurgitant jet velocity. Estimated PA systolic pressure equals $4V^2$ where V is the maximal tricuspid regurgitant jet velocity. Normally, the estimated right atrial pressure based on IVC characteristics is added to this value to estimate the PA systolic pressure.

An additional finding often seen with acute RV dysfunction is McConnell sign, which refers to hypokinesis or akinesis of the mid RV free wall and hyperkinesis of the apex. This sign is best seen in the A4C and S4C views. It is not specific for pulmonary embolism and can be seen in ARDS or other conditions associated with acute RV strain.

The ultrasound findings of RV dysfunction are used together with other standard clinical assessments (history, examination, EKG findings, BNP, troponin, lactate, Chest CT, DVT screen) in patients with evolving acute cor pulmonale from pulmonary embolism. This added risk stratification which ultrasound provides allows for a reasoned approach to the use of anticoagulation, thrombolytic therapy, inotropic support, and fluid administration.

Deep Vein Thrombosis

- Traditional duplex and triplex vascular studies include a combination of compression, color, and spectral doppler.
- Most point-of-care evaluations of DVT used in emergency and critical care settings use the compression portion of the exam only.
- Proximal deep veins of the LE include the external iliac, common femoral, deep femoral, superficial femoral, and popliteal veins.
- The reader is encouraged to learn the venous anatomy of the lower extremity from a standard anatomy text in order to perform DVT screening.

Image Acquisition

- A high frequency transducer is used (5 to 12 MHz).
- Compared to veins, arteries appear more round, thick walled, pulsatile, smaller, and require substantial pressure to be compressed. Venous structures generally compress with gentle pressure.
- Ideal patient position is supine with leg externally rotated and knee flexed.
- Start with transducer in transverse position near the iliac artery. The external iliac vessels should be identified here.
- Normal veins should compress fully with complete collapse of the opposing walls. Firm downward pressure is required. Pressure needed to completely collapse the vein is much less than that needed to compress the adjacent artery. Failure to fully compress the vein suggests the presence of acute thrombus. Acute thrombi are often not visible with ultrasound. Subacute or chronic thrombi which are organized will be visible within the vessel lumen.

Common femoral vein: starting just proximal to the great saphenous vein, slide down the common femoral vein, compressing every 1 to 2 cm. Care must be taken to identify each branching point until just beyond the division into the superficial and deep femoral veins.

Popliteal: Place the transducer in the transverse plane within the popliteal fossa. The popliteal vein is superficial to the artery in the center of the fossa.

BASIC ABDOMEN

Key Points

FAST exam can detect as little as 100 to 260 mL of free peritoneal fluid. The type of fluid cannot be differentiated by ultrasound exam alone.

Sonographic appearance of injured liver or splenic tissue is subtle and difficult to appreciate. Presence of free peritoneal fluid is a surrogate marker for solid organ injury following trauma.

Hydronephrosis and bladder outlet obstruction can be rapidly diagnosed with the use of bedside ultrasound, expediting appropriate therapies.

Identification of renal cysts/masses or bladder masses require further evaluation and are beyond the scope of point-of-care ultrasound.

Free Peritoneal Fluid

The FAST exam evaluates gravitationally dependent areas in the RUQ, LUQ, and pelvis. This exam was developed to look for hemoperitoneum in trauma patients.

All types of free fluid, including blood, ascites, bile, lymph, and urine will appear black. Fluid with higher levels of protein (clotted blood, loculated fluid, pus) are more echogenic.

Both the curvilinear or phased-array probes may be used.

RUQ: evaluate the hepatorenal recess (Morrison's pouch), under the diaphragm, and the inferior pole of the kidney (right paracolic gutter).

Image Acquisition:

Place probe in coronal plane (indicator at 12 o'clock) in the mid axillary line at the level of the xiphoid.

Center the hepatorenal recess in the center of the screen.

- Fluid in the hepatorenal recess will appear as an anechoic space between the two organs.
- Tilt the probe anteriorly and posteriorly, making sure to evaluate the inferior pole of the kidney.
- Angle the transducer superiorly to image under the diaphragm.

2. **LUQ:** evaluate under the diaphragm, the spleen, the splenorenal space, and the left kidney (left paracolic space).

Image Acquisition:

- The left kidney is located more posterior and superior compared to the right kidney.
- Start with the probe in the posterior axillary line as close to the bed as possible (may help to have patient role into right decubitus position if possible).
- Once the left kidney is centered on the screen, fan the space above and below to evaluate the inferior pole and the splenorenal space.
- Angle superiorly to appreciate the area under the diaphragm.

3. **Pelvis:** fluid accumulates in the rectovesicular space or pouch of Douglas in men and women respectively.

Image Acquisition:

- Start with the transducer just above the pubic symphysis in the transverse plane with the indicator toward the patient's right.
- Tilt inferiorly until the bladder is visualized.
- Adjust depth so that the posterior part of the bladder is located in the top half of the image.
- Fan through the entire length of the bladder, from the fundus to the neck.
- Rotate 90 degrees and scan the entire bladder in the sagittal plane (Fig. 87.14).

Renal Ultrasound

- Normal kidney: Gerota's fascia creates a bright outline of the kidney. The underlying renal cortex appears grainy and is slightly less echogenic than surrounding liver or splenic tissue. The renal sinus, which contains the calyces and renal pelvis, appears hyperechoic due to the fat between the renal sinuses. The fluid-filled medullary pyramids and renal calyces appear black.

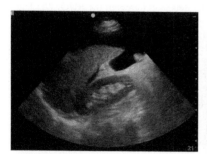 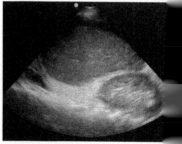

Figure 87.14. Free fluid in the right upper quadrant around the liver and within the hepatorenal space. Free fluid seen around the spleen under the diaphragm in the left upper quadrant (**right**).

- The kidneys are positioned slightly obliquely with the inferior poles more anterior and lateral. Imaging the full length of the kidney requires slight (15 to 30 degree) rotation of the transducer.
- In the longitudinal axis, the kidney appears in the shape of a football. In the transverse, view it is C-shaped.

Image Acquisition

- **Right Kidney:**
  - Place transducer in coronal plane in mid to anterior axillary line at the level of the xiphoid.
  - Aim the probe slightly posteriorly to visualize the kidney.
  - Center the kidney in the middle of the screen, then rotate counterclockwise 15 to 30 degrees to appreciate the longest axis.
  - Assess the entire kidney by tilting the probe anteriorly and posteriorly.
  - Rotate 90 degrees to evaluate the short axis.
  - Tilt to evaluate the superior and inferior pole.
- **Left Kidney:**
  - Start with the transducer in the posterior axillary line.
  - Center the kidney, rotate 15 to 30 degrees clockwise to find the longest axis, then fan through the kidney.
  - Rotate 90 degrees and tilt superiorly and inferiorly to evaluate the entire length of the kidney.

Hydronephrosis

Differentiated by mild, moderate, and severe:
- Mild: increased fluid within the calyces with preservation of renal papillae.
- Moderate: rounding of the calyces with ballooning of the papillae. Preservation of the outer cortex.
- Severe: large calyces and pyramids filled with fluid surrounded by thinned cortex.

Compared to renal cysts, in hydronephrosis, all dilated areas of fluid can be traced back to the collecting system.

Unilateral hydronephrosis is likely secondary to obstructive uropathy and may be associated with pyelonephritis. Differential for obstruction includes ureteral stone, or a retroperitoneal mass/adenopathy.

Bilateral hydronephrosis suggests bladder outlet obstruction and a sonographic bladder exam should be performed at a minimum (Fig. 87.15).

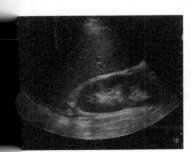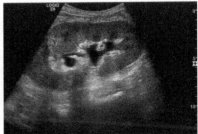

Figure 87.15. Normal kidney (**left**). Mild/moderate hydronephrosis (**right**).

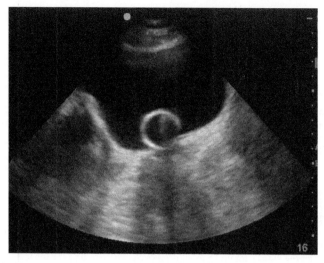

Figure 87.16. Transverse bladder view with distended bladder despite the presence of a Foley catheter (inflated catheter balloon visible).

Bladder Ultrasound

- Bladder ultrasound can evaluate for bladder distention and enables differentiation between true decreased urine production (empty decompressed bladder) versus postobstructive renal failure caused by urinary retention (Fig. 87.16).
- In patients with declining urine output, this is a very valuable test to make sure that the Foley catheter is not blocked and to verify the position of the Foley balloon within the bladder.
- Pelvic ascites can mimic the bladder.
- Bladder volume is calculated using measured height, width, and length:
  - Volume = $0.75 \times w \times h \times 1$
- Qualitative assessment: bladder dome is half way to the umbilicus in a distended bladder.

Image Acquisition

- Curvilinear probe is recommended since wider footprint allows for visualization the entire bladder.
- Place transducer in transverse plane just superior to the pubic symphysis and below the umbilicus.
- Aim transducer inferiorly to appreciate the anechoic, fluid-filled bladder.
- Measure width and length in the transverse plane.
- Rotate probe 90 degrees to evaluate the long axis.
- Measure height in the sagittal (long) axis.

SUGGESTED READINGS

Critical Care Ultrasound

Frankel HL, Kirkpatrick AW, Elbarbary M, et al. Guidelines for the appropriate use of bedside general and cardiac ultrasonography in the evaluation of critically ill patients-part i: general ultrasonography. *Crit Care Med.* 2015;43:2479–2502.

Evidence-based guidelines for appropriate use of ultrasonography in the ICU for diagnostic and therapeutic chest, abdomen, pelvic, neck and extremity exams. Key diagnostic recommendations include ruling-in pneumothorax, ruling-in pleural effusion and diagnosing DVT. Conditional recommendations include the diagnosis of calculous cholecystitis, renal failure and interstitial and parenchymal lung disease.

Levitov A, Frankel HL, Blaivas M, et al. Guidelines for the Appropriate Use of Bedside General and Cardiac Ultrasonography in the Evaluation of Critically Ill Patients-Part II: Cardiac Ultrasonography. *Crit Care Med.* 2016;44:1206–1227.

Consensus established guidelines for the use of cardiac ultrasonography in the ICU. Of the 45 statements considered, 15 were approved as conditional recommendations, and 24 as strong recommendations. Key strong recommendations include assessing preload responsiveness in mechanically ventilated patients, left ventricular systolic and diastolic function, acute cor pulmonale, pulmonary hypertension, symptomatic pulmonary embolism, right ventricular infarct, efficacy of fluid resuscitation and inotropic therapy, presence of RV dysfunction in septic shock, the reason for cardiac arrest to assist in CPR, left ventricular function status in ACS, presence of pericardial effusion, cardiac tamponade, valvular dysfunction, endocarditis, great vessel disease and injury, penetrating chest trauma and for use of contrast.

Mayo PH, Beaulieu Y, Doelken P, et al. American college of chest physicians/la société de réanimation de langue française statement on competence in critical care ultrasonography. *Chest.* 2009;135:1050–1060.

Consensus statement defining competence in critical care ultrasonography. Competence in general critical care ultrasound includes all aspects of pleural, lung, abdominal and vascular image acquisition (including ultrasound physics, machine controls, systematic scanning, and transducer manipulation), image interpretation, clinical applications and specific limitations. Specific technical (image acquisition) and cognitive (image interpretation) elements are described for each exam. Competencies for critical care echocardiography are divided into basic and advanced.

Physics

Aldrich JE. Basic physics of ultrasound imaging. *Crit Care Med.* 2007;35:S131–S137.

Introduction to physical principles of image generation and description of common artifacts.

Pulmonary/Respiratory Failure

Lichtenstein DA. BLUE-Protocol and FALLS-Protocol: Two Applications of Lung Ultrasound in the Critically Ill. *Chest.* 2015;147(6):1659–1670.

Provides an overview of the history of lung ultrasound and the ten classic signatures, followed by an excellent review of the BLUE-protocol to diagnose acute respiratory failure and the FALLs protocol to systematically rule out and effectively treat the various etiologies of shock.

Mayo PH, Doelken P. Pleural Ultrasonography. *Clin Chest Med.* 2006;27:215–227.

Provides an introduction to ultrasound physics, machine requirements, and normal pleural findings, and a thorough summary of the ultrasound characteristics of pleural effusions, solid pleural abnormalities, and pneumothoraces.

Volpicelli G, Elbarbary M, Blaivas M, et al. International evidence-based recommendations for point-of-care lung ultrasound. *Intensive Care Med.* 2012;38:577–591.

Multi-specialty, international, evidence-based guidelines on the clinical application of lung ultrasound. The following pathologies were specifically discussed: pneumothorax, interstitial syndrome, lung consolidation, monitoring lung diseases, and pleural effusion.

Focused Echo

Repessé X, Charron C, Vieillard-Baron A. Intensive care ultrasound: V. Goal-directed echocardiography. *Ann Am Thorac Soc.* 2014;11:122–128.

> Describes how to rapidly approach hemodynamically compromised patients using focused cardiac ultrasound.

Via G, Hussain A, Wells M, et al. International evidence-based recommendations for focused cardiac ultrasound. *J Am Soc Echocardiography.* 2014;27:683.e1–683.e33.

> *Guidelines from the first international conference on focused cardiac ultrasound (FoCUS) by The World Interactive Network Focused on Critical Ultrasound. An international multi-disciplinary panel developed comprehensive, evidence-based recommendations outlining the definition, applications, techniques, potential benefits, clinical integration education and certification processes for FoCUS.*

DVT

Kory PD, Pellecchia CM, Shiloh AL. Accuracy of ultrasonography performed by critical care physicians for the diagnosis of DVT. *Chest.* 2010;139:538–542.

> *Multicenter, retrospective study comparing intensivist-performed compression ultrasonography for diagnosing proximal lower extremity DVT to formal vascular studies. Intensivist performed exams yielded a sensitivity of 86% and specificity of 96% with a diagnostic accuracy of 95%. Study suggests that compression ultrasound is a rapid and accurate method for diagnosing proximal LE DVTs in the ICU.*

Volume Responsiveness

Lamia B, Ochagavia A, Monnet X, et al. Echocardiographic prediction of volume responsiveness in critically ill patients with spontaneous breathing activity. *Intensive Care Med.* 2007;3 1125.

> *Shows that transthoracic echo can predict volume responsiveness in spontaneously breathing critically ill patients by measuring change in cardiac output pre- and post leg raise maneuver.*

Abdominal

Kameda T, Taniguchi N. Overview of point-of-care abdominal ultrasound in emergency a critical care. *J Int Care.* 2016;4:1–9.

> *Review of abdominal ultrasonography in the evaluation of acute abdominal pain, hemoperitoneum, and renal dysfunction.*

Boniface KS, Calabrese KY. Intensive care ultrasound: IV. Abdominal ultrasound in critical ca *Ann Am Thorac Soc.* 2013;10:713–724.

> *Reviews focused trauma (eFAST), kidney and bladder, and abdominal aorta exams. Provi techniques for image acquisition, describes specific limitations, and shows examples normal and abnormal findings.*

88 Patient and Family Engagement, Goals of Care Communication, and End of Life Care in the Intensive Care Unit

Brian T. Wessman and Jonathan M. Green

INTRODUCTION

Despite individuals' stated preference to die at home, most deaths occur in institutions (hospital or nursing homes). Of those that expire in hospitals, many die in intensive care units (ICUs) having undergone high-burden interventions despite little likelihood of meaningful benefit. Medicare data shows that in the last 6 months of life, 1 in 5 beneficiaries will elect to undergo inpatient surgery and over one-third of patients will have received medical care in the ICU. A staggering 1 in 5 patients will die either while in the ICU or soon thereafter.

Many families of patients receiving critical care services hold overly optimistic expectations regarding survival, functional outcome status, and ultimately the quality of life that is likely to be achieved. Although physicians in general have more realistic attitudes, they often still overestimate both functional recovery and survival rates. Poor communication between the medical team and family exacerbates the disconnect between expectations and outcomes. This further complicates the decision-making process and makes it difficult to develop a plan of care likely to achieve the patient or families' expectations.

To address these problems, critical care providers must have the skills necessary effectively discuss end of life (EOL) issues with patients and families. Unfortunately, many clinicians are not adequately trained or skilled at discussing critically patients' preferences and goals regarding EOL situations. One study showed that though 80% of people say that if they were seriously ill they would want a conversation with their physician regarding EOL care, only 7% of patients actually have this type of conversation. The SUPPORT trial documented a number of deficiencies EOL care in ICUs, including poor communication between physician and patient about preferences for CPR, failure to write do not resuscitate (DNR) orders for patients that desire them, and inadequately treated pain and discomfort during the final days of life. Unfortunately, there is little evidence that these problems have been significantly reversed.

Effective EOL discussions can reduce both the incidence of aggressive interventions and the subsequent psychological stress among surviving family members. Furthermore, helping patients and families delineate life values and preferred care outcomes has been shown to reduce medical provider stress. Finally, the ICU physician needs to have at least a basic understanding of palliative care strategies as well as the skills and techniques to appropriately manage the dying patient. This chapter will review some basic medical ethics, discuss communication strategies to elicit patient-centered goals, delineate some basic palliative care terminology, explore care strategies to support the dying patient and their family, and review the concept of medical futility. While this chapter is focused on the unique aspects of the ICU and critical care patient population, the principles and techniques presented are applicable to all medical settings.

CORE ETHICAL PRINCIPLES

The four traditional pillars of medical ethics are respect for persons, beneficence, nonmaleficence, and justice (Table 88.1). One way physicians can demonstrate respect for persons is by facilitating their patient's ability to exercise their autonomy. Autonomy, derived from the Greek "autos," meaning self, and "nomos," meaning rule, acknowledges the fact that in general, patients are the best arbiters to determine which medical options promote their self-interest and values. An essential part of a physician's duty to respect persons is to provide accurate information and counsel to patients with regard their illness, potential treatment options, and outcomes. By doing so, the clinician promotes the individual's ability to make an autonomous decision.

Beneficence is the positive obligation of an individual to "do good," and requires the clinician to act in the patient's best interest. The idea of "what is best" for the patient should be defined from the patient's perspective and be informed by competent and complete information provided by the clinician. Beneficence does not always connote a need for intervention. When the benefit of the proposed therapy is not congruent with the patient's goals, beneficence may, in fact, require not intervening. A frequent source of conflict between caregivers and patients/families, and within families themselves, arises when there are significant differences in what each party feels represents the best interests of the patient. This is often most problematic when the patient is unable to participate in the decision-making process.

Nonmaleficence is the principle of "first do no harm." Virtually all therapies have the potential for adverse effects. Clinicians and patients should always carefully consider the relative harms and benefits of any intervention. This is especially relevant when providing treatments at the EOL as curative options are typically not feasible.

TABLE 88.1	Four Traditional Pillars of Medical Ethics

- Autonomy: The capacity to think, decide, and act on one's own free initiative.
- Beneficence: Promoting what is best for the patient.
- Non-maleficence: Do no harm.
- Justice: Resources are limited; patients in similar situations should have access to the same care.

Particular thought should be given when considering highly invasive, burdensome therapies, such as mechanical ventilation or hemodialysis, during the development of a plan for patients for whom death is imminent, such as someone with terminal widespread metastatic oncologic disease that presents with septic shock.

ICU beds are a scarce resource, and as such, intensivists are required to make decisions as to who will or will not be admitted to the critical care setting. Justice requires that this resource be allocated fairly, giving consideration to relevant factors only, including the condition of the patient, the capabilities of the ICU, and the likelihood that the patient will benefit from intensive care. A decision to provide care to one patient will inevitably have an impact on the ability to treat others. How to fairly allocate ICU resources is a highly controversial issue, a full discussion of which is beyond the scope of this chapter. Nonetheless, physicians should be cognizant of the issues, and avoid idiosyncratic decision-making when determining whether or not to admit a patient to the ICU.

Conflicts between these principles will inevitably arise during the care of patients, and these are often more pronounced when treating critically ill patients at the EOL. An understanding of the core ethical principles that underlie the practice of medicine can provide the physician with tools to navigate the difficult terrain of guiding patients and families through this highly stressful experience.

ESTABLISHING GOALS OF CARE

Establishing appropriate goals of care (GOC) is essential for all aspects of medical care however due to the acuity of the illness; it assumes even greater importance in the ICU setting. A goal of care is *NOT* the same as a code status or DNR order, but is a patient-centered value that may range from a desire for relief from pain to wishes such as "returning home to resume my gardening" or "being able to independently attend a baseball game." The objective of a GOC discussion is for the health care team to gain an understanding of the patient's values and preferences, and to provide the patient and/or family with accurate prognostic and treatment information. Ideally, together the physician and patient/family can develop an appropriate patient-centered treatment plan, including resuscitation status, that is congruent with this expressed personal quality of life goal.

Patients admitted to ICUs are at an increased risk of death and also face the prospect of being subjected to invasive procedures and treatments. Individual's preferences for intervention vary widely. Studies have demonstrated that as the potential for a good outcome declines, so does willingness to undergo highly burdensome treatment regimens. However, individual preferences are not uniform. In one study, % of those surveyed stated they strongly agreed with receiving ICU care despite an outcome predicted to be a persistent vegetative state or terminal illness. Conversely, between 1% and 2% did not wish to undergo ICU care even if they were to be returned to a fully functional health status. Given these data, it is essential for the health care provider to determine the patient's desire for aggressive care either prior to admission or early in the course of an ICU stay.

Upon admission to the ICU, the physician should ascertain whether a patient has previously appointed a Durable Power of Attorney for Health Care (DPOA) and/or completed an Advance Directive (AD) (Table 88.2). The DPOA appoints a specific individual to serve as proxy for the patient should they lose decision-making capacity, whereas the AD typically specifies the range of interventions that the patient

TABLE 88.2	Durable Power of Attorney for Health Care and Advanced Directive

- Durable Power of Attorney for Health Care (DPOA): The legal naming of a trusted person to oversee a patient's medical care and the legal ability to make health care decisions for that patient if they are unable to do so.
- Advance Directive (AD): Legal documents that allow a patient to preemptively spell out personal decisions about end-of-life care prior to critical illness. This legal document also serves as a way to document a patient's wishes for family, friends, and health care professionals with the goal of avoiding any confusion during critical illness.

would find acceptable and under what circumstances. If available, these documen should be obtained and the contents discussed with the patient/family. Ironicall several studies have shown that the presence of an AD had no association with th intensity of care at the EOL. Much of the value of the AD arises from the accomp nying discussion between the patient, family, and physician at the time it is writt as to the patients' preferences. Realistically, an AD *without* in-depth communicatic about what intensity of medical care each individual desires is of limited utility.

The majority of patients have neither document, and despite the presence life limiting illness, many will have not discussed EOL care with either their persor physician or family members. Thus, it may be that these difficult discussions a occurring in the ICU setting for the first time. If the patient is capable of parti pating, discussions to establish GOC should be held directly with him or her. T outcome of these discussions should then be shared by the patient and physici together with the patient's family and loved ones, as directed by the patient. If t patient is not decisional either due to the acute condition or previous underlyi disease, the discussion should be held with an appropriate surrogate (see *Surrog Decision-Making* section).

Due to their acute critical illness requiring an ICU admission, almost all patie admitted to the ICU should have an initial GOC conversation early in the cours that admission. The purpose of the initial discussion is to ascertain what the pati and family's expectations are for the acute hospitalization as well as for the underly disease process. The physician should elicit the values, preferences, and wishes of patient with respect to what they view as an acceptable outcome for their ICU s This may range from hope for cure, to a desire for a pain-free death, or anywher between. Often patients have multiple seemingly contradictory goals, in which the physician should take time to help in clarification and prioritization. It is equ important for the physician to provide prognostic information and advise the pati family as to what can reasonably be expected during this hospitalization.

Disparities between the patient/family's goals and physician's medical goals be a source of conflict in the ICU. If significant differences are identified, ong discussions to identify reasons for the disagreement and reach a consensus are cru This will often require multiple subsequent exploratory conversations. Possible sons may include misunderstandings on the part of the patient or family as to na of the disease or treatment options, or failure of the physician to appreciate cul differences or other values inherent to the individual patient. It is also impo to recognize that the goals/values may shift during the evolving course of an acute illness. Therefore, as the clinical scenario changes, ongoing discussions to reevaluate the GOC are necessary. As with any procedure, adequate documentation of these conversations in the medical record should be chronicled.

SHARED DECISION-MAKING

Shared decision-making (SDM) is of utmost importance when approaching a GOC discussion and for EOL decisions. The responsibility for most major medical decisions should be *shared* between the ICU team and the patient/surrogate. Ideally, the physician provides information about the disease state(s), current treatments, realistic medical feasibility, and prognosis, whereas the patient/surrogate informs the team about the patient's values, quality of life, and treatment preferences. This two-way information sharing should stimulate questions and conversation for both sides. Subsequently, this should lead to the joint deliberation and decision stage where both sides focus on the best available options for the patient, and together agree on a course of action.

The physician bears the responsibility to develop a plan of care that is medically feasible and congruent with the goals and values of the patient, and should not hesitate to make recommendations to the family. When discussing EOL care, and particularly resuscitation status, all too often physicians end the conversation with a question, such as "what do you want us to do" or "should we *do everything*." This unfairly burdens the family with having to make choices for which they may not be equipped or qualified. When discussing resuscitation status, they may feel they have to actively choose to end their loved one's life. Instead, by focusing on specific patient-centered values and goals, the physician can develop and recommend a treatment plan that may or may not include initiation of life-sustaining interventions or attempts at resuscitation. The plan should be clearly stated to the patient and/or family with sufficient probing to assure understanding. The family is then prompted to voice if they agree with the stated plan. In this way, the burden is shifted appropriately from the family to the physician. Remember, the goal is to communicate and jointly develop a critical care medical plan that best respects patient/family values in light of what is medically achievable.

SURROGATE DECISION-MAKING

Patients in the ICU are often unable to participate in decision-making due to either their acute illness or underlying disease process. In these instances, appropriate surrogates must be identified. If the patient has appointed a specific individual as DPOA, that individual should serve as the primary decision maker. Oftentimes, there is not a specific individual identified. Many, but not all, states have a legal order of surrogacy established (i.e., spouse or offspring). One should be familiar with the relevant laws of their state. A valid surrogate can be defined as an individual that can faithfully represent the goals, values, and wishes of the patient, act accordingly and in the patient's best interest. Typically, it is presumed that family members are best able to fill this role; however, persons not related to the patient may also be able to serve as a valid surrogate. As implied by the above definition, the role of the surrogate is to represent the patient's wishes. However, this is often a difficult task, and is almost

TABLE 88.3	Surrogate Decision-Making

Incapacitated patient's wishes are spoken through a surrogate.
- *Stated wishes:* treatment preferences previously expressed by the patient
- *Substituted judgment standard:* surrogate "dons the mental mantle of the patient" and assumes the voice for what the patient would want if they could speak themselves
- *Best interest standard:* surrogate offers thoughts on the treatment course with highest benefit for the patient based on prior interactions without clear knowledge of what the patient would want

always colored by the surrogate's own values and preferences. Studies of surrogate decision-making have shown that surrogates accurately represent the patient only 50% to 70% of the time.

The family may choose to appoint one person as spokesperson, or may prefer to decide as a group. Not infrequently, there is disagreement among them as to what the patient's wishes would be. It is important that the Intensivist works to guide the family and helps them reach consensus. The communication techniques discussed previously are essential in this process. Typically, a series of family meetings in which the disputed issues are explored will lead to consensus and resolution. It is often helpful to include nurses, social workers, chaplains, palliative care consultants, and other team members in these discussions.

The standards for surrogate decision-making are (1) stated wishes, (2) substituted judgment standard, and (3) best interest standard (Table 88.3). Stated wishes are exact verbatim treatment preferences the patient had previously expressed to the surrogate. The substituted judgment standard asks the surrogate to guide the team as to what decision the patient would make in this circumstance, essentially asking the surrogate to assume the voice for what the patient would want if they could speak for themselves. If the patient and surrogate have had specific discussions that inform this decision, then this approach may be reasonable. Often, however, no such discussion has taken place leaving the surrogate to speculate. The best interest standard asks the surrogate to help the physician determine whether the proposed treatment is in the best interest of the patient, weighing the potential benefits and burdens of the treatment with what is known about the goals and values of the patient. This standard can also be problematic, as in the absence of specific information; it is difficult to determine what an acceptable outcome is and what level of treatment burden the patient would tolerate for that outcome. Typically, both surrogates and caregivers *underestimate* the willingness of patients to undergo aggressive interventions, and *underestimate* the quality of life that patients deem to be acceptable. The Intensivist plays an active role in the process of arriving at a consensus medical plan as part of SDM.

COMMUNICATION STRATEGIES

Effective, compassionate communication is essential and can be thought of in the same way as an acquired procedural skill, with the language and terminology used being the instruments. As with any procedure, these skills are teachable, require practice to gain competency, and are of paramount importance for the Intensivist

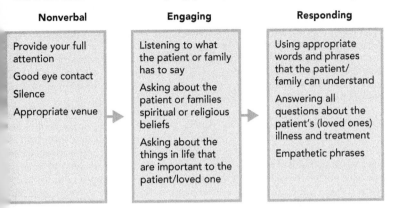

Figure 88.1. Communication is more than language.

Multiple studies have shown that communication with patients/families in the ICU is frequently inadequate. Physicians often dominate these conversations by speaking over 2/3 of the time, and use technical language that is not understandable by the listener. One study showed that during approximately 30% of family meetings, physicians miss the opportunity to listen, acknowledge, and address families' emotions, explore individual patient preferences/desires, and explain surrogate decision-making.

Language can be used in a constructive or destructive manner (Fig. 88.1). Expressions of compassion and empathy are particularly important. Use positive phrases emphasizing the things you *will do* and not what you *will not* do, such as you WILL provide comfort, WILL provide pain medications, WILL provide dignity, WILL respect the patient's autonomy," as opposed to "withdrawing care" or "we will not give vasopressors or attempt defibrillation." Phrases such as "Your loved one will not return to the way they were previously…" and "I wish (we could cure the cancer),…"
"I understand how hard this must be for you" help to convey clear meaning and show empathy. The authors of this chapter prefer the phrase "allow natural death" instead of the commonly employed "do not resuscitate (DNR)." This change in terminology can help shift the conversation as the family understands that the critical care team is allowing the natural progression of life into death.

It is essential to place the acute situation into the overall context of the patient's illness and life. The patient may have had a prolonged disease course, requiring multiple hospital admissions at increasing frequency over the past months or years. Placing the current acute illness in that context helps the family recognize and accept the inevitable death. In contrast, a previously healthy individual with little to no comorbidity experiencing an acute reversible critical illness is in a fundamentally different situation. Nonetheless, the same strategy and skills are applicable, and the GOC discussion will ideally clarify expectations and assist in the development of an appropriate plan of care.

SURGICAL AND PROCEDURAL CONSIDERATIONS

A patient for whom a DNR status has been established may require an invasive procedure for palliative purposes, such as relief of a bowel obstruction. A proceduralist, such as a surgeon, may be unwilling to intervene on a patient that is DNR unless this established code status is fully reversed. The rationale being that cardiac arrest during the procedure is often a consequence of the procedure itself or the accompanying anesthesia, and would typically be reversible with the appropriate intervention. Furthermore, an existing misconception is that a patient that undergoes a surgical intervention has subsequently agreed on treatment for any/all of the postoperative complications for at least 30 days in the postoperative period.

A patient that undergoes a surgical procedure does not suspend their autonomous right to a specific code status. If the patient requires an invasive or potentially dangerous procedure, the Anesthesiologist and the Surgeon/Proceduralist should hold a "Required Reconsideration" discussion with the patient. This discussion should define the goals of the surgical treatment, potential for resuscitative measures, and potential outcomes without resuscitation. If the patient decides to fully suspend a medical code status decision during the intraoperative/intraprocedure period, a specific timeframe should be defined for reinstating the preexisting code status in accordance with the patient's wishes. If there is any confusion, this should be addressed with the patient surrogate on arrival to the ICU setting by the critical care medicine team.

WITHDRAWING AND WITHHOLDING LIFE-SUSTAINING TREATMENTS

Critical care physicians are often faced with decisions to limit life-sustaining treatments (Table 88.4). In one large study of 851 patients admitted to a medical intensive care unit requiring mechanical ventilation, almost 20% had ventilatory support withdrawn. These decisions can be a source of distress and conflict for health care providers as well as patients and families. Family satisfaction regarding EOL care higher when families are encouraged to express their thoughts, support structures are in place, when families are assured that their loved one will not be abandoned, and are confident that their loved one will be kept comfortable and not suffer.

The ethical basis for withdrawal of life-sustaining treatments stems directly from the principle of respect for autonomy (see pillars of medical ethics section). It is widely accepted by the medical profession and society at large that an autonomous patient, and therefore by extension their surrogate, may make an informed decision to refuse any proposed treatment, even if the physician believes that such a decision is not in their best interest. From this, it follows directly that patients or their surrogates may opt to discontinue any treatment once initiated. If this were not the case, many patients might be reluctant to initiate potentially beneficial therapies for fear that

TABLE 88.4	Limiting Treatments at the End of Life

- Withholding: never starting a medical treatment or therapy
- Withdrawing: stopping a medical treatment or therapy that has already been initiated
- Euthanasia: the intentional killing of a patient (illegal in the United States)
- Physician-assisted suicide: a physician prescribes medication to the patient knowing that the patient intends to use it to commit suicide (legal in only a few states: Washington, Oregon, Vermont, Montana)

would not be permitted to stop at a later time. Conflicts may arise when the health care provider believes that discontinuation of life sustaining interventions violates the principles of beneficence and nonmaleficence, or because they feel such actions are in opposition to their own conscience. Alternatively, surrogates may wish to continue aggressive care despite the recommendation of the team that such treatments are only prolonging an inevitable death (see futility section).

Most commonly, withdrawal of life sustaining treatments is equated with discontinuation of mechanical ventilation. However, discontinuation of hemodynamic support, hemodialysis, enteral nutrition, transfusions, or other interventions should also be considered in this context. Once the decision to withdraw life-sustaining strategies has been made, all such therapies may be discontinued simultaneously. Alternatively, one published strategy is that of "stuttered withdrawal," or the staggered removal of life-sustaining treatments. In cases of family difficulty with EOL decisions, satisfaction was higher with stuttered withdrawal as it offered the family time to adjust to the decision. The decision to withdraw life-sustaining treatments should be approached in a manner similar to all other treatment decisions. While ultimate responsibility lies with the attending Intensivist physician, it is particularly important in these circumstances that the opinions of other health care providers are given voice and considered. The goal of withdrawal of life-sustaining interventions is to remove treatments that are no longer congruent with the patient's goals and values and are therefore no longer appropriate. If the patient is not decisional, it is essential that there has been prior discussion with the surrogate(s) and that they are in agreement with the proposed plan. This should be documented in the medical record.

In some appropriate cases, a terminal extubation may allow the patient a period of time to communicate or have meaningful interactions with their family members. Often times, the critical illness is too far advanced or the level of mechanical support too intense to allow this. Attention to the patient's comfort is paramount throughout the patient's ICU stay, but assumes particular importance during the process of withdrawal of life-sustaining treatments for the critically ill patient. Reluctance to administer adequate doses of analgesics and sedatives can result in undue and unacceptable levels of suffering to both the patient and surviving family members. There is ethical and legal consensus that although respiratory depression or hypotension may be a foreseeable consequence of these medications, if the intent is to relieve specific symptoms such as pain or dyspnea, it is essential to treat in adequate doses despite the possibility that death may be hastened. Ethically, the justification for this has been termed the principle of "double effect" (Table 88.5).

TABLE 88.5	The Principle of Double Effect

An action with two possible consequences, one good and one bad, is morally permissible if the action:

Is not in itself immoral.
Is undertaken only with the intention of achieving the possible good effect, without intending the possible bad effect, even though the bad effect may be foreseen.
The action does not bring about the good effect solely by means of the bad effect.
Is undertaken for a proportionately grave reason.

Palliative sedation is the goal of providing vigorous preemptive deep sedation to avoid patient suffering when death is imminent. Studies have repeatedly shown that there is no relationship with palliative sedation and "hastening of death." Doses of medication vary considerably depending upon the patient. Most commonly, narcotics such as morphine or fentanyl are given in combination with a benzodiazepine, typically either midazolam or lorazepam. The medications should be liberally administered initially as a bolus followed by continuous infusion. Each increase in infusion rate should be preceded by an appropriate bolus to allow for a rapid achievement of steady state levels. Individual patients may have greatly differing medication requirements, depending on their illness and previous exposure to the drugs. Therefore, the dosage needs to be titrated to individual patient needs. It is paramount to confirm patient comfort prior to proceeding with withdrawal of mechanical ventilation. Neuromuscular blocking agents should never be used (and train-of-four monitoring should be confirmed prior to withdrawal of mechanical ventilation if there was recent chemically induced paralysis), as they do not provide any palliative effect to the patient and make assessment of comfort impossible.

There should be frequent assessment by the nursing and medical staff for comfort as a patient approaches the end of life. Family members can be given the option of being present during the process, depending solely on their personal preference. If possible, the monitor screen in the patient's room should be turned off to allow the family to focus on the patient without distraction.

FUTILITY

The issue of medical futility has been a subject of prolonged and intense controversy. Typically, futility debates arise in the intensive care unit when the health care team believes that continued aggressive interventions are highly unlikely to lead to patient survival, yet the patient's surrogate insists that all measures continue. There are also times when disagreements between the various medical teams providing care for a patient occur. Frustration on the part of the physicians and other team members may result in the declaration that further treatment is futile, in an attempt to rationalize discontinuation of treatment and justify a unilateral decision. However, this is ethically problematic, and there remains no clear consensus on an approach to futility. Moreover, the vast majority of clinical situations in which these conflicts arise can be favorably resolved by improved communication between the physician, the various consulting services, and the family.

The concept of "futility" arises from the Latin *futilis*, meaning leaky. Greek mythology held that the daughters of Danaus were condemned in Hades to fill a large pond by transporting water in leaky buckets. Futile medical interventions serve no meaningful purpose, no matter how often they are repeated. Bernard Lo provides three specific conditions that define interventions that are futile in the strictest sense:

1. The intervention has no pathophysiologic rationale. An example of this would be the treatment of acute coronary syndrome with an antifungal medication.
2. Cardiac arrest occurs due to refractory hypotension or hypoxemia despite maximal supportive therapy. Performance of CPR in such a circumstance will be ineffective in restoring circulation.
3. The intervention has been tried and already failed in the patient.

Treatments that meet these strict criteria do not need to be provided. However, these are clearly the minority of clinical situations in which futility is discussed. Many other looser futility criteria have been proposed with concepts of quantitative, qualitative, and cost/benefit, however these concepts are problematic and should be discarded for these conversations. Most of these "futile definitions" rely on subjective determinations of what an acceptable probability of a favorable outcome is, or on determinations of quality of life. Instead of stating a "futile intervention," a preferred term in critical care medicine is "potentially inadvisable treatment."

Regardless, a strategy that focuses on process and conflict resolution rather than on absolute definitions is more likely to lead to a favorable outcome. Ultimately, it is the process of increased communication between the health care providers and family members that leads to the satisfactory resolution of these difficult situations. We highly discourage unilateral decision-making with regard to limiting life-sustaining care for critically ill patients using futility as a rationale for several reasons. First, the criteria are often incorrectly and inconsistently applied, and perhaps most importantly, such action can lead to extreme distress and anger among the surviving family members. This is not to imply that physicians need to be held hostage to unreasonable demands of unrealistic families, but that the focus of the Intensivist should be on continued communication to reach a plan of care that best represents patient and family values in light of what is medically achievable and acceptable to all parties. Policy statements, from medical organizations such as the American Medical Association (AMA), concerning due process in regards to resolving conflicts about inadvisable treatments do exist and we encourage the reader to review these individually for further guidance.

DEATH BY WHOLE BRAIN CRITERIA

Individuals that have sustained catastrophic head injuries or other causes of neurological devastation may be treated in ICUs and pose some unique challenges and issues for the Intensivist. As discussed below, these patients may meet the criteria for death; but appear to be alive to family members due to the presence of continued cardiac activity, ongoing monitoring devices, and other signs of organ function.

In 1981, the Presidents Commission for the Study of Ethical Problems in Medicine and Biomedical and Behavioral Research recommended a uniform standard for the determination of death. This stated that "An individual who has sustained either irreversible cessation of circulatory and respiratory functions, or (2) irreversible cessation of all functions of the entire brain, including the brainstem, is dead. A determination of death must be made in accordance with accepted medical standards." While death by cardiopulmonary criteria is understood and well accepted by physicians and lay people alike, declaration of death by whole brain criteria can be more problematic. Many families and religious groups are reluctant to accept this determination.

Determination of death by whole brain criteria requires examination by an experienced physician. Essential elements include that the patient is in deep coma, that brainstem function is documented to be absent, the cause of coma is established as sufficient to account for the loss of brainstem function, that the possibility of recovery of any brain function is excluded, and that cessation of all brain function exists for an appropriate period of observation and/or trial of therapy (Table 88.6). Implicit in this is that potentially reversible causes, such as drug intoxications, severe

TABLE 88.6	Whole Brain Criteria for Death: An Individual with Irreversible Cessation of All Functions of the Entire Brain, Including the Brainstem Is Dead

1. Cerebral functions are absent.
   a. Presence of deep coma, cerebral unreceptivity, and unresponsiveness.
2. Brainstem functions are absent.
   a. Absence of pupillary, corneal, oculocephalic, oculovestibular, oropharyngeal, and respiratory reflexes.
3. Irreversibility is recognized by;
   a. The cause of coma is established and is sufficient to account for the loss of brain function.
   b. The possibility of recovery of any brain function is excluded.
   c. The cessation of all brain functions persists for an appropriate period of observation and/or trial of therapy.

metabolic disturbances, infections, and hypothermia have been excluded as caus for the coma. The definition does not require the use of specialized testing, b in some instances cerebral perfusion scanning may be helpful to document t absence of cerebral blood flow. There are no published time intervals or "waitin periods" for brain death examinations (however hospitals may have their own inter guidelines).

After the determination of death, the family should not be told the patie is "brain dead" as this terminology is confusing to many. Instead, they should informed that the patient has been pronounced "dead" (similar to telling a family t someone is "dead" after a cardiac arrest). Families may become confused or angr discussions regarding withdrawal of support or medical therapies are initiated a declaration of death has occurred. All previously initiated life-sustaining treatmer such as mechanical ventilation and vasopressor support, should be withdrawn. T should be communicated to families prior to the formal brain death examinati In some circumstances, the clinician may elect to continue artificial support fo limited time to determine whether the patient wanted to be an organ donor or support organs that will be harvested for organ donation (however it should be m clear that the patient is dead and you are now providing organ supportive therapi It is not necessary to provide sedation or analgesia to the patient at this time as t have expired.

CONCLUSION

As Hippocrates taught, "the role of the physician is to cure sometimes, treat often, comfort always." Physicians caring for the critically ill will continue to face challe in providing appropriate care for the dying patient and by extension, their fami Many factors, including increases in technology and an aging population will alr certainly lead to greater numbers of patients dying in ICUs. A basic understanding application of the pillars of medical ethics is central to the knowledge of an Intens It takes time and practice to excel at the use of language required for compreher discussions about GOC and EOL issues. Enhanced communication between cri care providers, patients, and families at all stages of the illness is paramount to assuring that an acceptable outcome is achieved.

> "We only get 1 chance to do this well, and the family will always remember these last days…"
>
> —End-of-Life Nursing Education Consortium course

> "While as physicians and caregivers, we move on to care for the next patient, for the family, this is the only time their loved one will die"
>
> —Anonymous

SUGGESTED READINGS

Angus DC, Barnato AE, Linde-Zwirble WT, et al. Use of intensive care at the end of life in the United States: an epidemiologic study. *Crit Care Med.* 2004;32:638–643.

Beauchamp TL, Childress JF. *Principles of Biomedical Ethics.* New York, New York: Oxford University Press; 1994.

Blinderman CD, Krakauer EL, Solomon MZ, et al. Time to revise the approach to determining cardiopulmonary resuscitation status. *JAMA.* 2012;3079:917–918.

Chan JD, Treece PD, Engelberg RA, et al. Narcotic and benzodiazepine use after withdrawal of life support. *Chest.* 2004;126(1):286–293.

Cox CE, Martinu T, Sathy SJ, et al. Expectations and outcomes of prolonged mechanical ventilation. *Crit Care Med.* 2009;37(11):2888–2894.

Curtis J, Engelberg RA. What is the "Right" Intensity of Care at the End of Life and How Do We Get There? *Ann Intern Med.* 2011;154:283–284.

Curtis JR, Tonelli MR. Shared decision-making in the ICU: value, challenges, and limitations. *Am J Respir Crit Care Med.* 2011;183(7):840–841.

Cook D, Rocker G, Marshall J, et al. Withdrawal of mechanical ventilation in anticipation of death in the intensive care unit. *N Engl J Med.* 2003;349:1123–1132.

De Graeff A, Dean M. Palliative sedation therapy in the last weeks of life: a literature review and recommendations for standards. *J Palliat Med.* 2007;10(1):67–85.

Elpern EH, Patterson PA, Gloskey D, et al. Patients' preferences for intensive care. *Crit Care Med.* 1992;20:43–47.
    This study interviewed patients that had been in an ICU, and determined whether they would undergo ICU level care again given four specific outcome scenarios.

Fried TR, Bradley EH, Towle VR, et al. Understanding the treatment preferences of seriously ill patients. *N Engl J Med.* 2002;346:1061–1066.
    This study documents how patients modify their preferences in response to specific treatment strategies, weighing treatment burden against possible outcomes.

Gerstel E, Engelberg RA, Koepsell T, et al. Quality of Care and Timing of Withdrawal of Life Support in the ICU. *Am J Respir Crit Care Med.* 2008;178(8):798–804.

Halevy A, Brody BA. A multi-institution collaborative policy on medical futility. *JAMA.* 1996; 276:571–574.

Nua M, Wunsch W. Integrating palliative care in the ICU. *CO Crit Care.* 2014;20(6):673–680.

The Concept of Futility. SCCM Consensus Statement. *Critical Care Medicine.* 1997;25: 887–91.

Thompson AA, Davidson JE, Morrison W, Danis M, White DB. Shared Decision Making, A Consensus Statement. *Crit Care Med.* 2004;32:1781.

Lo B. *Resolving Ethical Dilemmas: A Guide for Clinicians.* Philadelphia, PA, Lippincott Williams and Wilkins; 2005.
    This is an outstanding text examining contemporary medical ethical issues in a practical way.

Murphy DJ, Barbour E. GUIDe (Guidelines for the Use of Intensive Care in Denver): a community effort to define futile and inappropriate care. *New Horiz.* 1994;2:326–331.

Nelson JE, Azoulay E, Curtis JR, et al. Palliative Care in the ICU. *J Palliat Med.* 2012;15(2): 168–174. Epub 2012 Jan 26.

Quill CM, Ratcliffe SJ, Harhay MO, et al. Variation on Decisions to Forgo Life-Sustaining Therapies in US ICUs. *Chest.* 2014;146(3):573–582.

Quill TE, Arnold R, Back AL. Discussing treatment preferences with patients who want everything. *Ann Intern Med.* 2009;151(5):345–349.

Scheunemann LP, Cunningham TV, Arnold RM, et al. How clinicians discuss critically ill patients' preferences and values with surrogates: an empirical analysis. *Crit Care Med.* 2015;43(4):757–764.

Shalowitz DI, Garrett-Mayer E, Wendler D. The accuracy of surrogate decision makers: a systematic review. *Arch Intern Med.* 2006;166:493–497.
   This study is a meta analysis demonstrating the difficulty in relying on surrogate decision makers to guide treatment plans.

Sheridan SL, Harris RP, Woolf SH; Shared Decision-Making Workgroup of the U.S. Preventive Services Task Force. Shared decision making about screening and chemoprevention. a suggested approach from the U.S. Preventive Services Task Force. *Am J Prev Med.* 2004;26: 56–66.

Support Principal Investigators. A controlled trial to improve care for seriously ill hospitalized patients. The study to understand prognoses and preferences for outcomes and risks of treatments (SUPPORT). *JAMA.* 1995;274:1591–1598.
   This large multicenter trial demonstrated significant gaps in communication about critical end of life issues in intensive care units. However, in a second, intervention phase, implementation of enhanced communication strategies failed to improve outcomes.

Teno J. Facts on Dying March 19, 2004. Center for Gerontology and Health Care Research, Brown University. Available at http://www.chcr.brown.edu/dying/2001DATA.HTM. Accessed October 2, 2006.

The Presidents Commission for the Study of Ethical Problems in Medicine and Biomedical and Behavioral Research. *Defining Death: Medical, Legal, and Ethical Issues in the Definition of Death.* Washington, DC: US Government Printing Office; 1981:159–166.

Truog RD, Cist AF, Brackett SE, et al. Recommendations for end-of-life care in the ICU: Ethics committee of SCCM. *Crit Care Med.* 2001;29(12):2332–2348.

Wessman B, Schallom M, Sona C. "Just Ask" for the ABCDEFG Campaign. *Crit Care Med.* 2015;43(12):e600–e601.

Wessman B, Sona C, Schallom M, et al. Improving caregivers' perceptions regarding patient goals of care/end-of-life issues for the multidisciplinary critical care team. *J Intensive Care Med.* 2015;32(1):68–76.

Wolf SM, Berlinger N, Jennings B. Forty years of work on end-of-life care– From patients' rights to systemic reform. *N Engl J Med.* 2015;372(7):678–682.

Zilberberg MD, Kramer AA, Higgins TL, et al. Prolonged acute mechanical ventilation: implications for hospital benchmarking. *Chest.* 2009;135(5):1157–1162.

Common Equations and Rules of Thumb in the Intensive Care Unit

Warren Isakow

PULMONARY EQUATIONS

Alveolar Gas Equation

$$PAO_2 = FIO_2 (PB - PH_2O) - PaCO_2/R$$

Where PAO_2 = alveolar partial pressure of oxygen,
   FIO_2 = fraction of inspired oxygen,
   PB = barometric pressure (760 mm Hg at sea level),
   PH_2O = water vapor pressure,
   $PaCO_2$ = partial pressure of carbon dioxide in the blood,
   R = respiratory quotient, assumed to be 0.8.

Alveolar-arterial Oxygen Gradient

$$PAO_2 - PaO_2$$

Normal value is between 3 and 15 mm Hg, and is influenced by age. In a healthy 40-year-old person, it may be as high as 28 mm Hg.
   For FiO_2 = 21%, should be 5 to 25 mm Hg
   For FiO_2 = 100%, should be <150 mm Hg

Partial Pressure of Arterial Carbon Dioxide

$$PaCO_2 = K \times VCO_2/\{(1 - Vd/Vt) \times VA\}$$

Where $PaCO_2$ = the partial pressure of carbon dioxide in the blood,
   K = constant,
   VCO_2 = carbon dioxide production,
   Vd/Vt = dead space ratio of each tidal volume breath,
   VA = minute ventilation.

Lung Compliance

$$Compliance_{static} = Tidal\ volume/\{Plateau\ pressure - PEEP\}$$

PEEP = positive end expiratory pressure
Normal compliance in an intubated patient = 0.05 to 0.07 L/cm H_2O

Airway Resistance

Airway Resistance = {Peak inspiratory pressure − Plateau pressure}/Peak inspiratory flow

Normal resistance in an intubated patient is 4 to 6 cm $H_2O \cdot L^{-1} \cdot sec^{-2}$.

ACID–BASE EQUATIONS

Acute Respiratory Acidosis or Respiratory Alkalosis

$$\Delta pH = 0.008 \times \Delta PaCO_2 \text{ (from 40)}$$

Chronic Respiratory Acidosis or Respiratory Alkalosis

$$\Delta pH = 0.003 \times \Delta PaCO_2 \text{ (from 40)}$$

Metabolic Acidosis

$$\text{Predicted PaCO}_2 = 1.5 \times [HCO_3^-] + 8 \ (\pm 2) \text{ (Winter's formula)}$$

$$\text{Bicarbonate deficit (mEq/L)} = [0.5 \times \text{body weight (kg)} \times (24 - [HCO_3^-])]$$

Metabolic Alkalosis

Predicted $PaCO_2 = 0.7 \times [HCO_3^-] + 21 (\pm 1.5)$ (when $[HCO_3^-]$ is <40 mEq/L)

Predicted $PaCO_2 = 0.75 \times [HCO_3^-] + 19 (\pm 7.5)$ (when $[HCO_3^-]$ is >40 mEq/L)

Bicarbonate excess $= [0.4 \times \text{body weight (kg)} \times ([HCO_3^-] - 24)]$

Validity of the Data, Henderson's Equation for Concentration of H⁺

$$[H^+] = 24 \times \frac{PaCO_2}{HCO_3^-}$$

pH	[H⁺] (mmol/L)
7.60	25
7.55	28
7.50	32
7.45	35
7.40	40
7.35	45
7.30	50
7.25	56
7.20	63
7.15	71

Anion Gap

$$\text{Anion Gap} = [Na^+] - ([CL^-] + [HCO_3^-]) = 10 \pm 4$$

The anion gap should be corrected for albumin, and for every decrease of 1 g/dl albumin, a decrease of 2.5 mmol in the anion gap will occur.

Delta Gap

$$\Delta gap = (AG - 12) - (24 - [HCO_3^-]) = 0 \pm 6$$

Positive delta gap signifies a concomitant metabolic alkalosis or respiratory acidosis. Negative delta gap signifies a concomitant normal anion gap metabolic acidosis or chronic respiratory alkalosis.

RENAL EQUATIONS

Calculated Osmolarity

$$\text{Osmolarity (mM)} = 2 \times [Na^+] + \frac{BUN \text{ (mg/dL)}}{2.8} + \frac{Glucose \text{ (mg/dL)}}{18} + \frac{ETOH}{4.8}$$

Where ETOH = alcohol.

Osmolar Gap

Osmolar gap = Measured osmolarity − calculated osmolarity. (Normal is <10 mOsm.)

Estimated Creatinine Clearance

Cockcroft-Gault CrCl = $(140 - age) \times (Wt \text{ in kg}) \times (0.85 \text{ if female})/(72 \times Cr)$

Creatinine Clearance

$$\text{Creatinine Clearance} = \frac{[\text{Urine creatinine (mg/dL)}] \times [\text{urine volume (mL/day)}]}{[\text{Plasma creatinine (mg/dL)}] \times (1440 \text{ min/day})}$$

Fractional Excretion of Sodium (FENa⁺)

$$FENa^+ = \frac{[\text{Urine Na}^+] \times [\text{Plasma Creatinine}]}{[\text{Urine Creatinine}] \times [\text{Plasma Na}^+]}$$

Fractional Excretion of Urea (FE urea)

$$FE \text{ Urea} = \frac{[\text{Urine Urea}] \times [\text{Plasma Creatinine}]}{[\text{BUN}] \times [\text{Urine Creatinine}]}$$

Correcting Sodium for Hyperglycemia

Corrected Na⁺ = 0.016 (Measured Glucose − 100) + Measured Na

Free Water Deficit

Free water deficit = TBW × (1 − {target sodium/measured sodium})

Where TBW (total body water in Liters) = coefficient × weight in kg
Use coefficient of 0.6 for men, 0.5 for nonelderly women and elderly men, for elderly women.

Useful Formula for Slowly Correcting Hyponatremia

Expected change in serum sodium with selected infusates

$$\Delta \text{ sodium} = \{\text{infusate sodium} + \text{infusate potassium} - \text{serum sodium}\}/(\text{TBW} + 1)$$

Where TBW (Total body water in Liters) = coefficient × weight in kg

Use coefficient of 0.6 for men, 0.5 for nonelderly women and elderly men, 0.4 for elderly women.

HEMODYNAMIC EQUATIONS

Mean Arterial Pressure (MAP) (70–100 mm Hg)

$$\text{MAP} = 1/3 \text{ (Pulse Pressure)} + \text{Diastolic BP (blood pressure)}$$

Where pulse pressure = systolic BP − diastolic BP

Arterial Oxygen Content (CaO$_2$) (18 to 21 mL O$_2$/dL)

$$\text{CaO}_2 = \{1.39 \times \text{Hb (g/dL)} \times \text{SaO}_2\} + (0.003 \times \text{PaO}_2)$$

Mixed Venous Oxygen Content (CvO$_2$) (14.5 to 15.5 mL O$_2$/dL)

$$\text{CvO}_2 = \{1.39 \times \text{Hb (g/dL)} \times \text{SvO}_2\} + (0.003 \times \text{PvO}_2)$$

Arterial-mixed Venous Oxygen Content Difference (3.5 to 5.5 mL O$_2$/dL)

$$\text{AVDO}_2 = \text{CaO}_2 - \text{CvO}_2$$

Cardiac Output (CO) (4 to 7 L/min)

$$\text{CO} = \text{heart rate} \times \text{stroke volume}$$

$$\text{CO (Fick principle)} = \text{Oxygen consumption}/\{\text{CaO}_2 - \text{CvO}_2\}$$

$$\text{CO in L/min (Fick principle)} = \text{Oxygen consumption}/\{13.4 \times \text{Hb} \times [\text{SaO}_2 - \text{SvO}_2]\}$$

Cardiac Index (CI) (2.5 to 4 L/min/m²)

$$\text{CI} = \text{CO/BSA}$$

Where Body Surface Area (BSA, in m²) = [height (cm)]$^{0.718}$ × [weight (kg)]$^{0.427}$ × 0.007449

Stroke Volume (SV) (50 to 120 mL per Contraction)

Stroke Volume Index (SVI) (35 to 50 mL/m²)

$$\text{SVI} = \text{SV/BSA}$$

Oxygen Delivery (mL/min) (1000 mL/min)

$$\text{O}_2 \text{ delivery} = \text{CO} \times \text{CaO}_2 \times 10$$

Systemic Vascular Resistance (SVR) (800 to 1200 dyne·s·cm^{-5})

$$\text{SVR (dyne·s·cm}^{-5}) = 80 \times \{(\text{MAP} - \text{RAP})/\text{CO}\}$$

Pulmonary Vascular Resistance (PVR) (120 to 220 dyne·s·cm^{-5})

$$\text{PVR (dyne·s·cm}^{-5}) = 80 \times \{(\text{mean PAP} - \text{PAOP})/\text{CO}\}$$

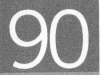

Drug–Drug Interactions

Paul Juang and Scott T. Micek

TABLE 90.1	Cytochrome P450 Enzyme Family Substrates, Inhibitors, and Inducers			
Substrates				
1A2	2C9	2C19	2D6	3A4
Acetaminophen	Celecoxib	Amitriptyline	Amitriptyline	Alprazolam
Caffeine	Ibuprofen	Citalopram	Aripiprazole	Aripiprazole
Cyclobenzaprine	Irbesartan	Clopidogrel	Carvedilol	Buspirone
Imipramine	Losartan	Cyclophos-	Codeine	Calcium chan-
Haloperidol	Phenytoin	phamide	Dextromethor-	nel blockers
Mexiletine	Sulfonylureas	Diazepam	phan	Carbamazepine
Olanzapine	Torsemide	Imipramine	Haloperidol	Conivaptan
Ondansetron	(S) Warfarin	Phenobarbital	Imipramine	Cyclosporine
Theophylline		Phenytoin	Lidocaine	Diazepam
Tizanidine		Proton pump	Metoprolol	Estradiol
(R) Warfarin		inhibitors	Metoclopra-	Fentanyl
		Voriconazole	mide	Haloperidol
			Mexiletine	Hydrocortisone
			Ondansetron	Lidocaine
			Paroxetine	Macitentan
			Propafenone	Midazolam
			Propranolol	PDE-5
			Risperidone	inhibitors
			Tramadol	Protease
			Venlafaxine	inhibitors
				Sirolimus
				Statins (except
				pravas-
				tatin and
				rosuvastatin)
				Tacrolimus
				Trazodone
				Zolpidem

(continued)

TABLE 90.1	Cytochrome P450 Enzyme Family Substrates, Inhibitors, and Inducers (*Continued*)

Inhibitors

(Increase the serum and tissue concentration of substrates)

1A2	2C9	2C19	2D6	3A4
Amiodarone	Amiodarone	Cimetidine	Amiodarone	Amiodarone
Cimetidine	Fluconazole	Fluoxetine	Bupropion	Aprepitant
Ciprofloxacin	Isoniazid	Fluvoxamine	Cimetidine	Cimetidine
Clarithromycin	Metronidazole	Isoniazid	Duloxetine	Clarithromycin
Efavirenz	Sulfamethox-	Ketoconazole	Fluoxetine	Conivaptan
Fluvoxamine	azole	Proton pump	Haloperidol	Diltiazem
	Voriconazole	inhibitors	Methadone	Erythromycin
		Voriconazole	Paroxetine	Itraconazole
			Quinidine	Ketoconazole
			Ritonavir	Netupitant
			Sertraline	Protease
				inhibitors
				Quinupristin-
				dalfopristin
				Verapamil
				Voriconazole

Inducers

(Decrease the serum and tissue concentration of substrates)

1A2	2C9	2C19	2D6	3A4
Carbamazepine	Bosentan	Bosentan	Dexametha-	Bosentan
Phenobarbital	Carbamaze-	Carbamaze-	sone	Carbamazepin
Rifampin	pine	pine	Rifampin	Efavirenz
Tobacco	Phenobarbital	Phenytoin		Glucocorticoid
	Phenytoin	Rifampin		Phenobarbital
	Rifampin			Phenytoin
				Rifabutin
				Rifampin
				St. John's wo

TABLE 90.2	Frequent Drug–Drug Interactions in Critically Ill Patients	
Medication	**Interacting Drug**	**Effect**[a]
Cardiac		
Amiodarone	2C9, 2D6, 3A4 substrates (Table 90.1)	↑ Substrate
	Digoxin	↑ Digoxin
Beta blockers	2D6 inhibitors (Table 90.1)	↑ Beta blocker
(2D6 substrates)	Carbamazepine	↓ Beta blocker
Carvedilol	Phenytoin	↓ Beta blocker
Metoprolol	Rifampin	↓ Beta blocker
Propranolol		
Digoxin	Amiodarone	↑ Digoxin
	Clarithromycin	↑ Digoxin
	Erythromycin	↑ Digoxin
	Esomeprazole	↓ Digoxin
	Quinidine	↑ Digoxin
	Verapamil	↑ Digoxin
Diltiazem/verapamil (3A4 inhibitors)	3A4 substrates (Table 90.1)	↑ Substrate
Lidocaine	Amiodarone	↑ Lidocaine
Antiepileptics		
Carbamazepine (enzyme inducer, 3A4 substrate)	1A2, 2C19, 3A4 substrates (Table 90.1)	↓ Substrate
		↑ Carbamazepine
	Clarithromycin	↑ Carbamazepine
	Diltiazem	↑ Carbamazepine
	Erythromycin	↑ Carbamazepine
	Quinupristin-dalfopristin	↑ Carbamazepine
	Verapamil	
Oxcarbazepine	Phenytoin	↑ Phenytoin
Phenytoin (enzyme inducer)	Verapamil	↓ Oxcarbazepine
	3A4 substrates (Table 90.1)	↓ Substrate
Antimicrobials		
Azithromycin	Antacids	↓ Azithromycin
	Cyclosporine	↑ Cyclosporine
	Digoxin	↑ Digoxin
	Tacrolimus	↑ Tacrolimus
Carbapenems	Valproic acid	↓ Valproic acid
Clindamycin	Aminoglycosides	↑ Nephrotoxicity
	Erythromycin	↓ Erythromycin
	Neuromuscular blocking agents	↑ Neuromuscular blockade
Ciprofloxacin (1A2 inhibitor)	1A2 substrates (Table 90.1)	↑ Substrate
	Cyclosporine	↓ Ciprofloxacin
	Sucralfate	↓ Ciprofloxacin
	Calcium, iron, antacids	↓ Oral ciprofloxacin

(continued)

TABLE 90.2	Frequent Drug–Drug Interactions in Critically Ill Patients (*Continued*)	
Medication	Interacting Drug	Effect[a]
Antimicrobials		
Clarithromycin (1A2, 3A4 inhibitor)	1A2, 3A4 Substrates (Table 90.1)	↑ Substrate
	Digoxin	↑ Digoxin
Colistin	Neuromuscular blocking agents	↑ Neuromuscular blockade
Linezolid	SSRIs	↑ Serotonin concentrations
	Tramadol	
	Tricyclic antidepressants	↑ Linezolid
	Methotrexate	↑ Linezolid
Piperacillin-tazobactam	3A4 substrates (Table 90.1)	↑ Methotrexate
Quinupristin-dalfopristin (3A4 inhibitor)		↑ Substrate
Vancomycin	NSAIDs	↑ Vancomycin
Antifungals		
Caspofungin	Carbamazepine	↓ Caspofungin
	Cyclosporine	↑ Caspofungin
	Dexamethasone	↓ Caspofungin
	Phenytoin	↓ Caspofungin
	Rifampin	↓ Caspofungin
	Tacrolimus	↓ Tacrolimus
Fluconazole, voriconazole (2C9, 3A4 inhibitor)	2C9, 3A4 substrates (Table 90.1)	↑ Substrate
Itraconazole	3A4 substrates (Table 90.1)	↑ Substrate
Ketoconazole (3A4 inhibitor)	Acid suppressants	↓ Oral capsule form itra/ketoconazole
Posaconazole	3A4 substrates (Table 90.1)	↑ Substrate
	Cimetidine	↓ Posaconazole (avoid concomitant use)
	Phenytoin	↓ Posaconazole (avoid concomitant use)
	Rifabutin	↓ Posaconazole (avoid concomitant use)
Antivirals		
Foscarnet	Ciprofloxacin	↑ Seizures

[a]↑, increase serum/tissue concentration; ↓, decrease serum/tissue concentration.
SSRIs, selective serotonin reuptake inhibitors; NSAIDs, nonsteroidal anti-inflammatory drugs.
From Baniasadi S, Farzanegan B, Alehashem M. Important drug classes associated with potentially drug–drug interactions in critically ill patients: highlights for cardiothoracic intensivists. *Ann Intensive Care.* 2015;5(1):44.

TABLE 90.3	Drugs Associated with QT-Interval Prolongation[a]

Antiarrhythmic Agents

Amiodarone	Ibutilide
Disopyramide	Procainamide
Dofetilide	Propafenone
Dronedarone	Quinidine
Flecainide	Sotalol

Antimicrobials

Azithromycin	Foscarnet
Azole antifungals	Levofloxacin
Chloroquine	Moxifloxacin
Ciprofloxacin	Pentamidine
Clarithromycin	Telavancin
Erythromycin	

Antidepressants

Amitriptyline	Fluoxetine
Citalopram	Imipramine
Desipramine	Sertraline
Doxepin	Venlafaxine
Escitalopram	

Antipsychotics

Aripiprazole	Paliperidone
Chlorpromazine	Quetiapine
Clozapine	Risperidone
Droperidol	Sertraline
Haloperidol	Thioridazine
Lithium	Ziprasidone

Other Agents

Buprenorphine	Ondansetron
Dolasetron	Ranolazine
Indapamide	Tacrolimus
Methadone	Tizanidine
Octreotide	Tyrosine kinase inhibitors

[a] The combination of these agents may increase the risk for adverse arrhythmic event including torsades de pointes.

From Li EC, Esterly JS, Pohl S, et al. Drug-induced QT-interval prolongation: considerations for clinicians. *Pharmacotherapy.* 2010;30(7):684–701.

TABLE 90.4	Drugs with Serotonergic Properties[a]	

Increased Release of Serotonin

Amphetamines and derivatives	MAOIs
Cocaine	Mirtazapine
Levodopa	

Inhibition of Serotonin Metabolism

Linezolid	Selegiline
MAOIs	St. John's wort

Impaired Presynaptic Reuptake

Amphetamines and derivatives	SNRIs
Bupropion	SSRIs
Cocaine	St. John's wort
Dextromethorphan	Tramadol
Fentanyl	Trazadone
Meperidine	Tricyclic antidepressants
Propoxyphene	

Enhance Serotonergic Effect

5-HT$_3$ receptor antagonists (i.e., ondansetron)

Direct Serotonin Receptor Agonism

5-HT$_1$ receptor agonists (i.e., sumatriptan)	Carbamazepine
Buspirone	Lithium

[a]The combination of these agents may increase the risk for serotonin toxicity manifested by a triad of symptoms including: (1) cognitive changes, (2) autonomic instability, and (3) neuromuscular excitability.

MAOIs, monoamine oxidase inhibitors; SSRIs, selective serotonin reuptake inhibitors.

From Taylor JJ, Wilson JW, Estes LL. Linezolid and serotonergic drug interactions: a retrospective survey. *Clin Infect Dis.* 2006;43(2):180–187, with permission.

91 | Common Drug Dosages and Side Effects

Mollie Gowan and Scott T. Micek

Toxicities were classified as "rare" and "common" in a relative fashion for each agent. This table does not include an exhaustive list of possible adverse effects.

TABLE 91.1	Shock		
Drug	Dosing	Rare Toxicities	Common Toxicities
Vasopressors/Inotropes			
Norepinephrine	0.02–3 mcg/kg/min	Tissue hypoxia, tachycardia, arrhythmias, myocardial ischemia, extravasation-associated tissue necrosis	Hyperglycemia
Epinephrine	0.01–0.1 mcg/kg/min	Tachycardia, arrhythmias, myocardial ischemia, splanchnic and renal hypoxia, lactic acidosis, extravasation-associated tissue necrosis	Tachycardia, hyperglycemia
Phenylephrine	0.5–10 mcg/kg/min	Bradycardia, reduced cardiac output, myocardial ischemia, extravasation-associated tissue necrosis	—
Dopamine	5–20 mcg/kg/min	Myocardial ischemia, tissue hypoxia, extravasation-associated tissue necrosis	Tachycardia, arrhythmias

(continued)

TABLE 91.1	Shock (*Continued*)		
Drug	Dosing	Rare Toxicities	Common Toxicities
Vasopressin	0.01–0.04 U/min	Reduced cardiac output, myocardial ischemia, hepatosplanchnic hypoperfusion, thrombocytopenia, hyponatremia, ischemic skin lesions	—
Dobutamine	2.5–20 mcg/kg/min	Arrhythmias	Tachycardia
Milrinone	50 mcg/kg bolus, then 0.25–0.75 mcg/kg/min	Thrombocytopenia, arrhythmias	Hypotension
Corticosteroids			
Hydrocortisone	200 mg/day in 4 divided doses	—	Short-term: hyperglycemia, mood changes, insomnia, gastrointestinal irritation, increased appetite Long-term: osteoporosis, acne, thin skin, fat redistribution, muscle wasting, cataracts HPA axis suppression, increased blood pressure, infection

HPA, hypothalamic–pituitary–adrenal; PO, by mouth; IV, intravenous.

TABLE 91.2	Respiratory Disorders		
Drug	**Dosing**	**Rare Toxicities**	**Common Toxicities**
ARDS, Status Asthmaticus, COPD Exacerbation			
Corticosteroids			
Methylpred-nisolone	1–2 mg/kg/day in 3–4 divided doses, tapering schedule dependent on disease process	—	Short-term: hyperglycemia, mood changes, insomnia, gastrointestinal irritation, increased appetite Long-term: osteoporosis, acne, thin skin, fat redistribution, muscle wasting, cataracts, HPA axis suppression, increased blood pressure, infection
Beta-agonists			
Albuterol	2–4 puffs BID to QID	Tachycardia, insomnia, irritability/nervousness, tremor, hyperglycemia, hypokalemia	—
Levalbuterol	0.63–0.125 mg TID		
Anticholinergics			
Ipratropium	2–4 puffs BID to QID	Dry mucous membranes, tachycardia	—
Pulmonary Hypertension			
Calcium channel blockers			
Diltiazem	Up to 720 mg/day in divided doses	Gingival hyperplasia, increased cardiovascular events	Peripheral edema flushing, headache, dizziness, hypotension
Nifedipine[a]	up to 240 mg/day in divided doses		

(continued)

TABLE 91.2 | Respiratory Disorders (*Continued*)

Drug	Dosing	Rare Toxicities	Common Toxicities
Prostacyclins			
Epoprostenol	2–50 ng/kg/min IV 5000–20,000 ng/mL continuous nebulization	bleeding	Jaw pain, nausea, headache, flushing, hypotension
Treprostinil	10–150 ng/kg/min SC* 3 inhalations (18 mcg) 4 times/day	bleeding	Jaw pain, nausea, headache, flushing, hypotension infusion-site pain*
Treprostinil Diolamine	0.375–0.5 mg/day PO in 2–3 divided doses	bleeding	Headache, diarrhea, nausea
Iloprost	2.5–5 mcg inhaled 6–9 times daily		Nausea, headache, flushing, hypotension, cough
Selexipag	200–1600 mcg bid	Hyperthyroidism	Jaw pain, nausea, headache, diarrhea
Endothelin antagonists			
Bosentan	62.5 mg PO bid × 1 month, then 125 mg PO BID, as tolerated	Anemia	Hepatotoxicity, headache, hypotension, flushing, peripheral edema
Ambrisentan	5–10 mg PO daily	Anemia	Peripheral edema, headache, cough
Macitentan	10 mg PO daily	Hepatotoxicity	Anemia, headache
PDE-5 inhibitors			
Sildenafil	20–40 mg PO TID	Vision changes, epistaxis	Headache, hypotension, flushing, dyspepsia
Tadalafil	40 mg PO daily		Headache, hypotension, flushing, dyspepsia
Soluble guanylate cyclase stimulator			
Riociguat	3–7.5 mg PO in 3 divided doses	Hypotension	Headache, dizziness, dyspepsia, nausea, diarrhea

(contin.

TABLE 91.2	Respiratory Disorders (*Continued*)		
Drug	Dosing	Rare Toxicities	Common Toxicities
Miscellaneous vasodilator			
Nitric oxide	5–40 parts per million	Methemoglobin-emia, elevated nitrogen dioxide	Hypotension
Pulmonary Embolism			
Unfrac-tionated heparin	80 U/kg bolus, then 18 U/kg/hr, adjust to aPTT 1.5–2.5 × control	Type II heparin-induced thrombo-cytopenia, hyperkalemia	Bleeding, type I heparin-induced thrombocytopenia bleeding
Alteplase	100 mg IV over 2 hr	—	Bleeding

[a]Immediate-release form.

HPA, hypothalamic–pituitary–adrenal; BID, twice daily; QID, four times a day; INR, international normalized ratio; IV, intravenous; SC, subcutaneously; PO, by mouth.

TABLE 91.3	Cardiac Disorders		
Drug	Dosing	Rare Toxicities	Common Toxicities
Acute Myocardial Infarction			
Antiplatelet agents			
Aspirin	160–325 mg PO daily	Tinnitus, anaphylaxis, gastritis	Bleeding, dyspepsia
Clopidogrel	600 mg PO loading dose, then 75 mg PO daily	Thrombotic thrombocytopenic purpura	Nausea, vomiting, diarrhea, bleeding
Prasugrel	60 mg PO loading dose, then 10 mg PO daily	Nausea, bradycardia, peripheral edema, leukopenia	Hypertension, hyperlipidemia, headache
Ticagrelor	180 mg PO loading dose, then 90 mg PO bid	Headache, dizziness, ventricular pause	Hyperuricemia, bleeding, dyspnea
Cangrelor	30 mcg/kg IV bolus prior to PCI, then 4 mcg/kg/min for ≥2 hours or duration of procedure		Bleeding
Abciximab	PCI: 0.25 mg/kg bolus, then 0.125 mcg/kg/min	Thrombocytopenia	Bleeding, hypotension, nausea
Eptifibatide	180 mcg/kg bolus, then 2 mcg/kg/min	Hypotension	Bleeding
Tirofiban	0.4 mcg/kg/min × 30 minutes, then 0.1 mcg/kg/min	Bradycardia	Bleeding
Beta-blockers			
Metoprolol	5 mg IV q5min × 3 dose 50–200 mg PO q12h	Heart block, bronchospasm, depression, nightmares, altered glucose metabolism, dyslipidemia, sexual dysfunction	Bradycardia, hypotension, fatigue, malaise, cold extremities

(continued)

TABLE 91.3	Cardiac Disorders (*Continued*)		
Drug	**Dosing**	**Rare Toxicities**	**Common Toxicities**
Esmolol	500 mcg/kg bolus, then 50–300 mcg/kg/min		
Nitrates			
Nitroglycerin	10–200 mcg/min	—	Headache, flushing, dizziness, hypotension, tachycardia
Isosorbide dinitrate	5–40 mg PO TID		
Isosorbide mononitrate	30–120 mg PO daily		
Fibrinolytics			
Alteplase	15 mg bolus, then 0.75 mg/kg (up to 50 mg) × 30 min, then 0.5 mg/kg (up to 35 mg) × 60 min (max, 100 mg over 90 min	—	Bleeding
Reteplase	10 mg IV, then 10 mg IV 30 min after first dose		
Tenecteplase	One-time bolus: ≤60 kg = 30 mg 61–70 kg = 35 mg 71–80 kg = 40 mg 81–90 kg = 45 mg ≥90 kg = 50 mg		
Streptokinase	1.5 million units over 2 hrs		
Anticoagulants			
Unfractionated heparin	60 U/kg bolus, then 12 U/kg/hr, adjust to aPTT 1.5–2.5 × control	Type II heparin-induced thrombocytopenia, hyperkalemia	Bleeding, type I heparin-induced thrombocytopenia bleeding
Enoxaparin	1 mg/kg SC q12h		Bleeding
Dalteparin	120 U/kg SC q12h		
Argatroban	PCI: 350 mcg/kg bolus, then 25 mcg/kg/min		Bleeding
Bivalirudin	PCI: 1 mg/kg bolus, then 2.5 mg/kg/hr		

(continued)

TABLE 91.3	Cardiac Disorders (*Continued*)		
Drug	Dosing	Rare Toxicities	Common Toxicities
Arrhythmias and Conduction Abnormalities			
Atropine	1 mg IV q3–5 min	—	Dry eyes, dry mouth, urinary retention, tachycardia
Epinephrine	1 mg IV q3–5min	—	Tachycardia, hypertension
Procain-amide	15–18 mg/kg bolus then 1–6 mg/min	Torsade de pointes	Diarrhea, nausea, vomiting
Lidocaine	1–1.5 mg/kg bolus (may repeat doses 0.5–0.75 mg/kg in 5–10 min up to max 3 mg/kg), then 1–4 mg/min	Confusion, drowsiness, slurred speech, psychosis, paresthesias, muscle twitching, seizures, bradycardia	—
Amiodarone	300 mg bolus, then 1 mg/min for 6 hrs, then 0.5 mg/min for ≥18 hrs	Heart block, pulmonary fibrosis, hypo/hyperthyroidism, blue-gray skin discoloration, torsade de pointes, corneal microdeposits, optic neuropathy	Bradycardia, hypotension, nausea
Calcium channel blockers			
Diltiazem	0.25 mg/kg bolus (may repeat 0.35 mg/kg bolus after 15 min), then 5–15 mg/hr	Heart block, heart failure, exacerbation	Bradycardia, hypotension, constipation (verapamil > diltiazem) headache, flushing edema
Verapamil	5 mg bolus (may repeat up to total 20 mg), then 5–15 mg/hr		
Adenosine	6 mg IV, if not effective in 1–2 min can give 12 mg, may repeat 12 mg	—	Flushing, lightheadedness, headache, nervousness/anxie

(contin

TABLE 91.3	Cardiac Disorders (*Continued*)		
Drug	**Dosing**	**Rare Toxicities**	**Common Toxicities**
Congestive Heart Failure			
Nesiritide	2 mcg/kg bolus, then 0.01–0.03 mcg/kg/min	—	Hypotension, increased serum creatinine
Digoxin	Load: 10–15 mcg/kg; give 50% of load in initial dose, then 25% at 6–12 hr intervals × 2 Maintenance: 0.125–0.5 mg/day (Dose should be reduced by 20–25% when changing from oral to IV)	Arrhythmias, heart block, visual disturbances (blurred or yellow vision), mental disturbances	Bradycardia
ACE inhibitors			
Captopril	6.25–50 mg PO TID	Anaphylaxis, angioedema	Cough, hyperkalemia, hypotension, renal insufficiency
Lisinopril	2.5–40 mg PO BID		
Enalapril	2.5–10 mg PO BID		
Ramipril	1.25–5 mg PO BID		
Aldosterone receptor antagonists			
Spironolactone	12.5–50 mg PO daily	Gynecomastia (spironolactone > eplerenone), hyponatremia	Hyperkalemia
Eplerenone	25–50 mg PO daily		
Loop diuretics[a]			
Furosemide	20–80 mg/day IV/PO in 2–3 divided doses	Ototoxicity	Hypokalemia, hypomagnesemia, hypocalcemia, orthostatic hypotension, azotemia
Torsemide	10–20 mg IV/PO daily		
Bumetanide	0.5–2 mg/day in 1–2 doses		

(*continued*)

TABLE 91.3	Cardiac Disorders (*Continued*)		
Drug	Dosing	Rare Toxicities	Common Toxicities
Hypertensive Emergencies			
Nitroprus-side	Usual, 0.25–3 mcg/kg/min Max, 10 mcg/kg/min	Muscle spasm	Nausea, vomiting, hypotension, tachycardia, thiocyanate, and cyanide toxicity
Nicardipine	3–15 mg/hr	—	Hypotension, tachycardia, headache, flushing, peripheral edema
Clevidipine	1–32 mg/hr	Headache, hyper-triglyceridemia	Atrial fibrillation, fever, nausea, insomnia
Labetalol	20–40 mg (max, 80 mg) as IV bolus at 10–20 min intervals, then 0.5–2 mg/min if needed	Heart block, bronchoconstriction	Hypotension, bradycardia, nausea, vomiting
Clonidine	0.1–0.3 mg PO BID–TID	—	Drowsiness, dizziness, hypotension, bradycardia, dry mouth
Hydralazine	10–40 mg IV q4–6h or 10–75 mg PO TID-QID	Drug-induced lupus-like syndrome, rash, peripheral neuropathy	Hypotension, tachycardia, flushing, headache
Enalaprilat	1.25–5 mg IV q6h	Anaphylaxis, angioedema	Hypotension, hyperkalemia, renal insufficiency

[a]Usual starting doses are listed for furosemide and torsemide; dosing is highly variable and much larger doses are often used.
PO, by mouth; IV, intravenous; TID, three times a day; STEMI, ST-segment elevation myocardial infarction; aPTT, activated partial thromboplastin time; PCI, percutaneous coronary intervention; BID, twice daily.

TABLE 91.4	Electrolyte Abnormalities		
Drug	Dosing	Rare Toxicities	Common Toxicities
Hyponatremia			
Conivaptan	20 mg IV bolus, then 0.8–1.6 mg/hr IV continuous infusion	—	Diarrhea, hypokalemia
Hyperkalemia			
Regular Humulin insulin	10–20 units IV (given with dextrose, every ~1 unit for 4–5 g dextrose)	Local skin reactions	Hypoglycemia, hypokalemia, weight gain
Sodium bicarbonate	1 mEq/kg IV	Extravasation-associated tissue necrosis	Metabolic alkalosis, hypernatremia, hypokalemia
Albuterol	10–20 mg nebulized over 30–60 min	Tachycardia, insomnia, irritability/nervousness tremor, hyperglycemia, hypokalemia	—
Calcium gluconate	1 gm IV over 2 min	Arrhythmias, phlebitis (chloride > gluconate)	Hypercalcemia, constipation (oral)
Hypercalcemia			
Bisphosphonates			
Pamidronate	60–90 mg IV bolus	Thrombophlebitis; bone, joint, muscle pain	Fever, fatigue
Zoledronic acid	4 mg IV bolus		
Calcitonin	Initial 4 U/kg IM q12h, up to 8 U/kg IM q6h	Allergic reaction	Facial flushing, nausea, vomiting
Denosumab	120 mg SC every 4 weeks	Hearing loss, osteonecrosis of jaw	Nausea, constipation, weakness, fatigue, hypophosphatemia
Hypophosphatemia			
Potassium phosphate	0.08–0.16 mmol/kg IV over 6 hrs	—	Hyperphosphatemia, Hypocalcemia.
Sodium phosphate			Hypomagnesemia, hyperkalemia, hypernatremia, diarrhea (oral)

Intravenously; IM, intramuscularly.

TABLE 91.5	Endocrine Disorders		
Drug	Dosing	Rare Toxicities	Common Toxicities
Hypothyroid			
Levothyroxine	Myxedema coma: 50–100 mcg IV q6–8h × 24 hrs, then 100 mcg IV q24h	Signs and symptoms of hyperthyroidism with excessive doses (tachycardia, angina pectoris, arrhythmias, myocardial infarction, heat intolerance, diaphoresis, hyperactivity)	—
Hyperthyroid			
Propylthiouracil*	Initial 300–600 mg/day in 3 divided doses q8h, maintenance 50–300 mg per day	Agranulocytosis, aplastic anemia, hepatotoxicity, lupus-like syndrome, hypoprothrombin-emia, polymyositis*	Rash, arthralgias, fever, leukopenia, nausea, vomiting
Methimazole	Initial 30–60 mg/day in 3 divided doses q8h, Maintenance 5–30 mg per day		
Propranolol	10–40 mg PO q6h	Heart block, bronchospasm, depression, nightmares, altered glucose metabo-lism, dyslipidemia, sexual dysfunction	Bradycardia, hypotension, fatigue, malaise, cold extremities
SS potassium iodide	1–2 drops PO q12h	Hypersensitivity reactions	Metallic taste, nausea, stomach upset, diarrhea, salivary gland swelling

(continued)

TABLE 91.5	Endocrine Disorders (*Continued*)		
Drug	Dosing	Rare Toxicities	Common Toxicities
Adrenal Insufficiency			
Hydrocortisone	100 mg IV q8h	—	Short-term: hyperglycemia, mood changes, insomnia, gastrointestinal irritation, increased appetite Long-term: osteoporosis, acne, thin skin, fat redistribution, muscle wasting, cataracts HPA axis suppression, increased blood pressure, infection
Dexamethasone	10 mg IV prior to ACTH stimulation test		
Fludrocortisone	50–200 mcg PO q24h	—	Increased blood pressure, edema, hypernatremia, hypokalemia
Insulin	—	Local skin reactions	Hypoglycemia, hypokalemia, weight gain

/, intravenous; PO, by mouth; ACTH, adrenocorticotropin hormone; HPA, hypothalamic—ituitary–adrenal; PRN, as needed; NSAIDs, nonsteroidal anti-inflammatory drugs; TID, three times day.

TABLE 91.6	Oncologic Emergencies		
Drug	Dosing	Rare Toxicities	Common Toxicities
Allopurinol	600–800 mg/day in 2–3 divided doses	Nausea, vomiting	Rash
Rasburicase	0.2 mg/kg/day or 3, 6, or 7.5 mg once	Hypersensitivity reactions, methemoglobinemia, hemolysis	Nausea, vomiting, fever, headache, rash, diarrhea, constipation

IV, intravenous; PO, by mouth; ACTH, adrenocorticotropin hormone; HPA, hypothalamic–pituitary–adrenal; PRN, as needed; NSAIDs, nonsteroidal anti-inflammatory drugs; TID, three times a day.

TABLE 91.7	Temperature Regulation		
Drug Class/ Prototypes	Dosing	Rare Toxicities	Common Toxicities
Acetaminophen	325–1000 mg PO q4–6h PRN	Hepatotoxicity	—
Ibuprofen	200–800 mg PO q3–6h PRN	Gastric ulceration, bleeding, acute renal failure, increased risk of cardiovascular events	Gastric irritation, nausea
Ketorolac	15–30 mg IM or 10 mg PO PRN		
Dantrolene	1–2.5 mg/kg IV; may repeat q5–10min to max cumulative dose 10 mg/kg	Hepatotoxicity, muscle weakness	Drowsiness, dizziness, diarrhea, nausea, vomiting
Bromocriptine	2.5–5 mg PO TID	—	Headache, dizziness, nausea, diarrhea, hypotension, nasal congestion

IV, intravenous; PO, by mouth; ACTH, adrenocorticotropin hormone; HPA, hypothalamic–pituitary–adrenal; PRN, as needed; NSAIDs, nonsteroidal anti-inflammatory drugs; TID, three tim a day.

TABLE 91.8	Toxicology		
Drug	Dosing	Rare Toxicities	Common Toxicities
Activated charcoal	25–100 g	Bowel obstruction	Vomiting, constipation, fecal discoloration (black)
Naloxone	0.4–2 mg IV q2min, up to 10 mg	Abrupt reversal may cause withdrawal symptoms (sweating, agitation, hypertension, tachycardia, nausea, vomiting, cardiovascular events, seizures) pulmonary edema	—
Flumazenil	0.2–0.5 mg IV q1min, up to 5 mg	Abrupt reversal may cause withdrawal symptoms (sweating, agitation, hypertension, tachycardia, nausea, vomiting, cardiovascular events, seizures)	—
N-Acetylcysteine	Oral 140 mg/kg loading dose, then 70 mg/kg q4h × 17 doses IV 150 mg/kg bolus, then 12.5 mg/kg/hr × 4 hrs, then 6.25 mg/kg/hr × 16 hrs	Anaphylactic reactions	Nausea, vomiting (oral), unpleasant odor (oral)

(continued)

TABLE 91.8	Toxicology (*Continued*)		
Drug	Dosing	Rare Toxicities	Common Toxicities
Deferoxamine	1 g IV bolus, then 500 mg IV q4h × 2 doses	Infusion-related reactions (hypotension, tachycardia, erythema, urticaria), anaphylactic reactions, acute respiratory distress syndrome	Urine discoloration (orange-red)
Fomepizole	15 mg/kg IV bolus, then 10 mg/kg IV q12h × 4 doses, then 15 mg/kg IV q12h until ethylene glycol or methanol level <20	—	—

IV, intravenous.

TABLE 91.9	Infectious Diseases		
Drug	Dosing	Rare Toxicities	Common Toxicities
Antibacterial Agents			
Penicillin			
Ampicillin	2–3 g IV q4–6h	Anaphylaxis, seizures, hemolytic anemia, neutropenia, thrombocytopenia, drug fever	Diarrhea, nausea, vomiting, rash
Aqueous penicillin G	2–4 million U IV q4h		
Antistaphylococcal Penicillins			
Nafcillin	2 g IV q4–6h	Anaphylaxis, neutropenia, thrombocytopenia, acute interstitial nephritis, hepatotoxicity	Diarrhea, nausea, vomiting, rash
Oxacillin	2 g IV q4–6h		
B-lactam/B-lactamase Inhibitors			
Amoxicillin/ clavulanate	975 mg PO BID	Anaphylaxis, seizures, hemolytic anemia, neutropenia, thrombocytopenia, *Clostridium difficile* colitis, cholestatic jaundice, drug fever	Diarrhea, nausea, vomiting, rash
Ampicillin/ sulbactam	1.5–3 g IV q6h		
Piperacillin/ tazobactam	3.375–4.5 g IV q6h		
Ticarcillin/ clavulanate	3.1 g IV q4–6h		
Cephalosporins			
Cefazolin	1–2 g IV q8h	Anaphylaxis, seizures, neutropenia, thrombocytopenia, drug fever	Diarrhea, nausea, vomiting, rash
Cefoxitin	1–2 g IV q4–8h		

(continued)

TABLE 91.9 Infectious Diseases (*Continued*)

Drug	Dosing	Rare Toxicities	Common Toxicities
Ceftriaxone	1–2 g IV q12–24h		Diarrhea, nausea, vomiting
Ceftaroline	600 mg IV q12h		
Cefepime	500 mg–2 g IV q8–12h		
Ceftazidime/ avibactam	2.5 g IV q8h		Nausea, headache
Ceftolozane/ tazobactam	1.5g IV q8h		
Carbapenems			
Imipenem	500 mg–1 g IV q6–8h	Anaphylaxis, seizures (imipenem > meropenem > ertapenem), *C. difficile* colitis, drug fever	Nausea, headache
Meropenem	1 g IV q8h		
Ertapenem	1 g IV q24h		
Doripenem			
Glycopeptides			
Vancomycin	500 mg IV q8h 15 mg/kg IV q12h	Ototoxicity, nephrotoxicity, Red-man syndrome (unlikely without concomitant nephrotoxins), thrombocytopenia	
Telavancin	7.5 mg/kg IV q 24h	Nephrotoxicity, QTc prolongation, nausea, vomiting, taste sense altered	
Dalbavancin	1000–1500 mg IV once, then 500 mg 1 week later		
Oritavancin	1200 mg IV once		

(continue

TABLE 91.9	Infectious Diseases (*Continued*)		
Drug	**Dosing**	**Rare Toxicities**	**Common Toxicities**
Oxazolidinones Linezolid	600 mg IV/PO q12h	More common with long-term use: peripheral and optic neuropathy, myelosuppression Possible with short-term use: lactic acidosis	Diarrhea
Tedizolid	200 mg IV/PO daily	Thrombocytopenia, anemia	Nausea, headache, diarrhea
Lipopeptides Daptomycin	4–6 mg/kg IV q24h	Myopathy, anemia	Diarrhea, constipation, vomiting
Streptogramin Quinupristin/ dalfopristin	7.5 mg/kg IV q8h	—	Arthralgia, myalgia, inflammation, pain, edema at infusion site, hyperbilirubin-emia
Aminoglycosides Amikacin	8 mg/kg IV q12h or 15 mg/kg extended interval	—	Nephrotoxicity, ototoxicity
Gentamicin	3 mg/kg bolus, then 2 mg/ kg IV q8h or 5–7 mg/ kg extended interval		
Tobramycin	See gentamicin		
Fluoroquinolones Ciprofloxacin	500–750 mg PO BID or 400 mg IV q8–12h	Anaphylaxis, QTc prolongation, joint toxicity in children, tendon rupture	Nausea, vomiting, diarrhea, photo-sensitivity, rash

(continued)

TABLE 91.9	Infectious Diseases (*Continued*)		
Drug	Dosing	Rare Toxicities	Common Toxicities
Levofloxacin	500–750 mg IV/ PO q24h		CNS stimulation, dizziness, somnolence
Moxifloxacin	400 mg IV/PO q24h		
Macrolides			
Azithromycin	250–500 mg IV/ PO daily	QTc prolongation (erythromycin > clarithromycin > azithromycin), cholestasis	Nausea, vomiting, diarrhea, abnormal taste
Clarithromycin	250–500 mg PO BID		
Erythromycin	250–500 mg PO qid or 0.5–1 g IV q6h		
Tetracyclines			
Tetracycline	250–500 mg PO q6h	Tooth discoloration and retardation of bone growth (in children), renal tubular necrosis, dizziness, vertigo, pseudotumor cerebri	Photosensitivity, diarrhea
Doxycycline	100 mg IV/PO q12h		
Minocycline	200 mg IV/PO, then 100 mg IV/PO q12h		
Other antibiotics			
Tigecycline	100 mg bolus, then 50 mg IV q12h	—	Nausea, vomitin diarrhea
Trimethoprim/ sulfamethoxazole	5 mg/kg IV q8h (based on the trimethoprim component)	Myelosuppression, Stevens–Johnson syndrome, hyperkalemia, aseptic meningitis, hepatic necrosis	Rash, nausea, vomiting, diarrhea

(contin

TABLE 91.9 Infectious Diseases (*Continued*)

Drug	Dosing	Rare Toxicities	Common Toxicities
Metronidazole	500 mg IV/PO q8h	Seizures, peripheral neuropathy	Nausea, vomiting, metallic taste, disulfiram-like reaction
Clindamycin	600–900 mg IV q8h	*C. difficile* colitis	Nausea, vomiting, diarrhea, abdominal pain, rash

Antifungal Agents
Azoles

Fluconazole	100–800 mg PO/IV daily	Hepatic failure, increased AST/ALT, cardiovascular toxicity, hypertension, edema, QTc prolongation (less with isavuconazonium)	Nausea, vomiting, diarrhea rash, visual disturbances, phototoxicity
Itraconazole	200 mg IV/PO q24h		
Voriconazole	4 mg/kg IV q12h or 200 mg PO BID		
Posaconazole	200–400 mg PO TID-BID		
Isavuconazonium	372 mg IV q8h × 6 doses, then 372 mg IV daily		

Amphotericin B products

Amphotericin B deoxycholate	0.3–1.5 mg/kg q24h	Nephrotoxicity (less common with lipid formulations), acute liver failure, myelosuppression	Acute infusion-related reactions, hypokalemia, hypomagnesemia
ABLC	5 mg/kg IV q24h		
ABCD	3–4 mg/kg IV q24h		
Liposomal amphotericin B	3–5 mg/kg IV q24h		

(continued)

TABLE 91.9 Infectious Diseases *(Continued)*

Drug	Dosing	Rare Toxicities	Common Toxicities
Echinocandins			
Caspofungin	70 mg IV bolus, then 50 mg IV q24h	Hepatotoxicity, infusion-related rash, flushing, itching	—
Micafungin	50–150 mg IV q24h		
Anidulafungin	200 mg IV bolus, then 100 mg IV q24h		
Other antifungal agents			
Flucytosine	25–37.5 mg/kg PO q6h	Myelosuppression, hepatotoxicity, confusion, hallucinations, sedation	Nausea, vomiting, diarrhea, rash
Antiviral Agents			
Nucleoside analogs			
Acyclovir	400 mg PO TID or 5 mg/kg IV q8h	Nephrotoxicity, rash, encephalopathy, inflammation at injection site phlebitis	Bone marrow suppression, headache, nausea, vomiting, diarrhea (with oral forms)
Valacyclovir	1000 mg PO q8h		
Ganciclovir	5 mg/kg IV q12hr		
Valganciclovir	900 mg PO daily–BID		
Neuraminidase inhibitors			
Oseltamivir	75 mg PO BID	Anaphylaxis	Nausea, vomiting,
Zanamivir	10 mg inhaled q12h	bronchospasm	Nausea, cough, local discomfort
Peramivir	600 mg IV once	Hyperglycemia, increased CPK, hepatotoxicity	Diarrhea, neutropenia

(continued)

TABLE 91.9	Infectious Diseases (*Continued*)		
Drug	Dosing	Rare Toxicities	Common Toxicities
Other antiviral agents			
Amantadine	100 mg PO BID	CNS disturbances (amantadine > rimantadine)	Nausea, vomiting, anorexia, xerostomia Nephrotoxicity, uveitis/iritis, nausea, vomiting
Rimantadine	100 mg PO BID		
Cidofovir	5 mg/kg IV weekly plus probenecid 2 g PO 3 hrs before the infusion and then 1 g at 2 and 8 hrs after the infusion	Anemia, neutropenia, fever, rash	
Foscarnet	60 mg/kg IV q8h or 90 mg/kg IV q12h	Seizures, anemia, fever	Nephrotoxicity, electrolyte abnormalities (hypocalcemia, hypomagnesemia, hypokalemia, hypophosphatemia), nausea, vomiting, diarrhea, headache

ntravenous; PO, by mouth; BID, two times a day; AST/ALT, alanine aminotransferase/aspartate notransferase; TID, three times a day.

TABLE 91.10	Hepatic Disorders		
Drug	**Dosing**	**Rare Toxicities**	**Common Toxicities**
Lactulose	20–30 g (30–45 mL) PO q2h until initial stool, then adjust to maintain 2–3 soft stools/day	—	Diarrhea, flatulence, nausea
Neomycin	500–2000 mg PO q6–12h	Nephrotoxicity, neurotoxicity	Nausea, vomiting, diarrhea, irritation or soreness of mouth or rectal area
Rifaximin	400 mg PO TID		Headache
Propranolol	20–80 mg PO q12h	Heart block, bronchospasm, depression, nightmares, altered glucose metabolism, dyslipidemia, sexual dysfunction	Bradycardia, hypotension, fatigue, malaise, cold extremities
Nadolol	20–80 mg PO q24h		
Spironolactone	12.5–100 mg PO q24h	Gynecomastia, hyponatremia	Hyperkalemia

PO, by mouth.

TABLE 91.11	Gastrointestinal Disorders		
Drug	Dosing	Rare Toxicities	Common Toxicities
Proton Pump Inhibitors			
Pantoprazole	20–40 mg PO q12–24h	Headache, dizziness, somnolence, diarrhea, constipation, nausea	—
Esomeprazole	20–40 mg PO q24h, 80 mg IV bolus, then 8 mg/hr × 72 hr		
Omeprazole	20–40 mg PO q12–24h		
Lansoprazole	30–60 mg PO q12–24h		
Other Agents			
Octreotide	25–50 mcg IV bolus, then 25–50 mcg/hr infusion	Arrhythmias, conduction abnormalities, hypothyroidism, cholelithiasis (long-term use)	Diarrhea, flatulence, nausea, abdominal cramps, bradycardia, dysglycemia

PO, by mouth; IV, intravenous.

TABLE 91.12	Neurologic Disorders		
Drug	Dosing	Rare Toxicities	Common Toxicities
Status Epilepticus			
Lorazepam	0.1 mg/kg at 2 mg/min up to 8 mg	Paradoxical excitation, hypotension, respiratory depression (high doses)	CNS depression
Midazolam	0.2 mg/kg bolus, then 0.75–10 mcg/kg/min		
Phenytoin	20 mg/kg IV bolus, then 5–7 mg/kg day	Idiosyncratic: rash, fever, bone marrow suppression, Steven–Johnson syndrome, hepatitis	Concentration-dependent: nystagmus, diplopia, ataxia, sedation, lethargy, mood/behavior changes, coma, seizures
Fosphenytoin	20-mg phenytoin equivalents/kg IV/IM bolus	Associated with chronic use: gingival hyperplasia, folic acid deficiency, hirsutism, acne, vitamin D deficiency, osteomalacia	IV form: hypotension, bradycardia, phlebitis
Phenobarbital	20 mg/kg IV bolus	Rash, bone marrow suppression	Sedation, nystagmus, ataxia, nausea, vomiting. IV form: hypotension, bradycardia, respiratory depression
Propofol	30–250 mcg/kg/min	Pancreatitis, propofol infusion syndrome	Hypotension, bradycardia, CNS depression, hypertriglyceridemia
Levetiracetam	500–1000 mg IV/PO q12h	Behavioral disturbances	Somnolence, nausea, vomiting

(continue

LE 91.12	Neurologic Disorders *(Continued)*		
	Dosing	Rare Toxicities	Common Toxicities
ฺate	1,000–2500 mg/ day IV/PO in 2–4 divided doses	Hepatotoxicity, pancreatitis, thrombocytopenia, hyperammonemia, rash	Somnolence, diplopia nausea, vomiting, diarrhea
ᴄranial Pressure Elevation			
ฺrtonic ᴉe (23.4% ᴉl)	For mannitol-refractory patients: 30–50 mL q3–6h as needed (central line only) 0.686 mL of 23.4% saline is equiosmolar to 1 g of mannitol	—	Hypernatremia, hyperchloremia
ฺitol	1–1.5 g/kg IV bolus, then 0.25–1 g/kg q3–6h as needed	—	Hypotension, acute renal failure, fluid and electrolyte imbalances
ฺᴋe			
ฺlase	Ischemic stroke: 0.9 mg/kg IV (NOT to exceed 90 mg), infused over 60 min with 10% of the dose given as an initial bolus over 1 min	—	Bleeding
ฺr VII	Hemorrhagic stroke: 1.2–4.8 mg IV	Thrombosis	Hypertension

(continued)

TABLE 91.12	Neurologic Disorders (*Continued*)		
Drug	Dosing	Rare Toxicities	Common Toxicities
ICU Delirium			
Haloperidol	2–80 mg IV/PO q6h	QTc prolongation, extrapyramidal side effects (dystonia, akathisia, pseudoparkinsonism, tardive dyskinesia), neuroleptic malignant syndrome	CNS depression, orthostatic hypotension
ICU Sedation			
Lorazepam	2–4 mg bolus, 0.5–4 mg/hr	Paradoxical excitation, hypotension, respiratory depression (high doses)	CNS depression
Midazolam	1–5 mg bolus, 1–10 mg/hr		
Propofol	25–100 mcg/kg/min	Pancreatitis, propofol infusion syndrome	Hypotension, bradycardia, CNS depression, hypertriglyceridemia
Dexmedetomidine	0.2–1.5 mcg/kg/hr	—	Hypotension, bradycardia

IV, intravenous; IM, intramuscular; PO, by mouth; ICU, intensive care unit.

TABLE 91.13	Hematopoeitic Disorders		
Drug	Dosing	Rare Toxicities	Common Toxicities
Argatroban	Initial 2 mcg/kg/min, adjust based on aPTT measurements		Bleeding
Warfarin	Initial 1–5 mg/day, adjust based on INR measurements	Skin necrosis, purple-toe syndrome	Bleeding
DDAVP	0.3 mcg/kg slow IV	Hyponatremia, hypotension, tachycardia, thrombosis	Facial flushing
Phytonadione (vitamin K)	1–10 mg q24h Can be given PO, SQ, or IV	IV form: anaphylaxis, hypotension	—
Kcentra	2500–5000 units IV	Hypotension, thrombosis	Headache

aPTT, activated partial thromboplastin time; IV, intravenous; PO, by mouth; SQ, subcutaneous; INR, international normalized ratio.

TABLE 91.14	Pregnancy		
Drug	Dosing	Rare Toxicities	Common Toxicities
Magnesium	4–6 g IV over 15–20 min, then 2 g/hr infusion	—	
Phenytoin	20 mg/kg IV bolus, then 5–7 mg/kg day	Idiosyncratic: rash, fever, bone marrow suppression, Steven-Johnson syndrome, hepatitis Associated with chronic use: gingival hyperplasia. folic acid deficiency. hirsutism, acne. vitamin D deficiency. osteomalacia Heart block, bronchoconstriction, drug-induced lupus-like syndrome, rash, peripheral neuropathy	
Labetalol	100–800 mg PO q8–12h, max 2.4 g/day		Hypotension, bradycardia. nausea, vomiting.
Hydralazine	10–40 mg IV q4–6h or 10–75 mg PO TID–QID		hypotension, tachycardia. flushing, headache

IV, intravenous; PO, by mouth; TID, three times a day; QID, four times a day.

Index

Note: Page numbers followed by a, f and t indicate algorithm, figure and table respectively.